Clinical Trials and Human Research

A PRACTICAL GUIDE TO REGULATORY COMPLIANCE

Fay A. Rozovsky
Rodney K. Adams

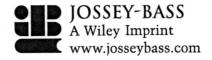

JOSSEY-BASS
A Wiley Imprint
www.josseybass.com

Copyright © 2003 by John Wiley & Sons, Inc. All rights reserved.

Published by Jossey-Bass
A Wiley Imprint
989 Market Street, San Francisco, CA 94103-1741   www.josseybass.com

Jossey-Bass books and products are available through most bookstores. To contact Jossey-Bass directly
call our Customer Care Department within the U.S. at 800-956-7739, outside the U.S. at 317-572-3993 or
fax 317-572-4002.

Jossey-Bass also publishes its books in a variety of electronic formats. Some content that appears in print
may not be available in electronic books.

Library of Congress Cataloging-in-Publication Data:
Rozovsky, F. A. (Fay Adrienne), 1950–
    Clinical trials and human research : a practical guide to regulatory compliance/Fay A.
Rozovsky, Rodney K. Adams.
      p. cm.
    Includes bibliographical references and index.
    ISBN 0-7879-6570-7
    1. Human experimentation in medicine. 2. Clinical trials. 3. Human experimentation in
medicine—Moral and ethical aspects. I. Adams, Rodney K., 1959-II. Title.

R853.H8R696 2003
619'.98—dc21

2003040074

FIRST EDITION
HB Printing   *10 9 8 7 6 5 4 3 2 1*

Clinical Trials and Human Research

Contents

Practical Tips . . . . *vii*

Foreword . . . . *ix*

About the Authors . . . . *xi*

Chapter 1   The Evolution of Human
             Experimentation Regulation 1

Chapter 2   Current Federal Regulations and
             Agencies Involved in Human Research 7

Chapter 3   State Regulation of Human Research 23

Chapter 4   Selection and Recruitment of Research Subjects 57

Chapter 5   Informed Consent in Clinical Trials 155

Chapter 6   Confidentiality of Clinical Trials Information 207

Chapter 7   The Investigator 221

Chapter 8   Research Protocols 239

Chapter 9   The Institutional Review Board 267

Chapter 10   Patient Safety in Clinical Trials Research 325

Chapter 11   Human Research Under the Food,
             Drug & Cosmetic Act 343

Chapter 12   Behavior Research 361

Chapter 13   Multisite and Collaborative Studies 365

Chapter 14   Medical Malpractice Liability in Human Research 391

Chapter 15   Quality Improvement, Accreditation, and Risk
             Management in Clinical Trials. 403

Chapter 16   Corporate Compliance and Human Research 443

Chapter 17 Ethics in Human Research 523

Chapter 18 International Research 535

Glossary *543*
Appendix *561*
Index *629*

Practical Tips

Chapter 2   Practical Tip for Managing Multiple Review
Requirements 11

Chapter 5   Fundamental Components That Are Important
to Consider in Setting the Content for Assent
Document, from a Risk Reduction Standpoint 160

Chapter 5   Revised Regulations 163

Foreword

Although steeped in corporate law, medical organizational requirements, reimbursement complexities, and regulatory schemes, this healthcare lawyer had no idea how difficult it would be to traverse the world of human subjects research without a guide. In the summer of 2001 following the tragic death of a healthy research volunteer, without warning, the Office of Human Research Protections (OHRP) suspended all research at The Johns Hopkins University School of Medicine. Although research was a joint enterprise between the University and the Johns Hopkins Hospital and related organizations, until 2001 management of the conduct of human subjects research had fallen principally to the university. In an instant, all hands were on board, including this hospital lawyer, and everyone needed to understand the research system that was, the research system that the regulators thought it should be, and the research system that realistically could work.

As the least-experienced member of the research team in the summer and fall of 2001, I searched for, but did not find, a simple, straightforward treatise on the fundamentals of human subjects research. Nor did I find a clear description of the OHRP and Food and Drug Administration regulations, the interplay of these agencies, the authority of each in compliance matters, and the interpretation of gray areas in all of these matters. Pieces of information were everywhere, but an authoritative source that discussed the context, current situation, and future challenges did not appear.

Now it has. In *Clinical Trials and Human Research: A Practical Guide to Regulatory Compliance,* Fay A. Rozovsky and Rodney K. Adams have compiled a resource for both experienced and not-so experienced lawyers, investigators, institutional review board members, and academic medical center administrators as they seek to comply with both the spirit and reality of the regulatory scheme.

Research is an amazing challenge when one thinks of it—seeking to advance the medical knowledge of mankind by using mankind to advance that knowledge. Research organizations and researchers must balance the risks and benefits in any given instance when necessarily the risks are not always zero. As the societal debate on human subjects research has been engaged over the past few years, I have been struck with view stated by so many that bad things should never happen in human research. They believe that if the research institutions are doing their jobs, and if the regulators are doing their jobs, no one should have an adverse reaction and certainly no one ever should die in human research.

Yet this unrealistic vision cannot be sustained. Medical breakthroughs often involve risk—appropriate, deliberate, minimized—but risk. Those volunteers who accept that risk are often heroic, dedicated, and high-minded. The research community must protect these volunteers and make sure they know exactly what may happen—but we must proceed responsibly and honestly in the research endeavor.

As I have learned more about human subjects research and about how carefully and seriously most investigators and IRB members take the balance that must be observed, I realize that there must be practical research tools for these busy people to use. As the reader will see when examining the carefully laid out chapters of this guide, the depth of background is there, but so is the practical view. How do I apply this rule? What problems has this posed? Where is this area likely to go in the future?

Let us hope that few bad things happen in human subjects research. The guide will ensure that those who pursue this course will understand, observe, and respect the balance.

Joanne E. Pollak
Vice President and General Counsel
Johns Hopkins Medicine
March 3, 2003

About the Authors

Fay A. Rozovsky, J.D., M.P.H., is senior vice president in the National Healthcare Practice of Marsh, Inc., based in Richmond, Virginia. Ms. Rozovsky has served as the adminstrator of an institutional review board and a member of human research committees in the United States and Canada. She is an affiliate associate professor in the Department of Legal Medicine, Medical College of Virginia, Virginia Commonwealth University, in Richmond.

Rodney K. Adams, J.D., LL.M., is an attorney in Richmond, Virginia, where he specializes in defending healthcare providers and patient care issues. He serves as an occasional reviewer of the *Journal of Health Politics, Policy and Law.* Mr. Adams is cochairman of the American Bar Association subcommittee on medical ethics and serves on the board of directors for the Richmond Bioethics Consortium. He also is adjunct assistant professor at University of Richmond, T.C. Williams College of Law, Richmond, Virginia.

1

The Evolution of Human Experimentation Regulation

The Forming of International Consensus on Human Rights 1
Efforts in the United States to Protect Research Participants 2
The Current Situation 3
How to Use This Book 4
References 4

National and international regulation of human experimentation is recent, compared with the centuries of scientific inquiry. The atrocities of World War II focused the world community on the rights and wrongs of using humans for research purposes. The recent surge of interest in protecting human research participants is often discussed in isolation from other key events, such as the national focus on fighting terrorism. Such discussions should consider the totality of the situation.

THE FORMING OF INTERNATIONAL CONSENSUS ON HUMAN RIGHTS

The Nuremberg War Crime Trials presented an unfortunate opportunity for modern thinking on human experimentation to be debated and synthesized. To their credit, the presiding judges developed *The Nuremberg Code* (1947) as part of their opinion in finding several German physicians guilty of crimes stemming from the use of prisoners in experimentation. The trial moved society to articulate clearly the ideas that scientific progress should not be to the detriment of the people subjected to the experiment and the participant must give voluntary informed consent. This was a tremendous shift in thinking from prior eras. The *Nuremberg Code* was incorporated as part of the Declaration of Human Rights and accepted in principle by each nation signing the charter of the United Nations. The Code of Ethics by the World Medical Association, known as the *Declaration of Helsinki: Recommendations Guiding Medical Doctors in Biomedical Research Involving Human Subjects* (1964) has further defined the international sense of propriety in human experimentation. The Declaration of Helsinki has been amended several times, as recently as 2000.

1

....

EFFORTS IN THE UNITED STATES TO PROTECT RESEARCH PARTICIPANTS

The United States, like most nations, has its own embarrassing history of exploiting human subjects in the name of scientific advancement. The famous Tuskegee Study of Untreated Syphilis in the Negro Male (commonly known as the Tuskegee Study) was started in 1932 by the Public Health Service (PHS) and ran for more than 40 years. Once viewed as a model of rigorous scientific study, it has come to be cited as a classic example of human rights abuse. Radiation experimentation, both in the military and among civilians, now regarded as unethical, had many episodes of using unwitting participants, including school children. The United States also has been sharply criticized for its complicity in not revealing or prosecuting the Japanese biological warfare research on prisoners in China during World War II (Veatch, 1989).

In 1953 the Clinical Center of the National Institutes of Health (NIH) generated the first federal policy for the protection of human subjects. Its major innovation was the prospective review of clinical research by an independent group of individuals. This was the beginning of the Institutional Review Board (IRB). The first federal statute requiring informed consent by participants receiving experimental drugs was enacted as part of the Drug Amendments of 1962 to the Food, Drug, and Cosmetic Act. Food and Drug Administration (FDA) regulations requiring informed consent were first issued in 1963 and tightened up in 1966. Since 1971, the FDA has required review of investigational drug protocols by IRBs. This was expanded to investigational device protocols in 1976. The Office for Protection from Research Risks (OPRR) was created in 1972 as part of NIH to ensure the safety of research participants in Department of Health and Human Services (HHS)-sponsored studies. OPRR was replaced by the Office of Human Research Protections (OHRP), which was moved from NIH to report to the secretary of the U.S. Department of Health and Human Services (HHS). However, before the metamorphosis of OPRR into OHRP, the former agency shocked the research community from its complacency by taking strong and public action against many highly regarded institutions, beginning with the Veteran's Administration Hospital in West Los Angeles and Duke University in 1999.

Even as recently as the 1970s, federal government agencies, such as the Central Intelligence Agency and the Department of Energy, conducted studies with potentially serious adverse effects on the participants without the participants' knowledge. The U.S. Congress undertook hearings and subsequent legislation to address the ethical and moral issues in human experimentation (The National Research Act of 1974). Requirements of informed consent and review by IRBs became part of research funded or conducted by the federal government. *The Belmont Report: Ethical Principles and Guidelines for the Protection of Human Subjects of Research* (1979), generated by the National Commission for the Protection of Human Subjects of Biomedical and Behavioral Research, has become a baseline for the regulation of human experimentation in the United States. The *Belmont Report* guides a clinician in distinguishing between therapeutic medicine and research, identifies fundamental ethical principles for protecting human subjects (respect for persons, beneficence, and justice), and illustrates how the ethical principles ought to be applied.

The President's Commission on Bioethics and the Office of Inspector General (OIG) at the Department of Health and Human Services continue to refine the government oversight of research activities. The Common Rule was issued by the Department of

Health and Human Services and most other federal agencies in 1991, after ten years of negotiation and coordination in the federal bureaucracy "Common Rule." This has been an attempt to standardize human research regulation among the many federal agencies. It formalized the responsibility of the researcher and the institution to protect human subjects. OPRR generated its landmark Institutional Review Board Guidebook in 1993. The FDA provided similar assistance in its Information Sheets, Guidance for Institutional Review Boards and Clinical Investigators, 1998 Update. Curiously, as of this writing, federal statutes do not extend directly to human research that is not conducted at an institution that receives federal research funds or that does not support an application to the FDA. This is in contrast to the tight regulation of all animal research under the Animal Welfare Act.

Nongovernmental organizations such as the American Medical Association (AMA) have maintained a Code of Ethics for many years. Although the focus of its Code of Ethics has been on clinical and professional relationships in the practice of medicine, the AMA has increasingly supplemented its Code of Ethics with regard to human research. Efforts have been made to standardize the regulation of human experimentation between nations. The International Conference on Harmonization developed the Guidelines for Good Clinical Practice (GCP). These mirror the U.S. regulations and are a good reference for any researcher, whether subject to federal or other oversight. Of course, for studies conducted in the United States, federal or state regulations take precedence over international guidance.

The regulatory environment of human research is complicated by other events in society. The national focus on fighting terrorism, as epitomized by the enactment of the Homeland Security Act, will have a tremendous impact on human subject research. For example, the new Department for Homeland Security is expected to have an enormous budget for funding research. What guidelines will be applied to its research? How will the rights of individuals be balanced with national security? Who will determine what research will be classified as secret? The dynamic of compensation for injury is being changed in relation to smallpox vaccine from manufacturer liability to a no-fault government scheme. Has sufficient testing on the impact of using smallpox vaccine in the general population been adequately studied?

Ongoing scandals in corporate accounting and short-term profiteering have led to a general mistrust of many industries. Deaths of research participants at prominent universities have grabbed newspaper headlines. The pressure continues to increase for clinical studies to be conducted with the utmost integrity and safeguards.

············

THE CURRENT SITUATION

Efforts are under way from several constituency groups to beef up protection for research participants. This has taken the form of continuing debate about the adequacy of current regulations and very public, very humiliating enforcement actions against prominent universities and other research organizations. The hundreds of federal and state regulations have been described as Byzantine by polite commentators and certainly far worse by many frustrated researchers and administrators. Pressure by the press has heightened the frequency and severity of investigations and sanctions by regulators. Unfortunately for physicians, scientists, IRB members, healthcare administrators, and others, there are too many references on regulation of human research (hundreds of government, association, and consultant Web sites) and yet too few resources that pull all of this information together in a comprehensive manual.

············

HOW TO USE THIS BOOK

The authors hope that they have addressed the dearth of practical guidance for those involved in human subject research. This book is intended to be an easy-to-read reference for physicians, scientists, IRB members, healthcare administrators, and others. The goal is not to attempt to answer every conceivable situation, but to address the common ones and give a framework for working through scenarios that are not directly addressed by statute or regulation. The authors have relied heavily on guidance from federal agencies such as the Food and Drug Administration, the Office of Human Research Protections, and the Office of Research Integrity (ORI). Every effort has been made to make the text of this book as close as possible to the exact language of regulations and official interpretations.

One emphasis of this book is the ethical and regulatory requirement for respect of the human subjects involved in research projects. To this end, "human participant" is often used in place of "human subject." Researchers should constantly consider what impact their work has on other people.

An important caveat of this and every book that discusses regulation of human research is that one must not only be cognizant of statutes and regulations but also an institution's policies and procedures, as well as the political environment in which the research will be conducted. The authors have always counseled clients that although an activity may be legal, it is better not to have to prove that at trial. In other words, working with government regulators, institutional officials, and community members can be as important as knowing the exact statutory text.

The second important caveat is that laws, regulations, and their interpretation are not static. Every effort has been made to make this book as current as possible. However, the authors have seen regulations and the positions of government agencies shift just during the time between completing the text and having it edited. To that end, readers should confirm with legal counsel the currency of any regulation cited in this book before embarking on a course of conduct based on the regulation.

The authors encourage readers to give them feedback. What sections need to be expanded? Do the recommended algorithms work? Have the authors missed an important point? The reader's input will make subsequent editions far more valuable to everyone.

References

American Medical Association, Code of Ethics.

The "Common Rule." U.S. Department of Health and Human Services regulations on human research, 45 CFR Part 46.

FDA, Information Sheets, Guidance for Institutional Review Boards and Clinical Investigators, 1998 Update. Available at [http://www.fda.gov/oc/oha/IRB/toc2.html#IRBOrg]

International Conference on Harmonization, Guidelines for Good Clinical Practice. [http://www.ifpma.org/ich5e.html#GCP]

National Commission for the Protection of Human Subjects of Biomedical and Behavior Research (1979). *The Belmont Report: Ethical Principles and Guidelines for the*

Protection of Human Subjects of Research. Washington, DC: U.S. Government Printing Office.

National Research Act of 1974, 42 USC 201 — 300aa-13.

OPRR, Institutional Review Board Guidebook, 1993. [http://ohrp.osophs.dhhs.gov/irb/irb_guidebook.htm]

The Nuremberg Code, 1947.

Veatch, Robert. (1989). *Medical Ethics.* Boston: Jones & Bartlett.

World Medical Association (1964). *Code of Ethics, Declaration of Helsinki: Recommendations Guiding Medical Doctors in Biomedical Research Involving Human Subjects.* Revised in 2000. [http://www.wma.net/e/policy/17-c_e.html]

2

Current Federal Regulations
and Agencies Involved
in Human Research

Introduction 7
The Federal Agencies That Fund Clinical Trials 8
The Regulatory Framework 9
The Common Rule in Clinical Trials Research 10
The Primary Elements of the Common Rule 10
The Common Rule and Review Under Multiple Regulations
and Private Contractual Requirements 11
   Practical Tip for Managing Multiple Review Requirements. 11
The FDA Regulations Compared with the Common Rule Provisions 11
The Role of the Office of Human Research Protections 12
The Role of the Office of Research Integrity 13
Medicare and Clinical Trials 13
The Health Insurance Portability and Accountability Act and Clinical Trials 15
The Fraud and Abuse Laws and Clinical Trials 16
Conclusion 17
References 20

INTRODUCTION

In June 1991, a Common Rule was adopted by a number of federal departments and Agencies that either conducted or funded human research (*Federal Register,* 1991). The Common Rule was first suggested by the President's Commission for the Study of Ethical Problems in Medicine and Biomedical and Behavioral Research. The President's Commission was asked to evaluate and make recommendations for action regarding the adequacy and uniformity of federal department and agency rules, regulations, and guidelines for the protection of human subjects. In 1982 the Federal Coordinating Council for Science, Engineering, and Technology appointed an ad hoc committee to study the recommendations of the President's Commission. Thereafter, the ad hoc committee agreed with the President's Commission recommendations to eliminate unnecessary rules and to encourage increased understanding and compliance by institutions carrying out federally supported or regulated human research trials. Once the ad hoc committee had finished its work, an Interagency Human Subjects Coordinating Council developed a proposed federal model policy for protection of human research subjects. From this effort emerged a proposed common rule that was published in November 1988; the final rule was published in the *Federal Register* in June 1991.

Of all the affected federal departments and agencies, only the FDA took a different approach. With the publication of the Common Rule, the FDA did make changes to its own regulations governing human research. Notwithstanding the FDA sharing a "common core" with the federal policy and the principles stated therein, the agency was seen as having unique requirements that formed the basis for differentiation from other federal departments and agencies (*Federal Register,* 1991).

Aside from the Common Rule and the FDA regulations, there are other federal requirements that control human research, including Medicare requirements for funding clinical trials that were first announced in 2000 (HCFA, 2000) and that were later incorporated into the Medicare Manual for Fiscal Intermediaries and Carriers (Medicare Manual, 2002). To be certain that potential subjects understood Medicare coverage for participation in clinical trials, the Center for Medicare and Medicaid Services (CMS, formerly the Health Care Financing Administration, "HCFA"), published a guide for recipients (HCFA, 2001).

Beyond Medicare and the Common Rule there is a set of federal requirements designed to curb financial fraud and abuse. The latter go well beyond the confines of clinical trials and extend to unlawful billing and coding practices (HCFA, 2001). The fraud and abuse requirements become relevant when so-called "double dipping" occurs in which a clinical trial funded by a private sponsor or a federal department or agency becomes the basis for unlawful billing for "services" under Medicare, Medicaid, or another Federal healthcare financial reimbursement program (HCFA, 2001) (discussed in Chapter Sixteen). More recently, federal rules were promulgated under the Health Insurance Portability and Accountability Act (HIPAA) dealing with confidentiality and privacy of individually identifiable information (*Federal Register,* 1996). These rules contain provisions that squarely address clinical trials providing yet another layer of federal protection for research subjects (see Chapter Six).

This chapter explores the scope of federal regulations involving clinical trials. It also discusses the impact of fraud and abuse laws. State-based laws and regulations are addressed in Chapter Three.

THE FEDERAL AGENCIES THAT FUND CLINICAL TRIALS

There are a number of federal departments and agencies that either conduct or fund clinical research. These include the following:

- Agency for International Development (AID)
- Department of Agriculture
- Department of Energy
- National Aeronautics and Space Administration
- Department of Commerce
- Consumer Product Safety Commission

- Department of Housing and Urban Development
- Department of Justice
- Department of Defense
- Department of Education
- Department of Veterans Affairs
- Environmental Protection Agency
- Department of Health and Human Services
- Food and Drug Administration
- National Science Foundation
- Department of Transportation

In addition, the National Science and Technology Council has a Human Subjects Research Subcommittee. The federal departments and agencies that follow the Common Rule are members of the subcommittee. Additional members include the Office for Human Research Protections of the Department of Health and Human Services, the Central Intelligence Agency, the Centers for Disease Control and Prevention, the National Institutes of Health, the Social Security Administration, and the Office of Science and Technology. The Secretary of State and Office of Management and Budget are ex officio members of the Subcommittee. The Human Subjects Research Subcommittee coordinates the implementation of federal policy for the protection of human subjects, an important responsibility in view of the underlying basis for the Common Rule to foster compliance with the federal rules.

············

THE REGULATORY FRAMEWORK

With few exceptions the Common Rule is followed by those federal departments and agencies that either conduct or fund human research. The FDA rules do take a different approach with respect to two provisions in the Common Rule. One relates to covered research conducted in foreign countries where the protections are at least equivalent to those of the department or agency. Under the Common Rule, a decision may be made to substitute the foreign procedures [e.g. 45 CFR §101[h]]. The second would permit an Institutional Review Board (IRB) to approve to alter or waive consent requirements in certain cases [§116[d]]. In both instances, the FDA chose to take a different approach. In the case of the consent provision, the FDA either does not regulate this type of research or an emergency treatment provision found in the FDA regulations addresses the issue. As to the foreign requirements, the FDA Modernization Act of 1997 (Public Law 105–115) and the FDA's participation in the International Conference on Harmonisation of Technical Requirements for Registration of Pharmaceuticals for Human Use are geared to a new way of recognizing drugs developed through clinical trials abroad. However, these developments came long after the FDA's decision not to follow the Common Rule on these issues. Under applicable provisions of the FDA regulations, the agency does provide criteria for accepting foreign clinical studies that are not done under an Investigational New Drug Application (21 CFR §812.1).

············

THE COMMON RULE IN CLINICAL TRIALS RESEARCH

In an effort to reduce confusion and streamline the review process for clinical trials research, the federal departments and agencies that conduct or fund human research developed a common federal policy. Termed the Common Rule, the federal policy is premised on the basic elements of the Department of Health and Human Services (HHS) for the protection of human subjects.

It is noteworthy that the Office of Inspector General (OIG) of the Department of Health and Human Services questions the wisdom of perpetuating the Common Rule. Concerned about protections for human research subjects, the OIG issued a number of recommendations to enhance review and oversight of clinical trials (IRB, 1998). However, under the Common Rule any of the changes recommended would have to be agreed upon by all the Federal Departments and Agencies who adhere to it. This is seen as a barrier to effective change and the basis for the OIG calling for change, possibly through legislation (OEI, 2000).

A list of the federal departments and agencies that follow the Common Rule is found at the end of the chapter. The list includes references to applicable parts of the Federal Code of Regulations (CFR) that address human research either conducted or supported by these federal departments and agencies.

············

THE PRIMARY ELEMENTS OF THE COMMON RULE

The Common Rule has largely achieved the goal of creating intergovernmental consistency in the definition and regulatory management of clinical trials. This is reflected in the criteria used by each agency or department to oversee human research subject clinical trials.

The Common Rule includes the following:

- Definitions
- Membership of the IRB
- Functions and Operations of the IRB
- Review of Research by the IRB
- Procedures for Expedited Review
- IRB Approval Criteria
- Review by Institution
- IRB Suspension or Termination of Research Approval
- Cooperative Research
- IRB Records
- Informed Consent
- Informed Consent Documentation
- Evaluation and Disposition Involving Applications or Proposals for Federally Conducted or Supported Research
- Use of Federal Funds
- Early Termination of Research
- Conditions

············

THE COMMON RULE AND REVIEW UNDER MULTIPLE REGULATIONS AND PRIVATE CONTRACTUAL REQUIREMENTS

Although the Common Rule does help to forge consistency among the federal departments and agencies involved with human research, principal investigators may still face some challenges. This is particularly the case when a research protocol must be reviewed under more than one federal department's or agency's regulations. The same can be said if a private sponsor sets review standards that differ from those of a federal entity or if the IRB must evaluate the protocol utilizing state legislative or regulatory requirements. Similar concerns may be raised if the research protocol must be reviewed under the laws or guideline.

Practical Tip for Managing Multiple Review Requirements

Satisfying multiple sets of review standards can prove time-consuming and tedious. From a practical standpoint, multiple standards of another jurisdiction should be anticipated. Standards review is a challenge that can be anticipated long before a protocol is submitted to an IRB for evaluation. The astute principal investigator will take steps to meet these multiple standards, and, when this cannot be achieved, provide an explanation to explain differences in the way the protocol is characterized under one set of regulations as compared with another.

One way to anticipate and overcome such difficulties is through the use of a matrix chart that provides a graphic representation or "crosswalk" between the differing requirements. Similarities might be portrayed by means of a check mark. Differences may be highlighted with an "x" and an explanation. This will save time for the IRB and help focus its examination. A cogent explanation of the differences can help to overcome perceived differences that might otherwise prolong the review process (see Multi-Review Matrix, page 22).

············

THE FDA REGULATIONS COMPARED WITH THE COMMON RULE PROVISIONS

There are several differences between the FDA regulations and the Common Rule requirements. Some bear particular attention, especially those that involve definitions, foreign clinical trials, and procedural or process requirements.

Here are some examples:

- *Foreign Clinical Trials*—The FDA regulations recognize foreign clinical studies not performed under an Investigational New Drug Application (IND). In contrast, under the Common Rule provisions, if procedures set forth by a foreign institution provide protections at least equivalent to the U.S. federal regulations, the department or agency head may approve the substitution of foreign procedures (21 CFR).

- *Definitions*—The FDA provisions define terms specific to the type of research covered by the FDA regulations such as the test article, application for research or marketing permit, and clinical investigation. In addition, the FDA provisions include a definition for emergency use. FDA adopted the Common Rule (21 CFR).

- *Reporting Obligation*—The Common Rule followed by HHS and other federal departments and agencies requires prompt reporting of unanticipated problems to the Secretary. By contrast, under the FDA regulations, the IRB must have and follow written procedures to make certain that unanticipated problems are reported by the sponsor and clinical investigator (21 CFR).

- *Confidentiality*—Unlike the departments and agencies that follow the Common Rule, the FDA does not permit an IRB to waive the requirement for signed consent when the principal risk is a breach of confidentiality. The rationale is that since the FDA does not regulate research protocols that would include this type of study, it need not made provision for it (21 CFR).

- *Behavioral Research*—Under the categories of research that may be reviewed using expedited review, HHS and other Common Rule departments and agencies include certain types of behavioral studies. These include research on characteristics of groups or individuals such as studies of perception, cognition, game theory, or test development. Since these studies are not regulated by the FDA, the agency chose not to make provision for such research in its regulations (21 CFR).

- *IRB Membership*—HHS and other departments and agencies under the Common Rule require the IRB to report changes in membership. Since the FDA is not required to follow this approach, no provision was made to notify the agency about changes in IRB membership (21 CFR).

- *Non-Compliance*—The FDA regulations includes sanctions for regulatory non-compliance. DHHS and other departments and agencies following the Common Rule allow termination of research support and evaluation of applications and proposals in view of prior non-compliance (21 CFR).

- *Inspection of Records*—The FDA requires that subjects be informed that the agency may inspect the records of the study. This is required since this may include examining a subject's medical records relevant to the study. By comparison, DHHS and the other departments and agencies following the Common Rule have the right to inspect records of studies they fund. However, they do not insist upon disclosure of this possibility as a consent requirement. They believe that such inspections occur so infrequently that there is no need to do so (21 CFR).

Beyond these provisions there are some similarities and differences with regard to informed consent. These requirements are discussed in Chapter Five.

. . . .

THE ROLE OF THE OFFICE OF HUMAN RESEARCH PROTECTIONS

In June 2000 The Secretary of the Department of Health and Human Services announced the creation of the Office of Human Research Protections (OHRP) to lead efforts for protecting human subjects in biomedical and behavioral research. The Office was recommended in 1999 by an advisory committee to the director of NIH. Located at the HHS department level, in the office of the Assistant Secretary for Health, it replaced the Office for Protection from Research Risks (OPRR), which was part of the National Institutes of Health (NIH) and had authority over NIH-funded research. Unlike its predecessor, which was responsible for both human and animal subjects, OHRP is focused on human research.

OHRP is supposed to provide leadership for the seventeen federal agencies that carry out research involving human subjects under a regulation known as the Common

Rule. At the same time, HHS also created a new National Human Research Protections Advisory Committee, to provide advice on patient protection and research needs. More information about the operational aspects of the OHRP can be found in Chapters Seven and Eight.

THE ROLE OF THE OFFICE OF RESEARCH INTEGRITY

The Department of Health and Human Services (HHS) has long had the authority to address misconduct in research conducted or funded by the department. Moreover, under federal criminal and civil fraud statutes, HHS has had authority to address research misconduct. The NIH Revitalization Act of 1993 (NIH Act) established the Office of Research Integrity (ORI) as an independent entity reporting to the Secretary of the Department of Health and Human Services. ORI was required to address research misconduct. Since other federal departments and agencies also face the potential for research misconduct, an initiative was started in 1996 to develop a definition of such for all federal agencies and the funded institutions. In May 1999, after an extensive agency review and clearance process, the proposed government-wide policy was put forward, consisting of a definition of research misconduct and guidelines for the handling of allegations of research misconduct.

Subsequently, in October 1999, HHS announced innovations to enhance its ability to respond to allegations of research misconduct and to promote research integrity. On December 7, 2000, ORI published a "Policy on Instruction in the Responsible Conduct of Research" (referred to as the "RCR" Policy), *Federal Register* 65. However, on February 21, 2001, the Policy was suspended in accordance with the President's Regulatory Review Plan of January 21, 2001. In particular, to be determined was "whether the document should have been issued as a regulation rather than a policy" (USDHHS, 2002). According to information found on the ORI Web site that was published in July 2002, the review process is nearing completion. ORI has indicated, however, that it intends to continue the development of its RCR Education Program "to encourage research organizations to do the 'right thing' for biomedical and behavioral research" (USDHHS, 2002).

Although the RCR Policy is currently suspended, it does provide very useful insights into research misconduct oversight, investigation, and resolution. In addition, the ORI has a number of other useful publications available from their Web site to assist healthcare entities and sponsors address the issue of research misconduct. These include the "Model Policy for Responding to Allegations of Scientific Misconduct" and the "Model Procedures for Responding to Allegations of Scientific Misconduct." In addition, the ORI has issued for public commentary *Guidelines for Assessing Possible Research Misconduct in Clinical Research and Clinical Trials* (ORI).

With the degree of regulatory scrutiny of clinical trials increasing, the work of the ORI may take on more prominence. Much depends on what is the outcome of the President's Regulatory Review and the approach of HHS on the subject.

MEDICARE AND CLINICAL TRIALS

For many years, Medicare did not cover items and services related to clinical trials. The rationale was quite simple: since beneficiaries would be involved in experimental programs, it was not a covered benefit. The result was that few beneficiaries could take part in clinical trials research. The exclusion of clinical trials from Medicare stood in stark contrast to the fact that senior citizens, the beneficiaries of the program, represented a segment of American society that utilized a large proportion of healthcare services. In June 2000, the president issued an Executive Memorandum directing the Secretary of Health and Human Services to authorize Medicare to pay for the routine care costs associated with beneficiaries taking part in clinical trials (Executive Memorandum).

HCFA (now known as the Centers for Medicare and Medicaid Services, CMS) was tasked with operationalizing the Executive Memorandum. Acting on authority found in the Social Security Act (1862 (a)(1)(e)), HCFA published a National Coverage Policy. The National Coverage Decision is applicable to Medicare Carriers, fiscal intermediaries, Peer Review Organizations (PROs, now known as Quality Improvement Organizations, QIOs), Health Maintenance Organizations (HMOs), Competitive Medical Plans, Health Care Prepayment Plans, and Medicare+Choice organizations. Effective September 19, 2000, the National Coverage Decision mapped out the scope of coverages (*Federal Register,* 2000). Thus Medicare will cover:

- Routine costs of "qualifying" clinical trials.
- Reasonable and necessary items and services to diagnose and treat clinical trials–related complications.

What constitutes routine costs? These are items or services that are typically not part of a clinical trial such as conventional care, items or services needed only for the investigational component such as a noncovered chemotherapeutic agent, monitoring of the effects of the investigational item, prevention of complications, and tests or services to diagnose or treat a complication stemming from the study.

HCFA also developed some qualifiers to make certain that only appropriate routine costs would be covered by Medicare:

1. The trial must evaluate an item or service that falls within a Medicare benefit category (physicians' service, durable medical equipment, diagnostic test) and is not excluded from coverage (such as cosmetic surgery, hearing aids).
2. The trial must have therapeutic intent.
3. Trials of therapeutic interventions must enroll patients with diagnosed disease and not healthy volunteers. However, diagnostic trials may enroll healthy patients in order to have a proper control group (CMS, 2000).

Beyond these three prerequisites, clinical trials should have a number of "desirable characteristics" such as the following:

1. The principal purpose of the trial is to test whether the intervention potentially improves the participants' health outcomes.
2. The trial is well supported by available scientific and medical information, or it is intended to clarify or establish the health outcomes of interventions already in common clinical use.
3. The trial does not unjustifiably duplicate existing studies.
4. The trial design is appropriate to answer the research question being asked in the trial.
5. The trial is sponsored by a credible organization or individual capable of executing the proposed trial successfully.

6. The trial complies with federal regulations for the protection of human subjects.

7. The trial is conducted in accordance with standards of scientific integrity.

A multiagency panel under the leadership of the Agency for Healthcare Research and Quality (AHRQ) developed the qualifying criteria. The panel included representatives from the Department of Health and Human Services research agencies (National Institutes of Health (NIH), Centers for Disease Control and Prevention (CDC), the Food and Drug Administration (FDA), and the Office of Human Research Protection), and the research arms of the Department of Defense (DOD) and the Department of Veterans Affairs (VA). Beyond studies that meet the qualifying criteria, some are considered "deemed trials," meaning that they are considered to automatically have the requisite desirable characteristics. According to the National Coverage Decision, Effective September 19, 2000, clinical trials that are deemed to be automatically qualified are:

1. Trials funded by NIH, CDC, AHRQ, HCFA, DOD, and VA.

2. Trials supported by centers or cooperative groups that are funded by the NIH, CDC, AHRQ, HCFA, DOD, and VA.

3. Trials conducted under an investigational new drug application (IND) reviewed by the FDA.

4. Drug trials that are exempt from having an IND under 21 CFR §312.2(b)(1) will be deemed automatically qualified until the qualifying criteria are developed and the certification process is in place. At that time the principal investigators of these trials must certify that the trials meet the qualifying criteria in order to maintain Medicare coverage of routine costs. This certification process will only affect the future status of the trial and will not be used to retroactively change the earlier deemed status (CMS, 2002).

The Medicare requirements bear careful review to make certain that a study does qualify and thereafter, to understand what costs will and will not be covered by Medicare. Some confusion can be anticipated from this relatively new approach to cover some of the costs of Medicare beneficiaries participating in clinical trials. It is an area that merits delineation of costs that are covered by the study and those that are not, as well as documentation to substantiate the determination process. In this way, should questions arise about the propriety of a Medicare treatment or service cost, there will be ample information for substantiating the coverage.

············

THE HEALTH INSURANCE PORTABILITY AND ACCOUNTABILITY ACT AND CLINICAL TRIALS

Under the final rules published on December 28, 2000, under the Health Insurance Portability and Accountability Act (Public Law 104–191), provision was made to address privacy and confidentiality of research subjects in clinical trials (*Federal Register,* 2000). Termed the "Standards for Privacy of Individually Identifiable Health Information," the regulation covers verbal, written, and electronic formats of such data. Encompassed within the rule are provisions that address clinical trials (45 CFR). The rule has undergone several revisions since it was first promulgated, with the final changes announced in August 2002 (HIPAA). Under the Final Rule announced in August 2002, there is one set of authorization requirements for uses and disclosures of protected health information for the purpose of research. Such an authorization may also be combined with a consent to take part in research (*Federal Register* 67). Provision is also made in the HIPAA Privacy Rule for waiver of an authorization, a step that can be taken by either an IRB or a Privacy Board consistent with the regulatory framework for doing so (HIPAA).

The new rule has been the subject of considerable public discussion (see Chapter Six). Many see it as too broad and burdensome. To ease implementation of the new Rule, the Office of Civil Rights of the Department of Health and Human Services has published guidance on the Privacy Standard (OCR Guidance, December 4, 2002). A Web site link to the guidance is found in the Appendix, and it is discussed in Chapter Six.

··············

THE FRAUD AND ABUSE LAWS AND CLINICAL TRIALS

There are several ways in which federal fraud and abuse laws relate to clinical research. For example, a study funded by a federal department or agency should not generate bills or claims for the same items covered in the research award. This is true even with respect to the Medicare clinical trials coverage, which is specifically designed to cover those items not included in the research grant or award. If done knowingly and wittingly with the intention of "double dipping"—getting funding twice—this could trigger the application of fraud and abuse provisions.

There are other ways in which fraud can be attempted in medical research: Once under way, a principal investigator may file reports suggesting that additional funding is needed to continue the study when in fact this is not the case. Alternatively, the investigator may misuse the funds received for medical research.

Research fraud and abuse can occur also in the way in which protocols are presented, such as false representations, falsified data, or manipulation of information used as the pretext to obtain research funding for a study that would otherwise be rejected.

Various parts of federal statutory law can be used to pursue those responsible for false claims. For example, the criminal provisions deal with false claims (U.S. Code). Under a separate provision, a civil cause of action can also be pursued for false claims (U.S. Code). As a practical matter, federal prosecutors usually seek criminal prosecutions for false claims or false statements and then civil fraud. Criminal prosecutions have occurred regarding medical research fraud. There are treatises on this subject that provide detailed insights for attorneys and corporate compliance officers (see Fabrikant, Kalb, Hopson, and Bucy).

Plagiarism and falsifying study results is yet another type of fraud. This type of misconduct comes within the domain of the Office of Research Integrity. Such an investigation and finding may result in exclusion from participating in federally funded research for a period of time or even permanently. Much depends upon the nature of the offensive behavior. Additionally, the name of the excluded individual and a summary of the reasons for this action are published in an exclusion list that appears in the *Federal Register.* The long-term consequences may bring an end to the career of a research scientist.

Fraud and abuse in clinical research should not be treated lightly. In an era of ever-increasing regulatory scrutiny, fraudulent practices may be detected as part of a review conducted as a result of a serious adverse event or a "whistleblower" claim of safety concerns. Research may be suspended pending a complete determination of the seriousness of the situation, and reputations and integrity can be called into question.

Compliance with federal requirements may necessitate significant corrective action, which can prove expensive for all concerned. As discussed in Chapter Fifteen, prevention is the best approach to avoiding such risk exposure.

············

CONCLUSION

There are several layers of federal statutory and regulatory requirements that control the conduct of clinical research trials. These rules go well beyond the elements of what is expected of an IRB. The requirements include laws dealing with research misconduct, privacy of individually identifiable data, and fraud and abuse.

For research officers, it is prudent to develop a comprehensive list of the federal requirements and to incorporate salient provisions into the framework for clinical research policy and procedure. Educational efforts for the IRB, research office, and principal investigators should include an overview of these laws and regulations. Taking these steps should help to avert situations in which research trials are undertaken that do not fit within the confines of applicable federal law.

Common Rule Departments and Agencies (Not Including the FDA) Including List of Contacts

Director, Office for Human Research Protections
Department of Health and Human Services
6100 Executive Boulevard, Suite 3B01
MSC-7507
Rockville, MD 20892-7507
301-435-5646
301-402-2071 fax
E-mail: koskig@od.nih.gov

AGENCY FOR INTERNATIONAL DEVELOPMENT

James D. Shelton, M.D.
Senior Medical Scientist
Office of Population
Agency for International Development
Washington, DC 20523-1819
202-712-0869
202-216-3404 fax
E-mail: jshelton@usaid.gov

CONSUMER PRODUCT SAFETY COMMISSION

Ms. Lori E. Saltzman
Director
Division of Health Sciences
Consumer Product Safety Commission
4330 East West Highway, Room 600B
Bethesda, MD 20814-4008
301-504-0477 x1203
301-504-0079 fax
E-mail: lsaltzman@cpsc.gov

DEPARTMENT OF AGRICULTURE

Dr. Michael Kiley
Research Program Safety Officer
United States Department of Agriculture
Building 005, Room 208, BARC-W
10300 Baltimore Ave.
Beltsville, MD 20705
301-504-6065
301-504-5467 fax
E-mail: mpk@ars.usda.gov

DEPARTMENT OF COMMERCE

Dr. Alan Cookson
Acting Deputy Director
Electronics and Electrical Engineering Laboratory
National Institute of Standards and Technology
100 Bureau Drive - Building 220, Room B358, MSC8100
Gaithersburg, MD 20899-8100
301-975-2220
301-975-4091 fax
E-mail: alan.cookson@nist.gov

DEPARTMENT OF DEFENSE

CDR C. Dougas Forcino, Ph.D.
Regulatory Affairs Project Officer
Office of the Director, Defense Research and Engineering
Bio-Systems Division
1777 N. Kent St., Suite 3020
Roslyn, VA 22209
703-601-1724
703-588-7560 fax
E-mail: cdforcino@us.med.navy.mil

DEPARTMENT OF EDUCATION

Ms. Blanca Rosa Rodriguez
Director
Grants Policy Oversight Staff
U.S. Department of Education
Office of Chief Financial Officer
Washington, DC 20202-4248
202-708-8263
202-205-0667 fax
E-mail: blanca_rodriguez@ed.gov

DEPARTMENT OF ENERGY

Susan L. Rose, Ph.D.
Manager, Human Subjects Program
Life Sciences Division, SC-72
Office of Biological and Environmental Research
Office of Science
U.S. Department of Energy
19901 Germantown Road
Germantown, MD 20874-1290
301-903-4731
301-903-8521 fax
E-mail: susan.l.rose@science.doe.gov

DEPARTMENT OF HOUSING AND URBAN DEVELOPMENT

Dr. Paul Gatons
Associate Deputy Assistant Secretary
for Research, Evaluation and Monitoring
U.S. Department of Housing and Urban Development
451 7th Street, S.W.
Room 8146
Washington, DC 20410
202-708-4230
202-619-8000 fax
E-mail: paul_k._gatons@hud.gov

DEPARTMENT OF JUSTICE

Dr. Donald Prosnitz
General Counsel
Science Advisor to the Attorney General
U.S. Department of Justice
810 Seventh St., N.W.
Washington, DC 20531

DEPARTMENT OF LABOR

Mr. Daniel Ryan
Labor Economist
Employment Training Administration
Office of Policy and Research
U.S. Department of Labor
200 Constitution Avenue, N.W.
Room N-5637
Washington, DC 20210
202-693-3649
202-693-2766 fax
E-mail: dryan@doleta.gov

DEPARTMENT OF TRANSPORTATION

Dr. David R. Hunter
Program Scientist
Biomedical and Behavioral Sciences Branch
Office of Aviation Medicine, AAM/240
Office of Associate Admin. for Aviation Standards
Federal Aviation Administration
U.S. Department of Transportation
800 Independence Avenue, S.W.
Washington, DC 20591
202-267-8345
202-493-5006 fax
E-mail: david.hunter@faa.gov

DEPARTMENT OF VETERANS AFFAIRS

James F. Burris, M.D.
Deputy Chief Research and Development Officer - 12A
Veterans Health Administration
Department of Veterans Affairs
810 Vermont Avenue, N.W.
Washington, DC 20204
202-273-8284
202-273-6526 fax
E-mail: james.burris@mail.va.gov

ENVIRONMENTAL PROTECTION AGENCY

Mr. Roger Cortesi
Peer Review Compliance Executive
U.S. Environmental Protection Agency
Office of Research and Development (8701R)
401 M Street, S.W.
Washington, DC 20460
202-564-6852
202-565-2444 fax
E-mail: cortesi.roger@epamail.epa.gov

NATIONAL AERONAUTICS AND SPACE ADMINISTRATION

Dr. Victor S. Schneider
Manager, Space Physiology and Countermeasures Program
National Aeronautics and Space Administration
300 E Street, S.W.
Mail Code UL
Washington, DC 20546
202-358-2204
202-358-4168 fax
E-mail: vschneider@hq.nasa.gov

NATIONAL SCIENCE FOUNDATION

Stuart Plattner, Ph.D.
Program Director for Cultural Anthropology
National Science Foundation
4201 Wilson Boulevard, Suite 995
Arlington, VA 22230
703-292-7315 or 8758
703-292-9068 fax
E-mail: splattne@nsf.gov

References

Federal Register: 56(117): 28004, et seq, June 18, 1991.

"Medicare Coverage Routine Costs of Beneficiaries in Clinical Trials," HCFA FACT SHEET, September 19, 2000.

Medicare Manual, Transmittal AB-01-103, "Revised Guidelines for Processing Claims for Clinical Trials Routine Care Services," effective, January 1, 2002.

"Medicare & Clinical Trials," HCFA Publication No. HCFA-02226-S, January, 2001.

"The Medicare Intergrity Program—Pay It Right!" CMS March Publication No. HCFA—02201, March, 2001.

Public Law 104-91 (1996). Title II, Preventing Health Care Fraud and Abuse; Administrative Simplification; Medical Liability Reform, is the part discussed in this book. It should be noted that the so-called "Privacy Standard" has undergone several changes since first proposed in November 1999. The history of the rule includes the following: The Final Rule, published on December 28, 2000, in the *Federal Register* 65: 82462, et seq. It was then opened for additional public commentary in March, 2001, *Federal Register* 66 12738. It was then made effective on April 14, 2001, *Federal Register* 65: 12433. Proposed changes were announced on March 27, 2002, *Federal Register* 67: 14776. The revised Final Rule was published on August 14, 2002, *Federal Register* 67(157): 53182, et seq.

Public Law 105-115.

21 CFR §812.1.

"Institutional Review Boards: A Time for Reform," OEI-01-97-00193, June 1998.

"Protecting Human Research Subjects: Status of Recommendations, OEI-01-97-00197, April 2000.

21 CFR §56.102 and §812.1 and also Common Rule Provision __§102.

21 CFR §56.102(i).

21 CFR §56.108 (FDA); and __§108 (under the Common Rule).

21 CFR §56.109 (FDA); and under the Common Rule _§109; __§117(c).

21 CFR §56.110 (FDA); and __§110 under the Common Rule.

21 CFR §56.115 (FDA); and Common Rule __§.115.

21 CFR §§56.120-124 (FDA); Common Rule __§.123.

21 CFR §50.25(a)(5) (FDA); Common Rule __§.116(a)(5).

Federal Register 65: 76647, et seq.

Office of Research Integrity, U.S. Department of Health and Human Services, "Responsible Conduct of Research Education Program Statement," July 31, 2002.

These and other ORI documents can be found at http://ori.dhhs.gov/html/programs/rcr.

Executive Memorandum June 7, 2000.

§1862(a)(1)(E).

Federal Register 65(212): 65318-65319, November 1, 2000.

"Final National Medicare Coverage Decision on Clinical Trials," and also, "Coverages Issues Manual Clinical Trials," CMS, 30-1, at cms.hhs.gov/manuals/06_cim/ci30.asp, August 20, 2002.

Public Law 104-191 (1996) (Hereinafter referred to as "HIPAA").

Federal Register: 65(250): 82462, et seq, December 28, 2000.

45 CFR §164.508(f); 45 CFR §164.512(i) 2000.

For a detailed discussion of the history of the HIPAA Privacy Rule see Note 8, supra. The revised Final Rule was published on August 14, 2002, *Federal Register* 67(157): 53182, et seq.

See, *Federal Register* 67(157): 53182, 53268-53269, August 14, 2002.

Federal Register 67(157): 53182, 53270, August 14, 2002. This is a part of the HIPAA Privacy Rule that was modified since it was first promulgated.

18 U.S. Code §287 and false statements 18 US Code §1001.

31 U.S. Code §3129, et seq.

See, for example, U.S. ex rel Condie v. Board of Regents of the University of California, 1993 WL 740185 (N.D. Cal. Sept. 7, 1993) (fraud involving research findings); U.S. v. University of Connecticut Health Center, No. 3: 96CVOOO288 PCD (D. Conn. 1997) (false representations in grant application) and Boerrigter v. Beth Israel Deaconess Medical Center, No. 97-11858 (D. Mass. 1998) (accepting funding even though researcher had left the United States).

R. Fabrikant, P. Kalb, M. Hopson, P. Bucy. *Health Care Fraud: Enforcement and Compliance,* New York: Law Journal Press, 2000.

OCR Guidance Explaining Significant Aspects of the Privacy Rule—December 4, 2002, Research, www.hhs.gov/ocr/hipaa/privacy.htm/

Clinical Trial Review/Oversight Criteria	Federal Requirements Specify ___ CFR___	Contractual Requirements Sponsor	Foreign Law/Guideline	Comment Section
• Definitions • IRB Composition • IRB Review Requirements • Expedited Review • IRB Approval Criteria • Institutional Review • Protocol Monitoring • IRB Suspension or Termination of Research Approval • Cooperative Research • IRB Records • Informed Consent • Informed Consent Documentation • Use of Federal Funds • Early Termination of Research • Privacy • Confidentiality • Conflict-of-Interest Statements • Safety/Security Specifications • Adverse Event Reporting • Continuity of Research-Enterprise Disruption • Insurance Coverages • Quality Management				

Multi-Review Matrix Instructions

Place an "x" for each category in which there is a multiple review. In the Commentary Section provide details regarding overlap or inconsistency and explain how it has been addressed.
If this requires a lengthy explanation, attach a separate sheet for referencing the applicable category.

3

State Regulation
of Human Research

Introduction 23
The Application of State Regulations to a Study 23
The Relationship of State and Federal Regulations 24
The Gordian Knot of State Regulations for a Multicenter Study 24
The Role of State Regulations in Federally Funded Studies 24
The Role of State Regulations in Privately Funded Studies 24
The Application of State Regulations Beyond Its Borders 24
How Do States Define *Experimentation?* 25
Table of State Statutes 25
Conclusion 25
References 56

INTRODUCTION

Keeping up with federal regulations is challenging enough, but the research community must also be aware of state statutes and regulations that must be observed. This can be a daunting proposition when research is being conducted at more than one site. Often state regulations are not well known in the research community until a problem develops. As with any endeavor, ignorance of the law makes a poor defense.

THE APPLICATION OF STATE
REGULATIONS TO A STUDY

Depending on the jurisdiction, a state's regulations may be far broader than the federal regulations. For example, Virginia statutes apply to all studies regardless of the funding source or purpose. Federal regulations do not explicitly preempt state regulations in the area of human research. In fact, federal regulations rely on state law for such important topics as informed consent and surrogate decision-making.

············

THE RELATIONSHIP OF STATE AND FEDERAL REGULATIONS

Compliance with federal regulations does not ensure compliance with state regulations. For example, California has very explicit requirements that must be met that are not set forth in federal regulations. The entire topic of informed consent is driven by state case law, statutes, and regulations. Failure to comply with a state's informed consent requirements can lead to federal sanctions.

············

THE GORDIAN KNOT OF STATE REGULATIONS
FOR A MULTICENTER STUDY

A multicenter study must be very careful in determining what state regulations may apply. The regulations of more than one state will frequently be applicable. The location of where the study occurs usually determines which state law applies. This may become complicated when a study may be managed from one location but portions of the study may occur at offices in another state. For example, a New York university may conduct a study in which it enrolls participants while they are patients in the university's hospital. Once the patients are discharged from the hospital, data are collected by the participants' physicians at their offices. Many of these offices may be in New Jersey or Connecticut. The laws of New York, New Jersey, and Connecticut may apply to the study.

············

THE ROLE OF STATE REGULATIONS
IN FEDERALLY FUNDED STUDIES

Whether a state's regulations will apply to a federally funded study depends on the state. Most states defer to federal oversight. However, others may contend that their more restrictive statutes further the federal goal and thus apply to even federally funded studies. The more prudent course is to assume that state regulations do apply to a federally funded study. State regulations usually do not apply to studies conducted solely within the confines of a federal institution, such as at a Veteran's Administration hospital.

············

THE ROLE OF STATE REGULATIONS
IN PRIVATELY FUNDED STUDIES

Even in cases in which a study is funded solely from private sources, state regulations usually apply even when federal regulations may not. State statutes and regulations do not distinguish among the sources of funding. However, different regulations may apply based on whether the study is funded by a state agency or not, as well as whether the study is being conducted in a state facility.

············

THE APPLICATION OF STATE REGULATIONS
BEYOND ITS BORDERS

A state's regulations may apply beyond its borders. For example, a study may be based in one state while participants are enrolled in another state. Depending on how the state's regulations are written, the law of the home state may apply as well as the law of the jurisdiction where the study participants take part.

HOW DO STATES DEFINE *EXPERIMENTATION?*

Most states use a definition of *experimentation* identical or similar to the federal definition. However, some states have used human subject research statutes to address pro-life and fetal tissue research issues. Many of these state research statutes have been attacked as being unconstitutionally vague because they use the term *experimentation*. For example, the Arizona statute prohibiting experimentation on fetal tissue was struck down as unconstitutional because it was too vague. If a technique is at some time clearly experimental, there is no definitive way to ascertain when it ceases to be experimental. *Experimentation* is an ambiguous term that lacks a precise definition, held the federal district court (*Forbes v. Woods*).

A treating physician should keep the distinction between the novel use of a therapy and clinical research in mind. Both may be categorized as *experimentation*. Usually the former is not considered research that triggers state or federal regulations. However, a plaintiff may use the term to bolster the allegations of a medical malpractice action. For example, in West Virginia, written informed consent is required when experimental therapy is proposed to a patient (West Va. Code 30-3-14(c)(14)). The West Virginia Supreme Court determined that "depossession therapy" by a psychiatrist was experimental and therefore required written informed consent (*Modi v. West Virginia Board of Medicine*).

CONCLUSION

State regulation can be the most difficult compliance issue facing a clinical investigator. Few comprehensive guides exist for the researcher to follow. The regulations often change with little public notice. Constant vigilance by the institution, its compliance officer, and the investigator are required. As such, this table is only offered as a guide for readers who should obtain specific legal advice with regard to state requirements impacting a research protocol.

TABLE OF STATE STATUTES

ALABAMA

1.	Is there clinical trials legislation?	No
2.	General provisions of legislation	—
3.	Provisions concerning minors	—
4.	Provisions concerning pregnant women	—
5.	Provisions concerning fetal research	—
6.	Provisions concerning in vitro procedures	—
7.	Provisions concerning prisoners	—
8.	Provisions concerning the developmentally disabled/mentally handicapped	—
9.	Provisions concerning the mentally ill	—
10.	Provisions concerning nursing home/long-term facilities residents	—

ALASKA

1.	Is there clinical trials legislation?	No
2.	General provisions of legislation	—
3.	Provisions concerning minors	—
4.	Provisions concerning pregnant women	—
5.	Provisions concerning fetal research	—
6.	Provisions concerning in vitro procedures	—

(Continued)

TABLE OF STATE STATUTES (*Continued*)

7. Provisions concerning prisoners — —
8. Provisions concerning the developmentally — —
   disabled/mentally handicapped
9. Provisions concerning the mentally ill — —
10. Provisions concerning nursing home/long-term — —
    facilities residents

ARIZONA

1. Is there clinical trials legislation?   Yes
2. General provisions of legislation   —
3. Provisions concerning minors   —
4. Provisions concerning pregnant women   —
5. Provisions concerning fetal research   —
6. Provisions concerning in vitro procedures   —
7. Provisions concerning prisoners

Any prisoner, with the written consent of the director and the chief of health services, may volunteer to participate in an approved program of medical research or plasmapheresis and whole blood program. (ARS §31-321(A)) Before consenting to participate in the program, the prisoner must be advised of the nature of the program and the dangers, if any, which may result by reason of such participation. (ARS §31-321(B)) The consent of any prisoner to participate in the program must be evidenced in writing, and, as a condition precedent to a prisoner's participation, the prisoner must release the state, the director and the chief of health services from liability. (ARS §31-321(C))

An approved program of medical research or plasmapheresis and whole blood program may provide for the payment of compensation to participating prisoners. (ARS §31-323(A)) Proceeds from prisoner participation will be paid into the trust fund or retention account established by the director. (ARS §31-323(B))

8. Provisions concerning the developmentally   —
   disabled/mentally handicapped
9. Provisions concerning the mentally ill   —
10. Provisions concerning nursing home/long-term   —
    facilities residents

ARKANSAS

1. Is there clinical trials legislation?   No
2. General provisions of legislation   —
3. Provisions concerning minors   —
4. Provisions concerning pregnant women   —
5. Provisions concerning fetal research   —
6. Provisions concerning in vitro procedures   —
7. Provisions concerning prisoners   —
8. Provisions concerning the developmentally   —
   disabled/mentally handicapped
9. Provisions concerning the mentally ill   —
10. Provisions concerning nursing home/long-term   —
    facilities residents

CALIFORNIA

1. Is there clinical trials legislation?   Yes
2. General provisions of legislation   Experimental drugs

Prior to prescribing or administering an experimental drug, consent to the use of the drug must be obtained in the method and manner specified in Chapter 1.3 (commencing

TABLE OF STATE STATUTES (*Continued*)

with Section 24170) of Division 20. (Cal Health & Saf Code §111525) Consent may be revoked at any time by either verbal or written communication to the practitioner supervising the administration of the drug. (Cal Health & Saf Code §111535)

Experimental subject's bill of rights

Except as otherwise provided in the informed consent provision (Health & Saf Code §24175), the bill of rights will include, but not be limited to, the subject's right to:

(a) Be informed of the nature and purpose of the experiment.

(b) Be given an explanation of the procedures to be followed in the medical experiment, and any drug or device to be utilized.

(c) Be given a description of any attendant discomforts and risks reasonably to be expected from the experiment.

(d) Be given an explanation of any benefits to the subject reasonably to be expected from the experiment, if applicable.

(e) Be given a disclosure of any appropriate alternative procedures, drugs or devices that might be advantageous to the subject, and their relative risks and benefits.

(f) Be informed of the avenues of medical treatment, if any, available to the subject after the experiment if complications should arise.

(g) Be given an opportunity to ask any questions concerning the experiment or the procedures involved.

(h) Be instructed that consent to participate in the medical experiment may be withdrawn at any time, and the subject may discontinue participation in the medical experiment without prejudice.

(i) Be given a copy of the signed and dated written consent form.

(j) Be given the opportunity to decide to consent or not to consent to a medical experiment without the intervention of any element of force, fraud, deceit, duress, coercion, or undue influence. (Cal Health & Saf Code §24172)

Informed consent required

Except as otherwise provided by statute, no person shall be subjected to any medical experiment, unless the informed consent of such person is obtained. (Cal Health & Saf Code §24175(a)) (As to definition of "informed consent," see Cal Health & Saf Code §24173.)

If a person is under a conservatorship of the person or of the person and estate, informed consent for a medical experiment involving such person must be obtained:

(1) As provided in Section 2354 of the Probate Code, if the person has not been adjudicated to lack the capacity to give informed consent for medical treatment.

(2) As provided in Section 2355 of the Probate Code, if the person has been adjudicated to lack the capacity to give informed consent for medical treatment. (Cal Health & Saf Code §24175(b))

If an adult person is gravely disabled and is under a conservatorship of the person or of the person and estate, informed consent for a medical experiment involving such person must be obtained from the person, unless the

(*Continued*)

TABLE OF STATE STATUTES (*Continued*)

	conservator has the right to consent to medical treatment on behalf of the conservatee. (Cal Health & Saf Code §24175(c))
	If an adult person is developmentally disabled and has no conservator and is mentally incapable of giving informed consent, informed consent must be obtained for a medical experiment involving such person, pursuant to subdivision (c) of Section 4655 of the Welfare and Institutions Code. (Cal Health & Saf Code §24175(d))
	Informed consent given by a person other than the human subject shall only be for medical experiments related to maintaining or improving the health of the human subject or related to obtaining information about a pathological condition of the human subject. (Cal Health & Saf Code §24175(e))
3. Provisions concerning minors	Notwithstanding the general informed consent provisions (Cal Health & Saf Code §24175), if the subject is a minor, consent must be provided by a parent or guardian of the subject and, if the subject is seven years of age or older, must also be provided by the subject. (Cal Health & Saf Code §111530(a)) Consent thus given shall only be for the prescribing or administering of an experimental drug that is related to (1) maintaining or improving the health of the subject, or (2) obtaining information about a pathological condition of the subject. (Cal Health & Saf Code §111530(b))
4. Provisions concerning pregnant women	—
5. Provisions concerning fetal research	—
6. Provisions concerning in vitro procedures	—
7. Provisions concerning prisoners	Behavioral research
	The Legislature affirms the fundamental right of competent adults to make decisions about their participation in behavioral research. (Cal Pen Code §3501) Behavioral research must be limited to studies of the possible causes, effects and processes of incarceration and studies of prisons as institutional structures or of prisoners as incarcerated persons which present minimal or no risk and no more than mere inconvenience to the subjects of the research. (Cal Pen Code §3505)
	Informed consent will not be required for participation in behavioral research, when the department determines that it would be unnecessary or significantly inhibit the conduct of such research. In the absence of such determination, informed consent will be required for participation in behavioral research. (Cal Pen Code §3505)
	Biomedical research
	No biomedical research shall be conducted on any prisoner in California. (Cal Pen Code §3502)
	Notwithstanding this prohibition, any physician who provides medical care to prisoners may provide a patient who is a prisoner with a drug or treatment available only through a treatment protocol or treatment IND (investigational new drug), if (1) the physician determines that access to that drug is in the best medical interest of the patient, and (2) the patient has given informed consent under Section 3521. (Cal Pen Code §3502.5(a)) Moreover, notwithstanding any other provision of law, neither a public entity nor a public employee shall be liable for any injury caused by the administration of a

TABLE OF STATE STATUTES (*Continued*)

drug pursuant to subdivision (a), where the administration is made in accordance with a treatment IND or a treatment protocol as defined in Section 312 of Title 21 of the Code of Federal Regulations. (Cal Pen Code §3502.5(b))

Informed consent

A prisoner will be deemed to have given informed consent only if all the following conditions are satisfied:

(a) Consent is given without duress, coercion, fraud, or undue influence.

(b) The prisoner is informed in writing of the potential risks or benefits, or both, of the proposed research.

(c) The prisoner is informed, orally and in writing in the language in which he or she is fluent, of each of the following:

(1) An explanation of the biomedical or behavioral research procedures to be followed and their purposes, including identification of any procedures which are experimental.

(2) A description of all known attendant discomfort and risks reasonably to be expected.

(3) A disclosure of any appropriate alternative biomedical or behaviorial research procedures that might be advantageous for the subject.

(4) The nature of the information sought to be gained by the experiment.

(5) The expected recovery time after completion of the experiment.

(6) An offer to answer any inquiries concerning the applicable biomedical or behavioral research procedures.

(7) An instruction that the person is free to withdraw his or her consent and to discontinue participation in the research at any time without prejudice. (Cal Pen Code §3521)

8. Provisions concerning the developmentally disabled/mentally handicapped	If an adult person is developmentally disabled and has no conservator and is mentally incapable of giving informed consent, informed consent must be obtained for a medical experiment involving such person, pursuant to the applicable consent provisions (Cal Wel & Inst Code §4655(c)). (Cal Health & Saf Code §24175(d))
9. Provisions concerning the mentally ill	—
10. Provisions concerning nursing home/long-term facilities residents	—

COLORADO

1. Is there clinical trials legislation?	Yes
2. General provisions of legislation	—
3. Provisions concerning minors	No developmentally disabled minor receiving services shall be subjected to any experimental research without the consent of his or her parent. Such consent may be given only after consultation with (1) the interdisciplinary team, and (2) a developmental disabilities professional not affiliated with the facility or community residential home in which the person receiving services resides. However, no developmentally disabled person of any age shall be subjected to experimental research, if said person implicitly or expressly objects to the procedure. (CRS §27-10.5-114(7))

(*Continued*)

TABLE OF STATE STATUTES (*Continued*)

4. Provisions concerning pregnant women	—
5. Provisions concerning fetal research	—
6. Provisions concerning in vitro procedures	—
7. Provisions concerning prisoners	—
8. Provisions concerning the developmentally disabled/mentally handicapped	No person receiving services will be subjected to any experimental research without the consent of such person, if the person is over eighteen years of age and is able to give such consent, or of the person's parent, if the person is under eighteen years of age, or of the person's legal guardian. Such consent may be given only after consultation with (1) the interdisciplinary team, and (2) a developmental disabilities professional not affiliated with the facility or community residential home in which the person receiving services resides. (CRS §27-10.5-114(7)) Consent will also require that the person whose consent is sought has been adequately and effectively informed as to the method of experimental research, the nature and consequence of such procedures, and the risks, benefits, and purposes of such procedures. (CRS §27-10.5-114((9)(a)) However, no such person of any age will be subjected to experimental research, if said person implicitly or expressly objects to the procedure. (CRS §27-10.5-114(7)) The consent of any person may be revoked at any time. (CRS §27-10.5-114(9)(b))
9. Provisions concerning the mentally ill	—
10. Provisions concerning nursing home/long-term facilities residents	—

CONNECTICUT

1. Is there clinical trials legislation?	Yes
2. General provisions of legislation	—
3. Provisions concerning minors	—
4. Provisions concerning pregnant women	—
5. Provisions concerning fetal research	—
6. Provisions concerning in vitro procedures	—
7. Provisions concerning prisoners	—
8. Provisions concerning the developmentally disabled/mentally handicapped	—
9. Provisions concerning the mentally ill	—
10. Provisions concerning nursing home/long-term facilities residents	There is a patients' bill of rights for any person admitted as a patient to any nursing home facility or chronic disease hospital, which provides that each such patient is afforded the opportunity to participate in the planning of his or her medical treatment and to refuse to participate in experimental research. (Conn. Gen. Stat. §19a-550(b)(3))

DELEWARE

1. Is there clinical trials legislation?	Yes
2. General provisions of legislation	—
3. Provisions concerning minors	Mental Health Hospital patients The hospital or residential center must require written, informed consent by a parent or legal guardian, for the use of research, investigational or experimental drugs or procedures. (16 Del. C. §5161(8)(d))
4. Provisions concerning pregnant women	—
5. Provisions concerning fetal research	—
6. Provisions concerning in vitro procedures	—

TABLE OF STATE STATUTES (*Continued*)

7. Provisions concerning prisoners	—
8. Provisions concerning the developmentally disabled/mentally handicapped	Mental Health Hospital patients The hospital or residential center must require written, informed consent by the patient, or, if the patient is a minor, a parent or legal guardian, for the use of research, investigational or experimental drugs or procedures. (16 Del. C. §5161(8)(d))
9. Provisions concerning the mentally ill	—
10. Provisions concerning nursing home/long-term facilities residents	The patient or resident must give prior informed consent to participation in any experimental research after a complete disclosure of the goals, possible effects on the patient, and whether or not the patient can expect any benefits or alleviation of the patient's condition. In any instance of any type of experiment or administration of experimental medicine, there must be written evidence of compliance with this section, including the signature of the patient, or the signature of the patient's guardian or representative if the patient has been adjudicated incompetent. A copy of signed acknowledgment or informed consent, or both when required, must be forwarded to each signer, and a copy must be retained by the facility. (16 Del. C. §1121(4))

DISTRICT OF COLUMBIA

1. Is there clinical trials legislation?	Yes
2. General provisions of legislation	—
3. Provisions concerning minors	—
4. Provisions concerning pregnant women	—
5. Provisions concerning fetal research	—
6. Provisions concerning in vitro procedures	—
7. Provisions concerning prisoners	—
8. Provisions concerning the developmentally disabled/mentally handicapped	Customers have a right not to be subjected to experimental research without the express and informed consent of the customer, or if the customer cannot give informed consent, of the customer's parent or guardian. (DC Code §6-1969)
9. Provisions concerning the mentally ill	—
10. Provisions concerning nursing home/long-term facilities residents	—

FLORIDA

1. Is there clinical trials legislation?	Yes
2. General provisions of legislation	Health care facility Each health care facility or provider must observe the following standards: Experimental research.—In addition to the provisions of the Florida Medical Consent Act (Fla. Stat. §766.103), a patient has the right to know if medical treatment is for purposes of experimental research and to consent prior to participation in such experimental research. For any patient, regardless of ability to pay or source of payment for his or her care, participation must be a voluntary matter; and a patient has the right to refuse to participate. The patient's consent or refusal must be documented in the patient's care record. (Fla. Stat. §381.026(4)(e))
3. Provisions concerning minors	Prior to instituting a plan of experimental medical treatment, express and informed consent must be obtained from the developmentally disabled client's parent or legal guardian. Information upon which the client shall make

(Continued)

TABLE OF STATE STATUTES (*Continued*)

	necessary treatment decisons will include, but not be limited to: (1) the nature and consequences of such procedures, (2) the risks, benefits, and purposes of such procedures, and (3) alternate procedures available. (Fla Stat §393.13(4)(c)(6))
4. Provisions concerning pregnant women	—
5. Provisions concerning fetal research	—
6. Provisions concerning in vitro procedures	—
7. Provisions concerning prisoners	—
8. Provisions concerning the developmentally disabled/mentally handicapped	Prior to instituting a plan of experimental medical treatment, express and informed consent must be obtained from the client, if competent, or the client's parent or legal guardian. Information upon which the client shall make necessary treatment decisons must include, but not be limited to: (1) the nature and consequences of such procedures, (2) the risks, benefits, and purposes of such procedures, and (3) alternate procedures available. (Fla Stat §393.13(4)(c)(6))
9. Provisions concerning the mentally ill	—
10. Provisions concerning nursing home/long-term facilities residents	—

GEORGIA

1. Is there clinical trials legislation?	Yes
2. General provisions of legislation	—
3. Provisions concerning minors	—
4. Provisions concerning pregnant women	—
5. Provisions concerning fetal research	—
6. Provisions concerning in vitro procedures	—
7. Provisions concerning prisoners	—
8. Provisions concerning the developmentally disabled/mentally handicapped	—
9. Provisions concerning the mentally ill	—
10. Provisions concerning nursing home/long-term facilities residents	Each resident must be free from experimental research or treatment, unless the informed, written consent of the resident or guardian is first obtained. (O.C.G.A. §31-8-108(c))

HAWAII

1. Is there clinical trials legislation?	No
2. General provisions of legislation	—
3. Provisions concerning minors	—
4. Provisions concerning pregnant women	—
5. Provisions concerning fetal research	—
6. Provisions concerning in vitro procedures	—
7. Provisions concerning prisoners	—
8. Provisions concerning the developmentally disabled/mentally handicapped	—
9. Provisions concerning the mentally ill	—
10. Provisions concerning nursing home/long-term facilities residents	—

IDAHO

1. Is there clinical trials legislation?	No
2. General provisions of legislation	—
3. Provisions concerning minors	—
4. Provisions concerning pregnant women	—
5. Provisions concerning fetal research	—
6. Provisions concerning in vitro procedures	—
7. Provisions concerning prisoners	—

TABLE OF STATE STATUTES (*Continued*)

8. Provisions concerning the developmentally disabled/mentally handicapped	—
9. Provisions concerning the mentally ill	—
10. Provisions concerning nursing home/long-term facilities residents	—

ILLINOIS

1. Is there clinical trials legislation?	Yes
2. General provisions of legislation	Any patient who is the subject of a research program or an experimental procedure, as defined under the rules and regulations of the Hospital Licensing Act (210 ILCS 85/1 et seq.), will have, at a minimum, the right to receive an explanation of the nature and possible consequences of such research or experiment before the research or experiment is conducted, and to consent to or reject it. (410 ILCS 50/3.1(a)) No physician may conduct any research program or experimental procedure on a patient without the prior informed consent of the patient or, if the patient is unable to consent, the patient's guardian, spouse, parent, or authorized agent. (410 ILCS 50/3.1(b)) However, these rules will not apply to any research program or medical experimental procedure for patients subject to a life-threatening emergency that is conducted in accordance with Part 50 of Title 21 of, and Part 46 of Title 45 of, the Code of Federal Regulations. (410 ILCS 50/3.1(c))
3. Provisions concerning minors	—
4. Provisions concerning pregnant women	—
5. Provisions concerning fetal research	No person is permitted to sell or experiment upon a fetus produced by the fertilization of a human ovum by a human sperm, unless such experimentation is therapeutic to the fetus thereby produced. This does not prohibit the performance of in vitro fetilization. (720 ILCS 510/6(7)) However, nothing prohibits the use of any tissues or cells obtained from a dead fetus or dead premature infant whose death did not result from an induced abortion, for therapeutic purposes or scientific, research, or laboratory experimentation, provided that written consent to such use is obtained from one of the parents of the fetus or infant. (720 ILCS 510/12.1)
6. Provisions concerning in vitro procedures	—
7. Provisions concerning prisoners	—
8. Provisions concerning the developmentally disabled/mentally handicapped	Intervention, treatment or aftercare services under Alcoholism and Other Drug Abuse and Dependency Act A patient must be permitted to refuse to participate in any experimental research or medical procedure without compromising his or her access to other, non-experimental services. Before a patient is placed in an experimental research or medical procedure, the provider must first obtain informed written consent or otherwise comply with the federal requirements regarding the protection of human subjects contained in 45 C.F.R. Part 46. (20 ILCS 301/30-5(q))
9. Provisions concerning the mentally ill	—
10. Provisions concerning nursing home/long-term facilities residents	No resident will be subjected to experimental research or treatment without first obtaining his or her informed, written consent. (210 ILCS 45/2-104(a))

(Continued)

TABLE OF STATE STATUTES (*Continued*)

The conduct of any experimental research or treatment must be authorized and monitored by an institutional review committee appointed by the administrator of the facility where such research and treatment is conducted. The membership, operating procedures and review criteria for institutional review committees will be prescribed under rules and regulations of the Department. (210 ILCS 45/2-104(a))

INDIANA

1.	Is there clinical trials legislation?	Yes
2.	General provisions of legislation	—
3.	Provisions concerning minors	—
4.	Provisions concerning pregnant women	—
5.	Provisions concerning fetal research	No experiments except pathological examinations may be conducted on any fetus abourt, nor may any fetus so aborted be transported out of Indiana for experimental purposes. (Burns Ind. Code Ann. §16-34-2-6)
6.	Provisions concerning in vitro procedures	—
7.	Provisions concerning prisoners	—
8.	Provisions concerning the developmentally disabled/mentally handicapped	—
9.	Provisions concerning the mentally ill	—
10.	Provisions concerning nursing home/long-term facilities residents	—

IOWA

1.	Is there clinical trials legislation?	No
2.	General provisions of legislation	—
3.	Provisions concerning minors	—
4.	Provisions concerning pregnant women	—
5.	Provisions concerning fetal research	—
6.	Provisions concerning in vitro procedures	—
7.	Provisions concerning prisoners	—
8.	Provisions concerning the developmentally disabled/mentally handicapped	—
9.	Provisions concerning the mentally ill	—
10.	Provisions concerning nursing home/long-term facilities residents	—

KANSAS

1.	Is there clinical trials legislation?	No
2.	General provisions of legislation	—
3.	Provisions concerning minors	—
4.	Provisions concerning pregnant women	—
5.	Provisions concerning fetal research	—
6.	Provisions concerning in vitro procedures	—
7.	Provisions concerning prisoners	—
8.	Provisions concerning the developmentally disabled/mentally handicapped	—
9.	Provisions concerning the mentally ill	—
10.	Provisions concerning nursing home/long-term facilities residents	—

KENTUCKY

1.	Is there clinical trials legislation?	Yes
2.	General provisions of legislation	—
3.	Provisions concerning minors	—
4.	Provisions concerning pregnant women	—

TABLE OF STATE STATUTES (*Continued*)

5. Provisions concerning fetal research	No person may sell, transfer, distribute, or give away any live or viable aborted child, or permit such child to be used for any form of experimentation. (KRS §436.026)
6. Provisions concerning in vitro procedures	—
7. Provisions concerning prisoners	—
8. Provisions concerning the developmentally disabled/mentally handicapped	—
9. Provisions concerning the mentally ill	—
10. Provisions concerning nursing home/long-term facilities residents	—

LOUISANA

1. Is there clinical trials legislation?	Yes
2. General provisions of legislation	—
3. Provisions concerning minors	—
4. Provisions concerning pregnant women	—
5. Provisions concerning fetal research	No person is permitted to experiment on an unborn child or on a child born as the result of an abortion, whether the unborn child or child is alive or dead, unless the experimentation is therapeutic to the unborn child or child. (La RS §40:1299.35.13)
6. Provisions concerning in vitro procedures	The use of a human ovum fertilized in vitro is solely for the support and contribution of the complete development of human in utero implantation. No in vitro fertilized human ovum will be farmed or cultured solely for research purposes or any other purposes. Furthermore, the sale of a human ovum, fertilized human ovum, or human embryo is expressly prohibited. (La RS §9:122)
7. Provisions concerning prisoners	—
8. Provisions concerning the developmentally disabled/mentally handicapped	—
9. Provisions concerning the mentally ill	—
10. Provisions concerning nursing home/long-term facilities residents	—

MAINE

1. Is there clinical trials legislation?	Yes
2. General provisions of legislation	—
3. Provisions concerning minors	—
4. Provisions concerning pregnant women	—
5. Provisions concerning fetal research	—
6. Provisions concerning in vitro procedures	—
7. Provisions concerning prisoners	—
8. Provisions concerning the developmentally disabled/mentally handicapped	Prior to instituting a plan of experimental medical treatment, express and informed consent must be obtained from the person with mental retardation or autism, unless the person has been found to be legally incompetent, in which case the person's guardian may consent. Before making a treatment decision, the person must be given information, including, but not limited to, (1) the nature and consequences of the procedures, (2) the risks, benefits and purposes of the procedures, and (3) the availability of alternate procedures. The person, or, if legally incompetent, that person's guardian, may withdraw consent at any time, with or without cause, before treatment. (34-B M.R.S. §5605(8)(G))
9. Provisions concerning the mentally ill	—

(*Continued*)

TABLE OF STATE STATUTES (*Continued*)

10. Provisions concerning nursing home/long-term facilities residents	—

MARYLAND

1. Is there clinical trials legislation?	Yes
2. General provisions of legislation	—
3. Provisions concerning minors	—
4. Provisions concerning pregnant women	—
5. Provisions concerning fetal research	—
6. Provisions concerning in vitro procedures	—
7. Provisions concerning prisoners	—
8. Provisions concerning the developmentally disabled/mentally handicapped	—
9. Provisions concerning the mentally ill	—
10. Provisions concerning nursing home/long-term facilities residents	The extended care facility must (1) have the informed consent of a resident before the resident participates in any experimental research, and (2) keep the resident's written acknowledgment of that consent. (Md Health-General Code Ann. §19.344)

MASSACHUSETTS

1. Is there clinical trials legislation?	Yes
2. General provisions of legislation	—
3. Provisions concerning minors	—
4. Provisions concerning pregnant women	—
5. Provisions concerning fetal research	Living fetus No one is permitted to use any live human fetus, whether before or after expulsion from its mother's womb, for scientific, laboratory, research or other kind of experimentation. However, this does not prohibit procedures incident to the study of a human fetus while it is in its mother's womb, provided that (1) in the best medical judgment of the physician, made at the time of the study, said procedures do not substantially jeopardize the life or health of the fetus, and (2) said fetus is not the subject of a planned abortion. In any criminal proceeding, a fetus shall be conclusively presumed not to be the subject of a planned abortion if the mother signed a written statement at the time of the study, that she was not planning an abortion. (Mass. Ann. Laws ch. 112, @ 12J(a)l) This does not prohibit or regulate diagnostic or remedial procedures the purpose of which is to determine the life or health of the fetus involved or to preserve the life or health of the fetus involved or the mother involved. (Mass. Ann. Laws ch. 112, §12J(a)l) Dead fetus No experimentation may knowingly be performed upon a dead fetus, unless the consent of the mother has first been obtained; however, that such consent is not required for a routine pathological study. In any criminal proceeding, consent will be conclusively presumed to have been granted for the purposes of this section by a written statement, signed by the mother who is at least eighteen years of age, to the effect that she consents to the use of her fetus for scientific, laboratory, research or other kind of experimentation or study; such written consent will constitute lawful authorization for the transfer of the dead fetus. (Mass. Ann. Laws ch. 112, §12J(a)ll)

TABLE OF STATE STATUTES (*Continued*)

Distribution
   No one is permitted to knowingly sell, transfer, distribute or give away any fetus for a use which is in violation of the governing statute. For purposes of this section, the word "fetus" will include also an embryo or neonate. (Mass. Ann. Laws ch. 112, §12J(a)IV)

6. Provisions concerning in vitro procedures — —
7. Provisions concerning prisoners — —
8. Provisions concerning the developmentally disabled/mentally handicapped

   Every patient or resident of a facility has the right to refuse to serve as a research subject and to refuse any care or examination when the primary purpose is educational or informational rather than therapeutic. (Mass. Ann. Laws ch 111 §70E)

9. Provisions concerning the mentally ill

   Every patient or resident of a facility has the right to refuse to serve as a research subject and to refuse any care or examination when the primary purpose is educational or informational rather than therapeutic. (Mass. Ann. Laws ch 111 §70E)

10. Provisions concerning nursing home/long-term facilities residents

   Every patient or resident of a facility has the right to refuse to serve as a research subject and to refuse any care or examination when the primary purpose is educational or informational rather than therapeutic. (Mass. Ann. Laws ch 111 §70E)

MICHIGAN

1. Is there clinical trials legislation?   Yes
2. General provisions of legislation   —
3. Provisions concerning minors   —
4. Provisions concerning pregnant women

   The statutory provisions concerning use of an embryo, fetus, or neonate in research do not prohibit or regulate diagnostic, assessment, or treatment procedures, the purpose of which is to determine the life or status or improve the health of the mother involved. (MCLS §333.2686)

5. Provisions concerning fetal research

   Living fetus
      A person is not permitted to use a live human embryo, fetus, or neonate for nontherapeutic research, if, in the best judgment of the person conducting the research, based upon the available knowledge or information at the approximate time of the research, the research substantially jeopardizes the life or health of the embryo, fetus, or neonate. Nontherapeutic research shall not in any case be performed on an embryo or fetus known by the person conducting the research to be the subject of a planned abortion being performed for any purpose other than to protect the life of the mother. (MCLS §333.2685(1)) (The embryo or fetus will be conclusively presumed not to be the subject of a planned abortion if, at the time of the research, the mother signed a written statement that she was not planning an abortion. (MCLS §333.2685(2)))

   Dead fetus
      Research may not knowingly be performed upon a dead embryo, fetus, or neonate, unless the consent of the mother has first been obtained. However, consent will not be required in the case of a routine pathological study. (MCLS §333.2688(1))

(*Continued*)

TABLE OF STATE STATUTES (*Continued*)

Consent will be conclusively presumed to have been granted by a written statement, signed by the mother, that she consents to the use of her dead embryo, fetus, or neonate for research. (MCLS §333.2688(2))

Written consent shall constitute lawful authorization for the transfer of the dead embryo, fetus, or neonate to medical research facilities. (MCLS §333.2688(3))

Research being performed upon a dead embryo, fetus, or neonate must be conducted in accordance with the same standards applicable to research conducted pursuant to part 101. (MCLS §333.2688(4))

Exception
These provisions do not prohibit or regulate diagnostic, assessment, or treatment procedures, the purpose of which is to determine the life or status or improve the health of the embryo, fetus, or neonate involved or the mother involved. (MCLS §333.2686)

Distribution
A person must not knowingly sell, transfer, distribute, or give away an embryo, fetus, or neonate for a use which is in violation of the applicable provisions. (MCLS §333.2690)

6. Provisions concerning in vitro procedures —
7. Provisions concerning prisoners —
8. Provisions concerning the developmentally disabled/mentally handicapped —
9. Provisions concerning the mentally ill —
10. Provisions concerning nursing home/long-term facilities residents —

MINNESOTA

1. Is there clinical trials legislation?   Yes
2. General provisions of legislation   —
3. Provisions concerning minors   —
4. Provisions concerning pregnant women   —
5. Provisions concerning fetal research

The use of a living human conceptus for research or experimentation which verifiable scientific evidence has shown to be harmless to the conceptus is permitted. (Minn Stat §145.422(subd. 2))

Whoever uses or permits the use of a living human conceptus for any type of scientific, laboratory research or other experimentation, except to protect the life or health of the conceptus, or except as provided by statute, shall be guilty of a gross misdemeanor. (Minn Stat §145.422(subd. 1))

6. Provisions concerning in vitro procedures   —
7. Provisions concerning prisoners   —
8. Provisions concerning the developmentally disabled/mentally handicapped

Written, informed consent must be obtained prior to a patient's or resident's participation in experimental research. Patients and residents have the right to refuse participation. Both consent and refusal must be documented in the individual care record. (Minn. Stat. §144.651(subd 13))

Services to mentally retarded
The consumer's protection-related rights include the right to give or withhold written informed consent to participate in any research or experimental treatment. (Minn. Stat. §245B.04(subd 3)(9))

TABLE OF STATE STATUTES (*Continued*)

9. Provisions concerning the mentally ill

Written, informed consent must be obtained prior to a patient's or resident's participation in experimental research. Patients and residents have the right to refuse participation. Both consent and refusal must be documented in the individual care record. (Minn. Stat. §144.651(subd 13))

10. Provisions concerning nursing home/long-term facilities residents

Written, informed consent must be obtained prior to a patient's or resident's participation in experimental research. Patients and residents have the right to refuse participation. Both consent and refusal must be documented in the individual care record. (Minn. Stat. §144.651(subd 13))

MISSISSIPPI
1. Is there clinical trials legislation? — No
2. General provisions of legislation — —
3. Provisions concerning minors — —
4. Provisions concerning pregnant women — —
5. Provisions concerning fetal research — —
6. Provisions concerning in vitro procedures — —
7. Provisions concerning prisoners — —
8. Provisions concerning the developmentally disabled/mentally handicapped — —
9. Provisions concerning the mentally ill — —
10. Provisions concerning nursing home/long-term facilities residents — —

MISSOURI
1. Is there clinical trials legislation? — Yes
2. General provisions of legislation — —
3. Provisions concerning minors — —
4. Provisions concerning pregnant women — —
5. Provisions concerning fetal research

No person shall use any fetus or child aborted alive for any type of scientific, research, laboratory or other kind of experimentation, either prior to or subsequent to any abortion procedure, except as necessary to protect or preserve the life and health of such fetus or child aborted alive. (RS Mo. §188.037)

6. Provisions concerning in vitro procedures — —
7. Provisions concerning prisoners — —
8. Provisions concerning the developmentally disabled/mentally handicapped — —
9. Provisions concerning the mentally ill

Each patient, resident or client will be entitled to not be the subject of experimental research without his prior written and informed consent or that of his parent, if a minor, or his guardian (except that no involuntary patient shall be subject to experimental research except as statutorily provided.—RS Mo. §630.115(1)(8)) A patient, resident or client also has the right to decide not to participate and may withdraw from any research at any time for any reason. (RS Mo. §630.115(1)(9))

10. Provisions concerning nursing home/long-term facilities residents

Each resident admitted to the facility must be fully informed by a physician of his health and medical condition unless medically contraindicated, as documented by a physician in his resident record, and is afforded the opportunity to participate in the planning of his total care and medical treatment and to refuse treatment, and participates in experimental research only upon his informed consent. (RS Mo. §198.088(1)(6)(c))

(*Continued*)

TABLE OF STATE STATUTES (*Continued*)

MONTANA

1. Is there clinical trials legislation?	Yes
2. General provisions of legislation	—
3. Provisions concerning minors	—
4. Provisions concerning pregnant women	—
5. Provisions concerning fetal research	—
6. Provisions concerning in vitro procedures	—
7. Provisions concerning prisoners	—
8. Provisions concerning the developmentally disabled/mentally handicapped	Residents of a residential facility have a right not to be subjected to experimental research without the express and informed consent of the resident, if the resident is able to give consent, and of the resident's parents or guardian or the responsible person appointed by the court after opportunities for consultation with independent specialists and with legal counsel. (Mont. Code Anno. §53-20-147)
9. Provisions concerning the mentally ill	Patients have a right not to be subjected to experimental research without the express and informed consent of the patient, if the patient is able to give consent, and of the patient's guardian, if any, and the friend of respondent appointed by the court after opportunities for consultation with independent specialists and with legal counsel. If there is no friend of respondent or if the friend of respondent appointed by the court is no longer available, then a friend of respondent who is in no way connected with the facility, the department, or the research project must be appointed prior to the involvement of the patient in any experimental research. At least 10 days prior to the commencement of experimental research, the facility must send notice of intent to involve the patient in experimental research to the patient, the patient's next of kin, if known, the patient's legal guardian, if any, the attorney who most recently represented the patient, and the friend of respondent appointed by the court. (Mont. Code Anno., @ 53-21-147(1))
	A patient has the right to appropriate protection before participating in an experimental treatment, including the right to a reasonable explanation of the procedure to be followed, expected benefits, relative advantages, and the potential risks and discomforts of any experimental treatment. A patient has the right to revoke at any time consent to an experimental treatment. (Mont. Code Anno., §53-21-147(3))
10. Provisions concerning nursing home/long-term facilities residents	—

NEBRASKA

1. Is there clinical trials legislation?	Yes
2. General provisions of legislation	—
3. Provisions concerning minors	—
4. Provisions concerning pregnant women	—
5. Provisions concerning fetal research	The knowing, willful, or intentional sale, transfer, distribution, or giving away of any live or viable aborted child for any form of experimentation is a felony. The knowing, willful, or intentional consenting to, aiding, or abetting of any such sale, transfer, distribution, or other unlawful disposition of an aborted child is a felony. This does not prohibit or regulate diagnostic or remedial procedures the purpose of which is to preserve the life or health of the aborted child or the mother. (RRS Neb. §28-342)

TABLE OF STATE STATUTES (*Continued*)

6. Provisions concerning in vitro procedures	—
7. Provisions concerning prisoners	—
8. Provisions concerning the developmentally disabled/mentally handicapped	—
9. Provisions concerning the mentally ill	—
10. Provisions concerning nursing home/long-term facilities residents	—

NEVADA

1. Is there clinical trials legislation?	No
2. General provisions of legislation	—
3. Provisions concerning minors	—
4. Provisions concerning pregnant women	—
5. Provisions concerning fetal research	—
6. Provisions concerning in vitro procedures	—
7. Provisions concerning prisoners	—
8. Provisions concerning the developmentally disabled/mentally handicapped	—
9. Provisions concerning the mentally ill	—
10. Provisions concerning nursing home/long-term facilities residents	—

NEW HAMPSHIRE

1. Is there clinical trials legislation?	Yes
2. General provisions of legislation	Hospital

2. (continued) Hospital

The patient must be given the opportunity to participate in the planning of his or her total care and medical treatment, to refuse treatment, and to be involved in experimental research upon the patient's written consent only. For the purposes of this paragraph, "health care provider" means any person, corporation, facility, or institution either licensed by this state or otherwise lawfully providing health care services, including, but not limited to, a physician, hospital or other health care facility, dentist, nurse, optometrist, podiatrist, physical therapist, or psychologist, and any officer, employee, or agent of such provider acting in the course and scope of employment or agency related to or supportive of health care services. (RSA §151:21(IV))

Home health care

The statement of rights must state that, at a minimum, the client has a right to be involved in experimental research only upon the client's voluntary written consent. (RSA §151:21-b(II)(e))

Right to information

The patient must be given the opportunity to participate in the planning of his or her total care and medical treatment, to refuse treatment, and to be involved in experimental research upon the patient's written consent only. (RSA §332-I:2)

3. Provisions concerning minors	—
4. Provisions concerning pregnant women	—
5. Provisions concerning fetal research	—
6. Provisions concerning in vitro procedures	—
7. Provisions concerning prisoners	—
8. Provisions concerning the developmentally disabled/mentally handicapped	—

(Continued)

TABLE OF STATE STATUTES (*Continued*)

9. Provisions concerning the mentally ill	—
10. Provisions concerning nursing home/long-term facilities residents	—

NEW JERSEY

1. Is there clinical trials legislation?	Yes
2. General provisions of legislation	—
3. Provisions concerning minors	No person receiving services for the developmentally disabled at any facility will be subjected to medical, behavioral, or pharmacological research without the express and informed consent of such person's guardian ad litem specifically appointed by a court for the matter of consent to these proceedings, if a minor. Such consent must be made in writing and placed in the person's record. (N.J. Stat. §30:6D-5(a)(4))
4. Provisions concerning pregnant women	—
5. Provisions concerning fetal research	—
6. Provisions concerning in vitro procedures	—
7. Provisions concerning prisoners	—
8. Provisions concerning the developmentally disabled/mentally handicapped	No person receiving services for the developmentally disabled at any facility will be subjected to medical, behavioral, or pharmacological research without the express and informed consent of such person, if a competent adult, or of such person's guardian ad litem specifically appointed by a court for the matter of consent to these proceedings, if a minor or an incompetent adult or a person administratively determined to be mentally deficient. Such consent must be made in writing and placed in such person's record. (N.J. Stat. §30:6D-5(a)(4)) Under no circumstances may a person in treatment be subjected to hazardous or intrusive experimental research which is not directly related to the specific goals of his or her treatment program. (N.J. Stat. §30:6D-5(a)(4))
9. Provisions concerning the mentally ill	Each patient in treatment has the right not to be subjected to experimental research, without the express and informed consent of the patient after consultation with counsel or interested party of the patient's choice. Such consent must be made in writing, a copy of which must be placed in the patient's treatment record. If the patient has been adjudicated incompetent, a court of competent jurisdiction shall hold a hearing to determine the necessity of such procedure, at which the client is physically present, represented by counsel, and provided the right and opportunity to be confronted with and to cross-examine all witnesses alleging the necessity of such procedures. In such proceedings, the burden of proof will be on the party alleging the necessity of such procedures. In the event that a patient cannot afford counsel, the court must appoint an attorney not less than 10 days before the hearing. An attorney so appointed shall be entitled to a reasonable fee to be determined by the court and paid by the county from which the patient was admitted. Under no circumstances may a patient in treatment be subjected to experimental research which is not directly related to the specific goals of his or her treatment program. (N.J. Stat. §30:4-24.2(d)(2))

TABLE OF STATE STATUTES (*Continued*)

Short term care facility

A patient in a short-term care facility has the right not to participate in experimental research without the express and informed, written consent of the patient. The patient shall have the right to consult with counsel or interested party of the patient's choice. A copy of the patient's consent must be placed in the patient's treatment record. If the patient has been adjudicated incompetent, a court of competent jurisdiction will hold a hearing to determine the necessity of the procedure. The patient must be physically present at the hearing, represented by counsel, and provided the right and opportunity to be confronted with and to cross-examine all witnesses alleging the necessity of the procedure. (N.J. Stat. §30:4-27.11d(a)(5)

Screening service

A patient in a screening service will have the following rights, which will apply during the first 24 hours of involuntary assessment and care provided at a screening service and which must not be denied under any circumstances. Included in these rights is the right not to be subjected to experimental research, without the express and informed, written consent of the patient. The patient shall have the right to consult with counsel or interested party of the patient's choice. A copy of the patient's consent shall be placed in the patient's treatment record. (N.J. Stat. §30:4-27.11e(a)(2))

10. Provisions concerning nursing home/long-term facilities residents	A resident has the right to refuse to participate in experimental research, but if he or she chooses to participate, informed written consent must be obtained. (N.J. Stat. §30:13-5)

NEW MEXICO

1. Is there clinical trials legislation?	Yes
2. General provisions of legislation	—
3. Provisions concerning minors	—
4. Provisions concerning pregnant women	No woman, known to be pregnant according to generally accepted medical standards, shall be involved as a subject in any clinical research activity unless:

(1) the purpose of the activity is to meet the health needs of the mother or the fetus and the fetus will be placed at risk only to the minimum extent necessary to meet such needs; or

(2) there is no significant risk to the fetus. (N.M. Stat. Ann. §24-9A-2(A))

Such activity may be conducted only if the mother is legally competent and has given her informed consent after having been fully informed regarding possible impact on the fetus. (N.M. Stat. Ann. §24-9A-2(B))

No clinical research activity involving pregnant women shall be conducted, unless:

(1) appropriate studies on animals and nonpregnant human beings have been completed;

(2) anyone engaged in conducting the research activity will have no part in: (a) any decisions as to the timing, method and procedures used to terminate the pregnancy; and (b) determining the viability of the fetus at the termination of the pregnancy; and

(3) no procedural changes which may cause significant risk to the pregnant woman will be introduced into the

(*Continued*)

TABLE OF STATE STATUTES (*Continued*)

procedure for terminating the pregnancy solely in the interest of the research activity. (N.M. Stat. Ann. §24-9A-5(A))

No consent to involve a pregnant woman as a subject in clinical research activity will be valid, unless the pregnant woman has been fully informed of the following:

(1) a fair explanation of the procedures to be followed and their purposes, including identification of any procedures which are experimental;

(2) a description of any attendant discomforts and risks reasonably to be expected;

(3) a description of any benefits reasonably to be expected;

(4) a disclosure of any appropriate alternative procedures that might be advantageous for the subject;

(5) an offer to answer any inquiries concerning the procedure; and

(6) an instruction that the person who gave the consent is free to withdraw his consent and to discontinue participation in the project or activity at any time without prejudice to the subject. (N.M. Stat. Ann. §24-9A-5(C))

5. Provisions concerning fetal research

Fetus

No fetus shall be involved as a subject in any clinical research activity, unless (1) the purpose of the activity is to meet the health needs of the particular fetus, and (2) the fetus will be placed at risk only to the minimum extent necessary to meet such needs, or no significant risk to the fetus is imposed by the research activity. (N.M. Stat. Ann. §24-9A-3(A)) Such activity shall be conducted only if the mother is legally competent and has given her informed consent. (N.M. Stat. Ann. §24-9A-3(B))

Live born infant

No live-born infant shall be involved as a subject in any clinical research activity, unless (1) the purpose of the activity is to meet the health needs of that particular infant, and (2) the infant will be placed at risk only to the minimum extent necessary to meet such needs, or no significant risk to such infant is imposed by the research activity. (N.M. Stat. Ann. §24-9A-4(A)) Such an activity shall be conducted only if (1) the nature of the investigation is such that adults or mentally competent persons would not be suitable subjects, and (2) the mother or father or the infant's legal guardian is mentally competent and has given his or her informed consent. (N.M. Stat. Ann. §24-9A-4(A))

Requirements

No clinical research activity involving fetuses or live born infants shall be conducted unless:

(1) appropriate studies on animals and nonpregnant human beings have been completed;

(2) anyone engaged in conducting the research activity will have no part in: (a) any decisions as to the timing, method and procedures used to terminate the pregnancy; and (b) determining the viability of the fetus at the termination of the pregnancy; and

(3) no procedural changes which may cause significant risk to the fetus or the pregnant woman will be introduced

TABLE OF STATE STATUTES (*Continued*)

into the procedure for terminating the pregnancy solely in the interest of the research activity. (N.M. Stat. Ann. §24-9A-5(A))

Inducements

No inducements, monetary or otherwise, shall be offered to any woman to terminate her pregnancy for the purpose of subjecting her fetus or live-born infant to clinical research activity. (N.M. Stat. Ann. §24-9A-5(B))

Consent

No consent to involve a fetus or a live born infant as a subject in clinical research activity will be valid, unless the pregnant woman has been fully informed of the following:

(1) a fair explanation of the procedures to be followed and their purposes, including identification of any procedures which are experimental;

(2) a description of any attendant discomforts and risks reasonably to be expected;

(3) a description of any benefits reasonably to be expected;

(4) a disclosure of any appropriate alternative procedures that might be advantageous for the subject;

(5) an offer to answer any inquiries concerning the procedure; and

(6) an instruction that the person who gave the consent is free to withdraw consent and to discontinue participation in the project or activity at any time, without prejudice. (N.M. Stat. Ann. §24-9A-5(C))

6. Provisions concerning in vitro procedures

No clinical research activity involving fetuses shall be conducted unless:

(1) appropriate studies on animals and nonpregnant human beings have been completed;

(2) anyone engaged in conducting the research activity will have no part in: (a) any decisions as to the timing, method and procedures used to terminate the pregnancy; and (b) determining the viability of the fetus at the termination of the pregnancy; and

(3) no procedural changes which may cause significant risk to the fetus or the pregnant woman will be introduced into the procedure for terminating the pregnancy solely in the interest of the research activity. (N.M. Stat. Ann. §24-9A-5(A))

"Clinical research" means any biomedical or behavioral research involving human subjects, including the unborn, conducted according to a formal procedure. The term is to be construed liberally to embrace research concerning all physiological processes in man and includes research involving human in vitro fertilization, but will not include diagnostic testing, treatment, therapy or related procedures conducted by formal protocols deemed necessary for the care of the particular patient upon whom such activity is performed and shall not include human in vitro fertilization performed to treat infertility; provided that this procedure shall include provisions to insure that each living fertilized ovum, zygote or embryo is implanted in a human female recipient, and no physician may stipulate that a woman must abort in the event the pregnancy should produce a deformed or handicapped child. Emergency medical procedures necessary to preserve the life or health of the mother or the fetus will not be considered to be clinical research. (N.M. Stat. Ann. §24-9A-1)

(*Continued*)

TABLE OF STATE STATUTES (*Continued*)

7. Provisions concerning prisoners	—
8. Provisions concerning the developmentally disabled/mentally handicapped	—
9. Provisions concerning the mentally ill	—
10. Provisions concerning nursing home/long-term facilities residents	—

NEW YORK

1. Is there clinical trials legislation?	Yes
2. General provisions of legislation	Informed consent

No human research may be conducted in the absence of the voluntary informed consent subscribed to in writing by the human subject. If the human subject is a minor, such consent must be subscribed to in writing by the minor's parent or legal guardian. If the human subject is otherwise legally unable to render consent, such consent must be subscribed to in writing by another person legally empowered to act on behalf of the human subject. No such voluntary informed consent shall include any language through which the human subject waives, or appears to waive, any of his legal rights, including any release of any individual, institution or agency, or any agents thereof, from liability for negligence. (NY CLS Pub Health §2442)

Conduct of human research

No one except a researcher is permitted to conduct human research. (NY CLS Pub Health §2443)

3. Provisions concerning minors	Informed consent

No human research may be conducted in the absence of the voluntary informed consent subscribed to in writing by the human subject. If the human subject is a minor, such consent must be subscribed to in writing by the minor's parent or legal guardian. (NY CLS Pub Health §2442)

4. Provisions concerning pregnant women	—
5. Provisions concerning fetal research	—
6. Provisions concerning in vitro procedures	—
7. Provisions concerning prisoners	—
8. Provisions concerning the developmentally disabled/mentally handicapped	—
9. Provisions concerning the mentally ill	Informed consent

No human research may be conducted in the absence of the voluntary informed consent subscribed to in writing by the human subject. If the human subject is otherwise legally unable to render consent, such consent must be subscribed to in writing by another person who is legally empowered to act on behalf of the human subject. (NY CLS Pub Health §2442)

10. Provisions concerning nursing home/long-term facilities residents	—

NORTH CAROLINA

1. Is there clinical trials legislation?	Yes
2. General provisions of legislation	—
3. Provisions concerning minors	—
4. Provisions concerning pregnant women	—
5. Provisions concerning fetal research	—
6. Provisions concerning in vitro procedures	—

TABLE OF STATE STATUTES (*Continued*)

7. Provisions concerning prisoners —
8. Provisions concerning the developmentally
    disabled/mentally handicapped —
9. Provisions concerning the mentally ill —
10. Provisions concerning nursing home/long-term
    facilities residents

The patient must give prior informed consent to participation in experimental research. (N.C. Gen. Stat. §131E-117(4))

NORTH DAKOTA
1. Is there clinical trials legislation? — Yes
2. General provisions of legislation —
3. Provisions concerning minors —
4. Provisions concerning pregnant women

The provision concerning use of a live fetus in research does not prohibit or regulate diagnostic or remedial procedures, the purpose of which is to preserve the life or health of the mother involved. (N.D. Cent. Code, §14-02.2-01(3))

5. Provisions concerning fetal research

Live fetus

A person may not use any live human fetus, whether before or after expulsion from its mother's womb, for scientific, laboratory, research, or other kind of experimentation. This does not prohibit procedures incident to the study of a human fetus while it is in its mother's womb, provided that (1) in the best medical judgment of the physician, made at the time of the study, the procedures do not substantially jeopardize the life or health of the fetus, and (2) the fetus is not the subject of a planned abortion. In any criminal proceeding, the fetus is conclusively presumed not to be the subject of a planned abortion if the mother signed a written statement at the time of the study, that the mother was not planning an abortion. (N.D. Cent. Code, §14-02.2-01(1))

A person may not use a fetus or newborn child, or any tissue or organ thereof, resulting from an induced abortion in animal or human research, experimentation, or study, or for animal or human transplantation. (N.D. Cent. Code, §14-02.2-01(2)) This does not prohibit or regulate diagnostic or remedial procedures, the purpose of which is to determine the life or health of the fetus involved or to preserve the life or health of the fetus involved, or of the mother involved. (N.D. Cent. Code, §14-02.2-01(3))

Dead fetus

An experimentation may not knowingly be performed upon a dead fetus resulting from an occurrence other than an induced abortion, unless the consent of the mother has first been obtained; provided, however, that the consent is not required in the case of a routine pathological study. In any criminal proceeding, consent is conclusively presumed to have been granted for the purposes of this section by a written statement, signed by the mother who is at least eighteen years of age, to the effect that she consents to the use of her fetus for scientific, laboratory, research, or other kind of experimentation or study. Such written consent constitutes lawful authorization for the transfer of the dead fetus. (N.D. Cent. Code, §14-02.2-02(1))

A person may not use a fetus or fetal organs or tissue resulting from an induced abortion in animal or human research, experimentation, or study, or for animal or human

(*Continued*)

TABLE OF STATE STATUTES (*Continued*)

	transplantation except for diagnostic or remedial procedures, the purpose of which is to determine the life or health of the fetus or to preserve the life or health of the fetus or mother, or pathological study. (N.D. Cent. Code, §14-02.2-02(2))
	Distribution
	A person may not knowingly sell, transfer, distribute, give away, accept, use, or attempt to use any fetus or fetal organs or tissue for a use that is in violation of this section. For purposes of this section, the word "fetus" includes also an embryo or neonate. (N.D. Cent. Code, §14-02.2-02(4))
6. Provisions concerning in vitro procedures	—
7. Provisions concerning prisoners	—
8. Provisions concerning the developmentally disabled/mentally handicapped	No person receiving services at any institution or facility for the developmentally disabled may be subjected to medical, behavioral, or pharmacological research, except in conformity with an order of a court of competent jurisdiction. Under no circumstances may a person receiving treatment be subjected to hazardous or intrusive experimental research which is not directly related to the specific goals of that person's treatment program. (N.D. Cent. Code, §25-01.2-09(4))
9. Provisions concerning the mentally ill	Each patient of a treatment facility retains the right not to be subjected to experimental research without the express and informed written consent of the patient or of the patient's guardian. (N.D. Cent. Code, §25-03.1-40(12))
10. Provisions concerning nursing home/long-term facilities residents	—
OHIO	
1. Is there clinical trials legislation?	Yes
2. General provisions of legislation	—
3. Provisions concerning minors	—
4. Provisions concerning pregnant women	—
5. Provisions concerning fetal research	—
6. Provisions concerning in vitro procedures	—
7. Provisions concerning prisoners	—
8. Provisions concerning the developmentally disabled/mentally handicapped	—
9. Provisions concerning the mentally ill	—
10. Provisions concerning nursing home/long-term facilities residents	The rights of residents of a home shall include, but are not limited to, the right to refuse, without jeopardizing access to appropriate medical care, to serve as a medical research subject. (ORC Ann. §3721.13(A)(12))
OKLAHOMA	
1. Is there clinical trials legislation?	Yes
2. General provisions of legislation	—
3. Provisions concerning minors	—
4. Provisions concerning pregnant women	—
5. Provisions concerning fetal research	No person shall sell a child, an unborn child or the remains of a child or any unborn child resulting from an abortion. No person shall experiment upon a child or an unborn child resulting from an abortion or which is intended to be aborted unless the experimentation is therapeutic to the child or unborn child. (63 Okl. St. §1-735(A)) No person shall experiment upon the remains of a child or an unborn child

TABLE OF STATE STATUTES (*Continued*)

resulting from an abortion. The term "experiment" does not include autopsies performed according to law. (63 Okl. St. §1-735(B))

 6. Provisions concerning in vitro procedures — —
 7. Provisions concerning prisoners — —
 8. Provisions concerning the developmentally disabled/mentally handicapped — —
 9. Provisions concerning the mentally ill — —
10. Provisions concerning nursing home/long-term facilities residents — —

OREGON
 1. Is there clinical trials legislation?   Yes
 2. General provisions of legislation   —
 3. Provisions concerning minors   —
 4. Provisions concerning pregnant women   —
 5. Provisions concerning fetal research   —
 6. Provisions concerning in vitro procedures   —
 7. Provisions concerning prisoners   —
 8. Provisions concerning the developmentally disabled/mentally handicapped   —
 9. Provisions concerning the mentally ill   —
10. Provisions concerning nursing home/long-term facilities residents

Each resident has the right to participate in planning medical treatment and to refuse experimental research. (ORS §441.605(3))

PENNSYLVANIA
 1. Is there clinical trials legislation?   Yes
 2. General provisions of legislation   —
 3. Provisions concerning minors   —
 4. Provisions concerning pregnant women   —
 5. Provisions concerning fetal research   Unborn or live child.

Any person who knowingly performs any type of nontherapeutic experimentation or nontherapeutic medical procedure (except an abortion as defined in this chapter) upon any unborn child, or upon any child born alive during the course of an abortion, commits a felony of the third degree. "Nontherapeutic" means that which is not intended to preserve the life or health of the child upon whom it is performed. (18 Pa.C.S. §3216(A))

Nothing shall be construed to condone or prohibit the performance of diagnostic tests while the unborn child is in utero or the performance of pathological examinations on an aborted child. Nor shall anything in this section be construed to condone or prohibit the performance of in vitro fertilization and accompanying embryo transfer. (18 Pa.C.S. §3216(C))

Dead child

No fetal tissue or organs may be procured or used without the written consent of the mother. No consideration of any kind for such consent may be offered or given. Further, if the tissue or organs are being derived from abortion, such consent will be valid only if obtained after the decision to abort has been made. (18 Pa.C.S. §3216(B)(1))

No person who provides the information required by section 3205 (relating to informed consent) shall employ the possibility of the use of aborted fetal tissue or organs as an inducement to a pregnant woman to undergo abortion,

(Continued)

TABLE OF STATE STATUTES (*Continued*)

except that payment for reasonable expenses occasioned by the actual retrieval, storage, preparation and transportation of the tissues is permitted. (18 Pa.C.S. §3216(B)(2))

No remuneration, compensation or other consideration may be paid to any person or organization in connection with the procurement of fetal tissue or organs. (18 Pa.C.S. §3216(B)(3))

No person who consents to the procurement or use of any fetal tissue or organ may designate the recipient of that tissue or organ, nor shall any other person or organization act to fulfill that designation. (18 Pa.C.S. §3216(B)(5))

Nothing shall be construed to condone or prohibit the performance of diagnostic tests while the unborn child is in utero or the performance of pathological examinations on an aborted child. Nor shall anything be construed to condone or prohibit the performance of in vitro fertilization and accompanying embryo transfer. (18 Pa.C.S. §3216(C))

6. Provisions concerning in vitro procedures	—
7. Provisions concerning prisoners	—
8. Provisions concerning the developmentally disabled/mentally handicapped	—
9. Provisions concerning the mentally ill	—
10. Provisions concerning nursing home/long-term facilities residents	—

RHODE ISLAND

1. Is there clinical trials legislation?	Yes
2. General provisions of legislation	—
3. Provisions concerning minors	—
4. Provisions concerning pregnant women	—
5. Provisions concerning fetal research	—
6. Provisions concerning in vitro procedures	—
7. Provisions concerning prisoners	—
8. Provisions concerning the developmentally disabled/mentally handicapped	Mentally disabled/group home Each resident has the right to not be the subject of experimental research without his or her prior written and informed consent. (R.I. Gen. Laws §40.1-24.5-5(11))
9. Provisions concerning the mentally ill	—
10. Provisions concerning nursing home/long-term facilities residents	If it is proposed that a patient be used in any human experimentation project, the patient must first be (1) thoroughly informed in writing of the proposal, and (2) offered the right to refuse to participate in the project. A patient who, after being thoroughly informed, wishes to participate, must execute a written statement of informed consent. The informed consent documentation must be maintained on file in the facility. (R.I. Gen. Laws §23-17.5-7)

SOUTH CAROLINA

1. Is there clinical trials legislation?	Yes
2. General provisions of legislation	—
3. Provisions concerning minors	—
4. Provisions concerning pregnant women	—
5. Provisions concerning fetal research	—
6. Provisions concerning in vitro procedures	—
7. Provisions concerning prisoners	—
8. Provisions concerning the developmentally disabled/mentally handicapped	—

TABLE OF STATE STATUTES (*Continued*)

9. Provisions concerning the mentally ill
10. Provisions concerning nursing home/long-term facilities residents

—

Each resident or the resident's legal guardian has the right to refuse to participate in experimental research. (S.C. Code Ann. §44-81-40(C)(5))

SOUTH DAKOTA

1. Is there clinical trials legislation?
2. General provisions of legislation
3. Provisions concerning minors

Yes

—

No person with a developmental disability is subject to any experimental research procedures without the consent of the parent or guardian of the person with a developmental disability, if the person with a developmental disability is less than eighteen years of age. (S.D. Codified Laws §27B-8-41)

4. Provisions concerning pregnant women
5. Provisions concerning fetal research

—

An unborn or newborn child who has been subject to an induced abortion, other than an abortion necessary to prevent the death of the mother or any tissue or organ thereof, may not be used in animal or human research or for animal or human transplantation. This may not be construed to preclude any therapy intended to directly benefit the unborn or newborn child who has been subject to the abortion. This provision does not prohibit the use for human transplantation of an unborn child or any tissue or organ thereof if removed in the course of removal of an ectopic or a molar pregnancy. (S.D. Codified Laws §34-23A-17)

6. Provisions concerning in vitro procedures
7. Provisions concerning prisoners
8. Provisions concerning the developmentally disabled/mentally handicapped

—

—

No person with a developmental disability is subject to any experimental research procedures without the consent of:

(1) The person with a developmental disability, if eighteen years of age or over and capable of giving informed consent. If any person's capacity to give informed consent is challenged, the person, a qualified mental retardation professional, physician, or interested person may file a petition with the court to determine competency to give consent;

(2) The guardian of the person with a developmental disability, if the guardian is legally empowered to execute such consent; or

(3) The parent or guardian of the person with a developmental disability, if the person with a developmental disability is less than eighteen years of age.

No person with a developmental disability who is subject to an order of guardianship may be subjected to experimental research without prior authorization of the circuit court. (S.D. Codified Laws §27B-8-41)

9. Provisions concerning the mentally ill

No adult person may be the subject of experimental research, experimental or procedures or interventions, unless written informed consent is obtained from the person. Informed consent may be withdrawn at any time, is effective immediately, and must thereafter be reduced to writing. If the attending physician determines that the person is incapable of exercising informed consent, such treatment may be provided only if ordered after a hearing before the circuit court. If the court finds that the person is incapable of consenting to such treatment because the person's judgment is so affected

(*Continued*)

TABLE OF STATE STATUTES (*Continued*)

	by the mental illness that the person lacks the capacity to make a competent, voluntary and knowing decision concerning such treatment, the court may exercise a substituted judgment on the administration of such treatment. The order may be made to extend for up to one year. (S.D. Codified Laws §27A-12-3.20)
10. Provisions concerning nursing home/long-term facilities residents	—

TENNESSEE

1. Is there clinical trials legislation?	No
2. General provisions of legislation	—
3. Provisions concerning minors	—
4. Provisions concerning pregnant women	—
5. Provisions concerning fetal research	—
6. Provisions concerning in vitro procedures	—
7. Provisions concerning prisoners	—
8. Provisions concerning the developmentally disabled/mentally handicapped	—
9. Provisions concerning the mentally ill	—
10. Provisions concerning nursing home/long-term facilities residents	—

TEXAS

1. Is there clinical trials legislation?	Yes
2. General provisions of legislation	—
3. Provisions concerning minors	—
4. Provisions concerning pregnant women	—
5. Provisions concerning fetal research	—
6. Provisions concerning in vitro procedures	—
7. Provisions concerning prisoners	—
8. Provisions concerning the developmentally disabled/mentally handicapped	—
9. Provisions concerning the mentally ill	—
10. Provisions concerning nursing home/long-term facilities residents	A resident has the right to refuse to participate in experimental research. (Tex. Health & Safety Code §242.501(a)(9))

UTAH

1. Is there clinical trials legislation?	No
2. General provisions of legislation	—
3. Provisions concerning minors	—
4. Provisions concerning pregnant women	—
5. Provisions concerning fetal research	—
6. Provisions concerning in vitro procedures	—
7. Provisions concerning prisoners	—
8. Provisions concerning the developmentally disabled/mentally handicapped	—
9. Provisions concerning the mentally ill	—
10. Provisions concerning nursing home/long-term facilities residents	—

VERMONT

1. Is there clinical trials legislation?	No
2. General provisions of legislation	—
3. Provisions concerning minors	—
4. Provisions concerning pregnant women	—
5. Provisions concerning fetal research	—
6. Provisions concerning in vitro procedures	—

TABLE OF STATE STATUTES (*Continued*)

7. Provisions concerning prisoners — —
8. Provisions concerning the developmentally — —
   disabled/mentally handicapped
9. Provisions concerning the mentally ill — —
10. Provisions concerning nursing home/long-term — —
    facilities residents

VIRGINIA

1. Is there clinical trials legislation? — Yes
2. General provisions of legislation — Informed consent

In order to conduct human research, informed consent must be obtained if the person who is to be the human subject is as follows:

(i) competent, then it shall be subscribed to in writing by the person and witnessed;

(ii) not competent at the time consent is required, then it shall be subscribed to in writing by the person's legally authorized representative and witnessed; or

(iii) a minor otherwise capable of rendering informed consent, then it shall be subscribed to in writing by both the minor and his legally authorized representative. No informed consent form shall include any language through which the person who is to be the human subject waives or appears to waive any of his legal rights, including any release of any individual, institution, or agency or any agents thereof from liability for negligence. (Va. Code Ann. §32.1-162.18(A))

Notwithstanding consent by a legally authorized representative, no person who is otherwise capable of rendering informed consent shall be forced to participate in any human research. In the case of persons suffering from organic brain diseases causing progressive deterioration of cognition for which there is no known cure or medically accepted treatment, the implementation of experimental courses of therapeutic treatment to which a legally authorized representative has given informed consent shall not constitute the use of force. (Va. Code Ann. §32.1-162.18(A)) A legally authorized representative may not consent to nontherapeutic research unless it is determined by the human research committee that such nontherapeutic research will present no more than a minor increase over minimal risk to the human subject. (Va. Code Ann. §32.1-162.18(B))

Alteration or waiver

The human research review committee may approve a consent procedure which omits or alters some or all of the basic elements of informed consent, or waives the requirement to obtain informed consent, if the committee finds and documents that (i) the research involves no more than minimal risk to the subjects; (ii) the omission, alteration or waiver will not adversely affect the rights and welfare of the subjects; (iii) the research could not practicably be performed without the omission, alteration or waiver; and (iv) after participation, the subjects are to be provided with additional pertinent information, whenever appropriate. (Va. Code Ann. §32.1-162.18(C)) The human research review committee may waive the requirement that the investigator obtain written informed consent for some or all subjects, if the committee finds that the only record linking the subject and the research

(Continued)

TABLE OF STATE STATUTES (*Continued*)

	would be the consent document and the principal risk would be potential harm resulting from a breach of confidentiality. The committee may require the investigator to provide the subjects with a written statement explaining the research. Further, each subject must be asked whether he wants documentation linking him to the research, and the subject's wishes will govern. (Va. Code Ann. §32.1-162.18(D))
	Applicability of federal policies 　Human research which is subject to policies and regulations for the protection of human subjects promulgated by any agency of the federal government will be exempt from the provisions of this chapter. (Va. Code Ann. §32.1-162.20) 　(As to categories of human research that are exempt from these provisions, see Va. Code Ann. §32.1-162.17.)
3. Provisions concerning minors	In order to conduct human research, informed consent must be obtained if the person who is to be the human subject is a minor otherwise capable of rendering informed consent, then it shall be subscribed to in writing by both the minor and his legally authorized representative. (Va. Code Ann. §32.1-162.18(A)) 　Notwithstanding consent by a legally authorized representative, no person who is otherwise capable of rendering informed consent will be forced to participate in any human research. (Va. Code Ann. §32.1-162.18(A))
4. Provisions concerning pregnant women	—
5. Provisions concerning fetal research	—
6. Provisions concerning in vitro procedures	—
7. Provisions concerning prisoners	Subject to the general provisions concerning experimental research (Chapter 5.1 (§32.1-162.16 et seq.) of Title 32.1), the Director may permit such prisoners as may volunteer to undergo experimental treatment or tests in state or federal medical research programs. (Va. Code Ann. §53.1-36)
8. Provisions concerning the developmentally disabled/mentally handicapped	Each person who is a patient, resident, or consumer in a hospital, other facility, or program operated, funded, or licensed by the Department of Mental Health, Mental Retardation and Substance Abuse Services, excluding those operated by the Department of Corrections, shall be assured his legal rights including the right not be the subject of experimental or investigational research without his prior written and informed consent or that of his legally authorized representative. No employee of the Department or a community services board, behavioral health authority, or local government department with a policy-advisory community services board; a community services board, behavioral health authority, or local government with a policy-advisory community services board contractor; or any other public or private program or facility licensed or funded by the Department shall serve as a legally authorized representative for a consumer being treated in any Department, community services board, behavioral health authority, local government department with a policy-advisory community services board or other licensed or funded public or private program or facility, unless the employee is a relative or legal guardian of the consumer. (Va. Code Ann. §37.1-84.1(A)(4))

TABLE OF STATE STATUTES (*Continued*)

9. Provisions concerning the mentally ill

Each person who is a patient, resident, or consumer in a hospital, other facility, or program operated, funded, or licensed by the Department of Mental Health, Mental Retardation and Substance Abuse Services, excluding those operated by the Department of Corrections, will be assured his legal rights, including the right not be the subject of experimental or investigational research without his prior written and informed consent or that of his legally authorized representative. No employee of the Department or a community services board, behavioral health authority, or local government department with a policy-advisory community services board; a community services board, behavioral health authority, or local government with a policy-advisory community services board contractor; or any other public or private program or facility licensed or funded by the Department shall serve as a legally authorized representative for a consumer being treated in any Department, community services board, behavioral health authority, local government department with a policy-advisory community services board or other licensed or funded public or private program or facility, unless the employee is a relative or legal guardian of the consumer. (Va. Code Ann. §37.1-84.1(A)(4))

10. Provisions concerning nursing home/long-term facilities residents — —

WASHINGTON
1. Is there clinical trials legislation? — Yes
2. General provisions of legislation — —
3. Provisions concerning minors — —
4. Provisions concerning pregnant women — —
5. Provisions concerning fetal research — —
6. Provisions concerning in vitro procedures — —
7. Provisions concerning prisoners — —
8. Provisions concerning the developmentally disabled/mentally handicapped — —
9. Provisions concerning the mentally ill — —
10. Provisions concerning nursing home/long-term facilities residents

The facility must insure that each resident and guardian, if any, gives informed, written consent before participating in experimental research. (ARCW §74.42.040(4))

WEST VIRGINIA
1. Is there clinical trials legislation? — No
2. General provisions of legislation — —
3. Provisions concerning minors — —
4. Provisions concerning pregnant women — —
5. Provisions concerning fetal research — —
6. Provisions concerning in vitro procedures — —
7. Provisions concerning prisoners — —
8. Provisions concerning the developmentally disabled/mentally handicapped — —
9. Provisions concerning the mentally ill — —
10. Provisions concerning nursing home/long-term facilities residents — —

WISCONSIN
1. Is there clinical trials legislation? — Yes
2. General provisions of legislation — —
3. Provisions concerning minors — —

(Continued)

TABLE OF STATE STATUTES (*Continued*)

4. Provisions concerning pregnant women	—
5. Provisions concerning fetal research	—
6. Provisions concerning in vitro procedures	—
7. Provisions concerning prisoners	—
8. Provisions concerning the developmentally disabled/mentally handicapped	Each patient shall have a right not to be subjected to experimental research without the express and informed consent of the patient and of the patient's guardian after consultation with independent specialists and the patient's legal counsel. Such proposed research must first be reviewed and approved by the institution's research and human rights committee and by the department before such consent may be sought. (Wis. Stat. §51.61(1)(j))
9. Provisions concerning the mentally ill	Each patient shall have a right not to be subjected to experimental research without the express and informed consent of the patient and of the patient's guardian after consultation with independent specialists and the patient's legal counsel. Such proposed research shall first be reviewed and approved by the institution's research and human rights committee and by the department before such consent may be sought. (Wis. Stat. §51.61(1)(j))
10. Provisions concerning nursing home/long-term facilities residents	—
WYOMING	
1. Is there clinical trials legislation?	Yes
2. General provisions of legislation	—
3. Provisions concerning minors	Training School A resident of the training school may not be denied the following rights, unless authorized by a court or his guardian, parent or guardian ad litem: The right to refuse to be subjected to experimental medical or psychological research without the express and informed consent of the resident or his parent or guardian if he is a minor. The resident or his parent or guardian may consult with independent medical or psychological specialists and his attorney before consenting or refusing. (Wyo. Stat. §25-5-132(d)(ii))
4. Provisions concerning pregnant women	—
5. Provisions concerning fetal research	—
6. Provisions concerning in vitro procedures	—
7. Provisions concerning prisoners	—
8. Provisions concerning the developmentally disabled/mentally handicapped	—
9. Provisions concerning the mentally ill	—
10. Provisions concerning nursing home/long-term facilities residents	—

References

Forbes v. Woods, 1999 U.S. Dist. LEXIS 17025 (D. Ariz. 1999).

Jane L. v. Bangerter, 61 F.3d 1493 (Tenth Cir. 1995) revised and remanded on other grounds sub nom. *Leavitt v. Jane L.*, 518 U.S. 137 (1996).

Margaret S. v. Edwards, 794 F.2d 994 (Fifth Cir. 1986).

Lifchez v. Hartigan, 735 F. Supp. 1361 (N.D. Ill. 1990) aff'd 914 F.2d 260 (Seventh Cir. 1990).

Modi v. West Virginia Board of Medicine, 195 W. Va. 230, 465 SE 2d 230 (1995).

4

Selection and Recruitment of Research Subjects

Introduction 57
Common Practices in Recruitment of Potential Subjects
for Participation in Clinical Trials 58
Incentives Used to Encourage Practicing Physicians to
Help Increase the Pool of Potential Research Subjects 58
Problems Reported with Current Recruitment Practices 59
Federal Guidelines for Selecting or Recruiting Research Subjects 60
National Standards for Selecting or Recruiting Research Subjects 60
Concern About Gender Disparity in the Selection of Research Subjects 60
What the IRB Can Do to Avoid Gender Bias: Strategies
for the Selection of Research Subjects 61
Racial and Ethnic Disparity in Subject Recruitment or Selection 63
Government Action to Reverse Racial and Ethnic Disparity
in Subject Recruitment 63
Practical Steps to Avoid Racial or Ethnic Discrimination Allegations
of Inappropriate Subject Recruitment and Selection 64
Cultural and Language Issues in Subject Recruitment or Retention 65
e-Recruiting Concerns 66
Concern About Discouraging the Use of Financial Incentives
in the Subject Recruitment Process 67
Conclusion 68
References 68

INTRODUCTION

In June 2000, the Office of Inspector General (OIG) of the U.S. Department of Health and Human Services published an interesting report on research subject recruitment (*Recruiting Human Subjects,* 2000a). It outlined concerns about industry practices, including possible erosion of the consent process, undue influence exerted by physicians who are trusted by patients, and breaches of confidentiality. In a companion report, the OIG provided sample guidance for proper recruitment of research subjects (*Recruiting Human Subjects,* 2000b).

Efforts to set ethically appropriate practice standards for recruiting research subjects are not restricted to the OIG. Several prominent medical groups have also put forward suggestions.

Beyond these attempts to ensure proper recruitment of research subjects, there remain important subject selection considerations. For example, one concern is how to achieve a balance in terms of gender, ethnic, and racial composition among subjects selected for a research study. Language and culture are also important considerations since an inability to explain the potential study and put it in a familiar context may impede the ability of recruiters to select eligible subjects.

This chapter explores the issue of subject recruitment and selection. Practice strategies are provided for purposes of regulatory compliance as well as maintaining the integrity of research design.

············

COMMON PRACTICES IN RECRUITMENT OF POTENTIAL SUBJECTS FOR PARTICIPATION IN CLINICAL TRIALS

According to the OIG report there are four primary ways subjects are recruited for industry-based trials:

1. Through the use of financial and non-financial incentives.
2. By physicians flagging patients in their practice through a chart review or when they appear for an appointment.
3. Obtaining subjects by furnishing trial information to other local clinicians or to disease advocacy and other groups.
4. Through advertising and promotion such as media ads, press releases, televised news segments, and speakers at local health fairs.

Admittedly, the OIG report restricted its perspective to industry-sponsored drug research trials (*Recruiting Human Subjects,* 2000) because drug research constitute the majority of clinical trials. Aware of the competition in industry to develop effective, profitable drugs, the OIG wanted to learn more about the issues stemming from their recruitment practices. However, the report did take note that government-sponsored research may also feel the effect of similar and additional pressures. It left open the possibility of doing a similar report on government-sponsored trials (*Recruiting Human Subjects,* 2000).

············

INCENTIVES USED TO ENCOURAGE PRACTICING PHYSICIANS TO HELP INCREASE THE POOL OF POTENTIAL RESEARCH SUBJECTS

Financial incentives are not the only types of encouragement used to entice physicians and other healthcare professionals to recommend patients for clinical studies. Other forms of encouragement include providing stipends for educational programs, office equipment, and even the possibility of being named an author on journal articles that present the findings of the clinical research.

Financial drivers sometimes involve "sign on" bonuses so that as the subject enrollment deadline approaches, physicians are offered a bonus for each subject entered into the study above and beyond the project budget. According to an OIG report, some industry trials also rely upon multicenter competition to enroll subjects on what it described as a first-come, first-serve basis (*Recruiting Human Subjects,* 2000).

....

PROBLEMS REPORTED WITH CURRENT RECRUITMENT PRACTICES

A number of concerns have been voiced about subject recruitment. The issues identified include misleading advertising recruitment, repetitive contacts with individuals to persuade them to participate in a study, and compelling a nursing home resident to enroll in a study or leave the facility (*Recruiting Human Subjects,* 2000).

The OIG report (*Recruiting Human Subjects,* 2000) noted that three areas of informed consent were affected in questionable recruitment practices for clinical research trials. The influence of misleading information was seen as possibly shaping a subject's judgment about participation in clinical trials. IRB officials and others noted that ads about investigational drugs misled individuals to believe that the study article was a treatment and not the subject of research. Videos were seen as misrepresenting the purpose of a study and the possible effect of the experimental article.

The ability of subjects to understand what is involved in a study may be obscured by the prospect of financial incentives. At the same time, while IRBs spend a lot of time reviewing the content of a consent document, few observe the consent process. Pressure to enroll subjects in a study was seen as possibly leading the investigator to distort the description of the study. The consent process in such cases is questionable since individuals cannot comprehend the purpose and scope of the study.

Another key component of consent—voluntariness—was also seen as in doubt when physician-investigators use their relationship to encourage patients to participate in research trials. Not wishing to contradict the doctor's suggestion by not participating in the study, the physician-patient relationship may impede the individual's ability to voluntarily decide about enrolling in a clinical trial. That doctors receive referral fees was seen as incentivizing doctors to encourage patients to enroll in research studies. Use of well-known and well-respected doctors to serve as spokespersons for clinical trials may alter the decision-making process since their involvement suggests that potential subjects view this as a worthy study. Using disease-support chat rooms to promote clinical trials research was seen as potentially influencing the subject's ability to make a voluntary decision.

Pressure to find suitable research subjects and the perceived inability of IRBs to control recruitment practices were seen as major concerns in the OIG report. At the same time, federal oversight was seen as inadequate in regard to recruitment practices. This was seen as a part of the clinical research area that could be improved by:

- Making clear the authority vested in IRBs to review recruitment practices.
- Providing guidelines for acceptable recruitment practices.
- Making certain that IRB members and investigators are educated about protections for human research subjects.
- Increasing federal oversight of IRBs.

....

FEDERAL GUIDELINES FOR SELECTING OR RECRUITING RESEARCH SUBJECTS

One of the findings of the OIG was that the Department of Health and Human Services provided little direction on acceptable recruitment methods. Although the FDA provides "Information Sheets" to IRBs that describe methods for recruiting subjects, the OIG found that these documents caused some confusion about acceptable recruitment practices in multisite trials. For example, one IRB might find a recruiting practice acceptable, yet another involved in the same multisite trial might reject it, and in such instances IRBs are uncertain what should be done. The absence of clear guidelines from HHS was also noted in the OIG report (*Recruiting Human Subjects,* June 2000).

In a companion report the OIG issued sample guidelines for recruiting research subjects (*Recruiting Human Subjects,* 2000b). Three issues were stressed in the new guidelines:

- Use of recruitment incentives.
- Management of the dual role of the physician-investigator.
- Confidentiality of medical records.

Nothing was included in the guidelines on advertising. The OIG reasoned that since the Department of Health and Human Services has explicit guidelines on the subject of advertising and subject incentives, it was unnecessary to provide sample guidance on the subject.

The sample guidelines provided by the OIG were drawn from prominent professional associations, leading teaching facilities, and the *Canadian Tri-Council Policy Statement on Ethical Conduct for Research Involving Humans.* The guidelines were not presented as being best practices; rather, the OIG suggested that the samples were a starting point for a discussion on the topic among key stakeholders.

....

NATIONAL STANDARDS FOR SELECTING OR RECRUITING RESEARCH SUBJECTS

According to an OIG report, numerous professional organizations have taken the initiative to set guidelines on the recruitment of research subjects (*Recruiting Human Subjects,* 2000b). Many of the guidelines address the use of incentives and management of the dual role held by some physician-investigators.

Others have more general practice guidelines or codes of ethics that offer direction on recruitment of research subjects. Some may be found on Web sites that include other components from their clinical research guidelines or manuals.

....

CONCERN ABOUT GENDER DISPARITY IN THE SELECTION OF RESEARCH SUBJECTS

Several reasons can be given for concern about gender disparities in research subject selection. First, lack of appropriate gender balance in selection processes might call into question the validity of the study, as could happen when one gender or the other is heavily weighted in the subject population. The absence of a balanced population might lead some to doubt that the positive effects of an investigational drug can cross gender lines.

Second, there may be a hesitancy to involve one gender based on concern about the effect of an investigational drug on reproductive capability or so-called "second-generation" consequences. Fearing potential liability for birth defects passed on to offspring, the stance is taken to preclude members of the at-risk gender from participating in the study. The result may be a well-documented research outcome that cannot and should not be generalized to cross gender lines in terms of efficacy or safety.

Third, the value of the investigational drug may be seen as only potentially benefiting one gender. The result may be that the study is well along before researchers discover the possible benefit across gender lines. As such, a new study may be needed that could delay an important drug being brought to the market for the "other" gender. It may also be a needless waste of money that could have been avoided with better study design.

....

WHAT THE IRB CAN DO TO AVOID GENDER BIAS: STRATEGIES FOR THE SELECTION OF RESEARCH SUBJECTS

Rather than being portrayed as an administrative nuisance, the IRB can take several steps to lessen the risk of selection bias. These steps include:

- Education.
- Development of decision trees to aid in sample selection.
- Thorough review of study design in the initial review of a research protocol.
- Documentation to substantiate proper selection.

Each of these points merits specific discussion:

- *Education*—Principal investigators, research study staff, and IRB members would benefit from practical instruction on subject recruitment and selection. Topics would include study design as it relates to subject selection, and such issues as the likelihood of benefit and risk for a particular test subject population, and considerations of fairness. For example, training should include discussion of study designs that over-protect a specific population to the point that the group is underrepresented in the study. The effect of such practices on the generalizability of the study would be an important topic. The requirements of applicable law and funding requirements would also be part of the instructional program. Thus participants would learn that women are singled out for some specific protections under federal regulations, in National Institutes of Health (NIH) Policy on population studies, and in the Public Health Service (PHS) grant application process. Under the federal regulations, the protections are related to pregnancy whereas the PHS and NIH considerations attempt to guard against under-representation of women as research subjects.

- *Decision Trees*—A practical tool that an IRB may wish to develop is a decision tree for subject recruitment and selection. Following the appropriate pathway or decision tree both the researcher and the IRB can decide quickly whether the subject selection process described in the study design is acceptable in terms of gender qualifications. For example, a pharmaceutical sponsor may want to test a new type of contraceptive on women between ages 24 and 36 years. The decision tree might look like Figure 4.1 and demonstrate why it *would not* be appropriate to include men in

FIGURE 4.1.   Decision Tree

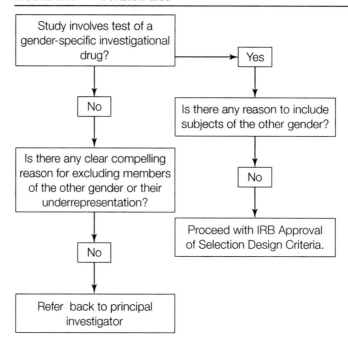

the study. However, as the decision tree points out, *if* a study does not demonstrate a need for gender exclusion or underrepresentation, it would be referred back to the principal investigator for reconsideration of study design.

Sample decision trees may be a useful tool for principal investigators. For many investigators and their staff, such a decision tree may facilitate inclusion of proper research subject selection critiera. For others, seeing such samples would help them explain the reasons for their study selection criteria or, in some cases, pinpoint the need to refine the protocol long before it is submitted to the IRB for consideration.

- *Thorough Review of Protocol Selection Criteria*—When reviewing a protocol that involves a single gender or an underrepresented gender, the IRB should carefully scrutinize the study design. The decision tree described earlier is one step in this process. Scientific design should be evaluated to determine if the study will yield valid, generalizable results or whether in trying to protect a "vulnerable" population, the study would do them a disservice by excluding them from participating in a valuable clinical trial. Epidemiologists, biostatisticians, study designers, ethicists, and others bring different perspectives to such a review. This multidisciplinary approach is useful in sorting out whether the study presents a good reason for its current design or whether opportunity exists to modify it to remove gender disparities.

- *Documentation*—For the benefit of all concerned, documentation is important in terms of substantiating the rationale for subject selection. The decision tree analysis, the study design, and the evaluation of it by the IRB can all be used to support an ethical and legal framework for the research project. By the same token, a rejection of a protocol based on study selection methodology requires a detailed review and analysis. When the IRB makes such a determination, objections can be expected from the researcher and the sponsor. To properly address these complaints, the IRB should delineate in writing the reasons for its decision. This can be done as part of the usual and customary business practice of the IRB in the preparation of meeting minutes. If the IRB provided recommended changes to the selection process that were rejected by the principal investigator or the sponsor, this too should be documented. By taking this step, the IRB can deflect possible claims of negligent deliberation, negligent decision-making, and acting in bad faith.

Should a complaint generate an inquiry by a federal or state oversight body, the documentation could serve to quickly end otherwise expensive, time-consuming investigations. Probes may come about either on claims of gender discrimination or assertions that the IRB was thwarting valid research. Regardless of the source of the complaint, a strong defense is a thoughtful process as evidenced in documentation.

RACIAL AND ETHNIC DISPARITY IN SUBJECT RECRUITMENT OR SELECTION

In the *IRB Guidebook* (1993) the point is made that both under-inclusion and over-inclusion of racial and ethnic minorities thwart important research. With over-inclusion, the concern is that racial and ethnic minorities bear a disproportionate share of the burden for research without obtaining any of the benefits of the results of these studies. Trying to protect racial and ethnic groups can have equally adverse outcomes in terms of precluding them from taking part in studies that could benefit such individuals.

Perhaps leery of being seen as spearheading a racially charged initiative or of being viewed as taking advantage of a vulnerable population, some investigators may not focus on a particular ethnic or racial group for important research endeavors. The impetus for such an attitude might be ascribed to the now infamous Tuskegee Study (Jones, 1993) in which a number of African-American men went untreated for syphilis in order to evaluate the course of the disease.

Important research needs to be done involving ethnic and racial minorities. Some of the research is of a broad-based population which demands recruitment and selection of individuals identified from ethnic and racial minority groups. Other studies may hone in on minorities as a whole or one particular group. To avoid allegations of racism or of taking advantage of vulnerable groups, care must be taken in designing an ethically sound research study. It is possible to do so, but the issue is "how" to do it.

GOVERNMENT ACTION TO REVERSE RACIAL AND ETHNIC DISPARITY IN SUBJECT RECRUITMENT

A number of initiatives have been launched to address racial and ethnic disparities not only in research but in healthcare (U.S. Dept. of Health and Human Services). These include initiatives developed by the Office of Minority Health of the U.S. Department of Health and Human Services. In addition, the National Institutes of Health (NIH) has issued guidelines on including minorities in clinical research and the Ethnic Outreach Program, a program to encourage minority participation in clinical trials.

The NIH Guidelines including women *and* minorities in the same segment demonstrates the definite parallels between racial and ethnic disparity in clinical research. To be certain that the NIH approach is clear, the guidelines issued by the Office of Extramural Research of NIH include a policy statement:

> It is the policy of NIH that women and members of minority groups and their sub-populations must be included in all NIH-supported biomedical and behavioral research projects involving human subjects, unless a clear and compelling rationale and justification establishes to the satisfaction of the relevant Institute/Center Director that inclusion is inappropriate with respect to the health of the subjects or the purpose of the research. Exclusion under other circumstances may be made by the Director, NIH, upon the recommendation of an Institute/Center Director based on a compelling rationale and justification. Cost is not an acceptable reason for exclusion except when the study would duplicate data from other sources. Women of child-bearing potential should not be routinely excluded from participation in clinical research. All NIH-supported biomedical and behavioral research involving human subjects is defined as clinical research. This policy applies to research subjects of all ages. The inclusion of women and members of minority groups and their subpopulations must be addressed in developing a research design appropriate to the scientific objectives of the study. The research plan should describe the composition of the proposed study population in terms of sex/gender and racial/ethnic group, and provide a rationale for selection of such subjects. Such a plan should contain a description of the proposed outreach programs for recruiting women and minorities as participants. [*NIH Guidelines on the Inclusion of Women and Minorities as Subjects in Research,* Policy III A 2000]

NIH did not stop at a policy statement. It published a useful text entitled, *Outreach Notebook for the NIH Guidelines on Inclusion of Women and Minorities as Subjects in Clinical Research.* Included in the Notebook are many practical suggestions that address study design, determinants for including women and minorities in research, and an entire appendix devoted to questions and answers on the subject. For its part, the Public Health Service (PHS) of the U.S. Department of Health and Human Services has included in its grant application (PHS 398) language that reinforces the NIH Policy.

....
PRACTICAL STEPS TO AVOID RACIAL OR ETHNIC DISCRIMINATION ALLEGATIONS OF INAPPROPRIATE SUBJECT RECRUITMENT AND SELECTION

Many practical steps can be taken to avoid allegations of racism or taking advantage of ethnic groups. These steps come back to the points raised earlier with respect to recruitment and selection of women for research trials. Many measures may be found in various federal documents, but some may come forth in other ways. For example

- *Specialized Training for Clinical Investigators*—Recruitment practices may vary with specific racial or ethnic groups. Knowing how to launch an effective recruitment campaign is critical, and obtaining effective training can eliminate barriers to success.

- *Specialized Training for IRBs*—To avoid a reaction based on paternalism, IRBs should receive appropriate training on the ethically and legally acceptable practices for minority subject recruitment. Once understood, protocols can be reviewed objectively and with a level of understanding that carefully weighs proposed recruitment practices against accepted standards and guidelines.

- *Involvement of Community Members in the Recruitment Process*—Although it may appear as tokenism, the involvement of credible individuals from racial or ethnic communities can help eliminate barriers to effective recruitment practices. Care must be exercised so that these individuals are not seen as misrepresenting or deceiving members of the community about the nature and purpose of the study or their proposed involvement. Rather, it is needed to build a bridge between the clinical investigators and the ethnic or racial groups from whom volunteers are sought for the study.

- *Involvement of Community Members on Study Design Evaluations or the IRB*— The insights of community members may be invaluable in terms of assessing study design or as voting members of the IRB. Once again, the inclusion of community members should not be seen as tokenism or as affording a false sense of security that "one of us" approved the study. Rather, community members must receive the same level of training as the other members of study design review panels or IRB, and they must be as qualified as anyone else in such important positions of responsibility.

- *Development of Specialized Review Tools*—As seen in the *Outreach Notebook for the NIH Guidelines on Inclusion of Women and Minorities as Subjects in Clinical Research,* rather specific questions can be asked in reviewing protocols impacting such specific populations. Other questions can be added to this list and formulated into a specialized review tool. Such a tool should include input from an ethical and legal standpoint to make certain that questions are addressed from key stakeholders. For example:

  → Has consideration been given to inclusion of all relevant racial and minority groups?

  → Have all the reasons been stated for singling out a small number of racial or minority groups in the study?

  → Is there a justification for a one-group study?

  → Is the study design ethically and legally sound?

  → Is the study design likely to generate statistically valid results?

  → Does the study design reflect consideration for recruitment of racial or ethnic minorities?

  → If so, what is included in the design for notifying the community about the study and its potential value to its members?

- *Monitoring of Recruitment Practices*—Once the study is approved and implemented, monitoring recruitment practices may reveal opportunities for improvement in seeking racial or ethnic minority members to participate in research. Unacceptable practices that are identified could lead to the IRB stopping the project or intervening to correct such practices. Information learned from the monitoring process might also reveal good practices for use in future studies involving racial or ethnic minorities.

··············

CULTURAL AND LANGUAGE ISSUES IN SUBJECT RECRUITMENT OR RETENTION

Cultural and linguistic barriers to subject recruitment may be as challenging as those found with racial and ethnic minorities. As noted in Chapter Five on consent, measures can be taken to address these issues for purposes of obtaining an authorization to participate in human research. The recruitment phase merits specific attention.

In some cultures, the gender of the person seeking to recruit a would-be subject may actually have a negative influence in the decision-making process. For example, it may be inappropriate for a woman to talk with a man about his possible involvement in a study to evaluate a new type of prostate marker. Offended by the very idea that a woman would speak to him, the man may refuse to participate in further discussion about the study. Cultural sensitivity is important in avoiding such situations.

Language is also important. Accommodation must be made for those sight-, hearing-, or speech-impaired participants. Not to do so could trigger difficulties under applicable federal laws such as the Americans with Disabilities Act (disability) or under Section 504 of the Rehabilitation Act of 1973 (handicap).

Beyond those with physiological challenges, there are other laws that protect those with a linguistic barrier. For example, recruitment practices should be fine-tuned to address the communication needs of someone with "Limited English Proficiency" (LEP). The failure to do so could pose difficulties under the 1964 Civil Rights Act and the "National Standards on Culturally and Linguistically Appropriate Services (CLAS) in Health Care," issued by the Office of Minority Health of the Department of Health and Human Services (2000). Policy guidance has been issued on the subject by the Office of Civil Rights of the U.S. Department of Health (Policy Guidance, 2000).

The fact that there is so much discussion in this arena reflects the nexus between culture and language in healthcare. When clinical trials recruitment involves individuals from diverse culture and language groups it is equally important to make certain that dialect and culturally specific needs are met. This can be accomplished through IRB policy and procedure, training, and monitoring practices.

. . . .

e-RECRUITING CONCERNS

The recruitment of research subjects via Internet or Web site advertising as well as by monitoring chat rooms is an evolving area of concern. Potential risks of these techniques include violation of Federal Trade Commission regulations, privacy rights, and Web site agreements. Before embarking on this route, the investigator would be well advised to consult experienced counsel as to the current state of the law. An IRB should also be sensitive to this new recruitment media as it impacts ethics and regulatory protections of participants.

Another area that merits close security is the recruitment of subjects and the impact of the Health Insurance Portability and Accountability Act (HIPAA). This is a minefield of regulatory interpretation that includes such questions as:

- Does recruitment of subjects from an investigator's private database require an HIPAA authorization?

- What steps need to be taken to use information in public databases or registries under HIPAA?

- What are the key elements for data management in HIPAA-protected subject recruitment practices?

- What are the core elements that should be included in a data use agreement to avert HIPAA problems?

- If a subject indicates that he does not want protected health information (PHI) to be warehoused in a databank for future research use, what systems are in place to prevent inadvertent entry of the information in the databank?

- How will the institution handle the matter of accounting of PHI in research?

Additional discussion of HIPAA and confidentiality is located in Chapter Six. The point here is that HIPAA should be considered in recruiting practices.

....

CONCERN ABOUT DISCOURAGING THE USE OF FINANCIAL INCENTIVES IN THE SUBJECT RECRUITMENT PROCESS

The use of financial incentives to recruit research subjects is one that has garnered much attention from IRBs. It has also captured the attention of the Office of Inspector General of the U.S. Department of Health and Human Services ("Offering Gifts and Other Inducements," 2002) The concern is that the amount of remuneration offered could interfere with the ability of potential research participants to make a voluntary choice regarding participation in research. This is particularly true for individuals with little or no health insurance. The prospect of regular medical attention, receipt of study drugs, special foods, and individualized attention may be so appealing that they cannot properly evaluate the risks of taking part in the study. Coupled with recruitment advertising that promises "receiving new treatment," vulnerable individuals may be ready to participate very quickly.

At the same time, IRB members recognize that some measure of financial incentives may be necessary to deal with such expenses as out-of-pocket costs and transportation. The same point is made in a Special Advisory Bulletin issued by the Office of Inspector of the U.S. Department of Health and Human Services ("Offering Gifts and Other Inducements," 2002). The key is to find the right amount of reimbursement or incentive that does not cloud the person's ability to make a clear decision. In this regard, the OIG may help further the discussion on the subject by proposing a new exception or safe harbor for government-sponsored clinical trials to permit free goods and services with respect to NIH- or HHS-sponsored human research ("Offering Gifts and Other Inducements," 2002). This is seen as an important consideration in view of the fact that since offering a Medicare or Medicaid beneficiary remuneration that is likely to influence the beneficiary's selection of a specific provider or service may be subject to civil monetary penalties (Social Security Act).

Currently, the *IRB Guidebook* (1993) offers some direction in this regard. There are no easy solutions. In fact, much will depend upon the type of study, its length, the level of participation of the subject, and geographic considerations. For example, if a study involves three blood tests per week for twelve weeks, the subject may be remunerated for travel costs and the inconvenience of having to get to a lab at 6:00 a.m. for each session. The financial incentive may be based on a per session basis or a twelve-week schedule.

The compensation rates and the extent of expense reimbursement may vary from community to community. In a largely rural area with limited public transportation, subjects may receive a reimbursement based on a mileage rate. In an urban location with readily accessible rapid transit, it may be the costs associated with using such public transportation. The compensation rate may vary as well.

From a practical standpoint, financial incentives may be part of the cost of clinical research—a reasonably monetary consideration may facilitate the individual staying within the study. However, the amount per subject should be reasonable and consistent with community standards.

There are some steps that IRBs can take to ensure ethically appropriate use of such incentives:

- Education for clinical investigators.
- Guidelines on acceptable rates of reimbursement and incentives.

- Recruitment disclosure provisions on what is reimbursable.
- Recruitment disclosure provisions on what subjects must do in order to receive incentives.
- Disclosure of the effect of study termination or removal from a study on receipt of incentives.
- Disclosure of what will happen to incentives when a subject withdraws from a study.
- Response to subject complaints about reimbursements and incentives withheld or not in keeping with the study schedule.
- Surveys of subjects from completed studies regarding the influence of reimbursement and incentives.
- Monitoring of recruitment discussions with respect to reimbursement and incentives.

············

CONCLUSION

As federal guidelines intensify on ethically responsible clinical trials, it is possible that additional standards will emerge on recruitment of research subjects. Some degree of change might be expected with regard to vulnerable subjects such as those with mental or behavioral challenges, the chronically ill, and individuals susceptible to undue influence of financial incentives. Research trials that include particularly serious risk, pain, or extensive changes in the daily lives of subjects may also give rise to a refinement of what is considered acceptable reimbursement and incentives. Recruitment practices are bound to change as these factors modify the context for clinical trials research. To assist IRBs and investigators in meeting the challenges of appropriate selection and recruitment practices included at the end of this chapter is the NIH *Outreach Notebook* that addresses the inclusion of women and minorities in clinical research. It provides useful information, including answers to commonly asked questions.

References

Americans with Disabilities Act of 1990, 42 U.S.C. §§12101 et seq.

Ethnic Minority Outreach Program, National Institutes of Health (NIH) Clinical Center.

Healthy People 2010. Office of Minority Health, U.S. Department of Health and Human Services. www.healthypeople.gov, November, 2002 update.

IRB Guidebook, 1993. Office of Human Research Protections, U.S. Department of Health and Human Services, Chapter III.

Jones, J. *Bad Blood: The Tuskegee Syphilis Experiment.* New York: Free Press, 1981, 1993.

"National Standards on Culturally and Linguistically Appropriate Services (CLAS) in Health Care." Office of Minority Health of the Department of Health and Human Services *Federal Register:* 65(247): 80865, December 22, 2000.

NIH Guidelines on the Inclusion of Women and Minorities as Subjects in Research. August 1, 2000, amended October, 2001.

Outreach Notebook for the NIH Guidelines on Inclusion of Women and Minorities as Subjects in Clinical Research. NIH Publication No. 97-4160, 1997.

"Policy Guidance" Office of Civil Rights. U.S. Department of Health and Human Services, *Federal Register:* 65(169): 52762, August 30, 2000.

Recruiting Human Subjects: Pressures in Industry-Sponsored Clinical Research. OEI-01-97-00195, June 2000a.

Recruiting Human Subjects: Sample Guidelines for Practice. OEI-01-97-00196, June 2000b.

Section 504 of the Rehabilitation Act of 1973, as amended 29 U.S.C. §794.

Social Security Act §1128A(a)(5).

U.S. Department of Health and Human Services. *Offering Gifts and Other Inducements to Beneficiaries.* Special Advisory Bulletin, August 2002.

OUTREACH NOTEBOOK

FOR THE NIH
GUIDELINES
ON INCLUSION OF WOMEN
AND MINORITIES
AS SUBJECTS IN
CLINICAL RESEARCH

NATIONAL INSTITUTES OF HEALTH
(NIH PUBLICATION NO. 97-4160)

·············?🐚·············

NIH Outreach Notebook Committee

Dr. Judith H. LaRosa, Co-Chair
Office of Research on Women's Health

Ms. Matilde Alvarado
*National Heart, Lung, and
Blood Institute*

Dr. Carlos Caban
Office of Extramural Research

Dr. George Counts
*National Institute of Allergy and
Infectious Diseases*

Dr. Mario de La Rosa
National Institute on Drug Abuse

Dr. Lawrence Friedman
*National Heart, Lung, and
Blood Institute*

Dr. Thomas Glynn
National Cancer Institute

Dr. Christine Grady
National Institute of Nursing Research

Dr. Robin Hill
*National Heart, Lung, and
Blood Institute*

Dr. Delores Parron, Co-Chair
National Institute of Mental Health

Dr. Jan Howard
*National Institute of Alcohol Abuse
and Alcoholism*

Dr. Melody Lin
Office of Protection from Research Risks

Dr. Margaret Mattson
National Institute on Drug Abuse

Ms. Rose Mary Padberg
National Cancer Institute

Dr. Belinda Seto
Office of Extramural Research

Ms. Pam Scanlan
*National Institute of Allergy and
Infectious Diseases*

Ms. Anne Thomas
Office of the Director

Dr. Donald Vereen
National Institute on Drug Abuse

Dr. Claudette Varricchio
National Cancer Institute

The committee wishes to extend its deepest appreciation to the NIH staff and those in the extramural community who contributed so much to the development of this notebook.

CONTENTS

INTRODUCTION 75

HOW TO USE THIS NOTEBOOK 76

FACTORS IN DETERMINING INCLUSION IN CLINICAL RESEARCH 77

DECISION TREE 78

ELEMENTS OF OUTREACH 81

    Understand the Study Population 82

    Establish Explicit Goals 86

    Achieve Agreement on Research Plans 88

    Design and Conduct Evaluations 89

    Establish and Maintain Communication 92

ETHICAL ISSUES 94

SEVEN POINTS OF CONSIDERATION FOR INSTITUTIONAL REVIEW BOARDS 96

WHERE DO I GO FOR HELP? 98

REVIEW CRITERIA FOR INCLUSION OF WOMEN AND MINORITIES 100

GLOSSARY 102

REFERENCES 104

APPENDIX A – "NIH Guidelines on the Inclusion of Women and Minorities as
    Subjects in Clinical Research," *Federal Register,* March 28, 1994 113

APPENDIX B – "Questions and Answers Concerning the 1994 NIH Guidelines
    on Inclusion of Women and Minorities as Subjects in Clinical Research" 125

INTRODUCTION

In March 1994, the National Institutes of Health (NIH) published its **NIH Guidelines on the Inclusion of Women and Minorities as Subjects in Clinical Research** in the *Federal Register.* These guidelines (Appendix A of this document), which address issues concerning the recruitment of women and minorities and their subpopulations in clinical research and especially clinical trials, were developed in response to requirements stated in Subtitle B of Part I of the NIH Revitalization Act of 1993 (Public Law 103-43). As part of these requirements, NIH must engage in efforts to recruit women and minorities into these studies. Section 131 of the Act states that:

The Director of NIH, in consultation with the Director of the Office of Research on Women's Health and the Director of the Office of Research on Minority Health, shall conduct or support outreach programs for the recruitment of women and members of minority groups as subjects in projects of clinical research.

The goal of this legislation is to increase the opportunities for obtaining critically important information with which to enhance health and treat disease among all Americans—and to detect and account for significant differences between genders or racial and ethnic groups where they exist.

In order to accomplish this task, investigators and their staffs must appropriately recruit and retain participants of both genders as well as diverse racial and ethnic groups in studies. The process of inviting individuals to participate and remain in a study requires a broad knowledge base encompassing behavior theory (Rimer et al. 1993, Green et al. 1980, von Winterfeldt and Edwards 1986). Investigators will therefore need to draw upon different theories, depending upon the nature of the research, the characteristics of the population of interest, and the settings in which they are encountered.

As part of its campaign to integrate these new guidelines into the biomedical and behavioral research infrastructure, the NIH has developed this notebook, a primer, outlining key issues in the recruitment and retention of individuals into studies. ***The suggestions presented in this notebook are not requirements that must be incorporated into research applications/ proposals.*** They are presented to provide guidance to investigators and their research teams as they consider the scientific question(s), study design, and methods to facilitate appropriate enrollment of study participants.

HOW TO USE THIS NOTEBOOK

The NIH recognizes that these guidelines will take some time to be understood and assimilated into the research community. This notebook is one step in that process and serves as a complement to the **NIH Guidelines on the Inclusion of Women and Minorities as Subjects in Clinical Research**.

Because participants are necessary for many different types of studies, outreach efforts necessarily span the entire clinical research spectrum, from the smallest observational studies and Phase I-II clinical trials, recruiting five or 10 participants, to the largest Phase III clinical trials enrolling thousands. Primary prevention studies involving apparently disease-free individuals, as well as secondary and tertiary intervention involving individuals with diagnosed disease are included, as are studies in which the unit of observation is the entire community.

The notebook does not tell investigators whether they need to enroll participants from various populations, nor is it a step-by-step guide through recruitment and retention. Rather, it furnishes advice on inclusion criteria in the form of a decision tree, provides an overview of key elements in the outreach process, and suggests a number of practical applications, including ethical considerations. Attention to these factors in the design of a research project will assist in the appropriate inclusion of women and minorities into studies. *The presentation of information and the suggestions included in the notebook are not requirements for grant or contract applications.*

For more information on outreach, readers should consult the Reference section at the end of this notebook. Because some important and relevant documents may have been missed, readers are urged to conduct their own search of the literature, and seek out other resources for guidance and expertise relevant to their particular study questions.

This primer is an evolving document that will be reviewed and revised in the future. Therefore, NIH staff welcome your comments for future editions of this notebook, particularly case studies that describe successful and effective strategies.

FACTORS TO CONSIDER IN DETERMINING INCLUSION OF WOMEN AND MINORITIES AND THEIR SUBPOPULATIONS IN CLINICAL RESEARCH

In deciding to what extent women and minorities should be included in a study and what outreach efforts are necessary to achieve appropriate participation, it is essential that the investigator carefully review the scientific question(s) or hypotheses. The need for incorporation of women and minority subpopulations will derive from the scientific question(s). As such, the investigator should consider the following questions.

❦ Is the scientific question or hypothesis applicable equally to both genders and to all minority groups and their subpopulations?

❦ Is the condition under study more prevalent or severe in one particular group?

❦ Have sufficient studies already been performed in one or more groups, leaving gaps that can be filled by focusing the research on certain population groups?

Having considered these questions, the investigator may next turn attention to the following questions.

❦ Can the need for appropriate diversity be met by obtaining access to participants from a single clinic or facility? Will oversampling of certain groups be possible?

❦ If a single clinic or facility is not adequate, can the needed participants be enrolled by going to hospitals or other clinical facilities in the nearby geographic region?

❦ If demographic limitations preclude answering scientific questions locally in the appropriate gender and minority groups, is it feasible or necessary to expand the geographic area, or to establish satellite centers?

A "decision tree" follows which may provide further guidance in determining inclusion for clinical research as well as Phase III clinical trials. To obtain a graphic interpretation of the decision tree, please address your requests to the senior extramural staff member of a particular NIH institute or center listed on page 14513 of the *Federal Register* (March 28, 1994), or to the Office of Research on Women's Health, or the Office of Research on Minority Health (page 14508 of the *Federal Register*). A copy of the *Federal Register* notice is reprinted in Appendix A of this notebook.

Decision Tree for Inclusion of Women and Minorities in Clinical Research*

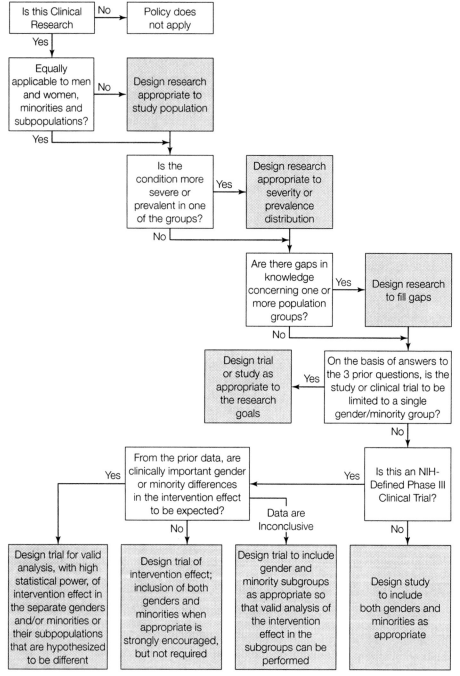

*Clinical Research is defined as all research involving human subjects. See policy for more detailed definition.

A DECISION TREE FOR THE
INCLUSION OF WOMEN AND MINORITIES
IN CLINICAL RESEARCH[1]

1. **Is this Clinical Research?** (Clinical Research is defined as all research involving human subjects. See policy for detailed definition.)

    ❧ If YES, proceed to the next question.

    ❧ If NO, the policy does not apply.

2. **Is the scientific question or hypothesis equally applicable to both men and women, and to minorities and their subpopulations?**

    ❧ If NO, design the research appropriate to the study population.
    Proceed to the next question.

    ❧ If YES, proceed to next question.

3. **Is the condition more severe or prevalent in one of the groups?**

    ❧ If YES, design the research appropriate to the severity or prevalence distribution.
    Proceed to the next question.

    ❧ If NO, proceed to next question.

4. **Are there gaps in knowledge concerning one or more population groups?**

    ❧ If YES, design the research to fill the gaps. Proceed to the next question.

    ❧ If NO, proceed to next question.

5. **On the basis of answers to questions 2,3, and 4, is the study or clinical trial to be limited to a single gender/minority group?**

    ❧ If YES, design the trial or study as appropriate to the research goals.

    ❧ If NO, proceed to next question.

---

[1]NOTE: *The text contained here is also available in a graphic decision tree. If the graphic is not included in this version of the notebook (e.g. obtained from the NIH Guide), you may obtain the graphic version of the decision tree by addressing your request to the senior extramural staff from one of the NIH Institutes or Centers listed at the end of the NIH Guidelines on page 14513 of the* Federal Register *(March 28, 1994), to the Office of Research on Women's Health, or to the Office of Research on Minority Health (page 14508 of the* Federal Register*); the* Federal Register *reprint is contained in Appendix A of this notebook.*

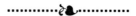

6. **Is this an NIH-Defined Phase III Clinical Trial?**

   ❧ If NO, design study to include both genders and minorities as appropriate.

   ❧ If YES, proceed to next question.

7. **From the prior data, are clinically important gender or minority differences in the intervention effect to be expected?**

   ❧ If YES, design trial for valid analysis, with high statistical power, of intervention effect in the separate genders and/or minorities or their subpopulations that are hypothesized to be different.

   ❧ If NO, design trial of intervention effect; inclusion of both genders and/or minorities when appropriate is strongly encouraged, but not required.

   ❧ If data are INCONCLUSIVE, design trial to include gender and minority subgroups as appropriate so that valid analysis of the intervention effect in the subgroups can be performed.

ELEMENTS OF OUTREACH

The five elements of outreach described below are based on reviews of the literature, ongoing NIH-sponsored studies, recent workshops, and numerous group discussions. These elements should be considered in the recruitment and retention of women and racial or ethnic groups into clinical studies across the entire spectrum of biomedical and behavioral research. The operational details may differ when individuals are recruited in hospitals, clinics, or other health care centers, rather than from the general community (work sites, schools, places of worship), but the underlying elements of understanding, communication, and evaluation are common to all successful outreach efforts.

1. **Understand the Study Population.** Identify the potential research participants, the medical settings in which they are found, and/or the community in which they reside. This may require an assessment of racial/ethnic characteristics, socioeconomic status, age, gender, family configuration, language, education/literacy levels, community structure, cultural norms, migration patterns, points of access (sites of intervention), and needs and values of the potential research participants, including reasons for seeking health care.

2. **Establish Explicit Goals.** Having determined the scientific question(s) for investigation and the study design, establish specific goals for recruiting and retaining study participants. Where possible, involve formal and informal decision makers, organizations, and institutions, as well as the main communication channels in each medical setting or community. Establish lines of communication and cooperation to promote continuing awareness of and trust in the project.

3. **Achieve Agreement on Research Plans.** Confirm that the investigators, medical and health care staff, and community all agree to the design, methodologies, implementation, and completion of the study.

4. **Design and Conduct Evaluations.** Design and implement an evaluation plan to assess the efficacy of recruitment and retention strategies. In cooperation with health care staff or community leaders and potential participants, pretest and periodically retest the recruitment and retention strategies—including resources, incentives, and problem-solving mechanisms—to ensure that they conform with the needs and values of the research participants and their communities. Monitor subject accrual on a frequent and regular basis and compare results with established goals.

5. **Establish and Maintain Communication.** Establish mechanisms for keeping all those involved in the study (research staff, health care providers, participants and their families and communities) apprised of progress and study findings. This will not only increase understanding and awareness of the project, but will also acknowledge the fact that the participants and their health care setting or community are valuable partners in the scientific process.

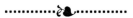

ELEMENT 1
UNDERSTAND THE STUDY POPULATION

Identify the potential research participants, the medical settings in which they are found, and/or the community in which they reside. This may require an assessment of racial/ethnic characteristics, socioeconomic status, age, gender, language, education/literacy levels, community structure, cultural norms, migration patterns, points of access (sites of intervention), and needs and values of the potential research participants, including reasons for seeking health care.

WHY IS THIS IMPORTANT?

Working in culturally diverse settings can be challenging for even the most experienced clinical investigator. One key to success is to learn as much as possible about the groups of interest. Gathering background information about the potential study populations and their communities is an essential first step, to be followed by periodic updates of this information (NHLBI, 1993a; Chen, 1993).

Hospitals and clinics represent a special type of community and should be approached as one would any community. There may be important differences, however. For example, research-based alcoholism after-care programs may have to compete with established service programs for the same population of patients—and their personal or insurance payments.

Background information on the potential study populations and their surroundings is important. *Investigators should note, however, that while suggestions are provided in a wide range of subpopulations, that the NIH Guidelines do not require that every study include each racial and ethnic group. The scientific question must determine the inclusion criteria.*

⧴   Considerable heterogeneity often exists within health care settings and communities. Socio-economic, cultural, and linguistic characteristics can vary widely, along with major differences in health beliefs and practices. Recruitment and retention strategies must therefore be based on the background information about the particular groups of interest. For example, the label "Southeast Asian" does not take into consideration the major differences among Filipino, Hmong, Laotian, Vietnamese, and Cambodian peoples. The term "Native Americans" is used to describe more than 500 federally recognized tribes. Similarly, "Hispanic/Latino" populations have different ethnic origins and racial characteristics and should not necessarily be considered as constituting a single subpopulation.

Country of origin, immigration status, language, and acculturation add to the wide diversity within racial and ethnic populations, and support the need to conduct a careful assessment of the population of interest (Johnson et al., 1992). Furthermore, in communities where individuals may be wary of free communication, such as those with illegal immigrants or where illegal activities are in evidence, investigators will need special skills to evaluate the population.

&. The successful recruitment and retention of women in studies requires consideration of several important factors. Women of childbearing potential must understand the requirements of the study and decide whether it is appropriate for them to participate (e.g., do the benefits outweigh the risks). Even with institutional review board approval, the research team must make special efforts to ensure that women who are considering participation fully understand the demands of the study and what they will be asked to do. Informed consent is essential. Indeed, issues of autonomy are paramount in the decision to participate. In some instances, women may wish to share their decision to participate in a study with family members or others in the community.

Other factors affect the ability of women of different ages and family statuses to participate and should be weighed when designing recruitment and retention strategies. Child care, location of the research site and ease of access and transportation, and time off work are only a few of these considerations.

&. If the research study requires the inclusion of individuals in a particular geographical region, investigators must know the infrastructure and the characteristics of the health care setting, the different communities within the region, and a perspective on the region itself. Is it a rural or an urban community? What are the various cultural groups living there? In which cities or neighborhoods does each ethnic or cultural group live? What are the structure and characteristics of local health care systems and settings?

&. Investigators also need to gain insights about how community residents, or hospital and clinic staff, perceive the research team and its home institution. Such information is crucial in identifying potential problems and finding ways to avoid or work through them early in the outreach efforts.

HOW DO I APPROACH IT?

Depending on the study questions and research setting, the assessment process requires data. A number of those components are presented here. Several sources describe orderly assessment procedures for learning about the individuals, health care settings, and communities of interest (NCI, 1992; NHLBI, 1993b; Braithwaite et al., 1989; Randall-David, 1989).

?• Identify characteristics of the potential participants and setting(s).

– *Individual characteristics:* age, gender, cultural norms, education, literacy, language, health awareness, reasons for seeking medical care, knowledge of available health care services, ideas and attitudes about disease, health beliefs and practices, beliefs in effectiveness of interventions, beliefs in susceptibility of disease, access to health care, sensitivity of health care providers, religious beliefs, sexual preferences, and acculturation patterns.

– *Family characteristics:* family structure, number and age of children and other family members, number of parents and head of household, socioeconomic level, beliefs and practices, cultural norms, education, literacy, language, health awareness, and access to health care.

– *Employment characteristics:* work patterns (daytime versus night-shift work), part versus full-time employment, willingness of employers to grant leave time for participation, and willingness of employees to take leave time for participation.

– *Community characteristics:* socioeconomic level, urban or rural background, migration patterns, racial and ethnic minority groups residing in the community, health care delivery systems, and business and community structure.

?• Identify contacts and points of access that potential participants might utilize.

– *Health care decision makers:* physicians (especially referring physicians), nurses, department chairs, hospital administrators, research committees, and institutional review boards (IRBs).

– *Community leaders:* not only political figures and government officials but also clergy, tribal leaders, teachers and principals, leaders of business and community groups, media personalities, sports figures, and youth leaders.

– *Community businesses and organizations:* schools, day-care centers, places of worship, colleges and universities (including fraternities and sororities), hospitals, clinics, nursing homes, women's and men's clubs, senior and community centers, and private organizations (e.g., American Heart Association, American Cancer Society), alumni associations, recreational facilities (e.g., gyms, local recreational centers) and work sites (including grocery and clothing stores, beauty parlors and barber shops, laundromats, restaurants, taverns, pharmacies, and fire and police stations).

— *Social service agencies:* public welfare, Women, Infants, and Children (WIC), tribal councils, community action agencies, public housing, community health clinics, mental health clinics, and drug treatment centers.

ﻹ Identify communication channels.

— *Formal interpersonal relationships:* health care providers, religious leaders, community leaders, and school teachers.

— *Informal interpersonal relationships:* family, friends, and those who are related by language or common origins, other researchers in the hospital or clinic, former students, and other contacts.

— *Mass media:* newspapers, magazines, films, radio, and television.

Language is a vital part of communication, and investigators from outside a particular community may not be familiar with the meaning of expressions common within a community or with the nuances of colloquial expressions. Another integral part of this process is a clear understanding of the literacy levels of participants. This literacy level must be ascertained for the individual in her or his first language and in English. As such, special efforts may be needed to develop and translate informational materials and other instruments so that they are sensitive to the linguistic and cultural differences among genders and subpopulations (e.g., Hispanic/Latino subpopulations and Asian subpopulations [Chen et al., 1992a,b]).

In general, the research staff and institution must be aware of their abilities and limitations working with the diversity of participants identified for the study (e.g., gays and lesbians, drug users and abusers, AIDS patients, older individuals, minorities [Giachello et al., 1992]).

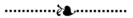

ELEMENT 2
ESTABLISH EXPLICIT GOALS

Having determined the scientific question(s) for investigation and the study design, establish specific goals for recruiting and retaining study participants. Where possible, involve decision makers, organizations, and institutions, as well as the main communication channels in each medical setting or community. Establish lines of communication and cooperation to promote continuing awareness of and trust in the project.

WHY IS THIS IMPORTANT?

The development and implementation of effective recruitment and retention strategies is a multidimensional and evolving process. Outreach strategies that are productive in one population or setting may be counterproductive in another. Consequently, it is essential to involve the health care setting and/or community early in the design of outreach strategies. Hospital and/or clinic staff and community leaders and organizations are important sources of perspective on potential participants. They can provide insights into problems in study design that would otherwise become barriers to the successful accrual of the participants. Forging linkages with these individuals and organizations will strengthen lines of communication, establish trust, and promote awareness (Mellins et al., 1992).

▪ Many people of color are skeptical about participating in clinical studies. Abuses of the past are well known and have been cited by individuals as reasons for refusing to take part in a clinical study. The Tuskegee Syphilis Study, for example, was a tragic deception well remembered even today. Opinion leaders can become the primary link to these groups and individuals, providing reassurance, and building trust.

▪ Leaders can inform investigators about the social and economic needs of the population. For example, the provision of basic social services has been shown to be an effective mechanism for overcoming barriers to the recruitment and retention of women and underserved populations in AIDS clinical trials in the inner cities. When payments or other incentives are offered, however, they should not be of such a magnitude as to be coercive. The level at which this occurs varies with the characteristics of the population.

▪ Consultation with hospital or clinic staff and formal and informal community leaders may allow investigators to "fine-tune" their recruitment and retention strategies to reflect differences among individuals and groups of interest. For example, Mexicans, Puerto Ricans, Cubans, and Central or South Americans may share a common language, but may differ in culture and values (Shumaker et al., 1992).

HOW DO I APPROACH IT?

Many mechanisms exist to establish explicit goals for appropriate recruitment and retention; several suggestions are presented here.

▸ Identify recruitment and retention goals as specifically and explicitly as possible, with the collaboration of hospital or clinic staff and community leaders.

▸ Involve hospital/clinic staff and/or community leaders and local organizations early in the process. For example, present the study plans to physicians and others in the health care settings. Consider creating an advisory board comprised of study staff, health care providers (where warranted), and participants and community members as soon as the study begins.

▸ Include one or more representative(s) from the hospital or clinic staff as members of the research team to serve as liaisons between the researchers, the staff, and the participants.

▸ Offer hospital or clinic staff and/or community organizations opportunities to participate at different levels of involvement, from establishing and taking part in focus groups, to providing sponsorship for the study, to assisting in recruiting, to contributing to the writing or reviewing of proposals.

▸ Recruit women and minority investigators and health care staff for the project. Consider subcontracting specific components of the research activities to hospital or clinic staff and/or community organizations.

▸ Ask advisory boards to review the research plans to ensure that incentives are appropriate for the individuals, that no undue coercion is used, and that materials are appropriate in terms of language and literacy levels.

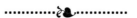

ELEMENT 3
ACHIEVE AGREEMENT ON RESEARCH PLANS

Confirm that the investigators, medical and health care staff, and/or community all agree to the design, methodologies, implementation, and completion of the study.

WHY IS THIS IMPORTANT?

Women and minorities must be included in clinical research if scientists are to make valid inferences about health and disease in these groups. It is essential that investigators strive to build the level of understanding and trust that will lead to a productive partnership and successful conduct of the research project.

HOW DO I APPROACH IT?

Many mechanisms exist to achieve agreement; several are presented here.

❧ Consult the hospital or clinic staff and/or the community at every stage of the study. It is much easier to achieve agreement on issues if all parties have been involved from the earliest stages. Mutually beneficial collaboration can be achieved, and maintained for many years, if the hospital's, clinic's, and community's needs, concerns, and recommendations are taken into account. Involve the hospital or clinic staff and/or community in the planning, as well as the conduct of the research. Understanding and responding to individual and group concerns can lead to more appropriate and useful results.

❧ Present the proposed study, complete with rationale and plans for implementing it, to those who are expected to recruit subjects or answer public questions. This can be accomplished through announcements in public forums in the hospital, clinic, or community, and through announcements in hospital and community newsletters and in special mailings. Do not use jargon in describing the proposed research.

❧ Create an advisory board that includes key members of hospital or clinic staff and community organizations. This can be a very effective mechanism for establishing and maintaining a functional study. Not only can an advisory board guide sensitive and sensible recruitment, it can also assist in understanding and reenlisting those who drop out of the study.

❧ Find ways of including and rewarding hospital or clinic staff so that they find the research to be a satisfying and interesting activity, rather than an additional burden.

ELEMENT 4
DESIGN AND CONDUCT EVALUATIONS

Design and implement an evaluation plan to assess how well the recruitment and retention strategies are working. In cooperation with community leaders, health care staff, and potential participants, pretest and periodically retest the recruitment and retention strategies—including resources, incentives, and problem-solving mechanisms—to ensure that they conform with the needs and values of the research participants and their communities. Monitor subject accrual on a frequent and regular basis and compare results with established goals.

Study design should include a process for systematically documenting the extent to which recruitment and retention objectives were accomplished during a defined period of time for a defined population. Such an evaluation will help investigators to (1) determine which strategies work well; (2) certify the degree of progress that has occurred; and (3) identify elements that are not working. Windsor et al. (1984) have identified several relevant forms of evaluation, including formative, process, short- and long-term outcome, and impact evaluation (see Glossary).

WHY IS THIS IMPORTANT?

Evaluation is an integral part of developing and planning the recruitment and retention strategies (NCI, 1992). As such, evaluation provides investigators with tools for the following tasks:

᠍᠍᠍ Addressing the issues of feasibility: Can the goals be accomplished with the existing staff and resources within the time frame specified?

᠍᠍᠍ Addressing the issues of accountability to the research institutions, research participants and their families, and the community.

᠍᠍᠍ Providing information to encourage the acceptance and response of the community and research participants involved.

᠍᠍᠍ Providing a feedback mechanism to guide changes in current strategies to avoid or counter participant drop out.

········.ક઼.···········

HOW DO I APPROACH IT?

Depending upon the type of evaluation being conducted, important elements form the basis for evaluation. Investigators wishing to learn more about any of the different types of evaluation are urged to consult the many texts prepared on the subject or to seek guidance from an expert. Because this can be a complex process, only the most general elements are presented here.

ક઼ Establish evaluation measures.

– *Study staff:* time-line schedules, work performed, and response to participants over time.

– *Media outreach:* publicity, promotion, type and extent of media coverage, estimated audience size and demographics, and materials planned and distributed.

– *Population response:* volume of inquiries, screening participation rates, and interviewees' perceptions of screening and proposed study and staff.

– *Enrollment rates:* proportion of eligible subjects who agree to participate.

– *Continuing functions and response:* number of phone calls or meetings with community-based organizations, advisory boards, focus groups, and other patient or participant groups.

– *Compliance:* participants' continuing responses to study protocols and demands.

– *Feedback:* consultation with and responses from research participants, community leaders, and hospital or clinic staff.

ક઼ Make use of the evaluation data to refine the recruitment and retention strategies.

– Are there objectives that are not being met? Why?

– Are there strategies or activities that are not succeeding? Why?

– Are more resources required, or can resources be used more efficiently?

– What are the strengths and weaknesses of the strategies or mechanisms for retaining study participants?

ક઼ Establish an ongoing, problem-solving mechanism. This should include not only regularly scheduled meetings with participant focus groups and hospital or clinic staff involved in the study, but also adequate mechanisms for tracking patients and investigating each patient withdrawal to determine if some aspect of the retention strategy is at fault. Investigators may also need to provide counseling to address the social needs that can impede the participation of women and members of minority groups in a clinicial study (e.g., child care, transportation costs, study site location, availability of parking). Above all, investigators must remain flexible within the constraints of the study goals and objectives.

Before initiating the full-scale project, investigators typically find it useful to conduct a pilot test of the proposed recruitment/retention strategies. This will allow the opportunity to test the feasibility of the planned approach and amend it according to feedback from the study population. Potential participants can contribute valuable information on the needs, cultures, and values of the population of interest and the community in which they reside. It is during this preliminary test period that the investigator can best determine the most cost-effective distribution of resources, including materials, equipment, personnel, and time. Based on this information, fiscal and budgetary planning can be finalized and problem-solving mechanisms can be put in place (Rand et al., 1992).

Pilot testing strategies can also provide feedback on proposed strategies and incentives, such as educational materials, hiring staff from the proposed study population, establishing a project office in the community, providing transportation, and other compensations (e.g., meals, food coupons, child care, or cash). Problem-solving mechanisms instituted following the pilot study can include regularly scheduled reviews to identify barriers that are interfering with compliance or continued participation.

Periodic retesting and refining of recruitment and retention strategies can also be important, for the following reasons.

⁊ Resources can vary during the course of the study, so it may be prudent to identify alternative mechanisms in advance. Should problems arise, local agencies or organizations may serve as backups. By the same token, members of the research team may need to take over some of the recruitment functions if they prove too time-consuming for hospital or clinic staff.

⁊ Community leaders and hospital or clinic staff can assist in determining the most appropriate distribution of resources—for example, instances where volunteers may be used in lieu of paid staff and the availability of bilingual and sign interpreters.

ELEMENT 5
ESTABLISH AND MAINTAIN COMMUNICATION

Establish mechanisms for keeping all those involved in the study (research staff, health care providers, participants and their families and communities) apprised of progress and, ultimately, study findings. This will not only increase understanding and awareness of the project, but will recognize the participants and their health care setting or community as valuable partners in the scientific process.

WHY IS THIS IMPORTANT?

Effective communication of study results is another important element in building trust in the community. Researchers must remember, however, that their professional priorities may conflict with the priorities of study participants. Specifically, publication of research results in scientific journals has little value to participants and could be perceived as exploitive unless the same results are also conveyed to the participants, and their communities, in a sensitive manner (Shumaker et al., 1992). Providing the community and the hospital or clinic staff with a detailed report on the progress of research is often the first step in developing a long-term relationship of trust and cooperation. Future relationships with these populations could depend on whether they perceive their role as that of partners in the research or merely "guinea pigs."

Communication of study results should therefore be among the ethical considerations of any research project (see below). Dissemination of research findings can also promote awareness of social, medical, and educational resources that have been made available a result of the project.

HOW DO I APPROACH IT?

The following avenues of communication can be used not only for announcing the study and recruiting participants, but also for disseminating study results (Rand et al., 1992). The important point is that participants, their health care providers, and their communities understand the outcome of the study and that their inestimable contribution is noted and appreciated.

ﻬ   Formal methods of communication can be used through the media, including radio (e.g., talk shows, ethnic language stations, and public service announcements), print (e.g., flyers, posters, hospital newsletters, and newspaper articles in language appropriate to the proposed study group), and television (e.g., talk shows, news shows, cable access channels, and ethnic language stations).

ﻬ   Informal methods of communication can be utilized by including personal contact (e.g., telephone, door-to-door, neighborhood events, schools, staff meetings) and multiple sites of intervention (e.g., health clinics, social service agencies, hospitals and clinics, places of worship, union halls, senior citizen centers, shelters, grocery stores, beauty shops, and day care centers).

ᖧ♠ At the conclusion of the study, the research team may wish to host a special presentation for participants, hospital or clinic staff, and community groups to discuss the outcome of the study and its subsequent application to health.

ᖧ♠ Feedback mechanisms can and should be utilized in the participants' language to ensure ongoing success and retention of participants and that follow-up questionnaires reach participants. Study results should also be provided at the completion of the study, along with the appreciation of the principal investigator and staff.

ᖧ♠ Consider employing an outreach educator, whose responsibilities might include:

– setting up monthly meetings with health care or community-based organizations and developing linkages to enhance research participation and to "trouble-shoot" problems;

– developing and preparing health care or community-oriented educational materials;

– attending health care or participant meetings, community health fairs or block parties to periodically disseminate study information;

– providing requested information about the research study to individuals and health care and/or community groups through educational presentations and workshops;

– providing in-service training and guidance to all investigative staff, to ensure that they are sensitive to the needs, attitudes, and concerns of study participants;

– providing education and training to health care and/or community leaders to ensure that they understand the benefits and demands of research and the role participants and their health care setting and/or communities play in such collaboration; and

– convening periodic meetings of scientific staff and health care and/or community leaders (or advisory board) to assess retention and to devise strategies for countering drop out and bolstering retention and protocol adherence.

ETHICAL ISSUES

Any research involving human subjects raises ethical issues that demand consideration and resolution. The requirement to include women and minorities may increase the difficulties presented by these issues, but this does not contravene the responsibility of investigators to anticipate and deal with ethical concerns. When studies are conducted in communities, community leaders, both formal and informal, should be consulted regarding the proposed study and its intended and unintended consequences. The procedures for seeking approval from the Institutional Review Board must be followed.

In interpreting the mandate for outreach in the recruitment and retention of women and racial and/or ethnic groups into clinical studies, investigators and their staff members must respect the three basic ethical principles established by the Belmont Report (National Commission, 1978):

1. **Respect for persons.** This principle incorporates two ethical convictions: first, individuals should be treated as autonomous agents; and second, persons with diminished autonomy are entitled to protection. When investigators conduct research involving human beings, respect for the rights of the individual requires that the participant enter into the research voluntarily and with adequate information.

2. **Beneficence.** This principle stipulates that persons are treated in an ethical manner not only by respecting their decisions and protecting them from harm, but also by making efforts to secure their well-being. Two complementary expressions of beneficent actions have been formulated: (1) do no harm; and (2) maximize possible benefits while minimizing possible harm.

3. **Justice.** This principle stipulates that injustice occurs when some benefit to which a person is entitled is denied without good reason, or when some burden is imposed unduly. When investigators recruit subjects for research, they should not systematically include some individuals or groups because of their easy availability, their compromised position, or their malleability. Rather, subjects should be recruited based on their relation to the problem being studied.

In short, while investigators should recruit participants who will provide the most useful, valid, and widely generalizable knowledge about the problem being studied, they should not recruit participants only because they are available, malleable, or in a compromised position. By the same token, however, participants should not be denied access for reasons unrelated to their health status or the purposes of the study.

It should also be assumed that all of the regulations of the NIH Office of Protection from Research Risks (OPRR) concerning ethical considerations in clinical and community trials apply to *all* individuals (human subjects) regardless of their gender, race, or ethnicity. However, successful implementation of these regulations depends on the ability of the research team to understand implications of conducting research in particular populations, settings, and trials.

Potential participants in clinical and community trials differ in ways that can affect their comprehension of the purpose, benefits, and risks of the study, as well as their capacity to adhere to the study protocol. Research has shown that a participant's understanding of design elements, such as randomization and placebo group, may be affected by race and educational level; other barriers to full participation (e.g., transportation costs, inflexible work schedules, availability of child care, literacy, and competency in English) may also present barriers to participation and require consideration. Issues of autonomy are paramount in the decision to participate. As such, allowing time for potential participants to become fully informed about what their participation entails is essential. Translators may be required, and potential participants may need several sessions to ask questions and understand procedures. In some instances, women may wish to share their decision to participate in a study with family members or others in the community.

Similarly, "coercion" requires interpretation in terms of a particular target population. Some participants may need reimbursement for costs incurred in the course of their participation, but the prospect of reimbursement should not become such an inducement that the potential participant feels compelled to participate for economic reasons.

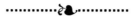

Seven Points of Consideration for Institutional Review Boards

To assist in consideration of ethical issues by Institutional Review Boards (IRBs), the Office of Protection from Research Risks recently released a document which listed seven key points (OPRR REPORTS, 1994).

Institutions and IRBs have the following responsibilities:

1. To help ensure that investigators understand the importance of inclusion of both genders and minorities in research and clearly delineate the expectations for the design and conduct of such research. They should assist in providing investigators with written guidance and educational opportunities for clarification.

2. To specify that, when scientifically appropriate, investigators cite evidence or lack of evidence if a health situation or intervention in the proposed research may affect one gender or minority group differently and describe how the proposed research addresses that evidence. Investigators should be prepared to describe the extent to which both genders and persons of various ethnic and racial backgrounds are or have been involved in similar research.

3. To help create guidelines for investigators to facilitate recruitment and retention of participants to ensure representation and sufficient involvement of targeted populations. The extent to which investigators are collaborating with researchers at other institutions that can involve increased numbers of men or women or populations from different minority groups must be part of the information the IRB reviews, particularly with regard to Phase III clinical trials.

4. To ensure that any special vulnerabilities of participants (e.g., educational level, socio-economic status) are accounted for and handled appropriately. The IRB should carefully consider if reimbursements (cash and material provisions) are appropriate to the context of the proposed research, with particular attention to ensure that these reimbursements do not promote coercion or undue influence to participate or remain in the study.

5. To safeguard the consent process and to promote open and free communication between the researcher and the participants. Investigators and IRBs must seek to understand cultural nuances and types of foreign languages inherent in the populations to be enrolled. The possibility of illiteracy among potential research participants must also be considered and assurances given that adequate provision has been made for the appropriate translations of the consent documents or the availability of translators.

6. To arrange for inclusion of women and members of minority groups on the IRB, especially if the nature and volume of the research to be conducted at the institution routinely includes these populations. IRBs should also consider consulting ad hoc advisors who could help with understanding the perspectives of various groups. Also, institutions and IRBs can encourage investigators to seek out such perspectives during the planning of research protocols.

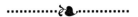

7. To specify that NIH-supported investigators provide details of the proposed involvement of humans in the research, including the characteristics of the subject population, anticipated numbers, age ranges, and health statuses. The proposed research should specify the gender and racial and/or ethnic composition of the subject population, as well as criteria for inclusion or exclusion of any subpopulation. If ethnic, racial, and gender estimates and continuing review numbers are not included in the background data for a protocol, the investigators must provide a clear rationale for exclusion of this information.

WHERE DO I GO FOR HELP?

⁊⁖ **START WITH A LITERATURE SEARCH.**

– Census data and other government reports and statistics can be helpful in identifying potential research participants, as well as the specific problems and needs potential participants may have in comparison with the general population. For example, the National Health Interview Survey (NHIS) and the National Health and Nutrition Examination Survey (NHANES), as well as several other national and periodic surveys, provide important and timely data on individuals and groups.

– Medical and public health references, especially epidemiology and health intervention articles, address issues of recruitment and retention for the specific group of interest in the research study. A sampling of such articles is included in the Reference section at the end of this notebook.

– Behavioral and social science literature focuses on intercultural and ethnic studies, including psychosocial, sociocultural, and anthropological references specific to various racial, ethnic, and cultural groups. Such information can be useful in providing a general understanding of various cultures' values, beliefs and practices, and historical experiences in the United States.

– Local newspapers are a good source of information about a community. The local news and editorial sections of newspapers can provide very specific information about a community (i.e., the issues community members consider most pressing, their concerns, and problems). These sources also provide listings of current and upcoming community events.

⁊⁖ **CONSULT WITH EXPERTS.**

– Other researchers who have investigated the same areas of scientific interest or who have personal experience with a specific ethnic and/or racial group or with women as study participants are invaluable sources of information and guidance.

– Health professionals or other persons working in similar communities or with similar problems can provide useful perspectives. Often such experts are available through local, regional, or national health-related and community organizations that have relevant experience with various groups.

– Individuals and groups from the place or community of interest can play crucial roles in helping to design, promote, and maintain interest in the research study.

ఇ▲ CONSIDER OTHER METHODS FOR UNDERSTANDING THE COMMUNITY.

– *Researcher observation.* The researcher can participate as an observer in a variety of community activities, such as organization meetings, community social gatherings, cultural ceremonies, and/or special celebrations.

– *Informal conversation.* This method allows the scientific team the opportunity to gather information in a less formal manner. Such encounters require thoughtful and careful listening to capture accurate information (history, anecdotes, perspectives) about the people and the community.

– *Case study or in-depth interview.* This method allows for more detailed information about a person's life, family, neighborhood, and community history and perspective.

– *Focus group and surveys.* While these two inquiries are quite different in the information produced, they are useful in developing culturally relevant strategies. Such inquiries can reveal the range of community attitudes and beliefs about a problem, people's perceived needs and priorities, and their preferences for strategies and formats.

ఇ▲ FEDERAL RESOURCES.

– Senior NIH extramural staff who can provide information about the relevant policies and programs in their respective institutes and centers are listed at the end of the *Federal Register* notice in Appendix A.

In addition, the Federal government has a number of agencies that maintain information and data bases: the Centers for Disease Control and Prevention, especially the National Center for Health Statistics, the Health Services and Resource Administration, the Agency for Health Care Policy and Research, the Health Care Financing Administration. These and other government resources can be accessed by calling a central information number or by writing to each agency.

NIH REVIEW CRITERIA FOR THE INCLUSION OF WOMEN AND MINORITIES INTO CLINICAL RESEARCH

In conducting peer review for scientific and technical merit, appropriately constituted initial review groups (including study sections and review committees), technical evaluation groups, and intramural review panels will be instructed to consider the following elements in the recruitment and retention of women and minorities in clinical research.

❧ Evaluate the proposed plan for the inclusion of women and minorities and their subpopulations for appropriate representation or evaluate the proposed justification when representation is limited or absent.

❧ Evaluate the proposed exclusion of women and minorities and their subpopulations on the basis that a requirement for inclusion is inappropriate with respect to the health of the subjects.

❧ Evaluate the proposed exclusion of minorities and women on the basis that a requirement for inclusion is inappropriate with respect to the purpose of the research.

❧ Determine whether the design of a clinical trial is adequate to measure potential differences.

❧ Evaluate the plans for recruitment, retention, and outreach for study participants.

These criteria, which apply to the full range of NIH-supported clinical research, are a part of the scientific assessment and will contribute to the assigned priority score.

The plans for recruitment and retention for study participants should be clearly presented in terms of the methods and mechanisms for outreach. Peer Review Group members will look for evidence that the investigator has addressed the inclusion of women and minorities and their subpopulations in a satisfactory manner.

Such evidence might include, for example, information on the population characteristics of the disease or condition under study; national and local demographics of the population; knowledge and understanding of the racial, ethnic, and cultural characteristics of the population and relevant scientific literature; prior experience, success, and collaborations in recruitment and retention of the populations and subpopulations to be studied; and the plans, arrangements, and letters of commitment from relevant community groups and organizations for the planned study. Plans should also consider appropriate staffing needs for recruitment, retention, and outreach plans.

The composition of any study group should be based on science, and not on the convenience of the investigator. It is not necessarily expected that every study will include representation from all racial or ethnic groups. For single hospital, clinic and university studies, it is important to distinguish between data on the characteristics of the population served by the site compared with the broader community or regional population. To avoid selection bias, planned enrollment should be viewed in terms of the demographics of the disease or condition in the broader community or regional or national population, rather than local demographics or referral patterns. For multicenter trials, the combined enrollment from all recruitment sites may achieve the appropriate gender and racial and/or ethnic composition for the study. Study designs involving oversampling to achieve the needed balance of groups may be appropriate in some circumstances.

Applicants must provide information using the summary table below for planned enrollment of women and minorities, and awardees will report annually on the planned enrollment for the approved project and the actual enrollment after receipt of the award and the start of the project.

TABLE 1: GENDER AND MINORITY INCLUSION (398/2590)

	American Indian or Alaskan Native	Asian or Pacific Islander	Black, not of Hispanic Origin	Hispanic	White, not of Hispanic Origin	Other or Unknown	Total
Female							
Male							
Unknown							
Total							

Note: (1) For planned studies, indicate the expected study composition using the categories noted in the table. If there is more than one study, provide a separate table for each study. In addition, report on the subpopulations which are included in the study. (2) For ongoing studies, provide the number of subjects enrolled in the study to date (cumulatively since the study began) according to the same categories and table format.

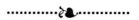

GLOSSARY

Acculturation: Degree to which people from a particular cultural or ethnic group display behavior that reflects the influence of pervasive, mainstream norms of behavior.

Assimilation: Extent to which an individual enters a new culture and becomes a part of it. Includes both the motivation of the individual to enter the mainstream culture and the extent to which members of the mainstream culture welcome or discourage the entry and inclusion of that person in the mainstream culture.

Clinical Trial, Phase III: A broadly based prospective clinical investigation for the purpose of evaluating an experimental intervention in comparison with a standard or control intervention or comparing two or more existing treatments. Often the aim of such investigation is to provide evidence leading to a scientific basis for consideration of a change in health policy or standard of care. The definition includes pharmacologic, non-pharmacologic, and behavioral interventions given for disease prevention, prophylaxis, diagnosis, or therapy. Community trials and other population-based intervention trials are also included.

Community-based organizations: Organizations that have their origins or basis within the community and which utilize some aspect of the community's goals, mandate, or objectives as part of their efforts.

Communication channels: The means by which a message gets from a source to a receiver. Mass media channels are more effective in making people aware of a new idea; interpersonal channels are more effective in persuading people to adopt a new idea.

Cultural competence: A set of academic and interpersonal skills that allows individuals to increase their understanding and appreciation of cultural differences and similarities within, among, and between groups. This requires a willingness and ability to draw on community-based values, traditions, and customs and to work with persons who are knowledgeable about and from the community in developing focused interventions, communications, and other supports.

Cultural diversity: Differences in race, ethnicity, language, nationality, or religion among various groups within a community, organization, or nation. A city is said to be culturally diverse if its residents include members of different racial and/or ethnic groups.

Cultural sensitivity: Respect for ethnic individuals and for their culture; the recognition that such individuals have cultural health beliefs and practices; the integration of those beliefs and practices in the overall treatment plan for the patient; and the ability to act on behalf of the individual to assure quality health care.

Formative evaluation: Collects information about the components of the recruitment and retention aspects of the research project. Information from this type of evaluation can be used to test messages, select communications channels, and revise the communication process.

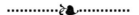

Impact evaluation: Focuses on the long-range results of the program and subsequent changes in health status. Impact evaluations are rarely possible because they are costly, involve extended commitment, and may depend upon other strategies in addition to the recruitment and retention component of the research project.

Mainstream: Used to describe the "general market," but usually refers to a broad population that, in the continental United States, is primarily white and middle class.

Multicultural: Designed for, or pertaining to, two or more distinctive cultures.

Outcome evaluation: Provides descriptive information on the project and can be used to document short-term results. Task-focused results describe the output of the activities (i.e., number of participants recruited as a result of a talk show in a local television station). Short-term results describe the immediate effects of the strategies on the target population (i.e., percentage of the target group that is participating in one of the research protocols).

Process evaluation: Documents the degree of implementation of the recruitment and retention activities. It describes how many items, of what materials, are provided to whom, by whom, and when and whether they responded. This type of evaluation may look at the origin of the research project, the methods used, the target population, program personnel/staff, and cost.

Race: A population of individuals who possess distinguishable physical characteristics that are genetically transmitted.

Site of intervention: A specific location used to establish contact with or gain access to subjects within the neighborhood or community in which they reside. Examples include schools, work sites, beauty shops, barber shops, ethnic grocery stores, small group meetings in people's homes, community clinics, hospitals, and day-care centers.

References

Agras WS, Bradford RH, eds. (1982). Recruitment to the Coronary Primary Prevention Trial: A Monograph. *Circulation* 66 (supp IV): 1–78.

American Cancer Society (1989). *The Culture of Poverty.* American Cancer Society: Atlanta, Ga. Pub. No. 89-1M-No. 2010.

–(1990). *Cancer and the Socioeconomically Disadvantaged.* American Cancer Society: Atlanta, Ga. Pub. No. 90-25M-No. 3350-PE.

–(1992). *Effective Approaches for Increasing Compliance with American Cancer Society Recommendations in Socioeconomically Disadvantaged Populations.* American Cancer Society: Atlanta, Ga. Pub. No. 92-50M-No. 3320.01-PE.

Ashery RS, McAuliffe WE, (1992). Implementation Issues and Techniques in Randomized Trials of Outpatient Psychosocial Treatments for Drug Abusers: Recruitment of Subjects. *Am J Drug Alcohol Abuse* 18: 305–29.

Barr D (1991). "Incorporating Community Input into AIDS Research: The Creation of the AIDS Clinical Trial Group Community Constituency Group." Presentation abstract in *Proceedings of the VII International Conference on AIDS,* Florence, Italy, June 16–21, 1991. 2: 39.

Basch CE, Shea S, and Zybert P (1994). The Reproducibility of Data from a Food Frequency Questionnaire Among Low-Income Latina Mothers and Their Children. *Am J Public Health.* 84(5): 861–64.

Bennett JC (1993). Inclusion of Women in Clinical Trials—Policies for Population Subgroups. *N Engl J Med* 329: 288–92.

Benson C (1989). Women with HIV Disease: Clinical Progression and Survival in a Cohort Followed at a University Medical Center. *Proceedings of the V International Conference on AIDS,* Montreal, Canada, June 4–9, 1989. 1: MO11.

Braithwaite R, et al. (1989). Community Organization and Development for Health Promotion Within an Urban Black Community: A Conceptual Model. *Health Education,* 1989, 20(5): 56–60.

Brisbane FL, Womble M (1992). *Working with African Americans.* Needham, MA: Ginn Press.

Brawley OW (1995). Response to inclusion of women and minorities in clinical trials and the NIH Revitalization Act of 1993—the perspective on NIH clinical trialists. *Controlled Clinical Trials* 16(5): 293–295 (October 1995).

Burhansstipanov L, Dresser C (1993). *Documentation of the Cancer Research Needs of American Indians and Alaska Natives.* Bethesda, MD: Cancer Control Science Program, DCPC, National Cancer Institute.

Bush PJ, et al. (1993). Surveying and Tracking Urban Elementary School Children's Use of Abusable Substances. In DeLaRosa MR and Recio JL, eds., *Drug Abuse Among Minority Youth: Advances in Research and Methodology* (NIDA Research Monograph 130, NIH Pub. No. 93-3479), pp. 280–97. Rockville, MD: National Institute on Drug Abuse.

Center for Drug Evaluation and Research (in press). *Guideline for the Study Of And Evaluation Of Gender Differences in the Clinical Evaluation of Drugs.* Washington, DC: U.S. Food and Drug Administration.

Chavez LR, Cornelius WA, Jones OW (1985). Mexican Immigrants and the Utilization of U.S. Health Services: The Case of San Diego. *Soc Sci Med* 21: 93–102.

Cheeseman S (1989). Compliance of HIV-Infected Intravenous Drug Users in Clinical Trials. June 4–9, 1989, p. 392. Poster abstract in *Proceedings of the V International Conference on AIDS,* Montreal, Canada, June 4–9, 1989, p. 392.

Chen M (1993). Cardiovascular Health Among Asian Americans/Pacific Islanders: An Examination of Health Status and Intervention Approaches. *Health Promotion* 7: 199–207.

Chen M, et al. (1992a). Recruitment of Minority Communities. *Health Behavior Research in Minority Populations: Access, Design, and Implementation* (NIH PubL. No. 92-2965). Bethesda, MD: National Institutes of Health.

Chen M, et al. (1992b). Lessons Learned and Baseline Data from Initiating Smoking Cessation Research with Southeast Asian adults. *Asian and Pacific Islander Journal of Health,* 1(2): 194–214.

Cotton D (1991). Participation of Women in a Multicenter HIV Clinical Trials Program in the United States. *Proceedings of the VII International Conference on AIDS,* Florence, Italy, June 16–21, 1991.

Council on Ethical and Judicial Affairs, American Medical Association (1991). Gender Disparities in Clinical Decision Making. *JAMA* 266: 559–62.

Craven DE, et al. (1990). AIDS in Intravenous Drug Users: Issues Related to Enrollment in Clinical Trials. *J Acquir Immune Defic Syndr* 3:(supp 2) S45–S50.

Currier J (1992). Women and Power: The Impact of Accrual Rates of Women on the Ability to Detect Gender Differences in Toxicity and Response to Therapy in Clinical Trials. Poster abstract in *Proceedings of the VIII International Conference on AIDS,* Amersterdam, Netherlands, July 15–24, 1992. 2:C329.

Debro J, Conley D (1993). School and Community Politics: Issues, Concerns and Implications When Conducting Research in Afro-American Communities. In DeLaRosa MR, Recio JL, eds, *Drug Abuse Among Minority Youth: Advances in Research and Methodology* (NIDA Research Monograph 130, NIH Pub. No. 93-3479). Rockville, MD: National Institute on Drug Abuse. pp. 298–307.

Debro JJ, Bolek CS (1991). *Drug Abuse Research Issues at Historically Black Colleges and Universities.* Atlanta, GA: Clark University and NIDA.

De La Cancela V (1989). Minority AIDS Prevention: Moving Beyond Cultural Perspectives towards Sociopolitical Empowerment. AIDS Educ Prev 1: 141–53.

DiClemente RJ, Boyer CB, Morales ES (1988). Minorities and AIDS: Knowledge, Attitudes and Misconceptions Among Blacks and Latino Adolescents. *Am J Pub Health* 78: 55–57.

Dressler WW (1992). Access Issues and Points of Entry. *Health Behavior Research in Minority Populations: Access, Design, and Implementation.* (NIH Pub. No. 92-2965). Bethesda, MD: National Institutes of Health.

El-Sadr W, Capps L (1992). The Challenge of Minority Recruitment in Clinical Trials for AIDS. *JAMA* 267: 954–57.

El-Sadr W, et al. (1992). The Challenge of Minority Recruitment in Clinical Trials for AIDS. *JAMA* 267: 7.

Eliason MJ (1993). Ethics and Transcultural Nursing Care. *Nurs Outlook* 41: 225–28.

Fairchild P (1989). Impediments to IVDA Enrollment in ACTG Clinical Trials. *Proceedings of the V International Conference on AIDS,* Montreal, Canada, June 4–9, 1989, p. 391.

Frank-Stromborg M, Olsen SJ, eds. (1993). *Cancer Prevention in Minority Populations.* St. Louis: Mosby.

Freedman LS, Simon R, Foulkes MA, Friedman L, Geller NL, Gordon DJ, Mowery R (1995). Inclusion of women and minorities in clinical trials and the NIH Revitalization Act of 1993—the perspective of NIH clinical trialists. *Controlled Clinical Trials* 16(5): 277–285.

Gans KM, et al. (1989). Measuring Blood Cholesterol in the Community: Participant Characteristics by Site. *Health Education Research* 4: 399–406.

Gath E (1991). The Merging of Public and Academic Institutions: A Model of Care for the HIV-Infected Child and Mother. Presentation abstract in *Proceedings of the VII International Conference on AIDS,* Florence, Italy, June 16–21, 1991. 1:51.

General Accounting Office (1992). *Women's Health: FDA Needs to Ensure More Study of Gender Differences in Prescription Drug Testing* (GAO/HRD-93-17). Washington, D.C.: U.S. Government Printing Office.

Giachello A, et al. (1992). Reconciling the Multiple Scientific and Community Needs. *Health Behavior Research in Minority Populations: Access, Design, and Implementation* (NIH Pub. No. 92-2965). Bethesda, MD: National Institutes of Health.

Glanz K, Lewis FM, Rimer BK, eds. (1990). *Health Behavior and Health Education: Theory, Research, and Practice.* San Francisco, CA: Jossey-Bass Publishers.

Glick R, Moore JW, eds. (1990). *Drugs in Hispanic Communities.* New Brunswick, NJ: Rutgers University Press.

Green LS, Kreuter MW, Deeds SG, Partridge KB (1980). *Health Education Planning: A Diagnostic Approach.* Palo Alto, CA: Mayfield Publishers.

Green LW, McAlister AL (1984). Macro-Intervention to Support Health Behavior: Some Theoretical Perspectives and Practical Reflections. Health Educ Q 11: 322–39.

Gritz, et al. (1992). Recruitment Through Schools and Churches. *Health Behavior Research in Minority Populations: Access, Design, and Implementation.* (NIH Pub. No. 92-2965). Bethesda, MD: National Institutes of Health.

Hamilton JA (1985). Guidelines for Avoiding Methodological and Policy-Making Biases in Gender-Related Health Research. In *Women's Health: Report of the Public Health Service Task Force on Women's Health Issues,* Vol 2. Rockville, Md.: Public Health Service, IV-54–IV-64.

Hamilton JA, Parry B (1983). Sex-Related Differences in Clinical Drug Response: Implications for Women's Health. *J Am Med Wom Assoc* 38: 126–32.

Hatch J, et al. (1993). Community Research: Partnership in Black Communities. *Community Research* pp. 27–31.

Hayunga EG, Rothenberg KH, Pinn VW (1996). Women of childbearing potential in clinical research: Perspectives on NIH policy and liability issues. *Food, Drug, Cosmetic and Medical Device Law Digest* 13: 7–11.

Hayunga EG, Pinn VW (1996). Including women and minorities in clinical research: Implementation of the 1994 NIH guidelines. *Applied Clinical Trials* (forthcoming, fall 1996).

Hayunga EG, Pinn VW (1996). Including women and minorities in clinical research: Responding to concerns of the research community. *Applied Clinical Trials* (forthcoming, fall 1996).

Hayunga EG, Costello MD, Pinn VW (1996). Including women and minorities in clinical research: Demographics of study populations. *Applied Clinical Trials* (forthcoming, fall 1996).

Hohmann A, Parron DL (1996). How the new NIH guidelines on inclusion of women and minorities apply: Efficacy trials, effectiveness trials, and validity. *Journal of Consulting and Clinical Psychology* 64 (in press).

Horgan J (1989). Affirmative Action: AIDS Researchers Seek to Enroll More Minorities in Clinical Trials. *Sci Am.* 261: 34.

Institute of Medicine (1993). *Forum on Drug Development: Women and Drug Development: Report of a Workshop.* Washington, D.C.: National Academy Press.

Jenkins RR, Parron D (1995). Guidelines for adolescent health research: Issues of race and class. *Journal of Adolescent Health* 17: 314–322.

Johnson K, et al. (1992). Access Issues and Points of Entry. *Health Behavior Research in Minority Populations: Access, Design, and Implementation.* (NIH Pub. No. 92-2965). Bethesda, MD: National Institutes of Health.

Kinney EL, et al. (1981). Underrepresentation of Women in New Drug Trials. *Ann Intern Med* 95: 409–99.

Kirschstein RL (1991). Research on Women's Health. *Am J Public Health* 81: 291–93.

Korvick J (1993). Women's Participation in AIDS Clinical Trials Group (ACTG) Trials in the USA—Enough or Still Too Few? Poster abstract in *Proceedings of the IX International Conference on AIDS,* Berlin, Germany, June 6–11, 1993. 1: 561.

Lacey L (1993). Cancer Prevention and Early Detection Strategies for Reaching Undeserved Urban, Low-Income Black Women. *Cancer* 72: 1078–83.

LaRosa JC, et al. (1994). Cholesterol Lowering in the Elderly. *Archiv Intern Med* 154: 529–39.

LaRosa JH, (1993). Building Women's Responsibility in Papanicolaou Screening. *The Female Patient* 18: 41–44.

LaRosa JH, Pinn VW (1993). Gender Bias in Biomedical Research. *J Am Med Wom Assoc* 48(5): 145–50.

LaRosa JH, Seto B, Caban CE, Hayunga EG. Including Women and Minorities in Clinical Research. *Applied Clinical Trials.* May 1995; 4:5: 31–38.

Lasater T, et al. (1992). Social marketing Planning Model: An Approach to Programs and Research for Groups from Diverse Backgrounds. *Health Behavior Research in Minority Populations: Access, Design, and Implementation* (NIH Pub. No. 92-2965). Bethesda, MD: National Institutes of Health.

Leader MA, Neuwirth E (1978). Clinical Research and the Noninstitutional Elderly: A Model for Subject Recruitment. *J Am Geriatr Soc* 26: 27–31.

Levine C (1992). Women as Research Subjects: New Priorities, New Questions. In Blank RH, Bonnicksen AL, eds., *Emerging Issues in Biomedical Policy: An Annual Review.* New York: Columbia University Press, 2: 169–88.

Levine RJ (1994). The impact of HIV infection on society's perception of clinical trials. *Kennedy Institute of Ethics* 4(2): 93–98.

Longorria JM, Turner NH (1991). Community Leaders Help Increase Response Rates in An AIDS Survey. *Am J Pub Health* 81: 654–55.

Lonner WJ, Berry JW, eds. (1986). *Field Methods in Cross-Cultural Research.* Newbury Park, CA: Sage Publications.

Mack E, et al. (1993). Reaching Poor Populations With Cancer Prevention and Early Detection Programs. *Cancer Practice* 1: 35–39.

Marin G, Marin BV (1982). Methodological Fallacies When Studying Hispanics. *Applied Social Psychology Annual* 99–117.

–(1991). *Research With Hispanic Populations.* Newbury Park, CA: Sage Publications.

Marin G, Marin BV (1990). Perceived Credibility of Channels and Sources of AIDS Information Among Hispanics. AIDS Education and Prevention 2: 154–161.

Marin G, et al. (1987). Development of a Short Acculturation Scale for Hispanics. *Hispanic Journal of Behavioral Science* 9(2): 183–205.

Mattson ME, et al. (1985). Participation in a Clinical Trial: The Patients' Point of View. *Controlled Clin Trials* 6: 156–67.

McCabe MS, Varricchio CG, Padberg RM (in press). State of the Art Care: Efforts to Recruit the Economically Disadvantaged to National Clinical Trials. *Semin Oncol Nurs.*

McCarthy CR (1994). Historical background of clinical trials involving women and minorities. *Academic Medicine* 69: 695–698.

Meisler A (1993). Adherence to Clinical Trials Among Women, Minorities, and Injection Drug Users. Poster abstract in *Proceedings of the IX International Conference on AIDS,* Berlin, Germany, June 6–11, 1993. 1: 558.

Mellins, et al. (1992). Recruitment from Hospitals and Clinics. *Health Behavior Research in Minority Populations: Access, Design, and Implementation* (NIH Pub. No. 92-2965). Bethesda, MD: National Institutes of Health.

Merkatz RB, et al. (1993). Women in Clinical Trials of New Drugs—A Change in Food and Drug Administration Policy. *N Engl J Med* 329: 288–86.

Millburn N, et al. (1991). Conducting Epidemiologic Research in Minority Communities: Methodological Considerations. *Journal of Community Psychology* 19: 3–12.

Millon-Underwood S, Sanders E, Davis M (1993). Determinants of Participation in State-of-the-Art Cancer Prevention, Early Detection/Screening, and Treatment Trials Among African-Americans. *Cancer Nurs* 16: 25–33.

Murphy TF (1991). Women and Drug Users: The Changing Faces of HIV Clinical Drug Trials. *QRB* 17: 26–32.

National Cancer Institute (1990). *Smoking, Tobacco, and Cancer Program: 1985–1989 Status Report* (NIH Pub. No. 90-3107). Bethesda, MD: National Institutes of Health.

–(1992). *Making Health Communication Programs Work* (NIH Publication No 92-1493). Bethesda, MD: Office of Cancer Communication, National Cancer Institute.

National Commission for the Protection of Human Subjects of Biomedical and Behavioral Research (1978). *The Belmont Report: Ethical Principles and Guidelines for the Protection of Human Subjects of Research.* Washington, DC: U.S. Government Printing Office.

National Heart, Lung, and Blood Institute (NHLBI) (1990). *Women's Health Issues.* Bethesda, MD: NHLBI.

–(1993a). *Proceedings of the Fourth National Minority Forum on Cardiovascular Health, Pulmonary Disorders, and Blood Resources, Minority Health Issues for an Emerging Majority. Bethesda,* MD: NHLBI.

–(1993b). *State Departments of Public Health: Contact List.* Bethesda, MD: NHLBI.

National Institute of Deafness and Other Communications Disorders (1991). *The Working Group on Research and Research Training Needs of Women and Women's Health Issues at the National Institute on Deafness and Other Communication Disorders.* Bethesda, MD: National Institutes of Health.

–(1992). *Research and Research Training Needs of Minority Persons and Minority Health Issues.*
Bethesda, MD: National Institutes of Health.

National Institute on Drug Abuse (NIDA) (1992). *Cultural Competence for Evaluators: A Guide for Alcohol and Other Drug Abuse Prevention Practitioners Working with Ethnic/Racial Communities* (DHHS Pub. No. [ADM] 92-1884). Rockville, MD: NIDA.

National Institutes of Health (NIH) (1992). *Health Behavior Research in Minority Populations: Access, Design, and Implementation* (NIH Pub. No. 92-2965). Bethesda, MD: NIH.

National Women's Health Network (1991). *Research to Improve Women's Health: An Agenda for Equity.*
Washington, DC: National Women's Health Network.

National Women's Health Resource Center (1991). *Forging a Women's Health Research Agenda.*
Washington, DC: National Women's Health Resource Center.

Negy C, Woods DJ (1992). The Importance of Acculturation in Understanding Research with Hispanic-Americans. *Hispanic Journal of Behavioral Science* 14: 224–47.

–(1990). *Delivering Preventive Health Care to Hispanics: A Manual for Providers.* Washington, DC: National Coalition of Hispanic Health and Human Services Organizations.

Office of Protection from Research Risks (OPRR) (1994). Inclusion of Women and Minorities in Research. *OPRR Reports* 94-01. Bethesda, MD: OPRR.

Olsen SJ, Frank-Stromborg M (1993). Cancer Prevention and Early Detection in Ethnically Diverse Populations. *Semin Oncol Nurs* 9: 198–209.

PEPI Trial Investigators (in press). The Recruitment of Postmenopausal Women for a Multicenter Trial: Experience of the Postmenopausal Estrogen/Progestin.

Perez-Stable EJ, et al. (1991). Evaluation of "Guia para Dejar de Fumar,"a Self-help Guide in Spanish to Quit Smoking. Public Health Rep 106: 564–70.

Petchers MK, Milligan SE (1988). Access to Health Care in a Black Urban Elderly Population. *The Gerontologist* 28: 213–17.

Pettiway E (1993). Identifying, Gaining Access To, and Collecting Data on Afro-American Drug Addicts. In DeLaRosa MR and Recio JL, eds., *Drug Abuse Among Minority Youth: Advances in Research and Methodology* (NIDA Research Monograph 130, NIH Pub No 93-3479), pp. 258–279. Rockville, MD: National Institute on Drug Abuse.

Pinn VW (1992). Women's Health Research: Prescribing Change and Addressing the Issues.
JAMA 268: 1921–22.

Ponterotto JG (1988). Racial/Ethnic Minority Research in the Journal of Counseling Psychology: A Content Analysis and Methodological Critique. *Journal of Counseling Psychology* 35: 410–18.

Porter PP, Villarruel AM (1993). Nursing Research with African American and Hispanic People: Guidelines for Action. *Nurs Outlook,* 41: 59–66.

Ramirez AG, et al. (1986). A media-based acculturation scale for Mexican-Americans: Application to Public Health Education Programs. Family Community Health 9: 63–71.

Ramirez AG, MacKellar DA, Gallion K (1988). Reaching Minority Audiences: A Major Challenge in Cancer Reduction. Cancer Bull 40: 334–43.

Rand, et al. (1992). Individual Recruitment. *Health Behavior Research in Minority Populations: Access, Design, and Implementation* (NIH Pub. No. 92-2965). Bethesda, MD: National Institutes of Health.

Randal-David E (1989). *Strategies for Working with Culturally Diverse Communities and Clients.* Washington, DC: Office of Maternal and Child Health, Bureau of Maternal and Child Health and Resources Development, U.S. Department of Health and Human Services.

Ray BA, Braude MC, eds. (1986). *Women and Drugs: A New Era for Research.* NIDA Research Monograph 65. Rockville, MD: National Institute on Drug Abuse.

Reinert BR (1986). The Health Care Beliefs and Values of Mexican-Americans. *Home Healthcare Nurse* 4: 23–31.

Resiman EK (1992). Products Liability—What Is The Current Situation and Will It Change (and How) When More Women Are Included In Studies? Presented at the Women in Clinical Trials of FDA-Regulated Products Workshop, Food and Drug Law Institute, Washington, DC.

Rimer BK (1993). Improving the Use of Cancer Screening for Older Women. *Cancer* 72: 1084–87.

Rogler LH (1989). The Meaning of Culturally Sensitive Research in Mental Health. *Am J Psychiatry* 146: 296–303.

Roman-Franco AA (1989). Some Thoughts on the Sociology of Cancer: A Hispanic Perspective. *Int J Cell Cloning* 8: 2–9.

Rothenberg KH, Hayunga EG, Rudick JE, Pinn VW (1996). The NIH inclusion guidelines: Challenges for the future. *IRB* (forthcoming, summer 1996).

Ruiz E, ed. (1989). *Hispanic Cancer Control Program.* Bethesda, MD: Special Populations Studies Branch, National Cancer Institute.

Samet, et al. (1988). Respiratory Diseases and Cigarette Smoking in a Hispanic Population in New Mexico. *Am Rev Respir Dis* 137: 815–819.

Schilling RF, et al. (1989). Developing Strategies for AIDS Prevention Research With Black and Hispanic Drug Users. *Public Health Rep* 104: 2–9.

Seminar On Women In Clinical Trials of FDA-Regulated Products (in press). *Food and Drug Law Journal.*

Sha B (1993). HIV Infection in Women: A Six Year Longitudinal, Observational Study. Poster Abstract in *Proceedings of the IX International Conference on AIDS,* Berlin, Germany, June 6–11, 1993. 1: 283.

Shea S, et al. (1992). Enrollment in Clinical Trials: Institutional Factors Affecting Enrollment in the Cardiac Arrhythmia Suppression Trial (CAST). *Controlled Clin Trials* 13: 466–86.

Shumaker, et al. (1992). Survey Measurement with Minority Populations. *Health Behavior Research in Minority Populations: Access, Design, and Implementation* (NIH Pub. No. 92-2965). Bethesda, MD: National Institutes of Health.

Spilker B (1991). *Guide to Clinical Trials.* Raven Press: New York.

Spilker B, Cramer J (1992). *Patient Recruitment in Clinical Trials.* Raven Press: New York.

Suarez L 1994. Pap Smear and Mammogram Screening in in Mexican-American Women: The Effects of Acculturation. *Am J Public Health* 84(5): 742–46.

Svensson CK (1989). Representation of American Blacks in Clinical Trials of New Drugs. *JAMA* 261: 263–65.

Thomas SB, et al. (1994). The Characteristics of Northern Black Churches with Community Health Outreach Programs. *Am J Public Health* 84: 575–79.

University of Nebraska Institutional Review Board (1990). *Policy for the Inclusion of Women of Child Bearing Potential in Clinical Research.* Omaha: University of Nebraska.

Von Winterfeldt D, Edwards W (1986). *Decision Analysis and Behavioral Research.* Cambridge, U.K.: Cambridge University Press.

West EA (1993). The Cultural Bridge Model. *Nurs Outlook* 41: 229–34.

Windsor R, et al. (1984). *Evaluation of Health Promotion and Education Programs.* California: Mayfield Publishing Company.

Zavertnik JJ (1993). Strategies for Reaching Poor Blacks and Hispanics in Dade County, Florida. *Cancer* 72: 1088–92.

NIH GUIDELINES

ON THE INCLUSION OF WOMEN AND MINORITIES AS SUBJECTS IN CLINICAL RESEARCH

[*Federal Register*, Vol. 59 No. 59 (March 28, 1994), pp. 14508–14513]

⁊

NATIONAL INSTITUTES OF HEALTH

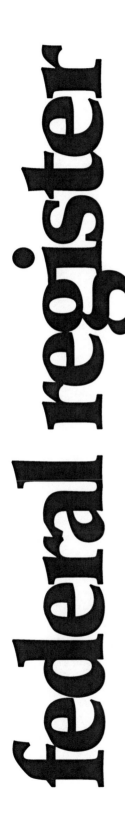

federal register

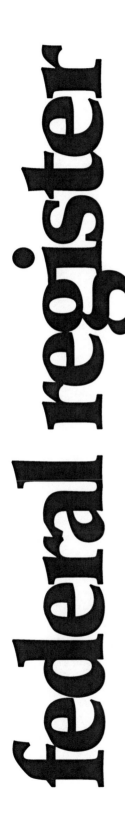 *(the vertical "federal register" masthead)*

.............ۿ.............

Monday
March 28, 1994

Part VIII

Department of Health and Human Services

National Institutes of Health

NIH Guidelines on the Inclusion of Women and Minorities as Subjects in Clinical Research; Notice

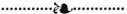
Department of Health and Human Services

National Institutes of Health

RIN 0905-ZA18

NIH Guidelines on the Inclusion of Women and Minorities as Subjects in Clinical Research

Editorial Note: This document was originally published at 59 FR 11146, March 9, 1994, and is being reprinted in its entirety because of typesetting errors.

AGENCY: National Institutes of Health, PHS, DHHS.

ACTION: Notice.

SUMMARY: The National Institutes of Health (NIH) is establishing guidelines on the inclusion of women and minorities and their subpopulations in research involving human subjects, including clinical trials, supported by the NIH, as required in the NIH Revitalization Act of 1993.

EFFECTIVE DATE: March 9, 1994.

ADDRESSES: Although these guidelines are effective on the date of publication, written comments can be sent to either the Office of Research on Women's Health, National Institutes of Health, Building 1, Room 203, Bethesda, MD 20892, or to the Office of Research on Minority Health, National Institutes of Health, Building 1, Room 225, Bethesda, MD 20892. During the first year of implementation, NIH will review the comments and experience with the guidelines in order to determine whether modifications to the guidelines are warranted.

FOR FURTHER INFORMATION CONTACT: Programmatic inquiries should be directed to senior extramural staff of the relevant NIH Institute or Center named at the end of this notice.

SUPPLEMENTARY INFORMATION: NIH Guidelines on the Inclusion of Women and Minorities as Subjects in Clinical Research.

I. Introduction

This document sets forth guidelines on the inclusion of women and members of minority groups and their subpopulations in clinical research, including clinical trials, supported by the National Institutes of Health (NIH). For the purposes of this document, clinical research is defined as NIH-supported biomedical and behavioral research involving human subjects. These guidelines, implemented in accordance with section 492B of the Public Health Service Act, added by the NIH Revitalization Act of 1993, Public Law. (Pub.L.) 103-43, supersede and strengthen the previous policies. NIH/ADAMHA Policy Concerning the Inclusion of Women in Study Populations, and ADAMHA/NIH Policy Concerning the Inclusion of Minorities in Study Populations, published in the NIH GUIDE FOR GRANTS AND CONTRACTS, 1990.

The 1993 guidelines continue the 1990 guidelines with three major additions. The new policy requires that, in addition to the continuing inclusion of women and members of minority groups in all NIH-supported biomedical and behavioral research involving human subjects, the NIH must:

- Ensure that women and members of minorities and their subpopulations are included in all human subject research;
- For Phase III clinical trials, ensure that women and minorities and their subpopulations must be included such that valid analyses of differences in intervention effect can be accomplished;
- Not allow cost as an acceptable reason for excluding these groups; and,
- Initiate programs and support for outreach efforts to recruit these groups into clinical studies.

Since a primary aim of research is to provide scientific evidence leading to a change in health policy or a standard of care, it is imperative to determine whether the intervention or therapy being studied affects women or men or members of minority groups and their subpopulations differently. To this end, the guidelines published here are intended to ensure that all future NIH-supported biomedical and behavioral research involving human subjects will be carried out in a manner sufficient to elicit information about individuals of both genders and the diverse racial and ethnic groups and, in the case of clinical trials, to examine differential effects on such groups. Increased attention, therefore, must be given to gender, race, and ethnicity in earlier stages of research to allow for informed decisions at the Phase III clinical trial stage.

These guidelines reaffirm NIH's commitment to the fundamental principles of inclusion of women and racial and ethnic minority groups and their subpopulations in research. This policy should result in a variety of new research opportunities to address significant gaps in knowledge about health problems that affect women and racial/ethnic minorities and their subpopulations.

The NIH recognizes that issues will arise with the implementation of these guidelines and thus welcomes comments. During the first year of implementation, NIH will review the comments, and consider modifications, within the scope of the statute, to the guidelines.

II. Background

The NIH Revitalization Act of 1993, PL 103-43, signed by President Clinton on June 10, 1993, directs the NIH to establish guidelines for inclusion of women and minorities in clinical research. This guidance shall include guidelines regarding—

(A) the circumstances under which the inclusion of women and minorities as subjects in projects of clinical research is inappropriate * * *

(B) the manner in which clinical trials are required to be designed and carried out * * *; and

(C) the operation of outreach programs * * * 492B(d)(1)

The statute states that

In conducting or supporting clinical research for the purposes of this title, the Director of NIH shall * * * ensure that—

A. women are included as subjects in each project of such research; and

B. members of minority groups are included in such research. 492B(a)(1)

The statute further defines "clinical research" to include "clinical trials" and states that

In the case of any clinical trial in which women or members of minority groups will be included as subjects, the Director of NIH shall ensure that the trial is designed and carried out in a manner sufficient to provide for valid analysis of whether the variables being studied in the trial affect women or members of minority groups, as the case may be, differently than other subjects in the trial. 492B(C)

Specifically addressing the issue of minority groups, the statute states that

The term "minority group" includes subpopulations of minority groups. The Director of NIH shall, through the guidelines established * * * defines the terms "minority group" and "subpopulation" for the purposes of the preceding sentence. 492B(g)(2)

The statute speaks specifically to outreach and states that

The Director of NIH, in consultation with the Director of the Office of Research of Women's Health and the Director of the Office of Research on Minority Health, shall conduct or support outreach programs for the recruitment of women and members of minority groups as subjects in the projects of clinical research. 492B(a)(2)

The statute includes a specific provision pertaining to the cost of clinical research and, in particular clinical trials.

(A)(i) In the case of a clinical trial, the guidelines shall provide that the costs of such inclusion in the trial is (sic) not a permissible consideration in determining whether such inclusion is inappropriate. 492B(d)(2)

(ii) In the case of other projects of clinical research, the guidelines shall provide that the costs of such inclusion in the project is (sic) not a permissible consideration in determining whether such inclusion is inappropriate unless the data regarding women or members of minority groups, respectively, that would be obtained in such project (in the event that such inclusion were required) have been or are being obtained through other means that provide data of comparable quality. 492B(d)(2)

Exclusions to the requirement for inclusion of women and minorities are stated in the statute, as follows:

The requirements established regarding women and members of minority groups shall not apply to the project of clinical research if the inclusion, as subjects in the project, of women and members of minority groups, respectively—

(1) Is inappropriate with respect to the health of the subjects;

(2) Is inappropriate with respect to purpose of the research; or

(3) Is inappropriate under such other circumstances as the Director of NIH may designate. 492B(b)

(B) In the case of a clinical trial, the guidelines may provide that such inclusion in the trial is not required if there is substantial scientific data demonstrating that there is no significant difference between—

(i) The effects that the variables to be studied in the trial have on women or members of minority groups, respectively; and

(ii) The effects that variables have on the individuals who would serve as subjects in the trial in the event that such inclusion were not required. 492B(d)(2)

III. Policy

A. Research Involving Human Subjects

It is the policy of NIH that women and members of minority groups and their subpopulations must be included in all NIH-supported biomedical and behavioral research projects involving human subjects, unless a clear and compelling rationale and justification establishes to the satisfaction of the relevant Institute/Center Director that inclusion is inappropriate with respect to the health of the subjects or the purpose of the research. Exclusion under other circumstances may be made by the Director, NIH, upon the recommendation of a Institute/Center Director based on a compelling rationale and justification. Cost is not an acceptable reason for exclusion except when the study would duplicate data from other sources. Women of childbearing potential should not be routinely excluded from participation in clinical research. All NIH-supported biomedical and behavioral research involving human subjects is defined as clinical research. This policy applies to research subjects of all ages.

The inclusion of women and members of minority groups and their subpopulations

must be addressed in developing a research design appropriate to the scientific objectives of the study. The research plan should describe the composition of the proposed study population in terms of gender and racial/ethnic group, and provide a rationale for selection of such subjects. Such a plan should contain a description of the proposed outreach programs for recruiting women and minorities as participants.

B. Clinical Trials

Under the statute, when a Phase III clinical trial (see Definitions, Section V-A) is proposed, evidence must be reviewed to show whether or not clinically important gender or race/ethnicity differences in the intervention effect are to be expected. This evidence may include, but is not limited to, data derived from prior animal studies, clinical observations, metabolic studies, genetic studies, pharmacology studies, and observational. natural history, epidemiology and other relevant studies.

As such, investigators must consider the following when planning a Phase III clinical trial for NIH support.

• If the data from prior studies strongly indicate the existence of significant differences of clinical or public health importance in intervention effect among subgroups (gender and/or racial/ethnic subgroups), the primary question(s) to be addressed by the proposed Phase III trial and the design of that trial must specifically accommodate this. For example, if men and women are thought to respond differently to an intervention, then the Phase III trial must be designed to answer two separate primary questions, one for men and the other for women, with adequate sample size for each.

• If the data from prior studies strongly support no significant differences of clinical or public health importance in intervention effect between subgroups, then gender or race/ethnicity will not be required as subject selection criteria. However, the inclusion of gender or racial/ethnic subgroups is strongly encouraged.

• If the data from prior studies neither support strongly nor negate strongly the existence of significant differences of clinical or public health importance in intervention effect between subgroups, then the Phase III trial will be required to include sufficient and appropriate entry of gender and racial/ethnic subgroups, so that valid analysis of the intervention effect in subgroups can be performed. However, the trial will not be required to provide high statistical power for each subgroup.

Cost is not an acceptable reason for exclusion of women and minorities from clinical trials.

C. Funding

NIH funding components will not award any grant, cooperative agreement or contract or support any intramural project to be conducted or funded in Fiscal Year 1995 and thereafter which does not comply with this policy. For research awards that are covered by this policy, awardees will report annually on enrollment of women and men, and on the race and ethnicity of research participants.

IV. Implementation

A. Date of Implementation

This policy applies to all applications/proposals and intramural projects to be submitted on and after June 1, 1994 (the date of full implementation) seeking Fiscal Year 1995 support. Projects funded prior to June 10, 1993, must still comply with the 1990 policy and report annually on enrollment of subjects using gender and racial/ethnic categories as required in the Application for Continuation of a Public Health Service Grant (PHS Form 2590), in contracts and in intramural projects.

B. Transition Policy

NIH-supported biomedical and behavioral research projects involving human subjects, with the exception of Phase III clinical trial projects as discussed below, that are awarded between June 10, 1993, the date of enactment, and September 30, 1994, the end of Fiscal Year 1994, shall be subject to the requirements of the 1990 policy and the annual reporting requirements on enrollment using gender and racial/ethnic categories.

For all Phase III clinical trial projects proposed between June 10, 1993 and June 1, 1994, and those awarded between June 10, 1993 and September 30, 1994,

Institute/Center staff will examine the applications/proposals, pending awards, awards and intramural projects to determine if the study was developed in a manner consistent with the new guidelines. If it is deemed inconsistent, NIH staff will contact investigators to discuss approaches to accommodate the new policy. Administrative actions may be needed to accommodate or revise the pending trials. Institutes/Centers may need to consider initiating a complementary activity to address any gender or minority representation concerns.

The NIH Director will determine whether the Phase III clinical trial being considered during this transition is in compliance with this policy, whether acceptable modifications have been made, or whether the Institute/Center will initiate a complementary activity that addresses the gender or minority representation concerns. Pending awards will not be funded without this determination.

Solicitations issued by the NIH planned for release after the date of publication of the guidelines in the Federal Register will include the new requirements.

C. Roles and Responsibilities

While this policy applies to all applicants for NIH-supported biomedical and behavioral research involving human subjects, certain individuals and groups have special roles and responsibilities with regard to the adoption and implementation of these guidelines.

The NIH staff will provide educational opportunities for the extramural and intramural community concerning this policy; monitor its implementation during the development, review, award and conduct of research; and manage the NIH research portfolio to address the policy.

1. Principal Investigators

Principal investigators should assess the theoretical and/or scientific linkages between gender, race/ethnicity, and their topic of study. Following this assessment, the principal investigator and the applicant institution will address the policy in each application and proposal, providing the required information on inclusion of women and minorities and their subpopulations in research projects, and any

required justifications for exceptions to the policy. Depending on the purpose of the study, NIH recognizes that a single study may not include all minority groups.

2. Institutional Review Boards (IRBs)

As the IRBs implement the guidelines, described herein, for the inclusion of women and minorities and their subpopulations, they must also implement the regulations for the protection of human subjects as described in title 45 CFR part 46, "Protection of Human Subjects." They should take into account the Food and Drug Administration's "Guidelines for the Study and Evaluation of Gender Differences in the Clinical Evaluation of Drugs," Vol. 58 Federal Register 39406.

3. Peer Review Groups

In conducting peer review for scientific and technical merit, appropriately constituted initial review groups (including study sections), technical evaluation groups, and intramural review panels will be instructed, as follows:

- To evaluate the proposed plan for the inclusion of minorities and both genders for appropriate representation or to evaluate the proposed justification when representation is limited or absent,
- To evaluate the proposed exclusion of minorities and women on the basis that a requirement for inclusion is inappropriate with respect to the health of the subjects,
- To evaluate the proposed exclusion of minorities and women on the basis that a requirement for inclusion is inappropriate with respect to the purpose of the research,
- To determine whether the design of clinical trials is adequate to measure differences when warranted,
- To evaluate the plans for recruitment/outreach for study, participants, and
- To include these criteria as part of the scientific assessment and assigned score.

4. NIH Advisory Councils

In addition to its current responsibilities for review of projects where the peer review groups have raised questions about the appropriate inclusion of women and minorities, the Advisory Council/Board of each Institute/Center shall prepare biennial reports, for inclusion in the overall

NIH Director's biennial report, describing the manner in which the Institute/Center has complied with the provisions of the statute.

5. Institute/Center Directors

Institute/Center Directors and their staff shall determine whether: (a) The research involving human subjects, (b) the Phase III clinical trials, and (c) the exclusions meet the requirements of the statute and these guidelines.

6. NIH Director

The NIH Director may approve, on a case-by-case basis, the exclusion of projects, as recommended by the Institute/Center Director, that may be inappropriate to include within the requirements of these guidelines on the basis of circumstances other than the health of the subjects, the purpose of the research, or costs.

7. Recruitment Outreach by Extramural and Intramural Investigators

Investigators and their staff(s) are urged to develop appropriate and culturally sensitive outreach programs and activities commensurate with the goals of the study. The objective should be to actively recruit the most diverse study population consistent with the purposes of the research project. Indeed, the purpose should be to establish a relationship between the investigator(s) and staff(s) and populations and community(ies) of interest such that mutual benefit is derived for participants in the study. Investigator(s) and staff(s) should take precautionary measures to ensure that ethical concerns are clearly noted, such that there is minimal possibility of coercion or undue influence in the incentives or rewards offered in recruiting into or retaining participants in studies. It is also the responsibility of the IRBs to address these ethical concerns.

Furthermore, while the statute focuses on recruitment outreach, NIH staff underscore the need to appropriately retain participants in clinical studies, and thus, the outreach programs and activities should address both recruitment and retention.

To assist investigators and potential study participants, NIH staff have prepared a notebook, "NIH Outreach Notebook on the Inclusion of Women and Minorities in Biomedical and Behavioral Research." The notebook addresses both recruitment and retention of women and minorities in clinical studies, provides relevant references and case studies, and discusses ethical issues. It is not intended as a definitive text on this subject, but should assist investigators in their consideration of an appropriate plan for recruiting and retaining participants in clinical studies. The notebook is expected to be available early in 1994.

8. Educational Outreach by NIH to Inform the Professional Community.

NIH Staff will present the new guidelines to investigators, IRB members, peer review groups, and Advisory Councils in a variety of public educational forums.

9. Applicability to Foreign Research Involving Human Subjects

For foreign awards, the NIH policy on inclusion of women in research conducted outside the U.S. is the same as that for research conducted in the U.S.

However, with regard to the population of the foreign country, the definition of the minority groups may be different than in the U.S. If there is scientific rationale for examining subpopulation group differences within the foreign population, investigators should consider designing their studies to accommodate these differences.

V. Definitions

Throughout the section of the statute pertaining to the inclusion of women and minorities, terms are used which require definition for the purpose of implementing these guidelines. These terms, drawn directly from the statute, are defined below.

A. Clinical Trial

For the purpose of these guidelines, a "clinical trial" is a broadly based prospective Phase III clinical investigation, usually involving several hundred or more human subjects, for the purpose of evaluating an experimental intervention in comparison with a standard or control intervention or comparing two or more existing treatments. Often the aim of such investigation is to provide evidence leading to a scientific basis for consideration of a change in health policy or standard of care. The definition includes pharmacologic, nonpharmacologic, and behavioral interventions given for disease prevention, prophylaxis, diagnosis, or therapy. Community trials and other population-based intervention trials are also included.

B. Research Involving Human Subjects

All NIH-supported biomedical and behavioral research involving human subjects is defined as clinical research under this policy. Under this policy, the definition of human subjects in title 45 CFR part 46, the Department of Health and Human Services regulations for the protection of human subjects applies: "Human subject means a living individual about whom an investigator (whether professional or student) conducting research obtains: (1) Data through intervention or interaction with the individual, or (2) identifiable private information." These regulations specifically address the protection of human subjects from research risks. It should be noted that there are research areas (Exemptions 1-6) that are exempt from these regulations. However, under these guidelines, NIH-supported biomedical and behavioral research projects involving human subjects which are exempt from the human subjects regulations should still address the inclusion of women and minorities in their study design. Therefore, all biomedical and behavioral research projects involving human subjects will be evaluated for compliance with this policy.

C. Valid Analysis

The term "valid analysis" means an unbiased assessment. Such an assessment will, on average, yield the correct estimate of the difference in outcomes between two groups of subjects. Valid analysis can and should be conducted for both small and large studies. A valid analysis does not need to have a high statistical power for detecting a stated effect. The principal requirements for ensuring a valid analysis of the question of interest are:

• Allocation of study participants of both genders and from different racial/ethnic groups to the intervention and control groups by an unbiased process such as randomization,

• Unbiased evaluation of the outcome(s) of study participants, and

• Use of unbiased statistical analyses and proper methods of inference to estimate and compare the intervention effects among the gender and racial/ethnic groups.

D. Significant Difference

For purposes of this policy, a "significant difference" is a difference that is of clinical or public health importance, based on substantial scientific data. This definition differs from the commonly used "statistically significant difference," which refers to the event that, for a given set of data, the statistical test for a difference between the effects in two groups achieves statistical significance. Statistical significance depends upon the amount of information in the data set. With a very large amount of information, one could find a statistically significant, but clinically small difference that is of very little clinical importance. Conversely, with less information one could find a large difference of potential importance that is not statistically significant.

E. Racial and Ethnic Categories

1. Minority Groups

A minority group is a readily identifiable subset of the U.S. population which is distinguished by either racial, ethnic, and/or cultural heritage.

The Office of Management and Budget (OMB) Directive No. 15 defines the minimum standard of basic racial and ethnic categories, which are used below. NIH has chosen to continue the use of these definitions because they allow comparisons to many national data bases, especially national health data bases. Therefore, the racial and ethnic categories described below should be used as basic guidance, cognizant of the distinction based on cultural heritage.

American Indian or Alaskan Native: A person having origins in any of the original peoples of North America, and who maintains cultural identification through tribal affiliation or community recognition.

Asian or Pacific Islander: A person having origins in any of the original peoples of the Far East, Southeast Asia, the Indian subcontinent, or the Pacific Islands. This area includes, for example, China, India, Japan, Korea, the Philippine Islands and Samoa.

Black, not of Hispanic Origin: A person having origins in any of the black racial groups of Africa.

Hispanic: A person of Mexican, Puerto Rican, Cuban, Central or South American or other Spanish culture or origin, regardless of race.

2. Majority Group

White, not of Hispanic Origin: A person having origins in any of the original peoples of Europe, North Africa, or the Middle East.

NIH recognizes the diversity of the U.S. population and that changing demographics are reflected in the changing racial and ethnic composition of the population. The terms "minority groups" and "minority subpopulations" are meant to be inclusive, rather than exclusive, of differing racial and ethnic categories.

3. Subpopulations

Each minority group contains subpopulations which are delimited by geographic origins, national origins, and/or cultural differences. It is recognized that there are different ways of defining and reporting racial and ethnic subpopulation data. The subpopulation to which an individual is assigned depends on self-reporting of specific racial and ethnic origin. Attention to subpopulations also applies to individuals of mixed racial and/or ethnic parentage. Researchers should be cognizant of the possibility that these racial/ethnic combinations may have biomedical and/or cultural implications related to the scientific question under study.

F. Outreach Strategies

These are outreach efforts by investigators and their staff(s) to appropriately recruit and retain populations of interest into research studies. Such efforts should represent a thoughtful and culturally sensitive plan of outreach and generally include involvement of other individuals and organizations relevant to the populations and communities of interest, e.g., family, religious organizations, community leaders and informal gatekeepers, and

public and private institutions and organizations. The objective is to establish appropriate lines of communication and cooperation to build mutual trust and cooperation such that both the study and the participants benefit from such collaboration.

G. Research Portfolio

Each Institute and Center at the NIH has its own research portfolio, i.e., its "holdings" in research grants, cooperative agreements, contracts and intramural studies. The Institute or Center evaluates the research awards in its portfolio to identify those areas where there are knowledge gaps or which need special attention to advance the science involved. NIH may consider funding projects to achieve a research portfolio reflecting diverse study populations. With the implementation of this new policy, there will be a need to ensure that sufficient resources are provided within a program to allow for data to be developed for a smooth transition from basic research to Phase III clinical trials that meet the policy requirements.

VI. Discussion—Issues in Scientific Plans and Study Designs

A. Issues in Research Involving Human Subjects

The biomedical and behavioral research process can be viewed as a stepwise process progressing from discovery of new knowledge through research in the laboratory, research involving animals, research involving human subjects, validation of interventions through clinical trials, and broad application to improve the health of the public.

All NIH-supported biomedical and behavioral research involving human subjects is defined broadly in this guidance as clinical research. This is broader than the definition provided in the 1990 NIH Guidance and in many program announcements, requests for applications, and requests for proposals since 1990.

The definition was broadened because of the need to obtain data about minorities and both genders early in the research process when hypotheses are being formulated, baseline data are being collected, and various measurement instruments and intervention strategies are being developed. Broad inclusion at these early stages of research provides valuable information for designing broadly based clinical trials, which are a subset of studies under the broad category of research studies.

The policy on inclusion of minorities and both genders applies to all NIH-supported biomedical and behavioral research involving human subjects so that the maximum information may be obtained to understand the implications of the research findings on the gender or minority group.

Investigators should consider the types of information concerning gender and minority groups which will be required when designing future Phase III clinical trials, and try to obtain it in their earlier stages of research involving human subjects. NIH recognizes that the understanding of health problems and conditions of different U.S. populations may require attention to socioeconomic differences involving occupation, education, and income gradients.

B. Issues in Clinical Trials

The statute requires appropriate representation of subjects of different gender and race/ethnicity in clinical trials so as to provide the opportunity for detecting major qualitative differences (if they exist) among gender and racial/ethnic subgroups and to identify more subtle differences that might, if warranted, be explored in further specifically targeted studies. Other interpretations may not serve as well the health needs of women, minorities, and all other constituencies.

Preparatory to any Phase III clinical trial, certain data are typically obtained. Such data are necessary for the design of an appropriate Phase III trial and include observational clinical study data, basic laboratory (i.e. in vitro and animal) data, and clinical, physiologic, pharmacokinetic, or biochemical data from Phase I and Phase II studies. Genetic studies, behavioral studies, and observational, natural history, and epidemiological studies may also contribute data.

It is essential that data be reviewed from prior studies on a diverse population, that is, in subjects of both genders and from different racial/ethnic groups. These data must be examined to determine if there are significant differences of clinical or public health importance observed between the subgroups.

While data from prior studies relating to possible differences among intervention effects in different subgroups must be reviewed, evidence of this nature is likely to be less convincing than that deriving from the subgroup analyses that can be performed in usual-sized Phase III trials. This is because the evidence from preliminary studies is likely to be of a more indirect nature (e.g. based on surrogate endpoints), deriving from uncontrolled studies (e.g. non-randomized Phase II trials), and based on smaller numbers of subjects than in Phase III secondary analyses. For this reason, it is likely that data from preliminary studies will, in the majority of cases, neither clearly reveal significant differences of clinical or public health importance between subgroups of patients, nor strongly negate them.

In these cases, Phase III trials should still have appropriate gender and racial/ethnic representation, but they would not need to have the large sample sizes necessary to provide a high statistical power for detecting differences in intervention effects among subgroups. Nevertheless, analyses of subgroup effects must be conducted and comparisons between the subgroups must be made. Depending on the results of these analyses, the results of other relevant research, and the results of meta-analyses of clinical trials, one might initiate subsequent trials to examine more fully these subgroup differences.

C. Issues Concerning Appropriate Gender Representation

The "population at risk" may refer to only one gender where the disease, disorders, or conditions are gender specific. In all other cases, there should be approximately equal numbers of both sexes in studies of populations or subpopulations at risk, unless different proportions are appropriate because

of the known prevalence, incidence, morbidity, mortality rates, or expected intervention effect.

D. Issues Concerning Appropriate Representation of Minority Groups and Subpopulations in All Research Involving Human Subjects Including Phase III Clinical Trials

While the inclusion of minority subpopulations in research is a complex and challenging issue, it nonetheless provides the opportunity for researchers to collect data on subpopulations where knowledge gaps exist. Researchers must consider the inclusion of subpopulations in all stages of research design. In meeting this objective, they should be aware of concurrent research that addresses specific subpopulations, and consider potential collaborations which may result in complementary subpopulation data.

At the present time, there are gaps in baseline and other types of data necessary for research involving certain minority groups and/or subpopulations of minority groups. In these areas, it would be appropriate for researchers to obtain such data, including baseline data, by studying a single minority group.

It would also be appropriate for researchers to test survey instruments, recruitment procedures, and other methodologies used in the majority or other population(s) with the objective of assessing their feasibility, applicability, and cultural competence/relevance to a particular minority group or subpopulation. This testing may provide data on the validity of the methodologies across groups. Likewise, if an intervention has been tried in the majority population and not in certain minority groups, it would be appropriate to assess the intervention effect on a single minority group and compare the effect to that obtained in the majority population. These types of studies will advance scientific research and assist in closing knowledge gaps.

A complex issue arises over how broad or narrow the division into different subgroups should be, given the purpose of the research. Division into many racial/ethnic subgroups is tempting in view of the cultural and biological differences that exist among these groups and the possibility that some of these differences may in fact impact in some way upon the scientific question. Alternatively, from a practical perspective, a limit has to be placed on the number of such subgroups that can realistically be studied in detail for each intervention that is researched. The investigator should clearly address the rationale for inclusion or exclusion of subgroups in terms of the purpose of the research. Emphasis should be placed upon inclusion of subpopulations in which the disease manifests itself or the intervention operates in an appreciable different way. Investigators should report the subpopulations included in the study.

An important issue is the appropriate representation of minority groups in research, especially in geographical locations which may have limited numbers of racial/ethnic population groups available for study. The investigator must address this issue in terms of the purpose of the research, and other factors, such as the size of the study, relevant characteristics of the disease, disorder or condition, and the feasibility of making a collaboration or consortium or other arrangements to include minority groups. A justification is required if there is limited representation. Peer reviewers and NIH staff will consider the justification in their evaluations of the project.

NIH interprets the statute in a manner that leads to feasible and real improvements in the representativeness of different racial/ethnic groups in research and places emphasis on research in those subpopulations that are disproportionately affected by certain diseases or disorders.

VII. NIH Contacts for More Information

The following senior extramural staff from the NIH Institutes and Centers may be contacted for further information about the policy and relevant Institute/Center programs:

Dr. Marvin Kalt, National Cancer Institute, 6130 Executive Boulevard, Executive Plaza North, Room 600A, Bethesda, Maryland 20892, Tel: (301) 496-5147.

Dr. Richard Mowery, National Eye Institute, 6120 Executive Boulevard, Executive Plaza South, Room 350, Rockville, Maryland 20892, Tel: (301) 496-5301.

Dr. Lawrence Friedman, National Heart, Lung and Blood Institute, 7550 Wisconsin Avenue, Federal Building, Room 212, Bethesda, Maryland 20892, Tel: (301) 496-2533.

Dr. Miriam Kelty, National Institute on Aging, 7201 Wisconsin Avenue, Gateway Building, Room 2C218, Bethesda, Maryland 20892, Tel: (301) 496-9322.

Dr. Cherry Lowman, National Institute on Alcohol Abuse and Alcoholism, 6000 Executive Boulevard, Rockville, Maryland 20892, Tel: (301) 443-0796.

Dr. George Counts, National Institute of Allergy and Infectious Diseases, 6003 Executive Boulevard, Solar Building, Room 207P, Bethesda, Maryland 20892, Tel: (301) 496-8214.

Dr. Michael Lockshin, National Institute of Arthritis and Musculoskeletal and Skin Diseases, 9000 Rockville Pike, Building 31, Room 4C32, Bethesda, Maryland 20892, Tel: (301) 496-0802.

Ms. Hildegard Topper, Bethesda, National Institute of Child Health and Human Development, 9000 Rockville Pike, Building 31, Room 2A-03, Bethesda, Maryland 20892, Tel: (301) 496-0104.

Dr. Earleen Elkins, National Institute of Deafness and Other Communication Disorders, 6120 Executive Boulevard, Executive Plaza South, Room 400, Rockville, Maryland 20892, Tel: (301) 496-8683.

Dr. Norman S. Braveman, National Institute on Dental Research, 5333 Westbard Avenue, Westwood Building, Room 509, Bethesda, Maryland 20892, Tel: (301) 594-7648.

Dr. Walter Stolz, National Institute of Diabetes and Digestive and Kidney Diseases, 5333 Westbard Avenue, Westwood Building, Room 657, Bethesda, Maryland 20892, Tel: (301) 594-7527.

Ms. Eleanor Friedenberg, National Institute on Drug Abuse, 5600 Fishers Lane, Parklawn Building, Room 10-42, Rockville, Maryland 20857, Tel: (301) 434-2755.

Dr. Gwen Collman, National Institute of Environmental Health Sciences, P.O. Box 12233, Research Triangle Park, North Carolina 27709, Tel: (919) 541-4980.

Dr. Lee Van Lenten, National Institute of General Medical Sciences, 5333 Westbard Avenue, Westwood Building, Room 905, Bethesda, Maryland 20892, Tel: (301) 594-7744.

Dr. Dolores Parron, National Institute of Mental Health, 5600 Fishers Lane, Parklawn Building, Room 17C-14, Rockville, Maryland 20857, Tel: (301) 443-2847.

Dr. Constance Atwell, National Institute of Neurological Disorders and Stroke, 7550 Wisconsin Ave., Federal Building, Room 1016, Bethesda, Maryland 20892, Tel: (301) 496-9248.

Dr. Mark Guyer, National Center for Human Genome Research, 9000 Rockville Pike, Building 38A, Room 605, Bethesda, Maryland 20892, Tel: (301) 496-0844.

Dr. Teresa Radebaugh, National Center for Nursing Research, 5333 Westbard Avenue, Westwood Building, Room 754, Bethesda, Maryland 20892, Tel: (301) 594-7590.

Dr. Harriet Gordon, National Center for Research Resources, 5333 Westbard Avenue, Westwood Building, Room 10A03, Bethesda, Maryland 20892, Tel: (301) 594-7945.

Dr. David Wolff, Fogarty International Center, 9000 Rockville Pike, Building 31, Room B2C39, Bethesda, Maryland 20892, Tel: (301) 496-1653.

Dated: March 3, 1994.

Harold Varmus,

Director, NIH.

[FR Doc. 94–5435 Filed 3–8–94; 8:45 am] BILLING CODE 1505-01-D

NIH Questions and Answers on Guidelines on Inclusion of Women and Minorities
···

A-123

QUESTIONS AND ANSWERS

CONCERNING THE 1994 NIH GUIDELINES ON INCLUSION OF WOMEN AND MINORITIES AS SUBJECTS IN CLINICAL RESEARCH

∂

NATIONAL INSTITUTES OF HEALTH

PREFACE

A s required by the National Institutes of Health (NIH) Revitalization Act of 1993, the NIH published **Guidelines on the Inclusion of Women and Minorities As Subjects in Clinical Research** in the *Federal Register* of March 28, 1994, (59 FR 14508-14513) and in the NIH *Guide for Grants and Contracts* of March 18, 1994. Research applications and proposals to be supported by NIH must comply with this policy as mandated by law.

This document contains a series of questions and answers to assist in the preparation of research applications and proposals in accordance with the 1994 NIH Guidelines. The questions cover many areas and are listed in a table of contents for ease in finding specific topics of interest. Although this document provides additional clarification and explanation, it is important to read the NIH Guidelines.

If there are questions about this policy, please contact the NIH representative from the appropriate Institute, Center or Division on the following pages (Question 36). This document will be updated as necessary should there be any significant changes in the NIH Guidelines as a result of comments received during the first year of implementation of the Guidelines.

This document is available electronically on the NIH Gopher (gopher.nih.gov 70) under 'From the Office of Extramural Research' and on the NIH Grantline (data line 301-402-2221; Dr. John James, moderator, 301-594-7270; jqj@cu.nih.gov). For additional information about online sources of documents about the extramural research programs of the NIH, refer to the NIH *Guide for **Grants** and **Contracts**,* Volume 23, Issue 23, June 17, 1994, or email questions to q2c@cu.nih.gov.

Note: This document replaces Appendix 5 of NIH Instruction and Information Memorandum OER 90-5.

CONTENTS

PREFACE

A. POLICY

What does the new policy say? B-131

What are the major differences between the 1990 policy and the Guidelines required
by the 1993 NIH Revitalization Act? B-131

What is the scientific basis of the policy? B-132

Who is responsible for implementation of the Guidelines? B-132

What is meant by minority groups and minority subpopulations? B-133

What is the NIH definition of clinical research? B-134

What is the NIH definition of a clinical trial? B-134

Are there special requirements for NIH-defined clinical trials? B-135

What do we mean by valid analysis? B-136

Is there a summary table to distinguish the inclusion requirements between clinical
research and clinical trials? B-136

Is there a decision tree available to help clarify the policy? B-137

B. APPLICATIONS

What information should applicants provide when justifying their choice of subjects in
a clinical study? B-137

What factors should be considered in determining inclusion of women and minorities
and their subpopulations? B-138

What type of information is required in describing the diversity of the composition
of the study population? B-138

Do all minority groups and subpopulations have to be included in each
study population? B-139

Does the policy permit a study population that contains only one gender or minority
group or subpopulation? B-140

What should applicants do if they are in a geographic area that does not offer a study
population with the diversity required by the policy? B-140

Can study populations in other related studies be used to justify a study population
that does not include both men and women or racial/ethnic minority groups? B-141

What is meant by outreach efforts to recruit and retain women and minorities
in studies? B-142

In multi-center clinical studies, must each study site meet the inclusion
requirements separately? B-142

Is increased cost an acceptable justification for not including women, minorities,
and minority subpopulations in clinical trials? B-143

Is it acceptable to use existing cohorts that are deficient in women or
minority participants? B-143

C. Exclusions/Justifications

What are the circumstances under which it is not necessary to include both women
and men, and minorities? B-143

What kinds of justifications are acceptable for not including adequate representation
of women or men? B-144

What kinds of justification are acceptable for not including adequate representation
of all racial/ethnic minorities and subpopulations? B-145

D. Peer Review

This policy appears to be based on political considerations. Why is it to be reviewed
as a part of the science by the Initial Review Groups? B-146

How will peer reviewers evaluate applications for compliance with this policy? B-146

The policy on inclusion of women and minorities is applied to research projects, rather
than applications or proposals. How is this dealt with in the IRG coding? B-148

If an application fails to include both genders or minority groups and this is not
appropriately justified, how much should the priority score be affected? B-148

How does the inclusion policy apply to research contract proposals and projects? B-149

E. Awards

How will conformance to this policy affect funding of projects? B-149

Does the policy apply to foreign projects funded by the NIH? B-149

How do the new Guidelines impact on Institutional Review
Boards (IRBs)? B-150

How do we report on inclusion of women and minorities? B-150

When does the policy begin to apply? B-151

Where can I obtain additional information? B-151

What are the initial review group codes for inclusion of women and
minorities in clinical research? B-153

Questions and Answers Concerning the 1993 NIH Guidelines on the Inclusion of Women and Minorities as Subjects in Clinical Research

A. Policy

1. What does the new policy say?

It is the policy of NIH that women and members of minority groups and their subpopulations must be included in all NIH-supported biomedical and behavioral research projects involving human subjects, unless a clear and compelling rationale and justification establishes to the satisfaction of the relevant Institute/Center Director that inclusion is inappropriate with respect to the health of the subjects or the purpose of the research. Exclusion under other circumstances may be made by the Director, NIH, upon the recommendation of an Institute/Center Director based on a compelling rationale and justification. Cost is not an acceptable reason for exclusion except when the study would duplicate data from other sources. Women of childbearing potential should not be routinely excluded from participation in clinical research. All NIH-supported biomedical and behavioral research involving human subjects is defined as clinical research. This policy applies to research subjects of all ages.

NIH funding components will not award any grant, cooperative agreement or contract or support any intramural project, to be conducted or funded in Fiscal Year 1995 and thereafter, that does not comply with this policy.

(See Sections III.A. and III.C. in the NIH Guidelines)

2. What are the major differences between the 1990 policy and the Guidelines required by the 1993 NIH Revitalization Act?

In addition to continuing the 1990 requirement to include women and minority groups in clinical research, the new Guidelines:

ઌ broaden the definition of clinical research to include all research involving human subjects;

ઌ direct that members of minority subpopulations be included in all human subject research;

ઌ require inclusion of women and minorities and their subpopulations in Phase III clinical trials such that valid analyses of differences in intervention effect can be accomplished;

    ᕒ promote development of outreach programs to recruit women and minorities and their subpopulations into clinical studies; and

    ᕒ do not allow cost as an acceptable reason for excluding these groups in clinical trials.

(See Section I. in the NIH Guidelines)

3. What is the scientific basis of the policy?

The guidelines and policy are *science driven* so that maximum information may be obtained to understand the implications of the research findings on the gender or minority group. As defined in Webster's dictionary, science is "systematized knowledge derived from observation, study and experimentation carried on in order to determine the nature or principles of what is being studied."

There is a need to obtain this systematized knowledge and data about minorities and both genders early in the research process when hypotheses are being formulated, baseline data are being collected, and various measurement instruments and intervention strategies are being developed. Broad inclusion at these early stages of research provides valuable information for informed decisions in designing subsequent broadly based Phase III clinical trials.

Research is a continuum of studies from basic laboratory to observational to clinical. Assessment of differential effects of an intervention or therapy on women, men, or members of minority groups and their subpopulations requires fundamental information on such groups. Therefore, at the earliest stages of research, investigators are encouraged to include individuals or tissues of both genders and diverse racial and ethnic groups in order to generate information necessary for the rational design of appropriate Phase III clinical trials. Investigators are encouraged to report results on gender and minority groups and their subpopulations, as appropriate.

Thus, this policy should result in a variety of new research opportunities to address significant gaps in knowledge about health problems that affect women and racial/ethnic minorities and their subpopulations.

(See Section VI.A. in the NIH Guidelines)

4. Who is responsible for implementation of the Guidelines?

The entire scientific community has a responsibility for implementing the policy as a partnership between research subjects, principal investigators, institutional review boards, peer review groups, NIH staff, NIH advisory councils, NIH Institute and Center Directors, and the NIH Director in fulfilling the intent of the law and ensuring that the results of research are broadly applicable to the entire population.

Principal investigators should assess the theoretical and/or scientific linkages between gender, race/ethnicity, and their topic of study in preparing their applications and conducting their research. Institutional review boards (IRBs) should review NIH protocols in terms of the NIH inclusion policy during their review for protection of human subjects. Peer review groups will include a scientific and technical merit evaluation of the proposed inclusion plan and assign appropriate scores. The Advisory Council/Board of each Institute/Center will prepare biennial reports describing the manner in which the Institute/Center has complied with the provisions of the statute.

The NIH staff will provide educational opportunities for the extramural and intramural community concerning this policy; monitor its implementation during the development, review, award and conduct of research; and manage the NIH research portfolio to address the policy. Research subjects will be involved as voluntary participants in NIH-supported research.

(See Section IV.C. in the NIH Guidelines)

5. What is meant by minority groups and minority subpopulations?

The following four racial/ethnic minority groups are those identified by the Office of Management and Budget for federal reporting: American Indian/Alaskan Native; Asian/Pacific Islander; Black, not of Hispanic Origin; and Hispanic. Caucasians, not of Hispanic Origin, are considered a majority group for the purposes of this policy. The classification of an individual is by self identification. This classification is for administrative purposes and is prevalent in the scientific and other literature and databases available for research. Data may be collected on subpopulations and persons of mixed race/ethnicity, but must be aggregated into these groups for reporting purposes to NIH. The OMB is currently evaluating whether there should be any modifications to these categories.

For scientific purposes, it may be necessary to deal with the very real biological and cultural differences that exist not only among these broad racial/ethnic groupings, but also within the groups because of their differing languages, cultural traditions, and biological characteristics; thus, variability is to be expected within the Asian or Pacific Island populations, the various American Indian tribes, groups of various Hispanic origins, etc.

In its Guidelines, NIH has defined a minority group as ". . . a readily identifiable subset of the U.S. population which is distinguished by either racial, ethnic, and/or cultural heritage." Each minority group contains subpopulations that may be defined for geographic origin, national origin, cultural differences, or mixed racial and/or ethnic parentage. The minority group or subpopulation to which an individual belongs is determined by self-reporting. For illustrative purposes, several major subpopulations for each United States (U.S.) minority group are listed below, although other examples of subpopulations may be used by investigators for their research projects:

American Indians/Alaskan Native
American Indian, specify tribe
Alaskan Eskimo
Aleut

Asian/Pacific Islander
Chinese
Filipino
Japanese
Asian Indian
Korean
Vietnamese

✦ **Black, not of Hispanic Origin**
Caribbean Black
African

✦ **Hispanic**
Mexican
Puerto Rican
Cuban
Other specific Central and South American origin
(OMB does not include Iberian peninsula natives as Hispanic.)

The NIH reporting requirements (see Question 34) also allow for those cases when the racial/ethnic group is "Other or Unknown."

The purpose of investigators routinely specifying the racial ethnic population(s) under investigation is to begin to systematically obtain data on the various minority groups and subpopulations to fill the gaps of health research information on those populations so that the study results may be optimally applicable to all citizens. Investigators may report their findings in the research literature consistent with the purpose of the research.

(See Section V.E.1. through V.E.3. in the NIH Guidelines)

6. What is the NIH definition of clinical research?

All research involving human subjects is considered clinical research for the purposes of this NIH policy. This includes both biomedical and behavioral research. Small scale, exploratory, or observational studies fall under this policy as well as large scale studies.

The policy is based on the definition in Federal regulations for human subjects: ". . . living individual(s) about whom an investigator conducting research obtains: (1) data through intervention or interaction with the individual; or (2) identifiable private information." [45 CFR §46.102(f)] However, research exempted from human subjects protection regulations as defined by 45 CFR §46.101(b) is not exempted from NIH policies on inclusion of both genders and of minorities in study populations and must be evaluated and coded. Thus, the inclusion covers individuals or tissues of both genders and diverse racial and ethnic groups.

The policy extends to all research involving the use of human organs, tissues, and body fluids from living individuals as well as to graphic, written, or recorded information derived from living individuals. Although the use of autopsy material or other material from deceased individuals is not specifically covered by the policy, the appropriate inclusion of both genders and minorities may still be relevant for scientific reasons indicated by the investigator or peer review group.

(See Section V.B. and VI.A. in the NIH Guidelines)

7. What is the NIH definition of a clinical trial?

NIH has developed a special definition for clinical trials as used in this policy to distinguish these trials from the other types of clinical research that NIH supports, and from other definitions, e.g., by the Food and Drug Administration (FDA). These clinical trials are an important subset of all clinical research projects.

For the purposes of the NIH policy, a clinical trial is a broadly based prospective Phase III clinical investigation that is designed to evaluate an experimental intervention in comparison with a standard or control intervention or to compare two or more existing treatments. Often the aim of such investigations is to provide evidence leading to a scientific basis for consideration of a change in health policy or standard of care. The definition includes pharmacological, nonpharmacological, and behavioral interventions given for disease prevention, prophylaxis, diagnosis or therapy. Community trials and other population-based intervention trials are also included.

Discussion

The NIH definition of a clinical trial is broad and includes the wide range of research that NIH sponsors. It differs from the FDA definition of Phase III clinical trials, which focuses primarily on clinical investigation of drugs, vaccines, biologics, and devices. The FDA defines Phase I, II, and III trials (21 CFR Section 312.21, 4-1-94 edition) as follows: "Phase 3 studies are expanded, controlled and uncontrolled trials. They are performed after preliminary evidence suggesting effectiveness of the drug has been obtained, and are intended to gather the additional information about effectiveness and safety that is needed to evaluate overall benefit-risk relationship of the drug and to provide an adequate basis for physician labeling. Phase 3 studies usually include from several hundred to several thousand subjects."

In determining whether a study fits the NIH definition of a clinical trial, an essential consideration is trial outcome—whether it would contribute to a change in the standard of care or contribute to a change in public health policy, regardless of the number of participants in the study.

(See Section V.A. in the NIH Guidelines)

8.   Are there special requirements for NIH-defined clinical trials?

YES. Applications for NIH-defined Phase III clinical trials must include a review of the available evidence to show whether or not clinically important gender or race/ethnicity differences in the response to the intervention are to be expected. The design of such trials must reflect the current state of knowledge about any such expected differences.

Evidence may include, but is not limited to, data from prior animal studies, clinical observations, metabolic studies, genetic studies, pharmacologic studies, and observational, natural history, epidemiologic, and other relevant studies. The nature of the evidence should be used to determine the extent to which women, men, and members of minority groups and their subpopulations must be included.

Three kinds of circumstances are described in the NIH Guidelines, based on the findings of the review of the prior data; in these cases, the terms "significant" and "valid analysis" are defined and used in a way that is different from the usual convention for clinical trials:

> ☙ If the data strongly indicate the existence of significant differences of clinical or public health importance in intervention effect among subgroups, the primary question(s) to be addressed by the trial must be designed for valid analysis, with high statistical power, of the intervention effect in the separate genders and/or minorities or their subpopulations that are hypothesized to be different. For example, if men and women are thought to

respond differently to an intervention, then the Phase III trial must be designed to answer two separate primary questions, one for men and the other for women, with adequate sample size for each.

• If the data strongly support no significant difference of clinical or public health importance in intervention effect between subgroups, then the trial is designed to measure the primary question of intervention effect; gender or race/ethnicity will not be required as subject selection criteria. However, the inclusion of gender or racial/ethnic subgroups is still strongly encouraged.

• If the data are inconclusive about potential differences, then the trial will be required to include sufficient and appropriate recruitment of gender and racial/ethnic subgroups, so that valid analysis of the intervention effect in subgroups can be performed. However, the trial will not be required to provide high statistical power for each subgroup. It should be recognized that the results of these types of subgroup analyses often provide the basis for doing additional studies to more fully examine subgroup differences. Existing data on the disease, disorder, or conditions under study should be used to guide the design of study populations for NIH-defined clinical trials. When these NIH-defined clinical trials are being designed, consideration should be given to using national statistics on the disease, disorder, or condition under study, as well as national population and subpopulation statistics.

(See Sections III.B. and VI.B. in the NIH Guidelines)

9. What do we mean by valid analysis?

The term "valid analysis" is defined in this policy as an unbiased assessment. Valid analysis can and should be conducted for both small and large Phase III clinical studies. A valid analysis does not necessarily need a high statistical power for detecting a stated effect. The principal requirements for ensuring a valid analysis of the question of interest are:

• allocation of study participants of both genders and from different racial/ethnic groups to the intervention and control groups by an unbiased process such as randomization,

• unbiased evaluation of the outcome(s) of study participants, and

• use of unbiased statistical analyses and proper methods of inference to estimate and compare the intervention effects among the gender and racial/ethnic groups.

(See Section V.C. in the NIH Guidelines)

10. Is there a summary table to distinguish the inclusion requirements between clinical research and clinical trials?

This table summarizes the inclusion requirements for clinical research on human subjects and for clinical trials.

	Include Women and Minorities	Include Minority Subpopulations	Required to Measure Differences
Clinical Research	✓	✓	—
Clinical Trial	✓	✓	✓

All studies involving human subjects must include women and minorities and minority subpopulations, subject to the justifications and exclusions noted previously.

Phase III clinical trials are, in addition, required to provide valid analyses to measure differences of clinical or public health importance in intervention effects based on gender or racial/ethnic subgroups when there is evidence supporting differences.

Note that Phase I and Phase II clinical trials, and many small studies, are included under "research involving human subjects" or "human studies" and are not required to be designed to measure differences of intervention effects. For such studies, the systematic inclusion and reporting of information on women and minorities will contribute to an increase in the scientific base of knowledge about them.

(See Sections III.A and B. in the NIH Guidelines)

11. Is there a decision tree available to help clarify the policy?

A "Decision Tree for Inclusion of Women and Minorities in Clinical Research" is available as a series of questions and instructions and as a graphic representation.

(See Page 78)

B. APPLICATIONS

12. What information should applicants provide when justifying their choice of subjects in a clinical study?

In addition to the usual information provided in a research application or proposal, applicants for clinical studies should discuss the following issues relevant to this policy:

    ❧ *Disease/disorder/condition characteristics*—Does the disease, disorder, or condition affect men and women, and racial/ethnic groups differently than the majority? Describe and provide known data, including references.

    ❧ *Treatment or intervention characteristics*—Do clinically important gender or racial/ethnic differences exist in the intervention effect? Describe and provide known data, including references.

This information will be especially important in determining whether the proposed study will be appropriately considered as an NIH-defined clinical trial, and whether the study design should evaluate different intervention effects by gender, race, and/or ethnicity.

(See Question 8 and Section IV.C.1. in the NIH Guidelines)

13. What factors should be considered in determining inclusion of women and minorities and their subpopulations?

In deciding to what extent women and minorities should be included in a study and, thus, what outreach efforts are necessary, it is essential that the investigator carefully review the scientific question or hypothesis proposed. The need for incorporation of women and minority subpopulations will derive from the scientific question. As such, the investigator should consider the following:

    ♣ Is the scientific question or hypothesis applicable equally to both genders and to all minority groups and their subpopulations?

    ♣ Is the condition under study more prevalent or severe in one particular group?

    ♣ Have sufficient studies already been performed in one or more groups, leaving gaps that can be filled by focusing the research on certain population groups?

Having considered these questions, the investigator should then ask:

    ♣ Can the need for appropriate diversity be met by obtaining access to participants from a single clinic or facility? Will oversampling of certain groups be possible?

    ♣ If a single clinic or facility is not adequate, can the needed participants be enrolled by going to hospitals or other clinical facilities in the nearby geographic region?

    ♣ If demographic limitations preclude answering scientific questions locally for the appropriate gender and minority groups, is it feasible or necessary to expand the geographic area or to establish satellite centers?

(See Question 11 and Section VI.D. in the NIH Guidelines)

14. What type of information is required in describing the diversity of the composition of the study population?

As stated in the policy: "The inclusion of women and members of minority groups and their subpopulations must be addressed in developing a research design appropriate to the scientific objectives of the study. The research plan should describe the proposed study population in terms of gender and racial/ethnic composition, and provide a rationale for selection of such subjects. Such a plan should contain a description of the proposed outreach programs for recruiting women and minorities as participants." (III.A.)

The grant application instructions (PHS 398) require this information in the Research Design and Methods section. The format for reporting is shown in Question 34. In addition, the "Human Subjects" section of the PHS 398 also requires applicants to do the following:

> ⇛ Describe the characteristics of the subject population, including their anticipated number, age range, and health status. Identify the criteria for inclusion or exclusion of any subpopulation.

> ⇛ Identify the sources of research material obtained from individually identifiable living human subjects in the form of specimens, records, or data. Indicate whether the material or data will be obtained specifically for research purposes or whether use will be made of existing specimens, records, or data.

> ⇛ Describe plans for the recruitment of subjects and the consent procedures to be followed.

The plans for recruitment and retention of study participants should be clearly presented in terms of the methods and mechanisms for outreach. Initial Review Group members look for various types of evidence that the investigator has addressed the inclusion of both women and men, and minorities and their subpopulations, in a satisfactory manner. Such evidence may include (but is not limited to), information on the population characteristics of the disease or condition under study; national and local demographics of the population; knowledge and understanding of the racial/ethnic/cultural characteristics of the population; prior experience and collaborations in recruitment and retention of the populations and subpopulations to be studied; and the plans, arrangements and letters of commitment from relevant community groups and organizations for the planned study. Justifications should also be made in support of appropriate staffing needs for outreach plans. Exclusion of any group should be based on scientific considerations, and not simply for the convenience of the investigator. For single hospital, clinic, and university studies, it is important to present data on the characteristics of the population served by the site compared to the broader community or regional population. Planned enrollment should be viewed in terms of the demographics of the disease or condition, rather than local demographics or referral pattern, in order to avoid selection bias. For multi-center trials, the combined enrollment from all recruitment sites may achieve the required gender and racial/ethnic composition for the study. Study designs involving oversampling may also be appropriately justified. See Question 30 for a further discussion of contract projects.

(See Section III.A. and IV.C.1. and C.3. in the NIH Guidelines)

15. Do all minority groups and subpopulations have to be included in each study population?

Investigators should decide which minority groups and subpopulations will be included in the study based on the scientific question under study. It is not expected that every minority group and subpopulation will be included in each study. Broad representation and diversity are strongly encouraged, even if multiple clinics and sites are needed to accomplish it. When determining the composition of the study population, scientific issues (e.g., high prevalence of a disease/condition in certain minority groups, health of the subjects, different disease characteristics, or gap(s) in knowledge in a minority subpopulation) should be considered. For smaller studies, investigators should discuss the proposed study population and provide a justification for the specific minority groups available, including those absent or in limited numbers.

(See Section II. [subsection on exclusions] and IV.C.1. in the NIH Guidelines)

16. Does the policy permit a study population that contains only one gender or minority group or subpopulation?

YES. If a study of only one gender or minority group or subpopulation is proposed, there must be a scientific justification for limiting the diversity of the study population, such as high prevalence of the condition, unique disease characteristics, or gaps in knowledge in the selected population. The review committee will include the adequacy and scientific appropriateness of the proposed study population, and any justification, among the criteria used in its determination of the priority score. Women of childbearing potential should not be routinely excluded from participation in clinical research.

(See Sections IV.C.3., VI.C. and VI.D. in the NIH Guidelines)

17. What should applicants do if they are in a geographic area that does not offer a study population with the diversity required by the policy?

Investigators based in areas of the country where the population is primarily majority, or of one racial/ethnic group, will have difficulty recruiting sufficient numbers of participants to represent all of the racial/ethnic groups that may be significantly affected by the condition, disorder, or disease of interest. Can geographic considerations justify limited representation? This question has been asked by investigators from several states (e.g., Vermont, New Hampshire, Iowa, Minnesota). If geography is the only basis for lack of representation, it cannot be used to justify limited representation.

Investigators have long been required by NIH to be inclusive in their study populations. The new guidelines expand on those previously in place. Applicants/offerors must select study participants in terms of the purpose of the research and other factors, such as prior research findings, the size of the study, relevant characteristics of and gaps in knowledge about the disease, disorder, or condition, and the feasibility of developing a collaboration or consortium or other arrangements to include minority groups.

Each investigator is given the opportunity to provide a clear and compelling description and rationale for the proposed study population and its appropriateness for the purpose of the research. When there is limited representation, the investigator must provide a justification satisfactory to the Institute or Center Director, based on the health of the participants and the scientific needs of the research being proposed.

The meaning of "adequate representation" is tied to the purpose of the research. It does not necessarily mean that all groups are to be included, nor does it mean that there must be sufficient numbers for separate analysis. For example, small, exploratory studies are not expected to have representation from all racial/ethnic groups. Single gender or minority subgroup studies are possible. However, Phase III trials, where gender, race or ethnic background can be a factor, must be inclusive and diverse and address racial/ethnic subgroup differences because these trials have broad societal impact on behavior or therapeutic interventions or standard of care.

When an investigator is aware of similar research completed or underway employing populations complementary to those available in his/her locale, this can be presented as a rationale for limited representation.

In other cases, if the appropriate participants are not available in the locale of the applicant institution, investigators are encouraged to seek collaborators in other geographic areas. Plans should be presented to recruit outside that area either by the investigator or through collaborative arrangements with investigators who do have access to more diverse populations. Particularly when multi-center clinical trials are proposed, the inclusion requirements may be met by combining recruitment from the multiple sites; in these trials, each clinical site must still describe its planned recruitment, and will be evaluated on that basis.

When adequate representation is not provided and is not adequately justified, it should have substantial negative impact on the evaluation of merit of an application. The NIH program staff is available to work with investigators whose study site(s) may not have adequate gender or minority representation (see Question 36).

Peer reviewers will consider the proposed study and any justifications provided for the applicant's choice of study population(s) using the required review criteria and their scientific judgment, as discussed below. When peer reviewers have identified concerns, NIH staff will work with investigators to resolve the concerns before any award is made. Furthermore, if an NIH Institute or Center chooses to fund a Phase III clinical study that is inconsistent with the Guidelines, it is the responsibility of the Institute or Center to either take administrative action to revise the pending trial or initiate complementary activity to address the gender or minority concern.

These Guidelines are in no way intended to discriminate against areas that do not have diverse populations, nor do we believe that they will have that effect. The NIH commitment is to ensure that medical knowledge from NIH research benefits the entire population.

(See Sections IV.C.3., V.G., and VI.D. in the NIH Guidelines)

18. Can study populations in other selected studies be used to justify a study population that does not include both men and women or racial/ethnic minority groups?

Investigators may propose that the planned study population composition has limited gender and/or minority representation, and is justified because the combination of the study population in their application and related past or ongoing studies provide the diversity required by the policy. Applicants should use published reports and discussions with NIH staff concerning ongoing research to identify studies that provide the appropriate diversity. In some cases, duplication of comparable data that include the excepted gender or population group may not be necessary.

(See Sections V.G. and III.A. in the NIH Guidelines)

19. What is meant by outreach efforts to recruit and retain women and minorities in studies?

Outreach efforts are attempts by investigators and their staff to recruit and retain women and minority populations in their studies. Such efforts could include involvement of organizations and persons relevant to the populations and communities of interest (e.g., religious organizations, community leaders, and public and private institutions) in order to develop appropriate and culturally sensitive outreach programs and activities for recruitment and retention of the most diverse study population, consistent with the purposes of the research project.

The research plan should contain a description of the proposed outreach programs for recruiting and retaining women and minorities as participants. Investigators should take precautionary measures to ensure that there is minimal possibility of coercion or undue influence in the incentives or rewards offered to prospective participants when recruiting or attempting to retain participants in studies.

The likelihood of success of the outreach plan will be evaluated as part of the peer review. Typically, peer reviewers use past experience and success as an indicator of an investigator's ability to mount and implement a successful outreach plan.

To assist investigators and potential study participants, NIH staff prepared this notebook, **Outreach Notebook for the NIH Guidelines on Inclusion of Women and Minorities as Subjects in Clinical Research.** It is not intended as a definitive text on this subject, but should assist investigators in their consideration of an appropriate plan for recruiting and retaining participants in clinical studies. The Office of Research on Women's Health also published *Recruitment and Retention of Women in Clinical Studies,* a report from a 1993 workshop identifying barriers for including women in clinical studies and providing recommendations to overcome these barriers.

(See Section IV.C.7. and V.F. in the NIH Guidelines)

20. In multi-center clinical studies, must each study site meet the inclusion requirements separately?

Each study site must describe its planned recruitment, retention and outreach plans, which will be evaluated as part of the initial review of the application.

The recruitment goals for women, men, and minorities may vary at different sites in multi-center clinical studies; however, the overall recruitment goals for the study may be met by combining recruitment from all sites. This could be acceptable if the women and minorities populations from the contributing centers do not have some relevant unique characteristics, other than being from those centers, that could limit the value of the study results. As part of its funding plan, the NIH may select recruitment sites with high minority enrollments for inclusion in multi-center studies to achieve inclusion of the most diverse study population. Annual reports on enrollment will be required for each site as well as for the overall study.

(See Section VI.B. in the NIH Guidelines)

21. Is increased cost an acceptable justification for not including women, minorities, and minority subpopulations in clinical trials?

NO. The legislation states unequivocally that the cost associated with increasing the diversity of a study population composition to include both women and men, minorities, and minority subpopulations is not an acceptable justification for excluding them from clinical trials. In other types of clinical research, cost is not an acceptable reason for exclusion except when the study would duplicate data from other sources.

(See Section I., II., III.A., and III.B. in the NIH Guidelines)

22. Is it acceptable to use existing cohorts that are deficient in women or minority participants?

Competitive continuation (type 2) applications or proposals that propose to complete a study or analyses of existing data bases are exempt from the new policy if they were initiated before June 1993. However, in new (type 1) applications or proposals, use of an existing cohort that lacks the diversity required by the new policy must be justified. The nature of the scientific question, a requirement for data provided by the cohort, or research portfolio balance may provide the basis of a justification. An NIH Institute or Center may also pursue other means of filling programmatic gaps due to the limitations of prior studies in meeting the new policy requirements.

(See Section IV.C.1., V.B., VI.A. and VI.B. in the NIH Guidelines)

C. EXCLUSIONS/JUSTIFICATIONS

23. What are the circumstances under which it is not necessary to include both women and men, and minorities?

The law allows for three circumstances. The requirements shall not apply when the inclusion of women and members of minority groups:

1. is inappropriate with respect to the health of the subjects;

2. is inappropriate with respect to the purpose of the research; or

3. is inappropriate under such other circumstances as the Director of NIH may designate.

The NIH Guidelines require a justification, to the satisfaction of an Institute/Center Director, when inclusion of both genders and minorities is not proposed for reasons (1) and (2) above.

(See Sections II. and III.A. in the NIH Guidelines)

24. What kinds of justifications are acceptable for not including adequate representation of women or men?

Depending on the specific research questions and design, one or more of the following possible acceptable justifications could apply:

> ❧ One gender (male or female) is excluded from the study because:
>
>> – inclusion of these individuals would be inappropriate with respect to their health (e.g., experimental procedures/treatment present unacceptable risk for women of childbearing potential. It should be noted, however, that women of childbearing potential should not be routinely excluded.);
>>
>> – the research question addressed is relevant to only one gender; or
>>
>> – evidence from prior research strongly demonstrates no difference between genders; or
>>
>> – sufficient data already exist with regard to the outcome of comparable studies in the excluded gender, and duplication is not needed in this study.
>
> ❧ One gender is excluded or severely limited because the purpose of the research constrains the applicant's selection of study subjects by gender (e.g., uniquely valuable stored specimens or existing datasets are single gender; very small numbers of subjects are involved; or overriding factors dictate selection of subjects, such as matching of transplant recipients, or availability of rare surgical specimens.)
>
> ❧ Gender representation of specimens or existing datasets cannot be accurately determined, (e.g., pooled blood samples, stored specimens, or datasets with incomplete gender documentation are used) and this does not compromise the scientific objectives of the research.
>
> ❧ The scientific question requires the use of the same or a comparable study population as that used in an earlier study and the potential gain in scientific knowledge outweighs the imbalance in the study population.
>
> ❧ Research is proposed with a pre-defined unique but underrepresented population (e.g., an extensive registry of patients with the condition of interest) and would not be feasible if a different sample were used.

Each of these justifications would be evaluated by Initial Review Groups in the context of the specific scientific goals and issues being addressed. Depending on the details, these justifications may or may not be considered adequate and compelling.

(See Section III.A. and VI.C. in the NIH Guidelines)

25. What kinds of justification are acceptable for not including adequate representation of all racial/ethnic minorities and subpopulations?

It is not anticipated that every study will include all minority groups and subgroups. The inclusion of minority groups should be determined by the scientific questions under examination and their relevance to racial/ethnic groups. Applications should describe the subgroups that will be included in the research. The investigator should address inclusion issues in terms of the size of the study, the relevant characteristics of the disease, disorder, condition, or phenomena under study, or the feasibility of making a collaboration or consortium or other arrangements to include representation.

Depending on the specific research questions and design, one or more of the following possible acceptable justifications could apply:

- ✒ Some or all minority groups or subgroups are excluded from the study because:

  – inclusion of these individuals would be inappropriate with respect to their health; or

  – the research question addressed is relevant to only one racial/ethnic group; or

  – evidence from prior research strongly demonstrates no differences between racial/ethnic groups on the outcome variables; or

  – a single minority group study is proposed to fill a research gap; or

  – sufficient data already exist with regard to the outcome of comparable studies in the excluded racial/ethnic group(s) and duplication is not needed in this study.

- ✒ Some minority groups or subgroups are excluded or poorly represented because the geographical location of the study has only limited numbers of these minority groups who would be eligible for the study, AND the investigator has satisfactorily addressed this issue in terms of the size of the study, the relevant characteristics of the disease, disorder, or condition, or the feasibility of making a collaboration or consortium or other arrangements to include representation.

- ✒ Some minority groups or subgroups are excluded or poorly represented because the purpose of the research constrains the applicant's selection of study subjects by race/ethnicity (e.g., uniquely valuable cohorts, stored specimens or existing datasets are of limited minority representation; very small numbers of subjects are involved; or overriding factors dictate selection of subjects, such as matching of transplant recipients, or availability of rare surgical specimens).

- ✒ Racial/ethnic origin of specimens or existing datasets cannot be accurately determined (e.g., pooled blood samples, stored specimens or datasets with incomplete racial/ethnic documentation are used), but this does not compromise the scientific objectives of the research.

Each of these justifications would be evaluated by Initial Review Groups in the context of the specific scientific goals and issues being addressed. Depending on the details, these justifications may or may not be considered adequate and compelling.

(See Section III.A. and VI.D. in the NIH Guidelines)

D. PEER REVIEW

26. This policy appears to be based on political considerations. Why is it to be reviewed as a part of the science by the Initial Review Groups?

The policy, while responsive to a Congressional mandate, has a scientific basis, as discussed in Question 3. In clinical research, the endpoint is to gain knowledge that will contribute to the health of the American public. To achieve this goal, research findings must be applicable generally to all of the people who may become or are affected by the conditions, disorders, or diseases that are the focus of the NIH research effort.

The scientific and technical merit of a research project depends, in part, on the appropriateness of the study population for the aims of the research. For example, if a clinical research study population does not include both men and women, the question must be asked: will the results be valid and useful to both men and women? If not, the scientific merit of the study may be diminished. In some circumstances, however, the assessment of scientific merit may not be affected by a more limited representation.

(See Sections V.A. and V.D. in the NIH Guidelines)

27. How will peer reviewers evaluate applications for compliance with this policy?

During initial review, peer reviewers will evaluate each project separately in terms of gender and minority representation and determine whether it is scientifically acceptable in regard to the inclusion policy. Their decision will be based on the proposed plans, any justifications provided, and the review criteria noted below. (See Question 30 for a further discussion of contract projects.)

For scientifically acceptable applications, gender representation proposed in the project may include both genders, only females, only males, or unknown gender. Minority representation proposed in the project may include both minority and non-minority subjects, only minority subjects, only non-minority subjects, or unknown minority representation in the subject population. Clinical trials will have additional criteria as discussed previously under Question 8. The quality of the inclusion plans will be factored into the priority score assigned by reviewers.

An application is judged to be unacceptable if it: fails to conform to NIH policy guidelines in relation to the scientific purpose and type of study; or fails to provide sufficient information; or does not adequately justify limited or lack of representation of one gender or minority groups; or does not realistically address recruitment and retention. The unacceptable inclusion plans should be reflected in a poorer priority score assigned by reviewers if the project is scored. (This "unacceptable" code constitutes a bar to funding unless or until resolved by NIH staff.)

Peer reviewers will be asked to evaluate whether the research plan in the application conforms to these policies, using questions such as the following:

> ❧ Is the proposed representation of women and men, and minorities and their subpopulations described?

> ❧ Is the proposed representation adequate with respect to the scientific questions under study?

> ❧ Have the subpopulations been appropriately identified and reported?

> ❧ Are the efforts being made to recruit and retain women and men, and minorities and their subpopulations adequately described and likely to accomplish the goals?

For a Phase III clinical trial: Has evidence been adequately evaluated in terms of whether clinically important gender or racial/ethnic differences in the intervention effect are to be expected? Has the planned trial been designed to take into account the inclusion requirements for the three options previously discussed under Question 8, including the need for valid analysis of the intervention effect in subgroups? Are sufficient numbers of men and women and minorities included to accomplish the valid analysis of differences of intervention effects?

If the proposed representation of women or minorities and their subpopulations is judged as unacceptable, it will be considered a scientific weakness or deficiency in the study design and will be reflected in assigning the priority score to the application.

Review Criteria

In conducting peer review for scientific and technical merit, appropriately constituted initial review groups (including study sections), technical evaluation groups, and intramural review panels will be instructed to consider the following elements in the recruitment and retention of women and minorities in clinical research.

> ❧ Evaluate the proposed plan for the inclusion of women and minorities and their subpopulations for appropriate representation or to evaluate the proposed justification when representation is limited or absent.

> ❧ Evaluate the proposed exclusion of women and minorities and their subpopulations on the basis that a requirement for inclusion is inappropriate with respect to the health of the subjects.

> ❧ Evaluate the proposed exclusion of minorities and women on the basis that a requirement for inclusion is inappropriate with respect to the purpose of the research.

> ❧ Determine whether the design of the study or clinical trial is adequate to measure differences when warranted.

> ❧ Evaluate the outreach plans for recruitment and retention of study participants.

These criteria, which apply to the full range of NIH-supported clinical research, will form part of the scientific assessment and assigned score.

Reviewers will assign codes, which correspond to the scientific and technical evaluation of the inclusion policy, to scored applications. The codes will be included in summary statements.

Note: Scientific Review Administrators of the Initial Review Groups (IRGs) will treat the evaluation of the representation of women and minorities and their subpopulations in a manner consistent with the evaluation of all other factors that contribute to the overall priority score. The Scientific Review Administrators will not routinely request written clarification from the applicant when the application does not describe and justify the gender or minority composition of the study population. If such information is not contained within the application, and it is not provided prior to the review meeting, the application will be reviewed by the IRG as submitted and the deficiencies will be reflected in the priority score. This procedure is consistent with review of all other parts of the application that contribute to the overall priority score.

(See Section IV.C.3. in the NIH Guidelines)

28. The policy on inclusion of women and minorities is applied to research projects, rather than applications or proposals. How is this dealt with in the IRG coding?

The clinical research project is the basic unit requiring compliance with the policy and it is characterized as a research activity focused on a particular problem, with a specific experimental design or protocol, and a particular study population. All research involving human subjects must be reviewed by an Institutional Review Board (IRB). Typically, an IRB examines each research activity involving a particular use of human subjects. Similarly, as a part of the NIH review, each such project will be reviewed and coded by the initial review group (IRG) for appropriate inclusion of both genders and minorities.

An application or proposal may consist of a single project (in which case it would be assigned the same codes as that project), or multiple projects. In addition to codes for each project, applications should be given an overall set of codes reflecting an evaluation of all of the activities being proposed, as indicated in the coding guidelines. In some cases, a series of related studies may involve varying one or more parameter(s) of interest with the same subject population, (e.g., dose-response studies or visual perception studies). Based on its merits and the IRG's judgment, such a series may be considered a single project or multiple projects and coded either as one or several studies.

29. If an application fails to include both genders or minority groups and this is not appropriately justified, how much should the priority score be affected?

The priority score is based on a scientific/technical evaluation, using published review criteria. The review criteria include not only the adequacy of plans to include both genders and racial/ethnic groups, but all of the standard criteria, such as adequacy of research plan, adequacy and appropriateness of training and experience of investigators and staff, and importance and scientific significance of the problem to be studied.

Because of the nature of scientific evaluation of grant and cooperative agreement applications, none of the review criteria is pre-assigned a specific weight, and reviewers are asked to weigh all of the criteria in the context of the research being proposed, giving each the importance appropriate for the specific work proposed. Any one criterion may be given a high or low weighting by each reviewer depending on its importance in the particular research being proposed.

(See Sections III.C. and IV.C.3. in the NIH Guidelines)

30. How does the inclusion policy apply to research contract proposals and projects?

The inclusion policy applies to NIH research and development contract projects as well as grant and cooperative agreement projects. However, there are some differences in procedures as a result of the federal acquisition regulations for contracting.

The description of the planned contract project is provided in the Request for Proposals (RFP), which includes the statement of work and the evaluation criteria. When planning and preparing the RFP, the NIH project officer must address many issues, including determining whether the project will be a clinical research project, and whether it will be an NIH-defined clinical trial; the study design, sample size issues, the inclusion requirements for both genders and minority groups, and outreach plans need to be addressed, and appropriate justifications provided when the requirement is for limited representation. The required review criterion should be included as part of the evaluation criteria published in the RFP.

The investigator responding to the RFP must address the inclusion policy as reflected in the RFP requirements and evaluation criteria. Peer reviewers will evaluate proposals, looking at plans for recruitment, retention and outreach for study participants, using the published review criteria.

(See Sections III.C., IV.A. and IV.G. in the NIH Guidelines)

E. Awards

31. How will conformance to this policy affect funding of projects?

Regardless of the priority score, percentile ranking or program relevance of the proposed research, the NIH funding components will not fund grants or award contracts that do not comply with this policy.

(See Section III.C. in the NIH Guidelines)

32. Does the policy apply to foreign projects funded by the NIH?

The NIH policy on inclusion of women in research conducted outside the United States is the same as that for research conducted in the United States. However, with regard to the population of the foreign country, the definition of the minority groups in foreign countries may be different than in the United States. If there is scientific rationale for examining subpopulation group differences within the foreign population, investigators should consider designing their studies to accommodate these differences.

(See Section IV.C.9. in the NIH Guidelines)

33. How do the new Guidelines impact on Institutional Review Boards (IRBs)?

IRBs have long had as part of their responsibilities examining ethical issues and determining equitable selection of subjects in accordance with the regulations for protection of human subjects [45 CFR §46.111(a)(3)]. The inclusion of both women and men and of minorities in research (intramural and extramural) is important, both to ensure that they receive an appropriate share of the benefits of research and that they do not bear a disproportionate burden. To the extent that participation in research offers direct benefits to the participants, underrepresentation of men, women, or minorities denies them the opportunity to receive this benefit. Moreover, for purposes of generalizing research results, investigators must include the widest possible range of population groups.

The Office for Protection from Research Risks has discussed the impact of this policy in OPRR Reports, Number 94-01, April 25, 1994, which has been distributed to IRBs. Seven points to consider in deliberations about appropriate selection of research participants are offered. IRBs are empowered (by 45 CFR Part 46, the DHHS assurances, and the NIH Guidelines) to approve, request modification of, or disapprove research based on their review. Copies of the OPRR Reports may be obtained from OPRR or your IRB.

(See Section IV.C.2. in the NIH Guidelines)

34. How do we report on inclusion of women and minorities?

Applicants will provide information in applications, proposals, and progress reports using the following summary table format for planned enrollment of women and minorities. Awardees will report annually on the actual enrollment for the approved project using the same format.

SUMMARY TABLE. GENDER AND MINORITY INCLUSION IN RESEARCH

Study title:

	American Indian or Alaskan Native	Asian or Pacific Islander	Black, not of Hispanic Origin	Hispanic	White, not of Hispanic Origin	Other or Unknown	Total
Female							
Male							
Unknown							
Total							

Note: For planned studies, indicate the expected study composition using the categories noted below. For ongoing studies, provide the number of subjects enrolled in the study to date (cumulatively since the most recent competitive award) according to the categories in the summary table. If there is more than one study, provide a separate table for each study. In addition, indicate the planned or actual minority subpopulations that are included in the study.

(See Section III.C. in the NIH Guidelines)

35. When does the policy begin to apply?

This policy applies to all applications, proposals, and intramural projects submitted on and after June 1, 1994, (the date of full implementation). Projects funded prior to June 10, 1993, must still comply with the 1990 policy and report annually on enrollment of subjects in contracts and in intramural projects using gender and racial/ethnic categories as required in the Application for Continuation of a Public Health Service Grant (PHS Form 2590).

(See Section IV.A. in the NIH Guidelines)

36. Where can I obtain additional information?

Additional information may be obtained from NIH staff identified in Request for Applications (RFAs), Program Announcements (PAs), or on awards. The following senior extramural staff from the NIH Institutes and Centers may be contacted for more information about the policy and relevant Institute/Center programs:

Dr. Marvin Kalt
National Cancer Institute
6130 Executive Boulevard
Executive Plaza North, Room 600A
Bethesda, Maryland 20892
Tel: (301) 496-5147

Dr. Ralph Helmsen
National Eye Institute
6120 Executive Boulevard
Executive Plaza South, Room 350
Bethesda, Maryland 20892-7164
Tel: (301) 496-5301

Dr. Lawrence Friedman
National Heart, Lung, and Blood Institute
6701 Rockledge Drive
2 Rockledge Center, MSC 7938
Bethesda, Maryland 20892
Tel: (301) 435-0422

Dr. Miriam Kelty
National Institute on Aging
7201 Wisconsin Avenue
Gateway Building, Room 2C218
Bethesda, Maryland 20892
Tel: (301) 496-9322

Dr. Cherry Lowman
National Institute on Alcohol
    Abuse and Alcoholism
6000 Executive Boulevard
Bethesda, Maryland 20892
Tel: (301) 443-0796

Dr. George Counts
National Institute of Allergy
    and Infectious Diseases
6003 Executive Boulevard
Solar Building, Room 4B04
Bethesda, Maryland 20892
Tel: (301) 496-8697

Dr. Julia Freeman
National Institute of Arthritis
    and Musculoskeletal and Skin Diseases
45 Center Drive, MSC 6500
Building 45, Room 5AS19F
Bethesda, Maryland 20892-6500
Tel: (301) 594-5052

Ms. Hildegard Topper
National Institute of Child Health
    and Human Development
9000 Rockville Pike
Building 31, Room 2A-03
Bethesda, Maryland 20892
Tel: (301) 496-0104

Dr. Craig Jordan
National Institute on Deafness
    and Other Communication Disorders
6120 Executive Boulevard
Executive Plaza South, Room 400C
Bethesda, Maryland 20892-7180
Tel: (301) 496-8693

Dr. Norman S. Braveman
National Institute on Dental Research
45 Center Drive
Building 45, Room 4AN24
Bethesda, Maryland 20892
Tel: (301) 594-2089

Dr. Paul Coates
National Institute of Diabetes
  and Digestive and Kidney Diseases
45 Center Drive
Building 45, Room 5AN24J
Bethesda, Maryland 20892
Tel: (301) 594-8805

Ms. Eleanor Friedenberg
National Institute on Drug Abuse
5600 Fishers Lane
Parklawn Building, Room 10-42
Rockville, Maryland 20857
Tel: (301) 443-2755

Dr. Gwen Collman
National Institute of Environmental
  Health Sciences
P.O. Box 12233
Research Triangle Park, North Carolina
27709
Tel: (919) 541-4980

Dr. Alison Cole
National Institute of General
  Medical Sciences
45 Center Drive, MSC 6200
Building 45, Room 2AS49K
Bethesda, Maryland 20892-6200
Tel: (301) 594-1826

Dr. Dolores Parron
National Institute of Mental Health
5600 Fishers Lane
Parklawn Building, Room 17C-14
Rockville, Maryland 20857
Tel: (301) 443-2847

Dr. Constance Atwell
National Institute of Neurological
  Disorders and Stroke
7550 Wisconsin Avenue
Federal Building, Room 1016
Bethesda, Maryland 20892-9190
Tel: (301) 496-9248

Dr. Mark Guyer
National Center for Human
  Genome Research
9000 Rockville Pike
Building 38A, Room 604
Bethesda, Maryland 20892
Tel: (301) 402-5407

Dr. Lynn M. Amende
National Institute of Nursing Research
45 Center Drive, MSC 6300
Building 45, Room 3AN12
Bethesda, Maryland 20892
Tel: (301) 594-5968

Dr. Harriet Gordon
National Center for Research Resources
6705 Rockledge Drive, MSC 7965
1 Rockledge Center, Room 6030
Bethesda, Maryland 20892-7965
Tel: (301) 435-0790

Johnnie Smith
Fogarty International Center
31 Center Drive, MSC 2220
Building 31, Room B2C39
Bethesda, Maryland 20892
Tel: (301) 402-9590

37. What are the initial review group codes for inclusion of women and minorities in clinical research?

The codes are as follows:

HEADER OUTPUT FOR SUMMARY STATEMENTS

࿊ Clinical Research

  (X) Clinical Trial, Gender, and Minority Codes not assigned*
     (for non-clinical research or non-scored applications)
  (Y) NIH-defined Phase III Clinical Trial*
  (N) Clinical Research—not an NIH-defined Phase III clinical trial*

࿊ Gender

  G1A Includes both genders, scientifically acceptable
  G2A Includes only women, scientifically acceptable
  G3A Includes only men, scientifically acceptable
  G4A Gender representation unknown, scientifically acceptable

  G1U Includes both genders, but scientifically unacceptable
  G2U Includes only women, scientifically unacceptable
  G3U Includes only men, scientifically unacceptable
  G4U Gender representation unknown, scientifically unacceptable

࿊ Minority

  M1A Includes minorities and non-minorities, scientifically acceptable
  M2A Includes only minorities, scientifically acceptable
  M3A Includes only non-minorities, scientifically acceptable
  M4A Minority representation unknown, scientifically acceptable

  M1U Includes minorities and non-minorities, but scientifically unacceptable
  M2U Includes only minorities, scientifically unacceptable
  M3U Includes only non-minorities, scientifically unacceptable
  M4U Minority representation unknown, scientifically unacceptable

these codes do not appear in header

5.

Informed Consent in Clinical Trials

Overview. 156
The Requirements for an Informed Consent to Participation in Clinical Trials 156
   Other Information That May Be Added by an IRB to the Consent Process 157
Parental Consent and Minors as Research Subjects 158
   Special Rules for Consent for Children as Research Subjects 158
   Determining When a Child Is Capable of Assenting to Participation in Clinical Trials 159
   Parental Consent to Participation of a Child in Clinical Trials 159
   Research Involving Children Who Have Been the Subject of Neglect or Abuse 159
   Documenting Permission and Assent to Participation in Research 159
   Special Requirements for Children Who Are Wards 160
Prisoners Participating in Clinical Research 161
Pregnant Women and Fetal and Neonatal Research 161
   Requirements for Securing Consent to Participate in Clinical Trials:
   Pregnant Women, Fetal, and Neonatal Research 161
   Federal Research Requirements That Address the Use of Placenta,
   Dead Fetuses, or Fetal Material 164
   The Opportunity for Studies Involving Pregnancy and Fetuses
   That Otherwise Does Not Meet the Requirements of the Regulations 164
Decisionally Incapable Research Subjects 164
   Securing Consent for Clinical Trials Research Participation
   for a Decisionally Incapable Subject 165
Linguistic, Cultural, and Communication Challenges to Consent in Clinical Trials 166
   Clinical Trials Involving Subjects with Limited English Proficiency 166
   Managing Consent and Cultural Differences with Potential Research Subjects 167
   Sight- and Hearing-Impaired Research Subjects and the Consent Process 167
   Overcoming Literacy Challenges to Effective Communication 167
Other Topics for Disclosure in Research Consents 168
   Anticipating Adverse Events in the Clinical Trials Consent Process 168
   Information Needed in the Consent Process Regarding Potential
   Commercial Value of Tissues or Cellular
   Material Discovered in the Course of Clinical Research 169
Emergency Research Consent Requirements 169
   Emergency Clinical Trials Research and Consent 169
Withdrawal of Consent. 172
   When a Subject Withdraws Consent to Participate in a Clinical Trial 173

Modifications and Waivers of Consent 173
    Modification to the Consent Requirements by an IRB 173
    When the Consent Requirements Can Be Waived by an IRB 174
Consent Documentation 174
    Documenting Consent to Participate in Clinical Trials 174
    Sample Consent Tools from Federal Departments 175
Conclusion: Practical Suggestions for Obtaining Consent to Participate in Clinical Trials . . . 175
References 176
OPRR Sample Short Form Written Consent Document for Subjects
Who Do Not Speak English 177
Informed Consent Checklist 178
Tips on Informed Consent 182
Informed Consent Recommendations: Appendices 3, 4, and 5 184
Informed Consent Template 187
Checklist for Evaluating Involvement of Decisionally
Incapable Persons in Clinical Trials 191
Part 2: Specific Tips for Trial Participants —
A Checklist of Questions to Ask the Research Team 192
Human Subject Regulations Decision Charts 194
The Office of Human Subjects Research (OHSR) National Institutes of Health 197
Common Concerns to Address in the Consent Process Sample: Cancer Trials 202

. . . .

OVERVIEW

Both federal and state laws emphasize the need for *informed* consent for participation in clinical trials. An agreement to participate in such endeavors is not the same as a patient authorizing a diagnostic test or medical treatment. This difference is made clear by the number of detailed specifications controlling consent especially for so-called vulnerable populations such as minors, prisoners, and pregnant women.

Participation in clinical trials does share a common bond with treatment authorizations for accepted therapy: consent is seen as a *process, not* a form. While acknowledging the importance of documenting the consent process, the laws and regulations that control clinical trials put forms in a practical context, using the documentation to signify completion of the steps necessary to properly secure the agreement of a research participant in a clinical investigation.

In this chapter, common questions are addressed regarding the consent process for clinical trials. Also considered are specific questions relating to consent documentation.

. . . .

THE REQUIREMENTS FOR AN INFORMED CONSENT TO PARTICIPATION IN CLINICAL TRIALS

The federal regulations set forth criteria for informed consent. These rules are published in the *Code of Federal Regulation* (Consent Regulations) with updates found in the *Federal Register.* Under the Common Rule, other federal agencies and departments follow very similar consent requirements. For purposes of this discussion, the example used will be the regulatory requirements promulgated by the U.S. Department of Health and Human Services (HHS).

The general consent requirements found in the Common Rule Code of Federal Regulations (Consent Regulations, 2001, with emphasis added) for the HHS specify the following parameters:

1. A statement that the study involves research, an explanation of the purposes of the research and the expected duration of the subject's participation, a description of the procedures to be followed, and identification of any procedures which are experimental;

2. A description of any reasonably foreseeable risks or discomforts to the subject;

3. A description of any benefits to the subject or to others which may reasonably be expected from the research;

4. A disclosure of appropriate alternative procedures or courses of treatment, if any, that might be advantageous to the subject;

5. A statement describing the extent to which *confidentiality* of records identifying the subject will be maintained;

6. For research involving more than minimal risk, an explanation as to whether any compensation and an explanation as to whether any medical treatments are available if injury occurs and, if so, what they consist of, or where further information may be obtained;

7. An explanation of *whom to contact for answers* to pertinent questions about the research and research subjects' rights, and whom to contact in the event of a *research-related injury* to the subject; and

8. A statement that *participation is voluntary,* refusal to participate will involve *no penalty or loss of benefits* to which the subject is otherwise entitled, and the *subject may discontinue participation at any time* without penalty or loss of benefits to which the subject is otherwise entitled.

Other Information That May Be Added by an IRB to the Consent Process

Under the consent provisions found in the Common Rule Code of Federal Regulations (Consent Regulations, 2001, with emphasis added), an IRB can require additional consent elements, including the following:

1. A statement that the particular treatment or procedure *may involve risks* to the subject (or to the embryo or fetus, if the subject is or may become pregnant) *which are currently unforeseeable;*

2. *Anticipated circumstances* under which the subject's *participation may be terminated* by the investigator without regard to the subject's consent;

3. *Any additional costs to the subject* that may result from participation in the research;

4. The *consequences of* a subject's *decision to withdraw from the research* and procedures for orderly termination of participation by the subject;

5. A statement that *significant new findings developed during the course* of the *research which may relate to the subject's willingness to continue participation* will be provided to the subject; and

6. The *approximate number of subjects* involved in the study.

············

PARENTAL CONSENT AND MINORS AS RESEARCH SUBJECTS

Under the federal regulations, minors are singled out for special protection. Seen as a vulnerable population, an entire subpart of the rules are devoted to safeguarding the well being of children as research subjects. As discussed in this part of the chapter, children are not asked to give or refuse consent. Rather, the rules grant certain responsibilities to parents or legal guardians. The federal rules suggest that in certain instances children may give their assent to take part in clinical trials.

Special Rules for Consent for Children as Research Subjects

The federal regulations map out a combination of "permission and assent" provisions involving children in clinical trials. The regulations define children as individuals who under pertinent state law have not attained the legal age to authorize treatment or participation in research.

The federal regulation divides up the analysis for children as research subjects into five groups, providing specific requirements relating to consent for each category:

- *When a clinical study does not involve greater than minimal risk to children—* The IRB must make certain that there are adequate provisions for obtaining the consent of the parents or guardian and seeking the assent of the child.

- *When research involving greater than minimal risk holds out the prospect of direct benefit to individual child research subjects*—The IRB must determine that the anticipated benefit to the research subjects justifies the risk involved and that the anticipated benefit is at least as favorable as available alternatives. In addition, there must be adequate provisions for the permission of the parents or guardian and the assent of the children.

- *When research involving greater than minimal risk* does not *hold out the prospect of direct benefit to individual child research subjects but is likely to result in generalizable knowledge about the individual's disorder or condition—* The IRB must determine that the risks involve only a minor increase over minimal risk. The research should involve experiences that are reasonably commensurate with those expected in medical, dental, psychological, or educational situations. Moreover, the generalizable knowledge to be obtained is of vital importance for either understanding or correcting the research subjects' disorder and condition. As with the other categories, permission must be obtained from the parents or guardian and the assent of the children.

- *Research involving a serious problem involving the health or welfare of children*—In this instance, the IRB must find the proposed research offers a "reasonable opportunity" to understand, prevent, or alleviate a serious problem to the health or welfare of children.

- *Otherwise nonapprovable research that offers the opportunity to understand, prevent, or alleviate a serious problem affecting the health and welfare of children*—This is the most restrictive category of research involving children. First, an IRB must determine that the research offers a reasonable opportunity to promote the stated goals of understanding, preventing, or alleviating a serious health or welfare problem involving children. In addition, a panel of experts must be consulted by the Secretary of Health and Human Services. They must advise that the proposed study either does satisfy the regulations or that beyond meeting the stated goals, the research will follow sound ethical principles and include provision for seeking permission of parents or guardians and the assent of children (Children as Research Subjects' Consent, 2001).

Determining When a Child Is Capable of Assenting to Participation in Clinical Trials

It is the responsibility of the IRB to determine whether children are capable of assenting to research. The criteria used involves the age, maturity, and psychological status of the proposed research subjects. The evaluation may be done for the entire pool of children or for each child. Notwithstanding this requirement, the assent component may be waived when the children cannot be consulted or the research holds direct benefit that is important to the health or well being of the children. Even when children are capable of assent, the IRB can apply the consent waiver provisions found in the Consent Regulations.

Parental Consent to Participation of a Child in Clinical Trials

One question that frequently comes up involves the need for both parents to give consent to their child participating in human research studies. The answer varies with the particular category of research in question. When research involves nothing greater than minimal risk and when research involves more than minimal risk that holds the prospect of direct benefit to the child, the IRB may determine that the permission of one parent is sufficient (Parental Consent Regulations, 2001).

However, when research is of greater than minimal risk and holds no prospect of direct benefit or might help to understand, prevent, or alleviate a serious health or welfare problem for children, the permission of *both* parents should be obtained. Exception is made for situations in which there is only one parent or the other parent is incompetent, unknown, or not reasonably available. The same pertains when one parent is solely responsible for the care and custody of the child (Parental Consent Regulations, 2001).

Research Involving Children Who Have Been the Subject of Neglect or Abuse

An IRB may waive the requirement for permission from a parent or guardian when it is not considered a reasonable requirement to safeguard the children. Cases of child neglect or abuse are illustrative in this regard. However, the regulations do require an appropriate mechanism to be in place to protect the children. The regulation is somewhat vague, indicating that such a mechanism will vary with what is involved in the clinical trial; the risks and anticipated benefits to the children; and the condition, age, maturity, and status of those who would be participants in the research (Parental Consent to Research, 2001).

Documenting Permission and Assent to Participation in Research

The federal rules that address the use of long-form and short-form consent apply to permission given by parents and guardians. This is a provision found in the general requirements for clinical trials research (Consent Regulations, 2001).

Interestingly, in the set of regulations governing minors as research subjects, the regulations do not delineate how assent is to be documented. This is a responsibility left to the IRB to determine (Parental Consent to Research, 2001). From a practical perspective, this increases the potential for wide variation in documentation requirements set by one IRB as compared to another. It could lead to disagreements, especially in multisite clinical trials. Practical strategies can be developed to avoid this problem. (See Tips Box below.)

TIP: Fundamental components that are important to consider in setting the content for assent document, from a risk reduction standpoint. These include the following:

- Name and age of minor
- Name(s) of parent(s) or guardians
- Name(s) and relationship if any of those in attendance during assent discussion (including whether or not the parent(s) or guardian were present)
- Date and time of assent discussion
- Condition of minor
  - Receiving pain medication—no influence on cognitive ability
  - Receiving other medication—not effective on cognitive ability
  - Minor developmentally challenged
- Description of clinical trial provided to minor
- Minor asked questions and received understandable answers
- Minor provided appropriate answers to questions posed that were designed to test understanding of nature, purpose, and role in clinical study
- Minor refused to give assent to participate in research
- Name and position of person facilitating assent discussion with minor

---

The strategies described above encourage development of a strong record of the assent discussion is the rationale for this type of documentation. It captures salient information about the ability of the minor to take part in the discussion. Further, it provides a description of information communicated to the minor. At a later time, this could prove important in the event that there is a challenge to the adequacy of the assent process.

Special Requirements for Children Who Are Wards

The rules do set forth specific requirements when the proposed research is of *greater than minimal risk* and there is *no prospect of direct benefit to children* who are wards. The same is true for those studies that might help to understand, prevent, or alleviate a serious health or welfare problem for children. In these instances, the research must be related to the individual's status as a ward and the activity must be performed in a setting in which the majority of the children involved as research subjects are not of a ward status (Research on Wards, 2001). Should an IRB approve such research, it must require the appointment of an advocate on behalf of a child involved in the study. The advocate must have sufficient experience to fulfill the role and must not be associated in any way with the research, the study investigators, or the guardian organization (Research on Wards, 2001).

············

PRISONERS PARTICIPATING IN CLINICAL RESEARCH

Additional safeguards are found in Subpart C of the Common Rule federal regulations relating to prisoners as research subjects. The rationale is to avoid the issue of incarceration affecting the ability of a prisoner to make a decision to participate in research voluntarily (Prisoner Research Regulations, 2001). To make certain that this stated purpose is achieved and that decisions are not coerced, the rules set forth very specific requirements. For example, at least one of the IRB members must be a prisoner or a prisoner representative. The proposed research must involve no more than minimal risk, and it should not entail more than an inconvenience to subjects. The studies conducted must be linked to incarceration or to prisoners as a class. Alternatively, research must be linked to innovative or accepted practices designed to improve the health or well being of prisoners (Prisoner Research Regulations, 2001).

To be certain that prisoners can make voluntary, informed choices, the rules specify that information must be provided in language understandable to the study population. Furthermore, prisoners must be informed in advance that taking part in the study will not affect their parole (Prisoner Research Regulations, 2001).

············

PREGNANT WOMEN AND FETAL AND NEONATAL RESEARCH

Over the last two decades, research involving pregnant women and fetuses has been one of the most hotly debated aspects of the clinical trials arena. In January 2001, the Clinton Administration promulgated a final rule that was designed to enhance the opportunity for pregnant women to take part in clinical trials (January, 2001 Rule). With the change in administration, the implementation of the new rule was delayed (Rule Delay).

The Final Rule was withdrawn in November 2001 and replaced with three changes dealing with parental consent to federally funded research directed solely at a fetus, a change in the definition of the term "fetus," and the involvement of neonates of "uncertain viability" in research (November, 2001 Rule). This section describes the new requirements.

Requirements for Securing Consent to Participate in Clinical Trials: Pregnant Women, Fetal, and Neonatal Research

The Rules are quite precise for research involving either pregnant women or fetuses, imposing considerable responsibility on the IRB to make certain that all of the required conditions are met in such studies. Given the precision of the regulatory requirements, it is useful to quote the provision in its entirety.

§46.204 Research Involving Pregnant Women or Fetuses. Pregnant women or fetuses may be involved in research if all of the following conditions are met:

(a) Where scientifically appropriate, preclinical studies, including studies on pregnant animals, and clinical studies, including studies on nonpregnant women, have been conducted and provide data for assessing potential risks to pregnant women and fetuses;

(b) The risk to the fetus is caused solely by interventions or procedures that hold out the prospect of direct benefit for the woman or the fetus; or, if there is no such prospect of benefit, the risk to the fetus is not greater than minimal and the purpose of the research is the development of important biomedical knowledge which cannot be obtained by any other means;

(c) <u>Any risk is the least possible</u> for achieving the objectives of the research;

(d) If the <u>research holds out the prospect of direct benefit to</u> the <u>pregnant woman</u>, the prospect of <u>a direct benefit both to the pregnant woman and the fetus</u>, or <u>no prospect of benefit for the woman nor the fetus when risk to the fetus is not greater than minimal</u> and the <u>purpose</u> of the research is the <u>development of important biomedical knowledge that cannot be obtained by any other means</u>, her consent is obtained in accord with the informed consent provisions of subpart A of this part;

(e) If the research holds out the <u>prospect of direct benefit solely to the fetus then the consent of the pregnant woman and the father is obtained</u> in accord with the informed consent provisions of subpart A of this part, <u>except that the father's consent need not be obtained if</u> he <u>is unable to consent because of unavailability, incompetence</u>, or <u>temporary incapacity or the pregnancy resulted from rape or incest</u>.

(f) Each individual providing consent under paragraph (d) or (e) of this section is fully informed regarding the reasonably foreseeable impact of the research on the fetus or neonate;

(g) <u>For children</u> as defined in Sec. 46.402(a) <u>who are pregnant</u>, assent and permission are obtained in accord with the provisions of subpart D of this part;

(h) No inducements, monetary or otherwise, will be offered to terminate a pregnancy;

(i) Individuals engaged in the research will have no part in any decisions as to the timing, method, or procedures used to terminate a pregnancy; and

(j) Individuals engaged in the research will have no part in determining the viability of a neonate. [November, 2001 Rule. Emphasis added]

A separate provision deals with neonates. It provides:

Sec. 46.205 Research involving neonates.

(a) <u>Neonates of uncertain viability and nonviable neonates</u> may be involved in research <u>if all of the following conditions are met</u>:

1. Where scientifically appropriate, <u>preclinical</u> and clinical studies have been conducted and provide data for assessing potential risks to neonates.

2. <u>Each individual providing consent</u> under paragraph (b)(2) or (c)(5) of this section is <u>fully informed regarding the reasonably foreseeable impact of the research on the neonate</u>.

3. Individuals engaged in the research will have no part in determining the viability of a neonate.

4. The requirements of paragraph (b) or (c) of this section have been met as applicable.

(b) <u>Neonates of uncertain viability</u>. <u>Until</u> it has been <u>ascertained</u> whether or not a <u>neonate is viable</u>, a <u>neonate may not be involved</u> in <u>research covered by this subpart unless</u> the following additional conditions are met:

1. The IRB determines that:
   (i) The <u>research holds out the prospect of enhancing the probability of survival of the neonate to the point of viability</u>, and <u>any risk</u> is the least <u>possible</u> for achieving that objective, or
   (ii) The <u>purpose</u> of the research is the <u>development of important biomedical knowledge which cannot be obtained by other means</u> and there will be <u>no added risk to the neonate</u> resulting from the research; and

2. The <u>legally effective informed consent of either parent</u> of the neonate <u>or</u>, if neither parent is able to consent because of unavailability, incompetence, or temporary incapacity, the legally effective informed <u>consent of either parent's legally authorized representative is obtained</u> in accord with subpart A of this part, <u>except that the consent of the father or his legally authorized representative need not be obtained if the pregnancy resulted from rape or incest</u>.

(c) <u>Nonviable neonates</u>. <u>After delivery</u> nonviable neonate <u>may not be involved in research</u> covered by this subpart <u>unless all of the following additional conditions are met</u>:

1. <u>Vital functions of the neonate will not be artificially maintained</u>;
2. The <u>research will not terminate the heartbeat or respiration</u> of the neonate;
3. There will be <u>no added risk to the neonate</u> resulting <u>from</u> the <u>research</u>;
4. The <u>purpose</u> of the research is the <u>development of important biomedical knowledge</u> that <u>cannot be obtained by other means</u>; and
5. The <u>legally effective informed consent of both parents</u> of the neonate is obtained in accord with subpart A of this part, <u>except</u> that the <u>waiver and alteration provisions of Sec. 46.116(c) and (d) do not apply</u>. However, <u>if either parent is unable to consent</u> because of unavailability, incompetence, or temporary incapacity, the <u>informed consent of one parent</u> of a nonviable neonate <u>will suffice</u> to meet the requirements of this paragraph (c)(5), <u>except that the consent of the father need not be obtained if the pregnancy resulted from rape or incest</u>. **The consent of a legally authorized representative of either or both of the parents of a nonviable neonate will not suffice to meet the requirements of this paragraph (c)(5).**

(d) Viable neonates. A neonate, after delivery, that has been determined to be viable may be included in research only to the extent permitted by and in accord with the requirements of subparts A and D of this part. [November, 2001 Rule. Emphasis added]

These changes took effect in December, 2001. From a practical standpoint, it is important for healthcare entities, IRBs, and clinical investigators to take steps to implement these revised regulations. Strategies for this purpose are provided in the Tips Box, below.

TIP: Revised Regulations

- Revision of current IRB protocol application for the three types of neonate research.
- Revision of consent policy and procedures to reflect research permission from both parents, one parent, or legally authorized representative. Note, however, that the legally authorized representative (as that term is used in this part of the regulation) is restricted for some types of research for nonviable neonates.
- Revise consent documentation to reflect research permission from one or both parents, and, where relevant, the legally authorized representative.
- Provide education for IRB, clinical investigators, and research staff.
- Monitor the "roll out" of the revised consent requirements with a view to modification as needed.

Federal Research Requirements That Address the Use of Placenta, Dead Fetuses, or Fetal Material

The federal rules permit research involving placenta, the remains of dead fetuses, and fetal material. This includes macerated fetal material, cells, tissues, and organs removed from a dead fetus. Such research, however, is subject to any applicable federal, state, or local laws. Some states have very precise requirements governing fetal research (see Chapter Three).

However, *if* this type of research information is linked with living persons who can be identified, they are considered research subjects, and all the relevant subparts of this regulation are applicable (November, 2001 Rule). Such identifier-linked research should also take into consideration the HIPAA Privacy Rule (see Chapter Six) and relevant state law.

The Opportunity for Studies Involving Pregnancy and Fetuses That Otherwise Does Not Meet the Requirements of the Regulations

For research involving pregnant women, neonates, and fetuses that does not fit within the categories outlined in the regulations for such research some latitude is granted the secretary of HHS to conduct or fund some studies. Such research must present an opportunity to understand, prevent, or alleviate a serious problem impacting either the health or welfare of pregnant women, fetuses, or neonates.

The secretary does not act unilaterally. Rather, the secretary must consult a multidisciplinary panel, and there must be a public review and comment that includes a public meeting. The determination to conduct or fund such research must find that the study satisfies the regulatory requirements for research involving pregnant women or fetuses, or

1. The research presents a reasonable opportunity to further the understanding, prevention or alleviation of a serious problem affecting the welfare of pregnant women, fetuses or neonates;

2. The research will be *conducted in accord with sound ethical principles;* and

3. *Informed consent will be obtained* in accordance with the informed consent provisions of subpart A and other applicable subparts of this part. [November, 2001 Rule, §46.207, emphasis added]

To satisfy this exceptional requirement, an investigator must surmount several challenges, which may prove to be a time-consuming task. There must be sufficient documentation to substantiate the regulatory requirements. Moreover, there must be an alignment of interests among the multidisciplinary panel and the public. For many researchers, this challenge may deter them from proceeding with such research pursuits in favor of those studies that fit within the existing regulatory framework with respect to pregnant women, neonates, and fetuses.

············

DECISIONALLY INCAPABLE RESEARCH SUBJECTS

Obtaining consent from someone with suspected Alzheimer's disease, other forms of dementia, or decisional incapability is a thorny issue in clinical research. No doubt research is needed to find ways to successfully manage or perhaps cure ailments that leave individuals unable to make treatment decisions for themselves. The problem is that these same individuals constitute a vulnerable population who may be seen as easy prey for those who would conduct needless or harmful research on them. This section examines the issue of consent from the standpoint of the decisionally incapable research subject.

Securing Consent for Clinical Trials Research Participation for a Decisionally Incapable Subject

In 1998 and 1999, the National Bioethics Advisory Commission (NBAC) issued a report and a series of commissioned papers on the subject of the decisionally incapable person who might be a candidate to participate in human research (NBAC Documents). The report contained a number of interesting recommendations including:

- Using Special Standing Panels, precluding research involving the use of decisionally incapable persons from research that could be done with other population groups.
- Expanding the authority of legally authorized representatives with regard to clinical research consents.
- Developing Prospective Authorization for participation in clinical trials.

Thus far, federal regulators have not acted on these recommendations. A report prepared by the Office of Extramural Research of NIH ("Questionable") did offer some thoughtful suggestions to assist IRBs in handling such research. One idea was to utilize advance directives in states in which enabling legislation includes clinical trials research within the scope of such decision-making tools. This is an important consideration since it would enable a person while capable of doing so to delineate the types of clinical trials research he or she would want to participate in when no longer able to make such choices in real time. It would also provide the person with the opportunity to delineate unacceptable types of research. From a practical perspective, this idea will take some legwork. It means working with the community, clinicians, members of the estate planning bar, and social service professionals to get the word out that research participation is a viable consideration in an advance directive. This may be a very meaningful opportunity for someone afflicted with early onset of Alzheimer's disease or Huntington's disease who wants to make a contribution to research. While capable of doing so, the afflicted individual can make such a choice and include it in the advance directive. As such, working with national, regional, and local support groups may be another vehicle for promoting inclusion of such language in an advance directive. The key is to make certain that the provisions of the advance directive are consistent with both applicable federal and state laws governing clinical trials research with a so-called vulnerable population. Given the importance of research with decisionally incapable persons, it should be anticipated that state laws will change to accommodate this new genre of advance directives.

It is important to remember that the basic requirements for informed consent to participate in clinical trials *do permit* the involvement of the decisionally incapable. In essence, the regulations, while protecting those who cannot look after themselves, also try to reach a balance so that such individuals are not discriminated against and left out from the potential pool of research subjects. A successful consent process can be completed with the subject's legally authorized representative (Consent Regulations, 2001). The legally authorized representative would be someone recognized as having not only such legal status but the statutory authority to consent to the subject being a participant in clinical trials. This requires a state-by-state analysis. States may have broad-based laws and regulations governing human research that address the consent requirements for the decisionally incapable. Other jurisdictions may address the issue in highly focused provisions for the mentally ill, mentally challenged, or developmentally disabled. Furthermore, even if a state permits a legally authorized representative to consent to involvement of an incapable person in research, there may be limits on the types of permissible research activities. These limits may be imposed by a private funding source or an IRB. Hence, IRBs and research investigators should familiarize themselves with the requirements in their jurisdiction.

If a research protocol involving decisionally incapable subjects crosses state lines, the IRB should be certain that consent and research parameters of the approved study are consistent with the laws in other jurisdictions. The failure to do so might render a study outside the scope of permissible laws and place the IRB under rigorous scrutiny for regulatory non-compliance. At the end of this chapter some useful checklist information is provided to help investigators and IRBs in making certain that such studies are within the parameters of applicable law.

. . . .

LINGUISTIC, CULTURAL, AND COMMUNICATION CHALLENGES TO CONSENT IN CLINICAL TRIALS

As noted in the chapter on selection and recruitment of research subjects, many individuals face challenges if they are viewed as candidates to participate in clinical trials. Barriers include limited English proficiency, cultural differences, and inherent communication barriers. The later may involve literacy or auditory or sight impairment. All these barriers are challenges that can be met if identified and addressed appropriately. These issues are addressed in this section of the chapter.

Clinical Trials Involving Subjects with Limited English Proficiency

The federal requirements make it clear that information needed for an informed consent must be provided in language that is understandable to the research subject. In most instances, the informed consent must be documented in writing. This means that a non-English speaking research subject should receive documentation written in the language that he or she can understand (Consent Regulations, 2001).

An option is recognized in which the informed consent information is provided verbally in association with a short form consent document that indicates the required elements of the consent have been presented verbally and a summary of the verbal communication. When this option is used, the short form consent document must be witnessed and the subject must receive copies of both the short form consent document and the summary. The witness should be fluent in both English and the language of conversation with the subject. When the services of a translator are used, this individual may serve as the witness.

Although a 1995 explanatory memo from OPRR permits the English language version of the informed consent document to serve as the summary, a prudent approach is to obviate the risk of misunderstanding and provide all documentation in the language used for the consent process. Thus, a computerized language template may be developed inexpensively for this purpose. In addition, the OPRR developed a model tool for the summary document, which can be found at the end of this chapter.

Aside from the OPRR guidance and the generalized statement on understandable language, it is important to remember that there are other federal laws governing limited

English proficiency. For example, in August 2000, the HHS issued policy guidance on meeting the needs of persons with Limited English Proficiency (LEP Guidance, 2000). Of concern to HHS was the potential for national origin discrimination under Title VI of the 1964 Civil Rights Act. The guidance is pertinent to hospitals, managed-care organizations, and health and social services research programs. It describes the ways in which such covered entities can meet their obligations in terms of furnishing interpreter and translated written materials (LEP Guidance, 2000). This is an important development for IRBs and clinical investigators. It necessitates a comparative analysis between the earlier OPRR guidance and this HHS Office of Civil Rights publication. The key is to develop practical translation practices that do not violate the discrimination provisions found in Title VI of the 1964 Civil Rights Act.

Managing Consent and Cultural Differences with Potential Research Subjects

Interestingly, there has not been any specific guidance on cultural issues and consent to clinical trials research. At the policy level, HHS has initiatives under way to deal with healthcare research disparities (CLAS Guidance, 2000). As with traditional treatment situations, sensitivity should be exerted when it comes to cultural aspects of consent to participate in clinical trials.

The specific needs of the multicultural service population can be discerned by talking with religious and cultural leaders. Indeed, taking a community-based approach might help to dispel myths and misunderstandings about the importance of multicultural involvement in clinical research trials. Oftentimes healthcare facility clergy and social service personnel can provide an introduction for this purpose. Bioethics committees can be equally useful in this regard.

Sight- and Hearing-Impaired Research Subjects and the Consent Process

Research subjects with visual or auditory disabilities are entitled to accommodation under the Americans with Disabilities Act (ADA). Similarly, Section 504 of the Rehabilitation Act of 1973 prohibits discrimination against those who are handicapped (Rehab Act). In practical terms this may mean providing disabled or handicapped subjects with language assistance. For those with auditory impairment this may mean using a sign language interpreter. With respect to the visually impaired, the assistance may come in the form of large-print documents, tapes, or braille.

Thinking in terms of regulatory compliance, when accommodation is necessary it is prudent to document that ancillary tools or services were used to obtain an effective consent. For example, if a sign interpreter is used with a group of deaf subjects, the name of the interpreter should be documented along with the type of sign language used in the consent process. Administratively there should be a demonstrated competency benchmark to make certain that interpreters are qualified to fulfill their responsibilities. Taking these additional steps eliminates possible questions about regulatory compliance. It also reduces the risk of claims based on negligent consent to research.

Overcoming Literacy Challenges to Effective Communication

Literacy can be a difficult hurdle to surmount for those with limited reading ability. It can be an arduous task for someone with a Grade 4 reading level to comprehend the content of a consent form or information sheet written at the level of a high school graduate.

Many would-be research subjects may be embarrassed to admit that they cannot read or don't read well.

Rather than taking the chance that a would-be subject does *not* understand, there are some practical steps that can be taken to overcome the challenge. For example:

- *Verify Comprehension Level Requirements*—The IRB can set standards for reading comprehension for all information and consent tools used with the research subject. If the documentation does not meet the specifications, it can reject the documents until such time as the principal investigator and research staff meet the requirements.

- *Assess Subject Reading Skill*—Even if bluntly asked, "Can you read?" a subject may be less than forthright in his or her answer. To avoid such embarrassing confrontations, a qualification may be put in place that requires each potential subject to read a paragraph tested as meeting the comprehension level set by the IRB. If the would-be subject cannot answer comprehension questions, it is an indicator that further inquiry is necessary. It may be that the subject is ill-suited for the study, particularly if the research requires a higher level of reading comprehension for protocol compliance. In other instances, it may mean revising the instructions and consent tools so that the information is meaningful and understandable.

....

OTHER TOPICS FOR DISCLOSURE IN RESEARCH CONSENTS

Beyond the realm of potential benefits and potential risks associated with a study there is other information that is pertinent to a potential research subject. This includes sharing information about adverse events and commercial use of valuable tissues and cells. These topics are addressed in this section of the chapter.

Anticipating Adverse Events in the Clinical Trials Consent Process

The HHS consent provisions do not address adverse events. Rather, the terminology is research-related injury. Indeed, one of the eight elements of an effective research consent focuses on this issue. Research subjects must be told whether compensation and medical treatments are available if injury should occur. The explanation should describe what is available and where additional information may be obtained. The name of the individual to contact in the event of a research-related injury should also be provided to subjects.

It is important to note that the regulations prohibit exculpatory language in the consent. This means that the research subject cannot be made to waive or appear to waive any legal rights, including the right to pursue litigation for negligence. The emphasis is definitely on informing subjects about their rights in the event that an injury takes place that is related to the study.

From a practical perspective, this could be part of a far more complex situation. A research subject may also be a patient for purposes of traditional therapy. When an injury occurs, it may not be clear whether it emanated from the research side or traditional treatment component of the clinical intervention. Under the Conditions of Participation for Hospitals in Medicare and Medicaid (Conditions of Participants, 1999), patients are entitled to file grievances and to obtain an explanation of the findings of the resulting investigation. It may be difficult to separate out the research component from the traditional therapeutic side of the grievance. This is especially important when the research protocol offers subjects compensation or medical care for injury related to the clinical trial. Absent good communication between clinical trial staff officials and facility-based risk management professionals, the opportunity may be missed for proper handling of such complex cases. The result may be regulatory scrutiny not only for failure to comply with research requirements but also the Conditions of Participation. This is a subject that merits careful attention in terms of informed consent. Subjects should know their rights regarding *both* research-related injury and the grievance process under the Conditions of Participation. From a practical perspective, it demonstrates the need for solid communication strategies between clinical research staff and the risk management department (see Chapter Fifteen).

Information Needed in the Consent Process Regarding Potential Commercial Value of Tissues or Cellular Material Discovered in the Course of Clinical Research

Following a highly publicized case involving a research subject with hairy cell leukemia, many IRBs refined their consent requirements to address commercial value material discovered in the course of a clinical trial ("Moe Cell Line Case," 1988). Many now require consent discussions and documentation to alert subjects to the fact that tissues or cellular material analyzed during a research trial may show indications that it has commercial value. For example, the subject may be informed that:

> It is possible that during the course of the research trial it may be determined that you have a commercially viable strain of cells or tissues. Should this be the case, you will be informed of this determination. You will then be asked whether this material may be removed for commercial purposes either with or without financial remuneration to you. The decision you reach will not influence your continued participation in the research study or any conventional treatment you are entitled to receive beyond the scope of the study.

There are two reasons for such a disclosure. First, it is important that the research subject does not feel coerced or influenced by the commercial viability issue. Second, it is to avoid the appearance of a conflict-of-interest on the part of the research investigator. Once a decision is made, the determination should be properly documented in accordance with established policy and procedure on clinical research consents.

EMERGENCY RESEARCH CONSENT REQUIREMENTS

Regulations promulgated by the FDA and a waiver by the HHS permit so-called consentless research. Some states have also followed suit by enacting similar laws. The exception permits consentless research in a limited number of situations and only *after* it is certain the IRB is satisfied that the protocol meets delineated criteria. The notion of research without consent presents a challenge to traditional views on involvement of subjects in clinical trials. It merits particular consideration, especially in view of other federal laws and practical considerations that seem to run contrary to the idea of consentless research.

Emergency Clinical Trials Research and Consent

The federal rule and waiver attempt to track the emergency exception to the rules of consent for use of generally recognized treatments or interventions. In nonresearch settings, an emergency involves a life-threatening or health-threatening event for which treatment is needed immediately. The patient is unable to participate in the consent process and there is no time to find and secure a treatment authorization from a duly authorized legal representative. In such instances the law implies that the person would consent to such treatment as is needed to alleviate the problem. Research consents are premised on the need for a detailed disclosure of information such that the subject or a legally authorized representative can voluntarily agree to the individual's participation in a research trial. Consentless human research marks a major shift in thinking in the arena of consent.

For the FDA, the requirements go beyond consent and include provisions that involve new drug applications (INDs) and investigational device exemptions (IDEs). When first published in the *Federal Register* in October 1996 (Emergency Rule), the preamble accompanying the FDA rule made it clear that the intent was to have consistency in application between the agency's new regulation and the waiver granted by HHS.

The FDA emergency exception (FDA Emergency Consent Regulation) includes a number of requirements. As indicated in the regulation the following criteria must be met:

1. The research subjects must be in a life-threatening situation and available treatments are unproven or unsatisfactory. The collection of valid scientific evidence is needed in order to ascertain the safety and effectiveness of specific interventions.

2. Obtaining informed consent is not feasible because the medical conditions of these subjects make them unable to give their informed consent and it is not feasible to secure the consent of legally authorized representatives prior to administering the investigatory intervention. Furthermore eligible subjects cannot be identified prospectively.

3. The subjects are facing a life-threatening situation that requires intervention. Based on the results of animal and pre-trial studies, the research holds out the prospect of direct benefit to individual subjects. The risks associated with the investigation are reasonable considering the risks and benefits of standard therapy, as compared to those involved in the proposed intervention.

4. Without a waiver the clinical investigation could not practicably be conducted by the clinical investigator.

5. The principal investigator has agreed to attempt to reach a legally authorized representative for each subject within the proposed therapeutic window, and, if possible, to seek the legally authorized representative's consent instead of proceeding without such an authorization. At the time of continuing review, the IRB must receive from the principal investigator a summary of the efforts made to contact legally authorized representatives.

6. The IRB has approved the informed consent procedures and document to be used with subjects or their legally authorized representatives in situations when the situation permits the use of such procedures and documentation. Moreover, the IRB has approved the procedures to be followed when offering a family member to object to an individual's involvement in the clinical study.

Aside from these requirements, there are additional protections found in the FDA regulations for emergency research subjects:

(i) Consultation (including, where appropriate, consultation carried out by the IRB) with representatives of the communities in which the clinical investigation will be conducted and from which the subjects will be drawn;

(ii) Public disclosure to the communities in which the clinical investigation will be conducted and from which the subjects will be drawn, prior to initiation of the clinical investigation, of plans for the investigation and its risks and expected benefits;

(iii) Public disclosure of sufficient information following completion of the clinical investigation to apprise the community and researchers of the study, including the demographic characteristics of the research population, and its results;

(iv) Establishment of an independent data monitoring committee to exercise oversight of the clinical investigation; and

(v) If obtaining informed consent is not feasible and a legally authorized representative is not reasonably available, the investigator has committed, if feasible, to attempting to contact within the therapeutic window the subject's family member who is not a legally authorized representative, and asking whether he or she objects to the subject's participation in the clinical investigation. The investigator will summarize efforts made to contact family members and make this information available to the IRB at the time of continuing review.

It is important to note that the IRB has the responsibility to make certain that procedures are in place to inform the subject or the legally authorized representative or family member of an incapacitated subject as soon as possible of the individual's involvement in the study. This includes information about the right to discontinue participation in the study without loss of benefits or any penalty.

For its part, the HHS waiver tracks the FDA regulation. In granting this waiver HHS indicated that it was intended for a narrow class of studies "involving human subjects who are in need of emergency medical intervention but who cannot give informed consent because of their life-threatening medical condition and who do not have available a legally authorized person to represent them" (*Federal Register:* 61(192): 51533, October 2, 1996).

Notwithstanding the FDA regulatory change and the HHS waiver, problems have persisted in terms of the operational aspects of emergency research. In 1998, almost two years after the revised rule took effect, FDA issued an information sheet entitled, "Emergency Use of an Investigational Drug or Biologic." This was seen as being needed to clear up confusion between the informed consent *exception* for "planned" emergency described earlier (21 CFR §50.24), and the emergency *exemption* from prospective IRB approval found in a different part of the regulations (21 CFR §104). The Information Sheet reinforced a key point: informed consent is needed prior to emergency use of a test article (21 CFR §50.23) unless the principal investigator believes immediate use is needed in order to preserve the subject's life. In such instances, a mechanism is in place for documenting and reporting such use of a test article.

In March 2000, the FDA published a draft guidance document to deal with relevant matters required for implementation of the emergency research regulation. The guidance has yet to be finalized by the FDA. Even this draft document fails to address some very practical issues surrounding emergency research. For example:

- *Community Notification*—It is laudable that the public is to be notified about IRB approved emergency research protocols. What this process does not contemplate is that many accident victims may not be from the community in which notification took place. The United States is a very mobile society. The person in a life-threatening situation may be a resident in a state hundreds of miles from the test facility. In effect, the geographic disparity nullifies the value of community notification.

- *Potential for Conflict with Advance Directives*—A research protocol may be incongruent with the express, written desires of a would-be test subject as articulated in an advance directive. If for example an advance directive states that the individual does not want to receive any heroic measures, it may be interpreted as precluding enrollment in emergency clinical trials. Failure to check for advance directives or acting against the express wishes of the declarant in an advance directive could prove embarrassing and potentially serve as the basis for litigation based on unauthorized interventions.

- *Conflict with the Emergency Medical Treatment and Active Labor Act (EMTALA)*—The EMTALA requirements include screening examinations, stabilization, and an informed consent process. It would appear that the FDA emergency research provision and the HHS waiver may at times conflict with EMTALA. This could result in burdensome federal investigations. If EMTALA is deemed to take precedence over the emergency research rule, a facility could be embroiled in significant regulatory problems.

- *Potential for Discrimination*—Those individuals in a life-threatening situation are particularly vulnerable. Unable to speak for themselves, they could be enrolled in a research intervention to which they would otherwise object. Is it not possible that an argument could be made that these provisions violate the Americans with Disabilities Act (ADA) and Section 504 of the Rehabilitation Act of 1973? Do the FDA and HHS emergency research provisions unlawfully discriminate on the basis of disability and handicap? This argument has yet to be tested, and for their part, the courts try their best to reconcile what appears to be conflicting federal laws. If such a challenge were successful, it would force the FDA and HHS to rethink the idea of an emergency research exception.

- *Denial of coverage*—While the emergency research phase of the protocol may cover related costs, this may not be true for longer-term follow-up treatment. Many healthcare plans stipulate that experimental or research interventions are not considered a covered benefit. Under nonemergent research, the consent process delves into expenses not covered by the study. Emergency research subjects do not have the benefit of such material information. In effect, the decision is being made for them by imputing their agreement to participate in research. Such an inference may not be warranted. If this is the case, who will pay for continued intervention? Can the research subject look to the investigator or the sponsor to cover these expenses? This too is ripe for a legal challenge.

These practical issues merit careful attention. Those concerns linked to EMTALA, the ADA, §504 of the Rehabilitation Act of 1973, and advance directives are particularly amenable to well-written policies, procedures, and practices. Education for personnel involved in emergency research is imperative as is the documentation process. On the latter point, this would include criteria for determining that the subject is unable to make a decision regarding involvement in the study, that it is not feasible to secure an authorization from a legally authorized representative, and that a reasonable effort was made to ascertain if the would-be subject possessed an advance directive in a wallet or articles of clothing.

WITHDRAWAL OF CONSENT

Just as there is a right to consent to participate in research, there is a right to withdraw from taking part in it. Like other consent situations, the focus should be on an informed withdrawal of consent. The subject should understand the actual and potential consequences of such a decision for himself and the study. In providing such information, the research investigator should not exert undue influence or appear coercive in explaining the consequences to the subject. It must be a balanced dialogue. Moreover, as suggested in this section, the discussion should be documented.

When a Subject Withdraws Consent to Participate in a Clinical Trial

The regulations provide for research subjects to be informed of their right to discontinue participation in the research study at any time without fear of penalty or loss of benefits to which they are entitled. In addition, investigators may be required by an IRB to disclose to subjects the consequences of withdrawing from the study and procedures for terminating their participation in the research (Consent Regulations, 2001).

Beyond these legal parameters there are very practical considerations when research subjects decide to withdraw. One is finding out why subjects want to leave the study. This can be done without running afoul of claims of intimidation, coercion, or undue influence. Asking some pertinent questions may reveal some lifestyle or transportation issues that can be addressed without "playing favorites" among the subject population. The second is to make certain that subjects understand the nature and consequences of their decisions to leave the study. Once again, it must be an honest disclosure free of language that might intimidate, coerce, or unduly influence them. Third, withdrawal from the study should be documented. Fourth, the number of subjects lost to follow-up should be tracked, as it may be evidence of a study design issue, a subject selection problem, or a communication issue that can be corrected before more individuals decide to leave the study.

....

MODIFICATIONS AND WAIVERS OF CONSENT

The federal requirements permit some alteration to the standard consent requirements. Such modification or waiver is carefully described in the federal rules. As described in this section, the IRB plays a pivotal role in such modification or waiver determinations.

Modification to the Consent Requirements by an IRB

In a number of circumstances alteration of the consent requirements is permitted under the federal requirements. This can be done upon a documented determination by an IRB that the research involved a project under the aegis or approval of a state or local government. In these projects the intent is to evaluate:

1. Public benefit or service programs.
2. Procedures for obtaining benefits or services under those programs.
3. Possible changes in or alternatives to those programs or procedures.
4. Possible changes in methods or levels of payment for benefits or services under those programs.

An important consideration for the IRB in these circumstances is a determination that the research could not practicably be carried out without the alteration to the consent requirements (Consent Regulations, 2001).

An IRB may also grant permission to alter the consent requirements in research that is not under the direction or approval of a state or local government. In these cases, the IRB must be satisfied that the research involves no more than minimal risk to subjects and altering the consent provisions will not adversely effect either the rights or welfare of these individuals. Moreover, it must be demonstrated that absent the alteration or a waiver of the consent provision it would not be practical to conduct the study. The IRB may also stipulate that whenever appropriate, the subjects will be provided with additional pertinent information after participation (Consent Regulations, 2001).

When the Consent Requirements Can Be Waived by an IRB

The federal requirements recognize two categories of research in which the consent requirements may be waived by an IRB. Specifically, the regulations state that this applies to research in which the only document linking the subject to the research would be the consent form and the primary risk would be a breach of confidentiality. In these cases, the research subject would be asked if he or she wants such documentation.

The other circumstance involves procedures with no more than minimal risk, and in the therapeutic treatment setting there ordinarily would be no requirement of a written informed consent for such care. It should be noted that the IRB may require the investigator to provide subjects with a written statement regarding the research.

The IRB should be familiar with the HIPAA waiver requirements when using the first type of confidentiality-based provision. This is a subject of discussion in Chapter Six.

············

CONSENT DOCUMENTATION

As is frequently acknowledged, consent is a process, *not* a form. However, some type of consent documentation is needed to provide evidence of successful completion of an authorization to participate in clinical trials research. In this section, the federal rules for documenting clinical trials consent are the focal point of discussion. Both the short form and long form consent methodologies are examined, and sample tools are provided for this purpose from federal resources.

Documenting Consent to Participate in Clinical Trials

Under the Code of Federal Regulations, there are basically two types of consent documentation methods recognized in clinical trials (Consent Documentation Regulation, 2001). One is a so-called long form consent document, and the other is a short form. The specific provision (emphasis added) states:

> A written consent document that embodies the elements of informed consent required by §46.116. This form *may be read to the subject* or the subject's legally authorized representative, but in any event, the investigator shall give either the subject or the representative *adequate opportunity to read it before it is signed;* or (2) A *short form written consent* document stating that the elements of informed consent required by §46.116 have been presented orally to the subject or the subject's legally authorized representative. When this method is used, *there shall be a witness to the oral presentation.* Also, the IRB shall approve a written summary of what is to be said to the subject or the representative. Only the short form itself is to be signed by the subject or the representative. However, the witness shall sign both the short form and a copy of the summary, and the person actually obtaining consent shall sign a copy of the summary. A copy of the summary shall be given to the subject or the representative, in addition to a copy of the short form.

From a practical standpoint, the IRB should give consideration to including the steps outlined in the documentation regulation in its policy and procedure on consent. Educational programs should provide clinical investigators and their staff members with flowchart diagrams that map out the necessary steps for documentation of the consent process. In this way, confusion regarding the long form and short form requirements can be avoided. Moreover, the educational program serves as a good opportunity to reinforce that the document is of the consent process and *not* a substitute for the communication that should take place between the clinical investigator and research subject (Rozovsky, 2000).

Sample Consent Tools from Federal Departments

A number of Federal Departments have prepared sample consent tools for clinical trials. These documents can be found on the Internet. Some of these tools can be found at the end of this chapter.

....

CONCLUSION: PRACTICAL SUGGESTIONS FOR OBTAINING CONSENT TO PARTICIPATE IN CLINICAL TRIALS

Beyond the sample tools made available by federal departments, there are a number of practical suggestions to facilitate obtaining a legally effective consent for clinical trial research. These include the following:

1. Develop a comprehensive research consent policy and procedure that anticipates problematic areas such as
   - Consent from those considered as vulnerable subjects (children, the decisionally incapable, pregnant women, prisoners, etc.)
   - Documentation
   - Emergency consents
   - Handicapped and disabled subjects
   - Legally authorized representatives
   - Limited English proficiency
   - Monitoring the consent process
   - Who may inform the subject
   - Who must secure consent to participate in the clinical trial
   - Withdrawal from a study
2. Train investigators on the proper methods to use in securing consent to participate in research.
3. Develop in-service programs that reinforce proper consent techniques in problematic areas or concerns identified in consent monitoring activities.
4. Manage the consent process for those who are both research subjects *and* recipients of conventional medical therapy.
5. Validate reading level of consent documentation.
6. Use confirmatory questions to verify that subjects understand the nature and purpose of the study, any anticipated benefits and risks, etc.

7. Avoid practices such as reliance on head nods in lieu of subjects answering questions, or providing responses to questions that are inconsistent with the query posed by the clinical investigator.

8. Manage consent with subjects receiving pain management.

9. Use interpreters, braille, sign language or other communications tools for consent to clinical research.

10. Coordinate the consent provisions with other relevant provisions such as the Emergency Treatment and Active Labor Act, the Patient Self-Determination Act, and applicable state laws such as those that encompass research authorizations in advance directives.

References

Americans with Disabilities Act of 1990, 42 U.S.C. §§ 12101 et seq.

Children as Research Subjects' and Consent, Subpart D, 45 CFR §46.401, et seq. (2001).

Code of Federal Regulations 45 CFR Part 46; revised 11/13/2001, Effective December 13, 2001.

Conditions of Participation for Hospitals in Medicare and Medicaid, Patients Rights Standards, Federal Register 64, (127). pp. 36069–36089, July 2, 1999.

Consent Documentation Regulation, 45 CGF §46.117 (2001).

Consent Regulations, 45 CFR §46.116 (2001).

Emergency Rule. *Federal Register:* 61(192): 51497, October 2, 1996.

EMTALA Section 1867 of the Social Security Act; 42 U.S.C. 1395dd.

FDA Emergency Research Regulation, Regulation 21 CFR Parts 50.56, 312, 314, 601, 812, and 814.

HHS Waiver 45 CFR Section 46.101(i).

LEP Guidance, "Limited English Proficient Persons; Civil Rights Act Title VI Prohibition Against National Origin Discrimination; Policy Guidance," Federal Register, 65(169); pp. 52762–52774, August 30, 2000. See also Department of Justice, "Guidance to Federal Financial Assistance Recipients Regarding Title VI Prohibition Against National Origin Discrimination Affecting Limited English Proficient Persons," April 12, 2002.

"Moe Cell Line Case," Moore v. Regents of Univ. of Cal., 249 Cal. Rptr. 494 (Cal.Ct.App. 1988); See also Office of Technology Assessment, *New Developments in Biotechnology: 1 Ownership of Human Tissues and Cells,* 1987.

National Bioethics Advisory Commission (NBAC), *Research Involving Persons with Mental Disorders That May Affect Decisionmaking Capacity Volume I December, 1998 and Volume II,* March, 1999.

National Standards on Culturally and Linguistically Appropriate Services (CLAS) in Health Care, *Federal Register* 65(247): pp. 80865, et seq. December 22, 2000. November 2001 Regulations, 42 CFR §§46.201-46.207 (2001).

Office of Extramural Research NIH, "Research Involving Individuals with Questionable Capacity to Consent: Points to Consider."

Parental Consent to Research, 45 CFR §46.405 (2001).

Prisoner Research Regulations, Subpart C, 45 CFR §301, et seq. (2001).

Research on Wards, 45 CFR §46.409 (2001).

Rozovsky, F. A. (2000) *Consent to Treatment A Practical Guide, Third Edition.* Gaithersburg, Maryland: Aspen Publishers (December, 2002 Supplement), Chapter 8.

Section 504 of the Rehabilitation Act of 1973, as amended 29 U.S.C. §794.

OPRR SAMPLE SHORT FORM WRITTEN CONSENT DOCUMENT FOR SUBJECTS WHO DO NOT SPEAK ENGLISH

THIS DOCUMENT MUST BE WRITTEN IN A LANGUAGE UNDERSTANDABLE TO THE SUBJECT

Consent to Participate in Research

You are being asked to participate in a research study.

Before you agree, the investigator must tell you about (i) the purposes, procedures, and duration of the research; (ii) any procedures which are experimental; (iii) any reasonably foreseeable risks, discomforts, and benefits of the research; (iv) any potentially beneficial alternative procedures or treatments; and (v) how confidentiality will be maintained.

Where applicable, the investigator must also tell you about (i) any available compensation or medical treatment if injury occurs; (ii) the possibility of unforeseeable risks; (iii) circumstances when the investigator may halt your participation; (iv) any added costs to you; (v) what happens if you decide to stop participating; (vi) when you will be told about new findings which may affect your willingness to participate; and (vii) how many people will be in the study.

If you agree to participate, you must be given a signed copy of this document and a written summary of the research.

You may contact _____ name _____ at _____ phone number _____ any time you have questions about the research.

You may contact _____ name _____ at _____ phone number _____ if you have questions about your rights as a research subject or what to do if you are injured.

Your participation in this research is voluntary, and you will not be penalized or lose benefits if you refuse to participate or decide to stop.

Signing this document means that the research study, including the above information, has been described to you orally, and that you voluntarily agree to participate.

_____
signature of participant

_____
date

_____
signature of witness
11/09/95

_____
date

§46.116 - Informed Consent Checklist—Basic and Additional Elements

	A statement that the study involves research
	An explanation of the purposes of the research
	The expected duration of the subject's participation
	A description of the procedures to be followed
	Identification of any procedures which are experimental
	A description of any reasonably foreseeable risks or discomforts to the subject
	A description of any benefits to the subject or to others which may reasonably be expected from the research
	A disclosure of appropriate alternative procedures or courses of treatment, if any, that might be advantageous to the subject
	A statement describing the extent, if any, to which confidentiality of records identifying the subject will be maintained
	For research involving more than minimal risk, an explanation as to whether any compensation, and an explanation as to whether any medical treatments are available, if injury occurs and, if so, what they consist of, or where further information may be obtained
( ) Research Qs	An explanation of whom to contact for answers to pertinent questions about the research and research subjects' rights, and whom to contact in the event of a research-related injury to the subject
( ) Rights Qs	
( ) Injury Qs	
	A statement that participation is voluntary, refusal to participate will involve no penalty or loss of benefits to which the subject is otherwise entitled, and the subject may discontinue participation at any time without penalty or loss of benefits, to which the subject is otherwise entitled
Additional elements, as appropriate	
	A statement that the particular treatment or procedure may involve risks to the subject (or to the embryo or fetus, if the subject is or may become pregnant), which are currently unforeseeable
	Anticipated circumstances under which the subject's participation may be terminated by the investigator without regard to the subject's consent
	Any additional costs to the subject that may result from participation in the research
	The consequences of a subject's decision to withdraw from the research and procedures for orderly termination of participation by the subject
	A statement that significant new findings developed during the course of the research, which may relate to the subject's willingness to continue participation, will be provided to the subject
	The approximate number of subjects involved in the study

§46.117 - **Documentation of Informed Consent Checklist**

a. Except as provided in paragraph "c" of this section, informed consent shall be documented by the use of a written consent form approved by the IRB, and signed by the subject or the subject's legally authorized representative. A copy shall be given to the person signing the form.	
WRITTEN	The consent form may be either of the following: 1. A **written consent** document that embodies the elements of informed consent required by §46.116. This form may be read to the subject or the subject's legally authorized representative, but in any event, the investigator should give either the subject or the representative adequate opportunity to read it before it is signed.
DONE ORALLY	2. A **short form written consent** document, stating that the elements of informed consent required by §46.116 have been presented **orally** to the subject or the subject's legally authorized representative. When this method is used, there shall be a **witness** to the oral presentation. Also, the IRB shall approve a **written summary** of what is to be said to the subject or the representative. Only the short form itself is to be signed by the subject or the representative. However, the witness shall sign both the short form and a copy of the summary, and the person actually obtaining consent shall sign a copy of the summary. A copy of the summary shall be given to the subject or the representative, in addition to a copy of the short form.
WAIVER of req't for signed form	c. An IRB may waive the requirement for the investigator to obtain a signed consent form for some or all subjects, if it finds either: 1. That the only record linking the subject and the research would be the consent document, and the **principal risk** would be potential harm resulting from a breach of confidentiality. Each subject will be asked whether the subject wants documentation linking the subject with the research, and the subject's wishes will govern; or 2. That the research presents **no more than minimal risk** of harm to subjects, and involves no procedures, for which written consent is normally required outside of the research context. In cases in which the documentation requirement is waived, the IRB may require the investigator to provide subjects with a written statement regarding the research.

IRB Latitude to Approve a Consent Procedure That Alters or Waives Some or All of the Elements of Consent

§46.116 - An IRB may approve a consent procedure, which does not include, or which alters, some or all of the elements of informed consent set forth in this section, or waive the requirements to obtain informed consent, provided the IRB finds and documents that:

	C: 1. The research or demonstration project is to be conducted by, or subject to the approval of, state or local government officials, and is designed to study, evaluate, or otherwise examine: (i) public benefit or service programs; (ii) procedures for obtaining benefits or services under those programs; (iii) possible changes in or alternatives to those programs or procedures; or (iv) possible changes in methods or levels of payment for benefits or services under those programs; and
	C: 2. The research could not practicably be carried out without the waiver or alteration.
	D: 1. The research involves no more than minimal risk to the subjects;
	D: 2. The waiver or alteration will not adversely affect the rights and welfare of the subjects;
	D: 3. The research could not practicably be carried out without the waiver or alteration; and
	D: 4. Whenever appropriate, the subjects will be provided with additional pertinent information after participation.

Special Requirements—45 CFR §46 Subpart D—Additional DHHS Protections for Children Involved as Subjects in Research	
Assent/Waiver	The IRB shall determine that adequate provisions are made for soliciting the assent of the children, when in the judgment of the IRB the children are capable of providing assent. If the IRB determines that the capability of some or all of the children is so limited that they cannot reasonably be consulted, or that the intervention or procedure involved in the research holds out a prospect of direct benefit that is important to the health or well-being of the children, and is available only in the context of the research, the assent of the children is not a necessary condition for proceeding with the research. Even where the IRB determines that the subjects are capable of assenting, the IRB may still waive the assent requirement under circumstances, in which consent may be waived in accord with §46.116 of Subpart A.
Parents	The IRB may find that the permission of **one** parent is sufficient for research to be conducted under §46.404 or §46.405.

Special Requirements (*Continued*)	
	Where research is covered by §46.406 and §46.407, and permission is to be obtained from parents, **both parents must give their permission**, unless one parent is deceased, unknown, incompetent, or not reasonably available, or when only one parent has legal responsibility for the care and custody of the child.
	If the IRB determines that a research protocol is designed for conditions or for a subject population, for which parental or guardian permission is not a reasonable requirement to protect the subjects (for example, neglected or abused children), it may waive the consent requirements in Subpart A of this part and paragraph (b) of this section, provided an appropriate mechanism for protecting the children who will participate as subjects in the research is substituted, and provided further that the waiver is not inconsistent with Federal, state or local law.

09/30/98

Policy and Assurances | OHRP Home Page

*If you have questions about human subject research, click   **ohrp@osophs.dhhs.gov***
*If you have questions/suggestions about this web page, click   **Webmaster***
Updated June 23, 2000

Office for Protection from Research Risks

TIPS ON INFORMED CONSENT

The process of obtaining informed consent must comply with the requirements of **45 CFR §46.116**. The documentation of informed consent must comply with **45 CFR §46.117**. The following comments may help in the development of an approach and proposed language by investigators for obtaining consent and its approval by IRBs:

- Informed consent is a process, not just a form. Information must be presented to enable persons to voluntarily decide whether or not to participate as a research subject. It is a fundamental mechanism to ensure respect for persons through provision of thoughtful consent for a voluntary act. The procedures used in obtaining informed consent should be designed to educate the subject population in terms that they can understand. Therefore, informed consent language and its documentation (especially explanation of the study's purpose, duration, experimental procedures, alternatives, risks, and benefits) must be written in "lay language", (i.e. understandable to the people being asked to participate). The written presentation of information is used to document the basis for consent and for the subjects' future reference. The consent document should be revised when deficiencies are noted or when additional information will improve the consent process.

- Use of the first person (e.g., "I understand that . . .") can be interpreted as suggestive, may be relied upon as a substitute for sufficient factual information, and can constitute coercive influence over a subject. Use of scientific jargon and legalese is not appropriate. Think of the document primarily as a teaching tool not as a legal instrument.

- **Describe the overall experience that will be encountered**. Explain the research activity, how it is experimental (e.g., a new drug, extra tests, separate research records, or nonstandard means of management, such as flipping a coin for random assignment or other design issues). Inform the human subjects of the reasonably foreseeable harms, discomforts, inconvenience and risks that are associated with the research activity. If additional risks are identified during the course of the research, the consent process and documentation will require revisions to inform subjects as they are recontacted or newly contacted.

- **Describe the benefits that subjects may reasonably expect to encounter**. There may be none other than a sense of helping the public at large. If payment is given to defray the incurred expense for participation, it must not be coercive in amount or method of distribution.

- **Describe any alternatives to participating in the research project**. For example, in drug studies the medication(s) may be available through their family doctor or clinic without the need to volunteer for the research activity.

- **The regulations insist that the subjects be told the extent to which their personally identifiable private information will be held in confidence**. For example, some studies require disclosure of information to other parties. Some studies inherently are in need of a Certificate of Confidentiality which protects the investigator from involuntary release (e.g., subpoena) of the names or other identifying characteristics of research subjects. The IRB will determine the level of adequate requirements for confidentiality in light of its mandate to ensure minimization of risk and determination that the residual risks warrant involvement of subjects.

- If research-related injury (i.e., physical, psychological, social, financial, or otherwise) is possible in research that is more than minimal risk (see 45 CFR §46.102[g]), an explanation must be given of whatever voluntary compensation and treatment will be provided. Note that the regulations do not limit injury to "physical injury". This is a common misinterpretation.

- The regulations prohibit waiving or appearing to waive any legal rights of subjects. Therefore, for example, consent language must be carefully selected that deals with what the institution is voluntarily willing to do under circumstances, such as providing for compensation beyond the provision of immediate or therapeutic intervention in response to a research-related injury. In short, subjects should not be given the impression that they have agreed to and are without recourse to seek satisfaction beyond the institution's voluntarily chosen limits.

- The regulations provide for the identification of contact persons who would be knowledgeable to answer questions of subjects about the research, rights as a research subject, and research-related injuries. These three areas must be explicitly stated and addressed in the consent process and documentation. Furthermore, a single person is not likely to be appropriate to answer questions in all areas. This is because of potential conflicts of interest or the appearance of such. Questions about the research are frequently best answered by the investigator(s). However, questions about the rights of research subjects or research-related injuries (where applicable) may best be referred to those not on the research team. These questions could be addressed to the IRB, an ombudsman, an ethics committee, or other informed administrative body. Therefore, each consent document can be expected to have at least two names with local telephone numbers for contacts to answer questions in these specified areas.

- The statement regarding voluntary participation and the right to withdraw at any time can be taken almost verbatim from the regulations (45 CFR §46.116[a][8]). It is important not to overlook the need to point out that no penalty or loss of benefits will occur as a result of both not participating or withdrawing at any time. It is equally important to alert potential subjects to any foreseeable consequences to them should they unilaterally withdraw while dependent on some intervention to maintain normal function.

- Don't forget to ensure provision for appropriate **additional requirements** which concern consent. Some of these requirements can be found in sections 46.116(b), 46.205(a)(2), 46.207(b), 46.208(b), 46.209(d), 46.305(a)(5-6), 46.408(c), and 46.409(b). The IRB may impose additional requirements that are not specifically listed in the regulations to ensure that adequate information is presented in accordance with institutional policy and local law.

Revised 3/16/93

Policy and Assurances | OHRP Home Page

If you have questions about human subject research, click ***ohrp@osophs.dhhs.gov***
If you have questions/suggestions about this web page, click ***Webmaster***
Updated June 23, 2000

Informed Consent Recommendations: Appendices 3, 4, and 5

APPENDIX 3: CHECKLIST FOR EASY-TO-READ INFORMED CONSENT DOCUMENTS[6,7,8,9]

TEXT

- Words are familiar to the reader. Any scientific, medical, or legal words are defined clearly.
- Words and terminology are consistent throughout the document.
- Sentences are short, simple, and direct.
- Line length is limited to 30-50 characters and spaces.
- Paragraphs are short. Convey one idea per paragraph.
- Verbs are in active voice (i.e., the subject is the doer of the act).
- Personal pronouns are used to increase personal identification.
- Each idea is clear and logically sequenced (according to audience logic).
- Important points are highlighted.
- Study purpose is presented early in the text.
- Titles, subtitles, and other headers help to clarify organization of text.
- Headers are simple and close to text.
- Underline, bold, or boxes (rather than all caps or italics) give emphasis.
- Layout balances white space with words and graphics.
- Left margins are justified. Right margins are ragged.
- Upper and lower case letters are used.
- Style of print is easy to read.
- Type size is at least 12 point.
- Readability analysis is done to determine reading level (should be eighth grade or lower).
- Avoid:
  - Abbreviations and acronyms.
  - Large blocks of print.
  - Words containing more than three syllables (where possible).

GRAPHICS

- Graphics are:
  - Helpful in explaining the text.
  - Easy to understand.
  - Meaningful to the audience.
  - Appropriately located. Text and graphics go together.
  - Simple and uncluttered.

- Images reflect cultural context.
- Visuals have captions.
- Each visual is directly related to one message.
- Cues, such as circles or arrows, point out key information.
- Colors, when used, are appealing to the audience.
- Avoid graphics that won't reproduce well.

---

[6]National Cancer Institute, *Clear and Simple,* 23.
[7]National Cancer Institute, *Making Health Communications Programs Work,* 37.
[8]C. Doak et al., *Teaching Patients With Low Literacy Skills* 2nd ed. (New York: Lippincott, 1996): 3.
[9]C. Meade, Consent forms, 1527.

APPENDIX 4: COMMUNICATION METHODS

The following communication methods may help to increase the potential research participant's comprehension of the informed consent document.

1. Time to Read and Discuss the Form

Researchers should encourage the potential research participant to thoroughly read and re-read the consent form and supplemental materials, if provided, and to discuss the proposed research with others before signing the consent form. This may require a delay between the describing of the study and the signing of the consent document.

2. Assess Understanding

It may be helpful for the researcher to ask the potential research participant short questions, after the research has been described and the consent form read, in order to assess that the potential research participant has at least a basic understanding of what the research involves.[10] Example questions include:

- Tell me in your own words what this study is all about.
- Tell me what you think will happen to you in this study.
- What do you expect to gain by taking part in this research?
- What risks might you experience by participating in the research?
- What are your alternatives (other choices or options to participating in this research)?

3. Communication Techniques

Videos, audiotapes, interactive computer programs, and discussions with qualified lay individuals may assist in educating the potential research participant about the clinical trial.

---

[10]S. Titus et al., "Do you understand? An ethical assessment of researchers' description of the consenting process," *J Clin Ethics* 7 (1996): 60-8.

APPENDIX 5: SUPPLEMENTAL MATERIALS

Information needs vary from person to person and it may be important to supplement the informed consent document with additional material that will increase the participant's understanding of the proposed study. The following list is intended to provide the clinical trial participant, as well as the clinical researcher, with an awareness of the cancer-related information that is available. It may be helpful to talk with local oncology professionals to learn of other resources, including published materials, videos, and Web-based documents.

Types of Information:

Clinical trial/disease information from national organizations

- therapeutic alternatives
- clinical trial information
- disease-specific booklets
- drug information
- nutrition booklets
- questions to ask your doctor
- symptom management

Information from local organizations

- clinical trials programs
- insurance programs/coverage
- Institutional Review Boards
- procedure information; e.g., bone marrow biopsy, insertion of a central line, etc.
- advocate/support programs

INFORMED CONSENT TEMPLATE

NOTE:

- Model text is in **bold.**
- Instructions are in *[italics]*.
- _____ Indicates that the investigator should fill in the appropriate information.

STUDY TITLE

This is a clinical trial (a type of research study). Clinical trials include only patients who choose to take part. Please take your time to make your decision. Discuss it with your friends and family.

[Attach <u>NCI booklet</u> "Taking Part in Clinical Trials: What Cancer Patients Need To Know"]

You are being asked to take part in this study because you have _____ (TYPE OF) cancer.

[Reference and attach information about the type of cancer (and eligibility requirements, if desired).]

WHY IS THIS STUDY BEING DONE?

The purpose of this study is to _____.

[Applicable text:]

Phase 1 studies:

Test the safety of _____ (DRUG/INTERVENTION) and see what effects (good and bad) it has on you and your _____ (TYPE OF) cancer.

or

Find the highest dose of a _____ (DRUG) that can be given without causing severe side effects.

Phase 2 studies:

Find out what effects (good and bad) _____ (DRUG/INTERVENTION) has on you and your _____ (TYPE OF) cancer.

Phase 3 studies:

Compare the effects (good and bad) of the _____

(NEW DRUG/INTERVENTION) with _____

(COMMONLY-USED DRUG/INTERVENTION) on you and your _____ (TYPE OF) cancer to see which is better.

This research is being done because _____

_____.

[Explain in one or two sentences. Examples are: **"Currently, there is no effective treatment for this type of cancer,"** *or* **"We do not know which of these two commonly-used treatments is better."***]*

HOW MANY PEOPLE WILL TAKE PART IN THE STUDY
[If appropriate:]

About _____ people will take part in this study.

WHAT IS INVOLVED IN THE STUDY?
[Provide simplified schema and/or calendar.]
[For randomized studies:]

You will be "randomized" into one of the study groups described below. Randomization means that you are put into a group by chance. It is like flipping a coin. Which group you are put in is done by a computer. Neither you nor the researcher will choose what group you will be in. You will have an _____ (EQUAL/ONE IN THREE/ETC.) chance of being placed in any group.

[For nonrandomized and randomized studies:]

If you take part in this study, you will have the following tests and procedures:

[List procedures and their frequency under the categories below. For randomized studies, list the study groups and under each describe categories of procedures. Include whether a patient will be at home, in the hospital, or in an outpatient setting. If objectives include a comparison of interventions, list all procedures, even those considered standard.]

* **Procedures that are part of regular cancer care and may be done even if you do not join the study.**
* **Standard procedures being done because you are in this study.**
* **Procedures that are being tested in this study.**

HOW LONG WILL I BE IN THE STUDY?
We think you will be in the study for _____ (MONTHS/WEEKS, UNTIL A CERTAIN EVENT).

[Where appropriate, state that the study will involve long-term followup.]

The researcher may decide to take you off this study if

_____.

[List circumstances, such as in the participant's medical best interest, funding is stopped, drug supply is insufficient, patient's condition worsens, new information becomes available.]

You can stop participating at any time. However, if you decide to stop participating in the study, we encourage you to talk to the researcher and your regular doctor first.

[Describe any serious consequences of sudden withdrawal from the study.]

WHAT ARE THE RISKS OF THE STUDY?
While on the study, you are at risk for these side effects. You should discuss these with the researcher and/or your regular doctor. There also may be other side effects that we cannot predict. Other drugs will be given to make side effects less serious and uncomfortable. Many side effects go away shortly after the _____ (INTERVENTION/DRUGS) are stopped, but in some cases side effects can be serious or long-lasting or permanent.

[List by regimen the physical and nonphysical risks of participating in the study in categories of "very likely" and "less likely but serious." Nonphysical risks may include such things as the inability to work. Do not describe risks in a narrative fashion. Highlight or otherwise identify side effects that may be irreversible or long-term or life threatening.]

Risks and side effects related to the _____ (PROCEDURES, DRUGS, OR DEVICES) **we are studying include:**

[List risks related to the investigational aspects of the trial. Specifically identify those that may not be reversible.]

Reproductive risks: Because the drugs in this study can affect an unborn baby, you should not become pregnant or father a baby while on this study. You should not nurse your baby while on this study. Ask about counseling and more information about preventing pregnancy.

[Include a statement about possible sterility when appropriate.]

[Attach additional information about contraception, etc.]

For more information about risks and side effects, ask the researcher or contact

_____.

[Reference and attach drug sheets, pharmaceutical information for the public, or other material on risks.]

ARE THERE BENEFITS TO TAKING PART IN THE STUDY?

If you agree to take part in this study, there may or may not be direct medical benefit to you. We hope the information learned from this study will benefit other patients with _____ (TYPE OF CANCER) **in the future.**

[For Phase 3 studies, when appropriate:]

The possible benefits of taking part in the study are the same as receiving _____ (STANDARD DRUG/INTERVENTION) **without being in the study.**

WHAT OTHER OPTIONS ARE THERE?

Instead of being in this study, you have these options:

[List alternatives including commonly-used therapy and "**No therapy at this time with care to help you feel more comfortable.**"*]*

[If appropriate (for noninvestigational treatments):]

You may get _____ (STUDY TREATMENTS/DRUGS AT THIS CENTER AND OTHER CENTERS) **even if you do not take part in the study.**

Please talk to your regular doctor about these and other options.

[Reference and attach information about alternatives.]

WHAT ABOUT CONFIDENTIALITY?

Efforts will be made to keep your personal information confidential. We cannot guarantee absolute confidentiality. Your personal information may be disclosed if required by law. Organizations that may inspect and/or copy your research records for quality assurance and data analysis include groups such as:

[List relevant agencies like the National Cancer Institute, Food and Drug Administration, study sponsor, etc.]

WHAT ARE THE COSTS?

Taking part in this study may lead to added costs to you or your insurance company. Please ask about any expected added costs or insurance problems.

In the case of injury or illness resulting from this study, emergency medical treatment is available but will be provided at the usual charge. No funds have been set aside to compensate you in the event of injury.

You or your insurance company will be charged for continuing medical care and/or hospitalization.

You will receive no payment for taking part in this study.
[If appropriate:]

If, during the study, the _____ (STUDY DRUG) becomes commercially available, you may have to pay for the amount of drug needed to complete the study.

WHAT ARE MY RIGHTS AS A PARTICIPANT?
Taking part in this study is voluntary. You may choose not to take part or may leave the study at any time. Leaving the study will not result in any penalty or loss of benefits to which you are entitled.

We will tell you about new information that may affect your health, welfare, or willingness to stay in this study.

[Or when a Data Safety and Monitoring Board exists:]

A Data Safety and Monitoring Board, an independent group of experts, will be reviewing the data from this research throughout the study. We will tell you about the new information from this or other studies that may affect your health, welfare, or willingness to stay in this study.

WHOM DO I CALL IF I HAVE QUESTIONS OR PROBLEMS?
For questions about the study or a research-related injury, contact the researcher _____ (NAME{S}) at _____ (TELEPHONE NUMBER).

For questions about your rights as a research participant, contact the_____ (NAME OF CENTER) Institutional Review Board (which is a group of people who review the research to protect your rights) at _____ (TELEPHONE NUMBER). *[And, if available, list patient representative (or other individual who is not on the research team or IRB).]*

WHERE CAN I GET MORE INFORMATION?
You may call the NCI's **Cancer Information Service** at
1 800 4 CANCER (1 800 422 6237) or **TTY: 1 800 332 8615**
Visit the NCI's Web sites

- **cancerTrials:** comprehensive clinical trials information/index.html.
- **CancerNet:** accurate cancer information including PDQ **http://cancernet.nci.nih.gov.**

You will get a copy of this form. You may also request a copy of the protocol (full study plan).

[Attach information materials and checklist of attachments. Signature page should be at the end of package.]

SIGNATURE
I agree to take part in this study.

Participant _____

Date _____

Checklist for Evaluating Involvement
of Decisionally Incapable Persons in Clinical Trials

■ Jurisdictions in which research is projected to be conducted:

State	State:
State	State:
State	State:
State	State:

■ It has been determined that the enumerated states permit involvement of decisionally incapable persons in clinical trials (yes) (no)

    If "no," this step must be completed before the IRB may consider the protocol.

■ For each of the named states, indicate if there are any restrictions on the types of research that may be conducted on decisionally incapable individuals:

State	State:
State	State:
State	State:
State	State:

■ Do any of the state restrictions preclude involvement of decisionally incapable individuals in the type of research involved in the proposed study?

    If "yes," the principal investigator and the IRB must be informed of this information so that the protocol can be changed to eliminate this jurisdiction and another comparable state can be included in the study at the request of the principal investigator.

This checklist was completed by _____ *on* _____, *2001.*

Part 2: Specific Tips for Trial Participants— A Checklist of Questions to Ask the Research Team

The following questions deal with many of the areas that should be covered in the informed consent document (see previous section). To double-check that you have all the information you need, consider printing out this checklist and bringing it to a meeting with the research team. You also may wish to fill it out as you read the informed consent document, both to ensure your own understanding of the trial and to create a ready reference written in your own words. Many of these questions are specific to treatment trials, but the checklist still should prove useful if you are considering a prevention, screening, or supportive care trial.

A CHECKLIST OF QUESTIONS

The Study

1. What is the purpose of the study?
2. Why do researchers think the approach may be effective?
3. Who will sponsor the study?
4. Who has reviewed and approved the study?
5. How are study results and safety of participants being checked?
6. How long will the study last?
7. What will my responsibilities be if I participate?
8. Whom can I speak with about questions I have during and after the trial? to find out the study results?
9. What steps will be taken to protect my privacy and the confidentiality of my medical records?

Possible Risks and Benefits

1. What are my possible short-term benefits?
2. What are my possible long-term benefits?
3. What are my short-term risks, such as side effects?
4. What are my possible long-term risks?
5. What other options do people with my risk of cancer or type of cancer have?
6. How do the possible risks and benefits of this trial compare with those options?

Participation and Care

1. What kinds of therapies, procedures and/or tests will I have during the trial?
2. Will they hurt, and if so, how long?
3. How do the tests in the study compare with those I would have outside of the trial?
4. Will I be able to take my regular medications while in the clinical trial?

5. Where will I have my medical care?
6. Will I have to be hospitalized? If so, how often and for how long?
7. Who will be in charge of my care?
8. What type of follow-up care is part of the study?

Personal Issues

1. How could being in the study affect my daily life?
2. Can I talk to other people in the study?

Cost Issues

1. Will I have to pay for any part of the trial such as tests or the study drug?
2. If so, what will the charges likely be?
3. What is my health insurance likely to cover?
4. Who can help answer any questions from my insurance company or health plan?
5. Will there be many travel or child care costs that I need to consider while I am in the trial?

last updated 02/05/99

HUMAN SUBJECT REGULATIONS DECISION CHARTS

The Office for Protection from Research Risks (OPRR) provides the following graphic aids to clarify portions of the Department of Health and Human Services (DHHS) human subject regulations at Title 45 Code of Federal Regulations Part 46 (45 CFR §46). These portions of the regulations are the subjects of frequent inquires to OPRR.

- **Chart 1: Definition of Human Subject at Section 46.102(f)**

  Is the definition of "human subject" at Section 46.102(f) met in this research activity?

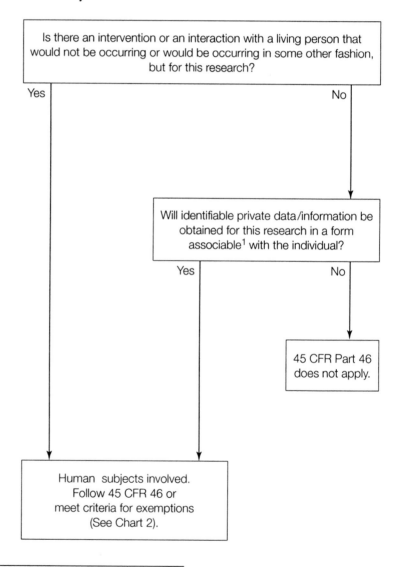

---

[1]That is, the identity of the subject is or may readily be ascertained or associated with information.

OPRR 10/01/98

- **Chart 2: Exemption at Section 46.101(b)(4)** regarding research involving the collection or study of existing data, documents, records, pathological specimens, or diagnostic specimens.

Is the research exempt in accordance with Section 46.101(b)(4)?
The regulations at 45 CFR Part 46 do not apply if the criteria for exemption under Section 46.101(b)(4) are met.

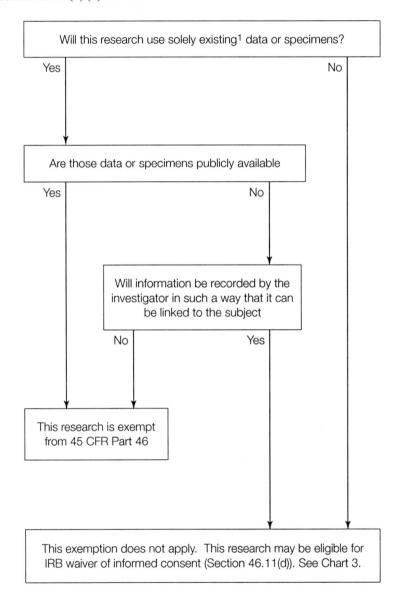

---

[1]"Existing" means collected (i.e., on the shelf) prior to the research for a purpose other than the proposed research. It includes data or specimens collected in research and nonresearch activities.

OPRR 10/01/98

- **Chart 3: Waiver or Alteration of Informed Consent under Section 46.116(d).**

Can the Institutional Review Board employ Section 46.116(d) to waive informed consent or alter informed consent elements?

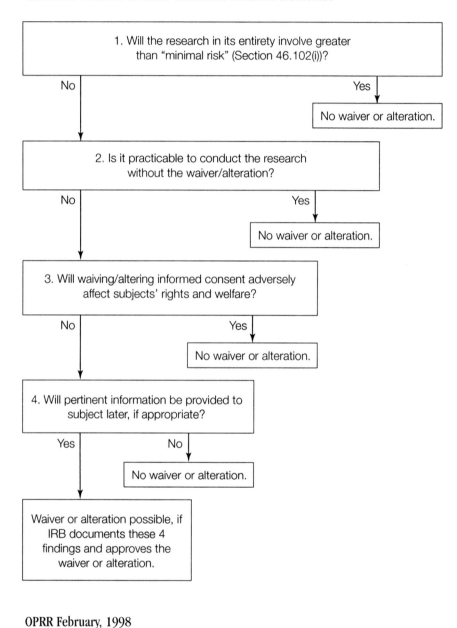

OPRR February, 1998

Policy and Assurances | **OHRP Home Page**

If you have questions about human subject research, click **ohrp@osophs.dhhs.gov**
If you have questions/suggestions about this web page, click **Webmaster**
Updated June 23, 2000

THE OFFICE OF HUMAN SUBJECTS RESEARCH (OHSR) NATIONAL INSTITUTES OF HEALTH

INFORMATION SHEET #6

GUIDELINES FOR WRITING INFORMED CONSENT DOCUMENTS

Revised 08/00

1. INTRODUCTION

The ethical principle of respect for persons requires that subjects be given the opportunity to choose what shall and shall not happen to them. Valid informed consent requires: (1) **Disclosure** of relevant information to prospective subjects about the research; (2) their **comprehension** of the information, and (3) their **voluntary agreement,** free of coercion and undue influence, to research participation.

Ideally, informed decision-making by research subjects is a process that generally includes discussion of the research study with the Principal Investigator (PI), and others as appropriate, and signing the written informed consent document. Depending on the nature, type and duration of the research, ongoing discussion with and education of subjects about the study may continue long after the informed consent document is signed.

A goal of the NIH is to assure that all written informed consent documents are complete and clearly written so as to promote informed decision-making by subjects participating in its research activities. This information sheet provides guidance to NIH clinical researchers and IRBs on the procedures and requirements for informed consent to research participation and the content and format of written consent documents.

2. REQUIREMENTS FOR INFORMED CONSENT

   a. General Procedures

   Unless otherwise waived by the IRB, NIH research investigators should obtain valid informed consent from all research subjects (or their legally authorized representatives) who participate in their research studies. Generally, after the Principal Investigator has explained the research study to the subject, the subject's informed consent is documented by signing the protocol's written consent document, which an IRB must have previously reviewed and approved. The NIH consent document form **NIH-2514-1** (Consent to Participate in a Clinical Research Study, Attachment A), obtainable from IRB Protocol Coordinators, is used for all subjects enrolled in research conducted at the Clinical Center. Form **NIH-2514-1** is also available from the Clinical Center's Website at (http://www.cc.nih.gov/ccc/protomechanics/index.html). The subject is given a copy of the signed document, and, when the research is conducted in the Clinical Center, the Principal Investigator ensures that the original signed consent document is filed in the subject's permanent medical record maintained by the Clinical Center's Medical Record Department. In cases where subject accrual occurs elsewhere, signed consent documents are retained according to the policies of the institution where the research is conducted.

b. <u>General Principles</u>

Unless otherwise authorized by an IRB, research investigators are responsible for ensuring that informed consent shall:

- be obtained in writing from the subject or the subject's legally authorized representative;

- be understandable to the subject or her/his representative. Suggestions for writing consent documents are provided in 3., below

- be obtained in circumstances that are not coercive and that offer the subject (or her/his representative) sufficient opportunity to decide whether she/he should participate. The consent document should not contain language that implies or suggests that the subject (or her/his representative) gives up any legal rights or releases research investigators or the NIH from liability for negligence.

c. <u>Basic Elements for Written Informed Consent Documents</u>

Unless otherwise authorized by an IRB, research investigators must provide the following information to each subject in writing:

The basic elements which have an asterisk (*) are incorporated in existing language printed on form NIH-2514-1 (Consent to Participate in a Clinical Research Study). Nevertheless, to enhance comprehension and readability, investigators are strongly urged to use a format in the body of the consent form that presents information in sections, introduced by headings, and that clearly and simply identifies and describes each of the elements to be discussed, even if the sections repeat information that appears on the printed form. An example of an effective way to use headings is attached (Attachment B).

- A statement that the study involves research;*

- An explanation of the purpose of the research and the expected duration of the subject's participation;

- A description of the procedures to be followed and identification of any procedures that are experimental;

- A description of any foreseeable risks or discomforts to the subject, an estimate of their likelihood, and a description of what steps will be taken to prevent or minimize them;

- A description of any benefits to the subject or to others that may reasonably be expected from the research. Monetary compensation is not a benefit. If compensation is to be provided to research subjects or healthy volunteers, the amount should be stated in the consent document;

- A disclosure of any appropriate alternative procedures or courses of treatment that might be advantageous to the subject;

- A statement describing to what extent records will be kept confidential, including a description of who may have access to research records;*

- For research involving more than minimal risk, an explanation and description of any compensation and any medical treatments that are available if research subjects are injured; where further information may be obtained, and whom to contact in the event of a research-related injury;*

- An explanation of whom to contact for answers to pertinent questions about the research and the research subject's rights (include the Clinical Center's Patient Representative and telephone number);* and
- A statement that participation is voluntary and that refusal to participate or discontinuing participation at any time will involve no penalty or loss of benefits to which the subject is otherwise entitled.*

d. Additional Elements

When appropriate, and required by the IRB, one or more of the following elements of information will also be provided to each research subject:

- If the subject is or may become pregnant, a statement that the particular treatment or procedure may involve risks, which are currently unforeseeable, to the subject or to the embryo or fetus;
- A description of circumstances in which the subject's participation may be terminated by the investigator without the subject's consent;
- Any costs to the subject that may result from participation in the research;
- What will happen if the subject decides to withdraw from the research and how withdrawal will be handled;
- A statement that the Principal Investigator will notify subjects of any significant new findings developed during the course of the study that may affect them and influence their willingness to continue participation;
- The approximate number of subjects involved in the study;
- When appropriate, a statement concerning an investigator's potential financial or other conflict of interest in the conduct of the study.

e. Waiver or Alteration of the Required Elements of Informed Consent

In certain circumstances prescribed by the Federal Regulations (45 CFR §46.116(d)), an IRB may waive the requirement to obtain informed consent, or may approve a consent process which does not include or alters some or all of the elements in (c) above. For more information, see the NIH Multiple Project Assurance G.3.

3. SUGGESTIONS FOR WRITING INFORMED CONSENT DOCUMENTS

When an investigator writes or reviews a research consent document, she/he should ask the following questions:

Question 1: Is it written at a reading level understandable to research subjects?

(a) A general rule of thumb is that consent documents should be written so that they are understandable to people who have not graduated from high school. The reading level of a document is more difficult if it contains: long sentences, words with more than two syllables, and continuous run-on text.

(b) Therefore, if possible use words with fewer than three syllables; use non-scientific/non-medical words; use short sentences, and break the text up into short sections.

Question 2: Is the document formatted well? Does it have headings which break the text into short sections (see Attachment B).

<u>Question 3:</u> Does the document contain the basic elements for informed consent and are they presented in a clear, easy-to-understand way? Even though the printed NIH consent form (Attachment A) incorporates some of the elements of consent, depending on the particular research study, it may be useful to include the information a second time but in a simpler form.

<u>Question 4:</u> Can the document be shortened without compromising clarity or other requirements?

Usually, before a person agrees to take part in a research study, he/she not only reads a written consent document but also discusses the study with a researcher. A suggestion when writing consent documents is to assume that prospective subjects will not talk to a researcher (or research nurse) at all about the study, and that all their information will come entirely from the consent document. If this approach is used the document is more likely to be clear, complete, devoid of medical/scientific terminology and able to "stand alone."

The Use of Headings to Format Informed Consent Documents

The use of headings in informed consent documents helps to ensure that all the basic elements of informed consent are conveyed to the prospective research subject in a simple, efficient way. Headings promote comprehension and readability. The number, order, and language of headings are left to the author of the informed consent document with the approval of the IRB. Some examples are:

Introduction:

Standard language printed at the beginning of NIH-2514-1

The purpose of this study:

Research tests or procedures for this study:

List each test separately and describe what it involves.

Research drugs or other treatments you will receive in this study:

Describe how the drug or treatment will be given (e.g., into a vein, injected under the skin), how long each drug administration will take, and how often they will be given, etc.

Risks and discomforts to you if you take part in this study:

For each procedure, test, treatment or drug, explain the risks, discomforts and inconveniences and provide an estimate of their likelihood. Describe the steps that will be taken to prevent, lessen or treat them.

The benefits to you of taking part in this study:

What other choices you have besides taking part in this study:

What will happen to the samples or information that are collected:

Other pertinent information:

The "standard language" on the last page of the CC consent document (see Attachment A) contains information about confidentiality, research related injuries, a general statement about payment to subjects, and whom to call with questions about the protocol. However, depending on the nature of the study, the PI may want to add additional information in the body of the consent document concerning these and other issues. For example, when appropriate, a PI may want to include the following, or other, headings:

- **How much you will be paid if you take part in this study**
- **Costs to you if you enter this study**
- **What to do if you decide you want to withdraw from the study**
- **Specific things you should understand about confidentiality**
- **Concerns about pregnancy and fertility or childbearing in the future**
- **How long this study will last and how many people will be enrolled.**

COMMON CONCERNS TO ADDRESS IN THE CONSENT PROCESS SAMPLE: CANCER TRIALS

The National Cancer Institute documents provide a strong backdrop for consent to participate in clinical trials. From a practical standpoint, the following questions may help the clinical investigator facilitate a solid consent dialogue. These questions are based on common concerns voiced by research subjects in clinical trials.

☐ Will I be physically ill for a long time?

☐ Will I be nauseous?

☐ Will I lose my hair? If so, how long will it take to grow back?

☐ Will my insurance cover a hairpiece for me?

☐ Will I lose my sexual reproductive capacity?

☐ Will I be left impotent by my cancer treatment?

☐ How long will I be unable to work?

☐ What is the likelihood of my cancer recurring with treatment? With the experimental protocol?

☐ Can I still consume alcoholic beverages when enrolled in the study?

☐ Can I still take over-the-counter medications (e.g., Tylenol, Ibuprofen, Sudafed, Benedryl) during my participation in the clinical trial?

NCI's recommendations for simplifying informed consent documents, with guidance on how to develop them.

Updated: 08/30/2001

English Informed Consent Template
NOTE:

Model text is in bold.
Instructions are in [italics].
_____ Indicates that the investigator should fill in the appropriate information.

STUDY TITLE

This is a clinical trial (a type of research study). Clinical trials include only patients who choose to take part. Please take your time to make your decision. Discuss it with your friends and family.

[Attach NCI booklet: "Taking Part in Clinical Trials: What Cancer Patients Need To Know"]

You are being asked to take part in this study because you have _____ (TYPE OF) cancer.

[Reference and attach information about the type of cancer (and eligibility requirements, if desired).]

WHY IS THIS STUDY BEING DONE?

The purpose of this study is to _____.
[Applicable text:]

Phase 1 studies:
Test the safety of _____ (DRUG/INTERVENTION) and see what effects (good and bad) it has on you and your _____ (TYPE OF) cancer. or

Find the highest dose of a _____ (DRUG) that can be given without causing severe side effects.

Phase 2 studies:
Find out what effects (good and bad) _____ (DRUG/INTERVENTION) has on you and your _____ (TYPE OF) cancer.

Phase 3 studies:
Compare the effects (good and bad) of the _____ (NEW DRUG/ INTERVENTION) with _____ (COMMONLY-USED DRUG/INTERVENTION) on you and your _____ (TYPE OF) cancer to see which is better.

This research is being done because _____.

[Explain in one or two sentences. Examples are: "Currently, there is no effective treatment for this type of cancer," or "We do not know which of these two commonly-used treatments is better."]

HOW MANY PEOPLE WILL TAKE PART IN THE STUDY?
[If appropriate:]

About _____ people will take part in this study.

WHAT IS INVOLVED IN THE STUDY?
[Provide simplified schema and/or calendar.]

[For randomized studies:]

You will be "randomized" into one of the study groups described below. Randomization means that you are put into a group by chance. It is like flipping a coin. Which group you are put in is done by a computer. Neither you nor the researcher will choose what group you will be in. You will have an _____ (EQUAL/ONE IN THREE/ETC.) chance of being placed in any group.

[For nonrandomized and randomized studies:]

If you take part in this study, you will have the following tests and procedures:

[List procedures and their frequency under the categories below. For randomized studies, list the study groups and under each describe categories of procedures. Include whether a patient will be at home, in the hospital, or in an outpatient setting. If objectives include a comparison of interventions, list all procedures, even those considered standard.]

Procedures that are part of regular cancer care and may be done even if you do not join the study.

Standard procedures being done because you are in this study.

Procedures that are being tested in this study.

HOW LONG WILL I BE IN THE STUDY?
We think you will be in the study for _____ (MONTHS/WEEKS, UNTIL A CERTAIN EVENT).

[Where appropriate, state that the study will involve long-term followup.]

The researcher may decide to take you off this study if

_____.

[List circumstances, such as in the participant's medical best interest, funding is stopped, drug supply is insufficient, patient's condition worsens, new information becomes available.]

You can stop participating at any time. However, if you decide to stop participating in the study, we encourage you to talk to the researcher and your regular doctor first.

[Describe any serious consequences of sudden withdrawal from the study.]

WHAT ARE THE RISKS OF THE STUDY?
While on the study, you are at risk for these side effects. You should discuss these with the researcher and/or your regular doctor. There also may be other side effects that we cannot predict. Other drugs will be given to make side effects less serious and uncomfortable. Many side effects go away shortly after the _____ (INTERVENTION/DRUGS) are stopped, but in some cases side effects can be serious or long-lasting or permanent.

[List by regimen the physical and nonphysical risks of participating in the study in categories of "very likely" and "less likely but serious." Nonphysical risks may include such things as the inability to work. Do not describe risks in a narrative fashion. Highlight or otherwise identify side effects that may be irreversible or long-term or life threatening.]

Risks and side effects related to the _____ (PROCEDURES, DRUGS, OR DEVICES) we are studying include:

[List risks related to the investigational aspects of the trial. Specifically identify those that may not be reversible.]

Reproductive risks: Because the drugs in this study can affect an unborn baby, you should not become pregnant or father a baby while on this study. You should not nurse your baby while on this study. Ask about counseling and more information about preventing pregnancy.

[Include a statement about possible sterility when appropriate.]

[Attach additional information about contraception, etc.]

For more information about risks and side effects, ask the researcher or contact

_____.

[Reference and attach drug sheets, pharmaceutical information for the public, or other material on risks.]

ARE THERE BENEFITS TO TAKING PART IN THE STUDY?
If you agree to take part in this study, there may or may not be direct medical benefit to you. We hope the information learned from this study will benefit other patients with _____ (TYPE OF CANCER) in the future.

[For Phase 3 studies, when appropriate:]

The possible benefits of taking part in the study are the same as receiving _____ (STANDARD DRUG/INTERVENTION) without being in the study.

WHAT OTHER OPTIONS ARE THERE?
Instead of being in this study, you have these options:

[List alternatives including commonly-used therapy and "No therapy at this time with care to help you feel more comfortable."]

[If appropriate (for noninvestigational treatments):]

You may get _____ (STUDY TREATMENTS/DRUGS AT THIS CENTER AND OTHER CENTERS) even if you do not take part in the study.

Please talk to your regular doctor about these and other options.

[Reference and attach information about alternatives.]

WHAT ABOUT CONFIDENTIALITY?

Efforts will be made to keep your personal information confidential. We cannot guarantee absolute confidentiality. Your personal information may be disclosed if required by law.

Organizations that may inspect and/or copy your research records for quality assurance and data analysis include groups such as:

[List relevant agencies like the National Cancer Institute, Food and Drug Administration, study sponsor, etc.]

WHAT ARE THE COSTS?

Taking part in this study may lead to added costs to you or your insurance company. Please ask about any expected added costs or insurance problems.

In the case of injury or illness resulting from this study, emergency medical treatment is available but will be provided at the usual charge. No funds have been set aside to compensate you in the event of injury.

You or your insurance company will be charged for continuing medical care and/or hospitalization.

You will receive no payment for taking part in this study.

[If appropriate:]

If, during the study, the _____ (STUDY DRUG) becomes commercially available, you may have to pay for the amount of drug needed to complete the study.

WHAT ARE MY RIGHTS AS A PARTICIPANT?

Taking part in this study is voluntary. You may choose not to take part or may leave the study at any time. Leaving the study will not result in any penalty or loss of benefits to which you are entitled.

We will tell you about new information that may affect your health, welfare, or willingness to stay in this study.

[Or when a Data Safety and Monitoring Board exists:]

A Data Safety and Monitoring Board, an independent group of experts, will be reviewing the data from this research throughout the study. We will tell you about the new information from this or other studies that may affect your health, welfare, or willingness to stay in this study.

WHOM DO I CALL IF I HAVE QUESTIONS OR PROBLEMS?

For questions about the study or a research-related injury, contact the researcher _____ _____ (NAME{S}) at _____ (TELEPHONE NUMBER).

For questions about your rights as a research participant, contact the_____ (NAME OF CENTER) Institutional Review Board (which is a group of people who review the research to protect your rights) at _____ (TELEPHONE NUMBER). [And, if available, list patient representative (or other individual who is not on the research team or IRB).]

WHERE CAN I GET MORE INFORMATION?

You may call the NCI's Cancer Information Service at:

1 800 4 CANCER (1 800 422 6237) or TTY: 1 800 332 8615

Visit the NCI Web site:

http://www.cancer.gov/

You will get a copy of this form. You may also request a copy of the protocol (full study plan).

[Attach information materials and checklist of attachments. Signature page should be at the end of package.]

SIGNATURE

I agree to take part in this study.

Participant _____

Date _____

6

Confidentiality of Clinical Trials Information

Overview 207
How the Common Rule Addresses Confidential Information in Human Research 209
   Individually Identifiable Information 209
   The Types of Research Studies That Are Exempt from the Basic Requirements
   for Maintaining Confidentiality in Clinical Trials 209
   The Role of the IRB with Regard to Confidentiality of Information 210
   Confidentiality and the Consent Requirements 210
   The "Waiver" of Consent Documentation for Purposes of Managing
   Research Subject Confidentiality 210
   HIPAA 211
   The Covered Entity 211
   The HIPAA Research Authorization 212
The Privacy Board 212
   The Composition of the Privacy Board 212
   The Role of the Privacy Board Relative to Clinical Research 213
   The Expedited Review Process for an Alteration or Waiver 214
   The IRB Waiver and the Privacy Board HIPAA Waiver 214
   Likely Difficulties in Terms of Waiver Provisions Between IRBs and Privacy Boards 214
State Law and Confidentiality in Clinical Trials 215
   How State Law Might Affect Confidentiality in Clinical Trials 215
Practical Considerations in Maintaining Confidentiality 216
   Giving Assurances of Confidentiality to Research Subjects 216
   The Confidentiality Pledge 216
   Practical Steps for Maintaining Confidentiality for Research Subject
   and Clinical Trial Information 217
Conclusion 218
References 218

OVERVIEW

The issue of confidentiality is important not only for research subjects but clinical investigators and sponsors. Whereas individuals provide information that is of a highly sensitive nature, the intellectual property gained in a research study can be worth large sums of money. Safeguarding such information is important for all concerned.

At some stage, confidentiality may have to give way for the benefit of the subject or identified individuals who may be potentially at risk. Thus a clinical investigator may be called upon to break code when a subject has experienced a life-threatening adverse reaction to a test article. In breaking code, the clinical investigator is asked to provide other information that may be important to treating the research subject.

For example, information that has been held in confidence until now, needs to be released to save the life of a research subject. Included in the release is the subject's list of therapeutic medications. The list contains a number of preparations associated with treatment of patients with HIV. Without actually saying so, the disclosure of the prescription drug list identifies the patient-research subject as being HIV positive. In the absence of an authorization to share such information, providing such details might be considered a breach of confidentiality under some state laws.

Consider a situation in which a research subject is enrolled in a study involving a test article for management of aggressive rage behavior. One individual is noncompliant. Rather than avoiding alcoholic beverages and attending adjunctive behavioral management sessions, the research subject boldly admits that he has been skipping therapy sessions to meet with friends at the local bar. He claims to be drinking an average of six beers each day. One day he arrives at the test center in a very hostile, aggressive mood. As he leaves the center he tells several staff members that he is going to kill his wife and his psychotherapist.

Fearful that the man will carry out his threat, the staff warns the man's wife and psychotherapist. Local police are also notified. Prior to reaching his home, the man is stopped by law enforcement authorities and arrested. Angry that the center staff squealed on him, the man shouts, "I will sue them for this! They had no right to tell anybody." Breaching research subject confidentiality is a serious matter. Is it justified in such a circumstance? Many would agree that it is appropriate when, as here, there are identifiable individuals at risk. Some states require such a breach of confidentiality under the so-called *Tarasoff* rule, referring to a landmark California ruling (Tarasoff v. Regents of University of California, 551 P.2d 334(1976)).

A researcher gets a very attractive offer and academic appointment at another institution. Now in the middle of a five-year grant, he wants to take the study with him. He claims that he can do so since the grant is in his name as principal investigator. However, support staff, facilities, and administrative assistance have been provided by his current employer. Moreover, the current employer claims that it has a faculty plan in place which gives it ownership of any patents that emerge from the study. Complicating the situation is the fact that the study has a number of local patient-subjects enrolled in the investigational trial. Can the researcher take the files with him? If so, what about the confidential research subject information? Moreover, is the confidential information the intellectual property of the institution? The principal investigator? Or both parties?

Aside from the foregoing confidentiality scenarios that are controlled by state law, there are federal regulations that govern the confidentiality of clinical trial information. A complicating factor is the HIPAA Privacy Rule. HIPAA stands for the Health Insurance Portability and Accountability Act (HIPAA). Several different regulations have been promulgated on the basis of rule-making authority under HIPAA. Of particular importance here is the Privacy Rule and those provisions that have a direct bearing on clinical trials. Also of importance are state laws dealing with confidentiality.

This chapter provides an understanding of the confidentiality requirements under existing regulations controlling clinical trials. The HIPAA provisions are also described along with the practical risk exposures that should be anticipated in trying to meet both sets of regulations. The topic of subject recruitment and HIPAA is discussed in Chapter Four.

············

HOW THE COMMON RULE ADDRESSES CONFIDENTIAL INFORMATION IN HUMAN RESEARCH

The Common Rule provides for the confidentiality of information about research subjects. It also includes exemptions and waiver provisions. These are separate from the HIPAA provisions discussed later in this chapter.

Individually Identifiable Information

As used in the Common Rule, confidentiality *involves identifiable private information* in human research (45 CFR §46.102(f)). It encompasses behavioral information "in a context in which an individual can reasonably expect that no observation or recording is taking place, and information which has been provided for specific purposes by an individual and which the individual can reasonably expect will not be made public (for example, a medical record)."

For *private information* to constitute human research data, it must be individually identifiable. This means that the research subject's identity can be readily ascertained by the investigator or linked with the information.

The Types of Research Studies That Are Exempt from the Basic Requirements for Maintaining Confidentiality in Clinical Trials

The Common Rule makes provision to *exempt* certain types of research activities from the confidentiality requirements of the federal rule. This typically involves the use of certain types of data such as the results of educational tests that measure cognitive, diagnostic, aptitude, and achievement. Similarly, research is exempted with respect to survey procedures and interview procedures, and observation of public behavior.

When, however, certain criteria are met, even these uses require confidentiality under the Common Rule (45 CFR §46.101(b)(2)). These include:

- Data that human subjects can be identified directly to or linked to the human research subjects.
- Disclosure of the individual's responses beyond the research setting that could reasonably place the subjects at risk of criminal or civil liability.
- Disclosure of the individual's replies outside the research context that could be damaging to the subjects' financial standing, employment, or reputation.

Additional categories of research that are exempt from the confidentiality requirements found in the Common Rule include:

(3) Research involving the use of educational tests (cognitive, diagnostic, aptitude, achievement), survey procedures, interview procedures, or observation of public behavior that is not exempt under paragraph (b)(2) of this section, if:

(i) The human subjects are elected or appointed public officials or candidates for public office; or (ii) federal statute(s) require(s) without exception that the confidentiality of the personally identifiable information will be maintained throughout the research and thereafter.

(4) Research, involving the collection or study of existing data, documents, records, pathological specimens, or diagnostic specimens, if these sources are publicly available or if the information is recorded by the investigator in such a manner that

subjects cannot be identified, directly or through identifiers linked to the subjects. [45 CFR §46.101(3)-(4)]

From a practical standpoint it is important for a clinical investigator to understand how to operationalize this set of criteria. Clinical research office personnel should be poised to assist in this regard.

The Role of the IRB with Regard to Confidentiality of Information

In approving a research protocol, the IRB must first decide that the study meets applicable regulatory standards. One provision squarely addresses the issue of confidentiality, providing the IRB with some latitude in this regard. As the regulation states, *"When appropriate,* there are adequate provisions to protect the privacy of subjects and to maintain the confidentiality of data" (45 CFR §46.111(a)(7)) (emphasis added).

Recognizing that in some instances a waiver may be granted from the confidentiality provisions, the regulation provides a degree of discretion for the IRB.

Confidentiality and the Consent Requirements

In the general criteria for consent to participate in human research, the regulations include a requirement that subjects be informed of the steps that will be taken to maintain the confidentiality of records identifying the individual (45 CFR.SL46.116(a)(5)). Notice, however, that this is not a guarantee that records will be maintained confidentially. Instead, the regulation requires a description of the steps, if any, that will be taken to accomplish this purpose.

As noted earlier, there is a rationale for this distinction. Latitude is accorded the IRB to alter some consent requirements including in certain instances those involving confidentiality. As the regulations indicate:

An IRB may approve a consent procedure which does not include, or which alters, some or all of the elements of informed consent set forth above, or waive the requirement to obtain informed consent provided the IRB finds:

- No more than <u>minimal risk</u> is involved for research subjects;
- Granting the modification or waiver <u>will not have an adverse affect</u> on either the rights or welfare of the research subjects;
- Without the modification or waiver the research <u>could not practicably be conducted</u>, and
- Following their participation and when it is appropriate to do so, research <u>subjects will be furnished with additional information</u> about their role in the study [45 CFR §46.116(c)].

The "Waiver" of Consent Documentation for Purposes of Managing Research Subject Confidentiality

Under the terms of the Common Rule an IRB has the prerogative to make inapplicable or waive the requirement to obtain a *signed* informed consent document from the research subject (see 45 CFR §46.117(c): (c)). In order to do so, the IRB must determine that this would be the *only record* that would link the subject to the research, and the principal risk would be possible harm stemming from a breach of confidentiality. In addition, research subjects must be asked whether they want documentation linking them with the research. It is the choice of each individual that governs in each case.

An IRB may also waive the signed consent document requirement in situations in which the study involves no more than minimal risk of harm and the research utilizes procedures for which written consent is normally not required outside of the research context.

Even though the signed consent document may be waived, the IRB can take measures to require documentation of another type. The IRB may require the investigator to provide research subjects with a written explanation of the nature of the study.

HIPAA

HIPAA is the acronym for the Healthcare Insurance Portability and Accountability Act of 1996 (Public Law 104-191). Under title II subtitle F of the 1996 law, Congress wanted measures taken to improve the efficiency and effectiveness of healthcare through a redesigned health information system. Through a series of regulations, the intent was to achieve administrative simplification. One factor in this process was to create a minimum National Standard for Privacy of Medical Information. The provisions dealing with privacy of individually identifiable information were first promulgated in December 2000 (*Federal Register* 65(250): 84261, et seq, December 28, 2000) and after delay, put into effect in April 2001.

The HIPAA regulation has gone through further revision. On March 27, 2002, the Department of Health and Human Services proposed some changes to the Privacy Rule (Federal Register 67: 14776). On August 14, 2002, the Department issued the revised Final Rule changes with regard to privacy under HIPAA (*Federal Register* 67(157): 53182, et seq.).

The HIPAA Privacy Rule addresses the use of "protected health information" by those termed "covered entities" under the Regulation. Under HIPAA, a covered entity includes health plans, healthcare clearinghouses, and health care providers who conduct certain financial and administrative transactions (45 CFR §160.103). It also addresses interaction with those termed "business associates," who in some instances may have access to protected health information under the terms of a "business associate agreement." Covered entities are expected to be in full compliance with the Privacy Rule by April 14, 2003. Additional time was built into the Rule for small health plans, a group granted until April 14, 2004, to achieve compliance. In the revised rule issued in August 2002, some changes were made to the time frame for the business associate agreement. A transition period was put in place to enable covered entities to operate under some existing contracts with business associates for one year after the expected compliance date of April 13, 2003. The transition period will enable covered entities to negotiate new contracts to achieve HIPAA Privacy Rule conformity by April 13, 2004, while still being in compliance under existing agreements. This transition period does not apply to small health plans as defined in the Privacy Rule.

The HIPAA Privacy Rule has a direct involvement in clinical research. As discussed above, this involves the use of research authorizations and waivers that be can granted by an IRB or a Privacy Board.

The Covered Entity

For purposes of the HIPAA Privacy Rule, the term "covered entity" includes health plans, healthcare clearinghouses, and healthcare providers who transmit any health information. This may be done verbally, electronically, or in written format.

From a practical standpoint, many of the projects conducted in human subjects research fit the definition of a covered entity. This fact is recognized by the way in which the HIPAA Privacy Rule addresses the need for authorizations for use of protected health information.

The HIPAA Research Authorization

The August 2002 revision to the HIPAA Privacy Rule streamlined what was seen as a cumbersome approach under the original version of the Regulation for obtaining permission to use protected health information. The new version of the Regulation eliminates the requirement of a consent for use of protected health information and replaces it with a Notice and Acknowledgement. Those who do choose to use a consent process are given considerable latitude in its design.

The "Authorization" includes a mechanism for uses and disclosure of protected health information for research purposes (*Federal Register* 67(157): 53182, 53225 (August 14, 2002)). The Privacy Rule permits a covered entity to combine an authorization with any other form of legal permission related to a research study, including a consent to participate in research (*Federal Register* 67(157): 53182, 53225 (August 14, 2002)).

The August 2002 revision to the Privacy Rule also eliminated inclusion of an expiration date for those authorizations given for research purposes (*Federal Register* 67(157): 53182, 53225 (August 14, 2002)). In doing so, however, the revised rule makes it clear that if there are no expiration dates, this information must be included in the authorization.

In most instances, patients may revoke their authorization for the use or disclosure of their protected health information for research purposes. The revised HIPAA Rule does, however, recognize a reliance exception. This exception allows covered entities to continue to use or disclose protected health information secured prior to the research subject revoking the authorization. The reliance exception applies to the extent that the covered entity relied on the authorization, and it is necessary in order to maintain the integrity of the research project (*Federal Register* 67(157): 53182, 53225 (August 14, 2002), referencing §164.508[b](5)).

••••••••••••

THE PRIVACY BOARD

A Privacy Board is recognized under the HIPAA rule as having the authority to alter or waive the need for an individual's authorization for use of or disclosure of protected health information for research purposes (45 CFR §164.512(1)(i)). The Privacy Board *does not* replace the IRB. As seen in this section, there is apt to be confusion about the role and responsibility of the Privacy Board and the IRB. Moreover, there is the potential for conflict between a Privacy Board and an IRB.

The Composition of the Privacy Board

The HIPAA regulation states that the Privacy Board should be composed of members with "varying backgrounds and appropriate professional competency as necessary to review the effect of the research protocol on the individual's privacy rights and related interests" (45 CFR §164.512(1)(i)(B)). The Regulation makes it clear that at least one member of the Privacy Board must be someone who is unaffiliated with the covered entity or with any entity either conducting or sponsoring the study, or not related to anyone who is associated with such entities. When a member of the Privacy Board has a conflict of interest, he or she must be precluded from participating in the review of the project.

The Role of the Privacy Board Relative to Clinical Research

Ordinarily under HIPAA, a written authorization must be obtained for the use of protected health information for research that includes treatment of the individual. As noted earlier, an authorization may be encompassed in a consent to participate in the research.

In some circumstances, the Privacy Board may waive the need for an authorization. There was much concern expressed about the waiver provisions included in the December 2000 version of the Privacy Rule. Many observers saw the waiver process as inconsistent, redundant, and confusing vis-a-vis the Common Rule, described earlier in this chapter.

The August 2002 version of the Privacy Rule incorporates a revised approach to the waiver process. The revamped rule states that:

A. The use or disclosure of protected health information involves no more than a minimal risk to the privacy of individuals, based on, at least, the presence of the following elements:
   1. An adequate plan to protect the identifiers from improper use and disclosure;
   2. An adequate plan to destroy the identifiers at the earliest opportunity consistent with conduct of the research, unless there is a health or research justification for retaining the identifiers or such retention is otherwise required by law; and
   3. Adequate written assurances that the protected health information will not be reused or disclosed to any other person or entity, except as required by law, for authorized oversight of the research study, or for other research for which the use or disclosure of protected health information would be permitted by this subpart;
B. The research could not practicably be conducted without the waiver or alteration; and
C. The research could not practicably be conducted without access to and use of the protected health information. [45 CFR § 164.512]

A majority of the Privacy Board must be in attendance to review the proposed waiver. Moreover, a majority of the board members present must approve the alteration or waiver. The rule also includes an expedited review procedure that does not require a majority of the members to be present.

The actions taken by the Privacy Board must be documented in accordance with the criteria set forth in the Final Rule. Thus, documentation must include:

- The date when the Privacy Board agreed to alter or modify the authorization requirement.
- A description of the action taken.
- The identity of the Privacy Board.
- A statement indicating that the Privacy Board decided that the action it took *met* the waiver criteria.
- A brief description of the protected health information for which it has been decided that either use or access was considered necessary.

- A statement indicating that the waiver granted was accomplished using either a normal or expedited review process.
- The waiver must be granted by the chair of the Privacy Board or another member designated to accomplish the task.

[45 CFR §164.512]

The Expedited Review Process for an Alteration or Waiver

The HIPAA rule permits the Privacy Board to conduct an expedited process when no more than *minimal risk* to individual privacy is involved in the research. When the expedited process is used by the Privacy Board, the review and approval of the alteration or waiver of authorization may be carried out by the chair of the Privacy Board, or by one or more members of the Privacy Board as designated by the chair.

The IRB Waiver and the Privacy Board HIPAA Waiver

In its commentary section preceding the actual text of the December 2000 version of the regulation, the Department of Health and Human Services rejected the idea that the waiver criteria found in the Common Rule should be allowed to be used instead of the waiver criteria found in the HIPAA regulation. As the Secretary of HHS stated:

> The Common Rule's waiver criteria were designed to protect research subjects from all harms associated with research, not specifically to protect individuals' privacy interests. We understand that the waiver criteria in the final rule may initially cause confusion for IRBs and researchers that must attend to both the final rule and the Common Rule, but we believe that the additional waiver criteria adopted in the final rule are essential to ensure that individuals' privacy rights and welfare are adequately safeguarded when protected health information about themselves is used for research without their authorization. [*Federal Register* 65(250): 826927, December 28, 2000]

With the publication of the revised Final Rule in August 2002, the changes described above were made in an attempt to avoid confusion and to better align the Privacy Rule with the Common Rule in this arena. Even with these changes, however, HHS has noted that the concerns expressed in the past may not be corrected by the changes made to this part of the Privacy Rule. The subject nature of the determinations is of particular concern. HHS believes that with the issuance of further guidance on the subject and experience, both IRBs and Privacy Boards will be able to make waiver decisions (*Federal Register* 67(157): 53182, 53230 (August 14, 2002)). To this end, the Office of Civil Rights (OCR) of the U.S. Department of Health and Human Services issued guidance on a number of components in the Privacy Standard (Medical Privacy—National Standards to Protect the Privacy of Personal Health Information, OCR Guidance Explaining Significant Aspects of the Privacy Rule, December 4, 2002).

Likely Difficulties in Terms of Waiver Provisions Between IRBs and Privacy Boards

In the commentary section prior to the Final Rule, HHS did acknowledge that there could be disputes. Indeed, HHS was quite emphatic on this point:

> We disagree with the comment that documentation of IRB or Privacy Board approval of the waiver of authorization should be given deference by other IRBs or

Privacy Boards conducting secondary reviews. We do not believe that it is appropriate to restrict the deliberations or judgments of Privacy Boards, nor do we have the authority under this rule to instruct IRBs on this issue. Instead, we reiterate that all disclosures for research purposes under §164.512[i] are voluntary, and that institutions may choose to impose more stringent requirements for any use and disclosure permitted under §164.512. [*Federal Register* 65 (250): 82692, December 28, 2000]

What are the implications of this statement? It is a reflection of the fact that Section 164.12 sets *minimum* documentation standards for covered healthcare providers and health plans when using or disclosing protected data for purposes of research. The regulatory minimum may not be enough. To an IRB at one facility, the minimal standards of a Privacy Board may lead to a rejection absent the researcher agreeing to meet the IRB's higher threshold. This is apt to have administrative ramifications for multicenter studies.

The Final Rule does not provide guidance as to which board would prevail. As HHS acknowledged:

The final rule requires covered entities to obtain documentation that one IRB or Privacy Board has approved of the alteration or waiver of authorization. The covered entity, however, has discretion to request information about the findings of all IRBs and/or Privacy Boards that have reviewed research protocols. [*Federal Register* 65 (250): 82692, December 28, 2000]

Although written in December 2000, the point remains valid even after the revisions made to the Final Rule in August 2002. Nowhere in the regulation does it set a requirement for the location or sponsorship of the IRB or Privacy Board. The researcher who believes that it will be difficult to obtain a waiver from a Privacy Board with a by-the-book reputation may try to get a waiver from another Privacy Board with a more liberal interpretation. The data authorization waiver, however, is but one part of the process. The IRB retains the right to dispute the Privacy Board on the subject. By trying to forum shop, the researcher may delay the approval process or thwart it from happening altogether if the investigator is insistent on using a waiver rejected by the IRB.

....

STATE LAW AND CONFIDENTIALITY IN CLINICAL TRIALS

Several states have enacted laws and promulgated regulations to address clinical trials. Three have very detailed laws: California, New York, and Virginia. Even in those states with less-detailed requirements, it is not uncommon to find laws that address privacy or confidentiality of individually identifiable healthcare information. Use of such identifier-linked information for research purposes may trigger the application of specific provisions.

How State Law Might Affect Confidentiality in Clinical Trials

Under HIPAA, a state can apply for a lifting of the federal preemption dealing with the protection, use, and disclosure of individually identifiable information. In order to secure it, the state must demonstrate that its law is more stringent than a standard, requirement, or implementation specification requirements dealing with the privacy of individually identifiable health information (45 CFR §160.203). For purposes of clinical research, the state would have to satisfy the requirements and the Secretary of Health and Human Services would have to decide if the state requirements provide greater protections for information waivers in clinical research than the HIPAA regulation.

The possibility does exist for a clash between state and federal provisions over a waiver for access to individually identifiable information for purposes of research. It remains to be seen how this situation will be resolved. For present purposes, it is important to understand how state law relates to federal requirements as a whole in terms of clinical trials. Particular attention should be paid to looking for state laws and regulations governing information privacy, confidentiality, and data access since these requirements may not be found in provisions labeled "human research." Once identified, matching up the HIPAA requirements with state law will be useful in developing an overall strategy for meeting pertinent requirements for purposes of clinical research and the use of individually identifiable data.

············

PRACTICAL CONSIDERATIONS IN MAINTAINING CONFIDENTIALITY

There are practical considerations that are generated by the HIPAA Privacy Rule and applicable state law. These considerations include the extent to which subjects should be assured of confidentiality, the use of a confidentiality pledge, effective policies and procedures, monitoring and oversight, and education. These practical considerations are described in this section.

Giving Assurances of Confidentiality to Research Subjects

Rather than create expectations that cannot be met, it is best to tell research subjects how individually identifiable information will be used and stored. The safeguards used to protect such information should be described as well.

Research information may be disclosed in ways not contemplated by study investigators. This could occur in civil litigation or in a federal investigation. Thus providing a blanket assurance that individual information will not revealed may create a false expectation.

Sometimes subjects are advised that individual information may be used in a published document. However, they are not told the extent to which this may occur. One can question whether it is sufficient to disclose that a subject's likeness may appear in a published study when in fact the subject's face is broadly displayed. Disclosure means providing the subject with an explanation in plain language that conveys exactly what is intended in terms of use of confidential or individually identifiable information.

The Confidentiality Pledge

Confidentiality pledges have been in use for many years by those involved in research administration. It is basically a document that is signed by research administrative staff, principal investigators and their team members, and IRB members. In signing it, they agree to maintain in a confidential manner any information learned about an individual or the clinical research trial.

The confidentiality pledge was designed to serve two purposes. One was to safeguard the research subject from revelations that could be embarrassing or that could jeopardize the individual in terms of employment, family or community relationships, and insurance coverage. The other was to protect the integrity of the research project and the intellectual property involved in the study.

In many instances, the confidentiality pledge was based on an honor system. However, this has not always been the case. In employee handbooks, for example, a breach of confidentiality usually is considered the basis for disciplinary action.

The Pledge of Confidentiality is different from the "Certificate of Confidentiality." The latter is issued to investigators by the Department of Health and Human Services under the authority granted by the Public Health Services Act (§301(d), 42 USC §241(d)). It authorizes them to withhold identifiable research participant information that may be summoned under federal or state judicial, administrative, or legislative proceedings.

The Certificate of Confidentiality is usually reserved for those instances involving sensitive data such as drug abuse, alcohol abuse, and mental health. According to a Draft Report from the National Bioethics Advisory Commission, it is thought that by issuing such certificates the pool of potential subjects can be increased (Draft Report: Ethical and Policy Issues in Research Involving Human Participants, December, 2000).

With the advent of HIPAA privacy, increased efforts may be expected in terms of serious consequences for non-compliance with policies and procedures designed to safeguard individually identifiable healthcare information.

Practical Steps for Maintaining Confidentiality for Research Subject and Clinical Trial Information

There are several steps to take in terms of maintaining confidentiality. Part of it involves study design and office management. Another part encompasses training. Yet another component involves surveillance and monitoring.

Many times confidentiality is taken for granted. The routine flow of information is slipshod, enabling unauthorized individuals to have access to individually identifiable information. Records or charts are left open in plain view. A subject's profile is left open on a computer screen. Idle chitchat in a hallway provides identifiers sufficient enough to link a research subject by name with an HIV protocol.

Here are some useful measures to address confidentiality in clinical trials:

- *Flowchart Information Management*—Identify unacceptable office management practices and inappropriate information flow patterns. It is useful to literally flowchart how the information is supposed to be transmitted and used and to contrast this expected standard with what is happening in a research setting. The variances are opportunities for breach of policy and procedure. If not resolved, such practices can lead to a claim of negligent breach of confidentiality. It is also an opportunity to improve practices to bring the system into compliance with expectations or to streamline current processes.

- *Need to Know Access*—Reduce the number of people who have access to information to those with a legitimate need to know. Position computer monitors in a way so that public view is impossible, and redesign information security to increase protection of individually identifiable data.

- *Education*—Provide staff with the knowledge they need to develop and achieve good practices in the management and use of confidential clinical trial information. Staff may be totally unaware that in public hallways they can be overheard talking about subjects who are easily linked by the conversation to a named study. The same may be said of discussions on elevators, in the cafeteria, or in audible phone conversations. Staff may also be unaware of the opportunities they provide for unauthorized personnel to view clinical research files. Where they place records is important. Through ongoing education, an awareness can be built up regarding information security and protecting individually identifiable research subject data. Soliciting input from staff for enhancing information protection is another way to obtain buy-in to a commitment to safeguarding individually identifiable data.

- *Monitoring and Surveillance*—Implement on-going reviews to reinforce good practices. Monitoring and surveillance also enable a research staff to identify unacceptable data security practices and take corrective action. Testing the system, especially computerized record security, is another useful tool in surveillance for would-be hackers.

- *Enlist Help from Key Stakeholders*—Utilize the expertise of the Chief Privacy Officer (CPO) in designing information systems to protect individually identifiable healthcare information in the research setting. Enlist the assistance of the Chief Information Security Officer to design data-hacking surveillance and firewall protections. Utilize material available from federal sources. For example, the Division of Compliance Oversight of the Office for Human Research Protections (OHRP) publishes a compendium of its compliance activities and guidance. Further, in *Protecting Data Privacy in Health Services Research: Committee on the Role of Institutional Review Boards in Health Services Research Data Privacy Protection* (2000) the Institute of Medicine issued ten recommendations that could facilitate development of best practices for maintaining data privacy. The IOM volume is instructive for those engaged in establishing systems and strategies for maximizing the use of individually identifiable data in clinical research while maintaining safeguards for protecting the information.

- *Develop an Interface Between Privacy and Intellectual Property*—Make certain policies and procedures governing migration of study-based intellectual property contemplates protection of health information collected or used in a research study. If the principal investigator leaves, the process should safeguard PHI.

CONCLUSION

The HIPAA Privacy Rule and the laws in several states address the uses and disclosure of individually identifiable health information for research purposes. Using the rules as a blueprint, policies and procedures can be developed that are practical and useful in safeguarding individually identifiable information in clinical trials. A related issue is safeguarding the intellectual property or work of a study investigator. The input of health information management experts, researchers, ethicists, and compliance officials will be invaluable in this regard. In the end, the result should be a very practical system that meets the needs of all concerned.

References

45 CFR §46.102 (f)

45 CFR §46.101 (b)

45 CFR §46.111 (a)

45 CFR §46.116 (c)

45 CFR §46.117 (c)

45 CFR §106.103

45 CFR §169.203

45 CFR §164.512(1)

Division of Health Care Services. (2000). *Protecting Data Privacy in Health Services Research.* Committee on the Role of Institutional Review Board in Health Services Research Data Protection. Washington, DC: National Academy Press.

Ethical and Policy Issues in Research Involving Human Participants, Draft Report, December 2000.

Federal Register 65(250) 4261, 82692, et seq., December 28, 2000.

Federal Register 67(157) 53182, 53225, et seq., August 14, 2002.

"OCR Guidance Explaining Significant Aspects of the Privacy Rule." December 4, 2002.

Public Health Services Act, 301(d), 42 USC 241(d)

Public Law 104-109

7

The Investigator

Overview. 222
Defining "Investigator" and "Investigations" 222
The Individual Patient As Research Participant 222
Qualifications to Conduct Research 222
   An Investigator's Qualifications to Conduct a Proposed Study. 223
   Educational Requirements for Clinical Investigators 223
   Other Educational Resources Available for Investigators 225
   Experience Requirements for Clinical Investigators 225
   Information That a Clinical Investigator Must Disclose About Himself 225
   A Clinical Investigator That Has a Financial Interest in a Study or a Sponsor
   Participating in the Study 226
   Determining Whether an Investigator Has Adequate Resources to Conduct
   a Clinical Investigation 227
Responsibility for the Protocol and Safety 227
   The Responsibility of an Investigator in Clinical Research 227
   The Responsibility of the Investigator for Following the Study Protocol. 228
   The Responsibility of the Investigator for Ensuring Human Participant Safety 228
   The Investigator's Obligations When Unexpected Findings Occur 228
   Defining an Adverse Event 228
   The Investigator's Responsibility to Comply with IRB Decisions and Procedures 228
   The Investigator's Responsibility for Control of an Investigational Drug. 229
   Records That the Investigator Must Maintain. 229
   The Investigator's Responsibility for Reports to the Sponsor. 229
   Common Examples of Investigator Noncompliance 229
   Defining Research Misconduct 230
   The Investigator's Obligations if He Realizes That a Staff Member Has Altered Records . . 230
   Protections for Whistleblowers 230
Corrective Actions Against Investigators 231
   The Steps to Be Taken if Research Misconduct Is Suspected 231
     Response of Institution 231
     Response of Federal Agency 232
     Response in Criminal or Civil Law 234
   FDA Monitoring Clinical Investigators 234
   FDA Procedure When a Problem Is Detected 235
   Other Actions That the FDA Can Take Against an Investigator, Institution, or Sponsor . . . 236
   Criminal Penalties Under the Food, Drug & Cosmetic Act 237

Civil Penalties Under the FDCA 237
Parties That Can Be Held Responsible for Violations of the FDCA 237
Parties Advised by the FDA When It Finds Investigator Misconduct 237
Conclusion 237
References 237

. . . .

OVERVIEW

Many people are surprised to learn that what they are doing is deemed human subject research and that they are therefore considered to be clinical investigators. With that title comes many responsibilities. This chapter will assist in identifying who is an investigator and what is expected of an investigator.

. . . .

DEFINING "INVESTIGATOR" AND "INVESTIGATIONS"

An investigator is the person responsible for conducting a research protocol. This can involve research in medicine, psychology, sociology, education, political science, or any other effort to organize data collected from human subjects. The FDA definition of clinical investigation, defined as "any experiment in which a drug is administered or dispensed to, or used involving, one or more human subjects" (21 CFR §312.3(b)), is only one aspect of the research that is governed by federal and state regulations. The more appropriate inquiry is the question: Is there an intervention or an interaction with a living person that would not be occurring or would be occurring in some other fashion but for this research? If so, then the investigator must determine if the research is subject to an institution's policies and procedures and to federal or state regulations. Making this determination is discussed in more detail in Chapter Eight, Research Protocols.

. . . .

THE INDIVIDUAL PATIENT AS RESEARCH PARTICIPANT

A single patient may be the subject of clinical trials research. The distinction is "if there is a clear intent before treating the patient to use systematically collected data that would not ordinarily be collected in the course of clinical practice in reporting and publishing a case study. Treating with a research intent should be distinguished from the use of innovative treatment practices" (OPRR, *Institutional Review Board Guidebook*).

. . . .

QUALIFICATIONS TO CONDUCT RESEARCH

Until recently, qualifications to conduct clinical investigations had been rarely articulated as even aspirational goals, let alone mandated. However, Ezekiel, Wendler, and Grady described the ideal training and skills of an investigator:

> Not only must clinical investigators be skilled in the appropriate methods, statistical tests, outcome measures, and other scientific aspects of clinical trials, they must have the training to appreciate, affirm, and implement these ethical requirements, such as the capacity and sensitivity to determine appropriate subject selection criteria,

evaluate risk-benefit ratios, provide information in an appropriate manner, and implement confidentiality procedures. [Ezekiel, Wendler, and Grady; 2000.]

An Investigator's Qualifications to Conduct a Proposed Study

An IRB should consider the following points in determining whether an investigator is qualified to conduct an investigation (ICH, *Guideline for Good Clinical Practice*):

- The investigator(s) is qualified by education, training, and experience to assume responsibility for the proper conduct of the trial, meets all the qualifications specified by the applicable regulatory requirement(s), and has provided evidence of such qualifications through an up-to-date curriculum vitae and/or other relevant documentation;

- The investigator is thoroughly familiar with the appropriate use of the investigational product(s), as described in the protocol, in the current Investigator's Brochure, in the product information and in other information sources provided by the sponsor;

- The investigator is aware of, and agrees to comply with, . . . the applicable regulatory requirements, and the institution's policies and procedures;

- The investigator affirms that he will permit monitoring and auditing by the sponsor, the IRB, and appropriate regulatory authority(ies);

- The investigator has identified appropriately qualified persons to whom the investigator has delegated significant trial-related duties; and

- The investigator is able to demonstrate that he has adequate resources available to safely and efficiently conduct the proposed study.

The qualifications and experience of an investigator should be considered by an IRB and weighed against the complexity of the protocol and risk to human subjects. An IRB can require a less-experienced investigator to be sponsored by more seasoned researchers. Proposals that require skills beyond those held by the investigator should be modified to meet the investigator's skills, have additional qualified personnel added, or be rejected by the IRB (OPRR).

Educational Requirements for Clinical Investigators

Currently, federal agencies have not enacted mandatory educational requirements for all investigators. The OIG has recommended that standards for education be established, and it has expressed frustration that federal agencies have not done so (OIG, April 2000). OPRR recommended that: "Personnel involved in the conduct of research should receive additional training in institutional expectations and specific regulations pertaining to research. Training designed to enhance the development of high quality proposals should be encouraged" (OPRR, *Institutional Review Board Guidebook*). HHS has proposed regulations that would require investigators to participate in educational programs concerning financial conflict of interest issues (HHS, 2000).

Researchers conducting human-subject research on the NIH campus are required to complete a Web-based tutorial (http://helix.nih.gov:8001/ohsr/newcbt). As of October 1, 2000 NIH requires education on protection of human research participants for all investigators submitting NIH applications for grants, contracts, or awards involving human participants. Investigators must provide a description of education completed in the protection of human subjects for each key personnel in the research proposal. Key personnel include all individuals responsible for the design and conduct of the study. This includes key personnel of foreign awards or foreign subcontractors. It does not include key personnel that are not involved with the human subjects portion of the project. The description should be submitted in a cover letter that accompanies the description of other support, IRB approval, and other information in accordance with just-in-time procedures. The documentation is part of the document to be signed by an institutional official. This description also must be contained in annual progress reports. The training of new key personnel added during the course of a project does not need to be reported to NIH until the annual progress report. NIH does not intend to endorse education programs but does point out that its Internet-based tutorial is available at http://ohsr.od.nih.gov/cbt. NIH has also developed a Web site containing bioethics resources for investigators (www.nih.gov.sigs/bioethics/). It is anticipated that its policy will eventually be superceded by the Office of Research Integrity's institutional assurance on the Responsible Conduct of Research.

The Office of Research Integrity issued a final Public Health Service Policy on Instruction in the Responsible Conduct of Research (RCR) on December 1, 2000. (This was subsequently suspended on February 20, 2001. 66 Fed. Reg. #35, pp. 11032–33.) Under the PHS Policy, an institution receiving PHS funds must assure ORI by October 1, 2001 that it has a program of instruction that complies with the RCR policy. The RCR requirements are to be fully implemented (all staff members fully trained) by an institution receiving PHS funds by October 1, 2003. RCR covers nine core instructional areas:

1. Data acquisition, management, sharing and ownership
2. Mentor/trainee responsibilities
3. Publication practices and responsible authorship
4. Peer review
5. Collaborative science
6. Human subjects
7. Research involving animals
8. Research misconduct
9. Conflict of interest and commitment

ORI allows some flexibility for an institution to exercise reasonable discretion to require the education of research staff members on pertinent topics among these nine core instructional areas. The exact content, length, level, and method of instruction is for the institution to determine. ORI has stated that a three-hour course would be sufficient (ORI, "Frequently Asked Questions for the PHS Policy on Instruction in the Responsible Conduct of Research"). Anyone who follows OHRP requirements on educating research staff automatically complies with RCR requirements as to protection of human subjects. "Research staff" is defined as:

> staff at the institution who have direct and substantive involvement in proposing, performing, reviewing, or reporting research, or who receive research training, supported by PHS funds or who otherwise work on the PHS-supported research project even if the individual does not receive PHS support. The institution may make reasonable determinations regarding which research staff fall within this definition. [ORI, 2000, p. 3]

Most academic institutions are moving toward minimum educational standards. Research sponsors are likely to follow suit.

Other Educational Resources Available for Investigators

Many universities are developing Internet-based educational programs for its faculty and staff. For example, University of California-Davis requires a researcher to complete both the NIH tutorial (http://ohsr.od.nih.gov/cbt) and the University of California-Irvine tutorial (http://tutorials.rgs.uci.edu). Government agencies have developed similar Web sites. For example, NIH has a continuing education program on the protection of human participants in research, now available online at http://cme.nci.nih.gov. The FDA has information for clinical investigators at http://www.fda.gov/cder/about/smallbiz/clinical_investigator.htm. Unfortunately, few comprehensive reference texts exist for an investigator.

Experience Requirements for Clinical Investigators

Federal regulations do not set any minimum experience requirements for an investigator. However, one function of an IRB is to determine that an investigator has adequate expertise and experience to ensure that human subjects are not exposed to unnecessary risk. To this end, the IRB should inquire as to what role an investigator has played in previous studies as well as his clinical experience with the object of the study (for example, a medication).

Information That a Clinical Investigator Must Disclose About Himself

In addition to responding to the inquiries of an IRB as to experience and expertise, an investigator has an ethical duty to identify any potential conflicts of interest. This includes a financial interest in the medication or device that is being studied or in the sponsoring company. Not only should this be required by an IRB in submitting a research protocol, an IRB should require that the investigator disclose this to potential participants during the informed consent process.

HHS has proposed regulations that conflict of interest information should be obtained from all clinical investigators according to institutional policies and procedures. HHS's draft regulations require that all financial relationships between an investigator and sponsor, whether or not directly related to the particular study, should be considered. (HHS, 2000).

The FDA requires that investigators submit financial information to the study sponsor who in turn completes FDA Financial Disclosure Form 3454 (certifying the absence of financial interests and arrangements) or Form 3455 (disclosing the financial interests and arrangements and steps taken to minimize the potential for bias) (21 CFR Part 54. Financial Disclosure by Clinical Investigators (FDA)). The burden is on the investigator to provide the sponsor with the required information. The FDA interprets financial disclosure by the investigator to include his or her spouse and each dependent child (FDA, 1999). The investigator must also advise the sponsor of pertinent changes in financial interests during the study and for up to one year afterward.

An application for an IND or IDE must advise the FDA of the following information about financial interests of clinical investigators, using Form 3455 (FDA, 21 CFR §54.4):

1. Any financial arrangement entered into between the sponsor of the covered study and the clinical investigator involved in the conduct of a covered clinical trial, whereby

the value of the compensation to the clinical investigator for conducting the study could be influenced by the outcome of the study;

2. Any significant payments of other sorts from the sponsor of the covered study, such as a grant to fund ongoing research, compensation in the form of equipment, retainer for ongoing consultation, or honoraria;

3. Any proprietary interest in the tested product held by any clinical investigator involved in a study;

4. Any significant equity interest in the sponsor of the covered study held by any clinical investigator involved in any clinical study; and

5. Any steps taken to minimize the potential for bias resulting from any of the disclosed arrangements, interests, or payments.

A complete copy of the FDA regulations regarding financial disclosure can be found at http://www.access.gpo.gov/nara/cfr/waisidx_98/21cfr54_98.html.

A Clinical Investigator That Has a Financial Interest in a Study or a Sponsor Participating in the Study

An investigator with a conflict of interest should not be permitted to directly engage in parts of the study where the conflict of interest could have a detrimental effect on human participants, such as design of the trial, monitoring of the trial, obtaining the informed consent, adverse event reporting, or analyzing data (HHS, 2000). However, an investigator is permitted to perform functions in a study where a conflict of interest can have no material impact on the human participants. (See 42 CFR Part 50, Subpart F. Responsibility of Applicants for Promoting Objectivity in Research for Which PHS Funding is Sought and 45 CFR Part 94.) If the financial interests of an investigator raise a serious question about the integrity of data submitted to the FDA, the agency will take any action it deems necessary to ensure that the data are reliable. Examples of actions it might take include:

• Initiating audits of the data derived from the investigator;

• Requesting that the sponsor submit further analyses of the data. For example, the FDA may ask for an evaluation of the effect of the investigator's data on the overall study outcome;

• Requesting that the sponsor conduct additional independent studies to confirm the results of the questioned study;

• Refusing to treat the covered clinical study as providing data on which the FDA can take action.

The following guidelines have been proposed to the Association of American Medical Colleges (Mangan, 2001):

1. Institutions should clearly specify what activities are and are not permitted;

2. Staff members and students, as well as faculty members, should be required to report potential conflicts of interest;

3. Restrictions on industry ties for clinical trials, which involve humans, should be stricter than those for basic laboratory research;

4. Specific rules should set forth types of financial involvement, such as fees, honoraria, gifts, and stock options;

5. Researchers should be required to disclose such financial ties when submitting articles for publication.

[Mangan, "Medical Educators Propose Guidelines to Strengthen and Clarify Conflict-of-Interest Policies," The Chronicle of Higher Education (http://chronicle.com), 2/9/2001].

Determining Whether an Investigator Has Adequate Resources to Conduct a Clinical Investigation

An IRB should consider whether an investigator has organized appropriate resources to conduct his proposed study (ICH, Guidelines for Good Clinical Practice). For example:

- Has the investigator demonstrated (based on retrospective data) a potential for recruiting the required number of suitable participants within the proposed recruitment period?
- Does the investigator have sufficient time to properly conduct and complete the trial within the proposed trial period?
- Does the investigator have available an adequate number of qualified staff and adequate facilities for the foreseen duration of the trial to conduct the trial properly and safely?
- Has the investigator ensured that all persons assisting with the trial are adequately informed about the protocol, the investigational product(s), and their trial-related duties and functions?

....

RESPONSIBILITY FOR THE PROTOCOL AND SAFETY

The Responsibility of an Investigator in Clinical Research

An investigator has the obligation to comply with the protocol, IRB directives, institutional policies and procedures, and applicable regulations (ICH, *Guidelines for Good Clinical Practice*):

- The investigator should conduct the trial in compliance with the protocol agreed to by the sponsor and, if required, by the regulatory authority(ies) and which was given approval by the IRB. The investigator and the sponsor should sign the protocol, or an alternative contract, to confirm agreement.
- The investigator should not implement any deviation from, or changes of the protocol without agreement by the sponsor and prior review and documented approval by the IRB of an amendment, except where necessary to eliminate an immediate hazard(s) to trial participants, or when the change(s) involves only logistical or administrative aspects of the trial (e.g., change in monitor(s), change of telephone number(s)).
- The investigator, or person designated by the investigator, should document and explain any deviation from the approved protocol.
- The investigator may implement a deviation from, or a change of, the protocol to eliminate an immediate hazard(s) to trial subjects without prior IRB approval. As soon as possible, the implemented deviation or change, the reasons for it, and, if appropriate, the proposed protocol amendment(s) should be submitted:
  a. to the IRB for review and approval,
  b. to the sponsor for agreement and, if required,
  c. to the regulatory authority(ies).

The Responsibility of the Investigator for Following the Study Protocol

Most institutions, via its IRB, and sponsors will mandate that the investigator is responsible for fastidious compliance with the study protocol. Likewise, federal regulations hold the investigator responsible for how a study is conducted. In clinical trials subject to FDA regulation, a clinical investigator signs an investigator agreement that attests to his knowledge of and agreement with his responsibilities under FDA regulations as a researcher and within the approved protocol (21 CFR §312.60).

The Responsibility of the Investigator for Ensuring Human Participant Safety

The investigator has primary responsibility for the safety of participants in any study he is conducting. This requires that the investigator have active involvement in all phases of a study, particularly during any interactions with human participants. The investigator will be held accountable for reporting and acting on any adverse events. He does not have the option of delegating this to a staff member.

The Investigator's Obligations When Unexpected Findings Occur

An investigator must inform research participants of any important new information that might affect their willingness to continue participation in a study (45 CFR §46.116(b)(5)). An investigator has the obligation to keep his IRB advised of unexpected findings involving risk and any occurrence of serious harm to research participants (45 CFR §46.103(b)(5)). The IRB can be helpful to an investigator in determining when new information should be disclosed to current or prospective participants. Likewise, most sponsors mandate that they be kept apprised of findings, especially adverse events.

Defining an Adverse Event

Investigators engaged in IND or IDE protocols must tell the FDA about problems that are serious, unexpected, and possibly related to an experimental treatment. A separate report is required each time such an incident occurs. Less serious events can be summarized in an annual report to the FDA. In contrast, NIH and other agencies following the Common Rule require that an investigator promptly send all reports of unanticipated problems to the IRB. Interpreting the meaning of "adverse event" can be difficult for both the investigator and those who review reports.

The Investigator's Responsibility to Comply with IRB Decisions and Procedures

The investigator is primarily responsible for seeking and obtaining IRB approval of a proposed study (21 CFR §312.66). In addition, the researcher is responsible for complying with all IRB decisions, conditions, and requirements. The investigator is responsible for reporting the progress of the research to the IRB and/or appropriate institutional officials as often and in the manner prescribed by the IRB but at least once per year (OPRR, *Institutional Review Board Guidebook*).

The Investigator's Responsibility for Control of an Investigational Drug

An investigational drug should only be administered under the personal supervision of the investigator or a subinvestigator responsible to the investigator (21 CFR §312.61). The investigator is responsible for the secure storage of an investigational drug, if it is subject to the Controlled Substances Act (21 CFR §312.69). He or she is also responsible for disposing of unused supplies of the investigational drug or returning it to the sponsor (21 CFR §312.59).

Records That the Investigator Must Maintain

In FDA-regulated studies, the investigator must maintain adequate records to track the disposition of an investigational drug, including dates, quantity, and use by human subjects. Unused supplies must be accounted for at the end of a study and returned to the sponsor or destroyed. The investigator also must draft and maintain case histories that record all observations and other data pertinent to the study for each participant in the investigation. The case history usually consists of the case report and supporting data as well as a file that includes the signed informed consent documents, progress notes, and other medical records. The investigator must keep these records for two years following the date that a marketing application for the investigational drug is approved. If approval is not sought, the records must be maintained for two years after the study is terminated and the FDA is notified (21 CFR §312.62).

The Investigator's Responsibility for Reports to the Sponsor

The investigator must supply any reports to the sponsor that may be part of the contract agreement between the sponsor and the investigator. At a minimum, the investigator must provide progress reports, safety reports, and a final report to the sponsor for investigational drug studies. The investigator's progress reports are used by the sponsor to submit a mandated annual report to the FDA on the progress of a clinical investigation. Safety reports are required with regard to any adverse events that are reasonably regarded as caused by or probably caused by the investigational drug. As discussed elsewhere, such reports should be made timely. Shortly after completion of the investigator's participation in a study, the investigator is required to provide a final report to the sponsor (21 CFR §312.64).

Common Examples of Investigator Noncompliance

The most common errors by investigators are failing to report changes in protocols, misuse or nonuse of informed consent documents, and failure to submit protocols to the IRB in a timely fashion (OPRR, *Institutional Review Board Guidebook*). Occasionally, an investigator will either avoid or ignore an IRB. "When unapproved research is discovered, the IRB and the institution should act promptly to halt the research, assure remedial action regarding any breach of regulatory or institutional human participant protection requirements, and address the question of the investigator's fitness to conduct human subject research" (OPRR, *Institutional Review Board Guidebook*). Any serious or continuing noncompliance with HHS human subject regulations must be promptly reported to OHRP (OPRR, *Institutional Review Board Guidebook*).

Defining Research Misconduct

Pursuant to a final rule dated December 6, 2000, research misconduct is now more easily sanctioned where the federal government funds or directly conducts research (65 Fed. Reg. 76260-76264). Fabrication, falsification, or plagiarism in proposing, performing, or reviewing research, or in reporting research results as well as unethical treatment of participants come under this rule. The government policy gives the following definitions:

• Fabrication is making up data or results and recording or reporting them.

• Falsification is manipulating research materials, equipment, or processes, or changing or omitting data or results such that the research is not accurately represented in the research record.

• Plagiarism is the appropriation of another person's ideas, processes, results, or words without giving appropriate credit.

Research misconduct does not include honest error or differences of opinion. Under the federal rule, a finding of research misconduct requires:

• A significant departure from accepted practices of the relevant research community has occurred.

• The misconduct was committed intentionally, knowingly, or recklessly.

• The allegation is proven by a preponderance of evidence.

The Investigator's Obligations if He Realizes That a Staff Member Has Altered Records

If an investigator determines that records have been altered, he should immediately report it to the institution's compliance officer and the private or government study sponsor (if there is one). A private sponsor may need to report the problem to the FDA if any potential exists that data supporting a submission to the FDA is suspect. If the alterations could in any way compromise human subject safety, the investigator must take any steps necessary to protect the participants and notify the IRB. Corrective actions with the staff member should be undertaken pursuant to the institution's policies.

Protections for Whistleblowers

The Office of Research Integrity (ORI) has proposed a "whistleblower protection" rule (November 28, 2000), based on the Public Health Service Act that requires DHHS to "establish regulatory standards for preventing and responding to occurrences of retaliation taken against whistleblowers by entities which have a research misconduct assurance under Section 493 and by those entities' officials and agents" (65 Fed. Reg. 70830-70841). The proposed rule prohibits an organization, its officials, or agents from retaliating against an employee who has in good faith (1) made an allegation that the organization, its officials, or agents have engaged in, or failed to respond adequately to, an allegation of research misconduct, or (2) cooperated with an investigation of such an allegation.

Under the proposed rule, a whistleblower must file a retaliation complaint with the institution within 180 days. The retaliation must have occurred within one year of the whistleblower's original misconduct allegation or cooperation with an investigation. The whistleblower and the institution have thirty days to negotiate a resolution of the retaliation complaint. The parties may also agree to extend this time period up to an additional 60 days. A settlement cannot prohibit the whistleblower from making future allegations of research misconduct or cooperating with future investigations. After the negotiation period, the whistleblower may elect to use an organization's administrative proceeding process or "any other available remedy provided by law" (65 Fed. Reg. 70830).

....

CORRECTIVE ACTIONS AGAINST INVESTIGATORS

The Steps to Be Taken if Research Misconduct Is Suspected

Allegations of research misconduct can be investigated and sanctions can be imposed by the investigator's institution, by a government agency, or by the courts. Research misconduct is defined by the Office of Research Integrity (ORI) as fabrication, falsification, or plagiarism in proposing, performing, or reviewing research, or in reporting research results.

Response of Institution   The ORI contends that while federal agencies have ultimate oversight authority for federally funded research, an institution has the primary responsibility for prevention and detection of research misconduct and for the inquiry, investigation, and adjudication of research misconduct alleged to have occurred in association with their own institution (ORI, Guidelines). An institution should have policies and procedures in place to investigate allegations of research misconduct. Analogous to medical staff privilege corrective actions, the institution should have a process in place for allegations to be investigated and adjudicated in a fair, impartial, and timely manner. The process should include:

1. An inquiry: the assessment of whether the allegation has substance and if an investigation is warranted.

2. An investigation: the formal development of a factual record, and the examination of that record leading to dismissal of the case or to a recommendation for a finding of research misconduct or other appropriate remedies.

3. Adjudication: the opportunity for hearing of evidence and appropriate, if any, corrective actions are imposed.

4. Appeal: the opportunity for the investigator to seek a further impartial review of the evidence and conclusions considered by the trial-level panel.

The investigation and adjudication should be conducted in a manner that is transparently fair and just. For example, the individuals appointed to investigate the allegations should be as independent from the investigator and the institution as possible. No one should be able to credibly allege that the motivation of anyone involved in the process is anything but honorable. Reasonable time limits, with the opportunity for reasonable extensions of time, for each phase of the investigative and adjudicative process should be set forth in the institution's policies and procedures. ORI has developed a Model Policy and Procedure for Responding to Allegations of Scientific Misconduct. (See Chapter Sixteen.)

Whistleblowers must be protected from retaliation. They should be assured that good-faith concerns will be objectively considered and that they will not suffer harm for raising such concerns. Likewise, the investigator should be assured that the mere allegation of misconduct will not halt all of his research projects or derail his career. The investigator should be given a timely written statement detailing the nature of the allegations against him, access to any information pertaining to the allegations, and the opportunity to substantively refute the allegations. The investigation and adjudication should be undertaken in as confidential of a manner as possible. Many states have confidentiality statutes specific to medical peer review actions which may be applicable to such a review if the investigation and adjudication processes are structured to come under such peer review laws and regulations. On the other hand, the institution should have well-defined and severe sanctions for fraud, fabrication, plagiarism, or other misconduct. These sanctions must be applied objectively and evenly (42 CFR Part 50, Subpart A. Responsibility of PHS Awardee and Applicant Institutions for Dealing with and Reporting Possible Misconduct in Science).

An institution must notify a government agency that is funding the research at issue of any research misconduct allegations if:

1. The allegations involve federally funded research (or an application for federal funding) and meet the federal definition of research misconduct given above.
2. If the institution's inquiry into the allegations determines there is sufficient evidence to proceed to an investigation.

The institution must notify the funding agency immediately if:

1. Public health or safety is at risk;
2. Agency resources or interests are threatened;
3. Research activities should be suspended;
4. Possible violations of civil or criminal law are reasonably indicated;
5. Federal action is required to protect the interests of those involved in the investigation;
6. The research institution believes the inquiry or investigation may be made public prematurely so that appropriate steps can be taken to safeguard evidence and protect the rights of those involved, and,
7. The research community or public should be informed.

The institution should forward the following to the funding agency:

- A copy of the evidentiary record.
- The investigative report.
- Recommendations made to the institution's adjudicating official.
- The researcher's written response to the recommendations (if any).
- The adjudicating official's decision.
- Corrective actions, if appropriate, taken or planned.

The federal directive is not very clear as to when these items are to be forwarded to the funding agency. The better course would be to provide each one to the agency as it is completed.

Response of Federal Agency   A federal agency (such as NIH or DOE) will usually rely on the investigator's institution to make the initial response to allegations of research misconduct against an investigator. Allegations made directly to a federal agency will usually be referred to the institution for investigation (42 CFR §50.101). However, an agency can initiate its own investigation at any time. Examples of when a federal agency may not defer to the institution include the following:

- The agency determines the institution is not prepared to handle the allegation in a manner consistent with this policy.

- Agency involvement is needed to protect the public interest, including public health and safety.

- The allegation involves an entity of sufficiently small size (or an individual) that it cannot reasonably conduct the investigation itself.

Once the federal agency receives the results of the institution's investigation and adjudication (or if the agency initiates its own investigation), the agency will determine if any further action is appropriate. The agency will notify the investigator and the institution of its conclusion. If the agency decides that administrative sanctions should be entered against the investigator, the agency will follow the steps for administrative hearings and appeals. A Departmental Appeals Board (DAB) hears appeals.

The Office of Research Integrity (ORI) has adopted the following target time line to complete misconduct cases involving PHS-supported research within 480 days:

Inquiry	60 days
Investigation	120 days
ORI Oversight Review	240 days
ASH Review	60 days
Total	480 days

This does not take into consideration a subsequent appeal to the DAB, which has a target of completing a hearing in nine months.

In determining the appropriate administrative action, the federal agency will consider "the seriousness of the misconduct, including, but not limited to, the degree to which the misconduct was knowing, intentional, or reckless; was an isolated event or part of a pattern; or had significant impact on the research record, research subjects, other researchers, institutions, or the public welfare" (ORI, Model Policy). If misconduct is proven by a preponderance of the evidence, a federal agency may take the following actions:

- Appropriate steps to correct the research record.

- Letters of reprimand.

- The imposition of special certification or assurance requirements to ensure compliance with applicable regulations or terms of an award.

- Suspension or termination of an active award.

- Suspension and debarment of the investigator in accordance with applicable government-wide rules on suspension and debarment.

The U.S. General Services Administration identifies investigators that are suspended or debarred on the public List of Parties Excluded from Federal Procurement and Nonprocurement Programs.

The foregoing discussion is separate and apart from any investigation that the Office of Inspector General or a law enforcement agency may undertake.

While a researcher may feel singled out and even treated unfairly, he does not have a right to be free from being investigated by a federal agency, to have an investigation be conducted on a confidential basis, or to have an investigation reach a particular result. Federal officials are entitled to qualified immunity in conducting such activities. Damage to one's reputation or prospects for employment do not give rise to a constitution-based action against the federal government or its employees, even when the researcher finally prevails in the administrative hearing process. *Popovic v. U.S.,* 997 F. Supp. 672 (D. Md. 1998) applying *Bivens v. Six Unknown Named Agents of Federal Bureau of Narcotics,* 403 U.S. 388 (1971); *Harlow v. Fitzgerald,* 457 U.S. 800 (1982); and *Anderson v. Creighton,* 483 U.S. 635 (1987).

Response in Criminal or Civil Law   If an institution believes that a crime has occurred, it should immediately notify the local law enforcement authorities. A sponsor or a funding federal agency may seek compensation for fraud through a civil law action. Human subjects may also seek compensation if they have been injured by the investigator's misconduct. As will be discussed elsewhere, a *qui tam* action may be filed against an investigator alleging that false data and false claims were submitted to obtain federal funds. For example, *United States v. Regents of Univ. of Minnesota,* 154 F.3d 870 (Eighth Cir. 1998). A determination by ORI is not controlling as to a finding that misconduct did or did not occur. *United States v. Regents of Univ. of California,* 912 F. Supp. 868, 880 (D. Md. 1995).

FDA Monitoring Clinical Investigators

The FDA Bioresearch Monitoring Program may inspect a clinical investigator with a focus toward a specific study or toward the investigator in regard to multiple studies. FDA oversight of clinical investigators has been primarily by retrospective review of clinical trials. In 1999, the FDA inspected only 468 clinical investigators of nearly 14,000 clinical investigators. Three-quarters of these inspections were initiated as part of the FDA's application review process and thus were not due to any suspicion of wrongdoing. FDA monitoring has been primarily focused on verifying data. The OIG has criticized this as not protecting human subjects during the research process. The OIG also criticized the FDA for not having written criteria for selection of investigators for inspection (OIG, June 2000).

A study-oriented investigation, says the FDA, has two components. The first is a review of the study by examining:

- Who did what.
- The degree of delegation of authority.
- Where specific aspects of the study were performed.
- How and where data were recorded.
- How test article accountability was maintained.
- How the monitor communicated with the clinical investigator.
- How the monitor evaluated the study's progress.

The second component is an audit of the study data. This is a detailed comparison of the information submitted to the FDA and the sponsor with all available data. A review of medical records during the study period, prior to the study period, and for a reasonable period after the completion of the study may be utilized as part of the audit. An investigator-oriented inspection, says the FDA, may be undertaken because:

- An investigator conducted a pivotal study that merits in-depth examination because of its singular importance in product approval or its impact on medical practice.
- A sponsor has reported concerns to the FDA about an investigator, such as difficulty getting case reports or receiving data inconsistent with other research sites.

- A participant complains to the FDA about violation of the protocol or his rights.
- An investigator has participated in a large number of studies or has done work outside of his specialty area.

In addition, a clinical investigator may be selected for inspection based on the FDA's application review process, a complaint, observations during previous inspections, or analysis of data submitted to the FDA (OIG, June 2000). A sponsor must notify the FDA when a clinical investigator's participation in a study has been terminated for non-compliance. However, many sponsors are reluctant to make such a report and can avoid doing so by terminating the clinical investigator for administrative reasons (OIG, June 2000). Once an investigator has been selected for inspection, an Office of Regulatory Affairs (ORA) investigator conducts the inspection. The inspection may involve interviews with the clinical investigator and study staff as well as review of the clinical investigator's processes, records, data, and documentation.

The investigative procedure for an investigator-oriented inspection is almost identical to a study-oriented inspection. However, the scrutiny is likely to be more in-depth and may cover more than one study.

At the end of an inspection, the FDA inspector will conduct an exit interview with the clinical investigator and will usually issue a written Form FDA-483 (Inspectional Observations) to the clinical investigator. The FDA inspector will also submit a written report to FDA headquarters for evaluation.

FDA Procedure When a Problem Is Detected

Based on the information contained in Form FDA-483 (OIG, 2000), the inspection is classified as:

- "No action indicated:" Few or no objectionable conditions or practices; the investigator is not required to make any changes or respond to the FDA.
- "Voluntary action indicated:" The clinical investigator is asked to make voluntary changes. A letter requesting voluntary action does not necessarily require a response from the clinical investigator; or
- "Official action indicated:" In the vast majority of cases, two official actions are taken. Where violations appear less serious, a Warning Letter is issued outlining violations and requesting a response. The response should include specific steps that the clinical investigator plans to take to correct the violations and prevent recurrence. The FDA may also elect to not allow the clinical investigator's data to be included in the application.

The FDA can place a "clinical hold" on a study if it finds that a clinical investigator has committed serious violations of FDA regulations. A clinical hold is an order that immediately suspends or imposes restrictions on an ongoing or proposed clinical study (21 CFR §312.42). A clinical hold may be complete or partial. A complete clinical hold is the delay or suspension of a study. A partial clinical hold is the delay or suspension of only part of a study. In contrast to the disqualification of an investigator, which is discussed next, a clinical hold can be imposed any time that the FDA finds that study participants are or would be exposed to an unreasonable and significant risk of illness or injury (21 CFR §312.42; also see FDA, April 2002).

The FDA can initiate the process for disqualification of the clinical investigator from future clinical research of FDA-regulated drugs or devices. First, a Notice of Initiation of

Disqualification Proceedings and Opportunity to Explain is issued. The investigator is offered the chance to meet informally with the FDA at a mutually convenient location to discuss violations found during the inspection or to respond in writing. The investigator may be represented by counsel, and a transcript may be made of the hearing. If the FDA is satisfied after the meeting that the clinical investigator is taking appropriate corrective action, the process may be terminated. If the FDA is not satisfied by the investigator's explanation or the investigator fails to respond, the next step is to issue a Notice of Opportunity for Hearing (also referred to as a "Part 16 hearing," from 21 CFR part 16). Third parties under the Freedom of Information Act can obtain the notice. The FDA may also notify other federal agencies of its preliminary findings with the caveat that a final decision on disqualification has not yet been made.

At a Part 16 hearing conducted at FDA headquarters, both the investigator, who can be represented by counsel, and the FDA present their case. The FDA gives the investigator notice of the matters to be considered. This includes a comprehensive statement of the basis for the proposed disqualification of the investigator and a general summary of the information that will be presented. The FDA and the investigator will exchange written notices of articles or written information to be relied on at the hearing. If a document is not available to one party, the other party must supply it. Either the investigator or the FDA may file a motion for summary decision, a finding based solely on the submitted written record. Oral and written evidence can be received at the hearing. The hearing officer from the Office of Health Affairs makes a recommendation to the Commissioner, who reviews the file and makes a decision.

The Part 16 hearing process can take several years, during which the clinical investigator can continue to conduct clinical research. At any point, the clinical investigator can agree to be disqualified or restricted by signing a consent agreement. Such a consent agreement can be drafted on any terms to which the FDA and the investigator agree. It is usually an agreement by the investigator to either (1) refrain from further studies with FDA regulated test articles; or (2) follow specific restrictions in the use of investigational products, such as oversight by an individual acceptable to both the investigator and the FDA. The FDA has stated that most disqualification actions are resolved by consent agreements.

A clinical investigator can be disqualified from receiving investigational drugs or devices when the FDA determines that he has repeatedly and deliberately failed to comply with the requirements for the conduct of clinical trials or submitted false information. The OIG has criticized the FDA's failure to define what "repeatedly" or "deliberately" mean or what the thresholds are for these terms (OIG, June 2000).

The FDA will also review data submitted by a sanctioned clinical investigator in other studies (OIG, June 2000).

Other Actions That the FDA Can Take Against an Investigator, Institution, or Sponsor

The FDA may take one or more of the following actions if it believes that the Food, Drug & Cosmetic Act (FDCA) has been violated:

- Obtain a court order (an injunction) directing the violator to cease violating the Act (21 USC §332).
- Charge the violator with a crime, seeking fines or imprisonment (21 USC §333).
- Seize the goods that violate the Act (21 USC §334).

- Bar the violator from participating in future new drug applications (21 USC §335a).
- Impose a civil monetary penalty (21 USC §335b).
- Issue a written notice or warning (21 USC §336).

Criminal Penalties Under the Food, Drug & Cosmetic Act

Conviction for violation of the Food, Drug & Cosmetic Act can lead to imprisonment for up to one year, a fine up to $100,000, or both. A second conviction or a finding of an intent to defraud increases the potential penalty up to three years, a fine up to $250,000, or both (21 USC §333, 18 USC §3559(a), 18 USC §3571(b)(1)).

Civil Penalties Under the FDCA

A civil action brought by the Attorney General can result in a fine up to $250,000 against individuals and up to $1,000,000 against other entities (21 USC §333). The important distinction between civil penalties and criminal penalties is that civil penalties do not require as high of a standard of proof by the government.

Parties That Can Be Held Responsible for Violations of the FDCA

In addition to individuals, corporations and its officers can be held responsible for violations by employees (*United States v. Dotterweich,* 320 US §277 (1943)). Corporate officers not only have a duty to seek out and remedy violations, but they also have an affirmative duty to implement measures that will ensure violations never occur (*United States v. Park,* 421 US 658).

Parties Advised by the FDA When It Finds Investigator Misconduct

The FDA now informs sponsors and IRBs associated with an investigator that it has found evidence of misconduct (OIG, April 2000). The FDA maintains a list of disqualified or restricted clinical investigators on its Internet home page. As of January 2000, the list had information on 133 clinical investigators. Even if a restriction or disqualification is lifted, the investigator's name remains on the list with a note that the sanction has been repealed.

············

CONCLUSION

With the title of investigator comes many responsibilities. The golden era of being identified and paid as an investigator simply as figurehead has passed. The investigator must be actively involved in every phase of a clinical study and is directly responsible for everything occurring in it. Failure to do so can cost a scientist his reputation, his wealth, and his freedom.

References

Anderson v. Creighton, 483 U.S. 635 (1987).

Bivens v. Six Unknown Named Agents of Federal Bureau of Narcotics, 403 U.S. 388 (1971).

Ezekiel, Wendler, & Grady. "What Makes Clinical Research Ethical?," *JAMA*. 2000; 283: 2701–2711.

FDA. Form FDA-3454 (Certifying the Absence of Financial Interests and Arrangements).

FDA. Form FDA-3455 (Disclosing the Financial Interests and Arrangements and Steps Taken to Minimize the Potential for Bias).

FDA. Form FDA-483 (Inspectional Observations).

FDA. Guidance for Industry and Clinical Investigators: The Use of Clinical Holds Following Clinical Investigator Misconduct (Draft Guidance). April 2002.

FDA. Guidance for Industry Financial Disclosure by Clinical Investigators, Draft Guidance, October 25, 1999.

FDA. Information for Clinical Investigators: http://www.fda.gov/cder/about/smallbiz/clinical_investigator.htm.

Harlow v. Fitzgerald, 457 U.S. 800 (1982).

HHS, Financial Relationships in Clinical Research: Issues for Institutions, Clinical Investigators, and IRBs to Consider when Dealing with Issues of Financial Interests and Human Subject Protection, Draft Interim Guidance, Jan. 2000.

ICH. *Guidelines for Good Clinical Practice*, 1996.

IOM, "Integrity in Scientific Research: Creating an Environment That Promotes Responsible Conduct." 15 July 2002.

Mangan, "Medical Educators Propose Guidelines to Strengthen and Clarify Conflict-of-Interest Policies." The Chronicle of Higher Education (http://chronicle.com), February 2, 2001.

NIH. Bioethics Resources for Investigators: www.nih.gov.sigs/bioethics/.

NIH. Continuing Education Program on the Protection of Human Participants in Research, http://cme.nci.nih.gov.

NIH. Investigator Training Tutorial, http://helix.nih.gov:8001/ohsr/newcbt.

NIH. Investigator Tutorial, http://ohsr.od.nih.gov/cbt.

OIG. "FDA Oversight of Clinical Investigators." June 2000, OEI-05-99-00350.

OIG. "Protecting Human Research Subjects: Status of Recommendations." April 2000, OEI-01-97-00197.

OPRR. *Institutional Review Board Guidebook* 1993. Chap II, see A.ii, #27.

ORI. Frequently Asked Questions for the PHS Policy on Instruction in the Responsible Conduct of Research.

ORI. Model Policy and Procedure for Responding to Allegations of Scientific Misconduct.

ORI. Public Health Service Policy on Instruction in the Responsible Conduct of Research (RCR). December 1, 2000. (This was subsequently suspended on 2/20/2001. 66 Fed. Reg. #35, pp. 11032–33).

Popovic v. U.S., 997 F. Supp. 672 (D. Md. 1998) applying *Bivens v. Six Unknown Named Agents of Federal Bureau of Narcotics*, 403 U.S. 388 (1971).

United States v. Dotterweich, 320 U.S. 277 (1943).

United States v. Park, 421 U.S. 658.

United States v. Regents of Univ. of California, 912 F. Supp. 868, 880 (D. Md. 1995).

United States v. Regents of Univ. of Minnesota, 154 F.3d 870 (Eighth Cir. 1998).

8.

Research Protocols

Introduction 239
  The Fundamental Methodology of Scientific Study 240
The Basic Elements of a Research Protocol 240
  The Investigator's Brochure 243
The General Issues to Be Considered by an IRB in Reviewing a Proposed Study 248
  Review of the Underlying Science of a Proposed Study by the IRB 249
  Considerations in Advertising for Research Participants 249
  Records to Be Maintained About a Study 250
Types of Studies and Issues Related to Each 254
  An Observational Study 254
    Record Review or Historical Study 254
    Surveys, Questionnaires, or Interviews 254
    Epidemiologic Studies 255
    Case-Control Study 255
    Prospective Study 256
    Clinical Trial 256
  IRB Considerations in Reviewing and Approving a Clinical Trial 256
    Randomization of the Patients 256
    Placebos 257
  The Phases of Clinical Trials 257
  Important Considerations with the Various Phases of Clinical Trials 258
  Charging Study Participants for Investigational Products Used in a Study 259
  Special Concerns of Vaccine Trials 259
  Special Concerns of a Study Using Radioactive Materials or X Rays 261
  Special Concerns in HIV-Related Research Protocols 263
  Special Concerns in Organ Transplant Studies 264
Compliance Issues in Research Protocols 265
Conclusion 265
References 265

INTRODUCTION

Many institutions have developed a template for research protocols. In the pharmaceutical industry, most clinical trials proceed in a standard fashion under FDA guidelines. This chapter is intended to assist a researcher who must develop his own protocol from a blank sheet as well as assist an IRB in evaluating research protocols that may come from many sources and have varying goals.

A research protocol should address the following seven ethical requirements: value, validity, fair participant selection, favorable risk-benefit ratio, respect for participants, informed consent, and independent review (Ezekiel, Wendler, and Grady, 2000). In addition, the research protocol or related policies and procedures should ensure compliance with rules and regulations effecting the provision of the services that will be part of the protocol. For example, clinical laboratory studies are subject to federal oversight under the Clinical Laboratory Improvement Act of 1976 (CLIA), Pub. L. No. 90-174, sec. 5.81. The research plan must also address quality assurance standards set by the institution as well as external entities.

The Fundamental Methodology of Scientific Study

Objective and systematic observation of physical events and analytic reasoning are the heart of scientific inquiry. Objective observation is directly experienced and can be repeated, making it possible for scientists to verify others' work. Systematic observation is done under clearly specified, and where possible, controlled conditions that can be quantified and evaluated. A research protocol should clearly describe the process by which the investigator intends to make objective and systematic observations, also known as empirical data, and how the investigator will analyze this data.

To organize empirical data, a scientist attempts to explain the causal factors underlying the data. This is a scientific theory. The internal consistency, ability to account for existing data, and ability to predict future events determine the usefulness of a theory. A hypothesis is a prediction of what can be tested empirically. A scientific theory or hypothesis can never be proven to be true. The test of either is whether available data supports (confirms) or not (disconfirms) the hypothesis or theory.

············

THE BASIC ELEMENTS OF A RESEARCH PROTOCOL

Regardless of the type of research being considered, the following outline from the International Conference on Harmonization, Good Clinical Practices (GCP) is an excellent starting point for ensuring that key issues are addressed in a research proposal:

6.1   General Information

6.1.1   Protocol title, protocol identifying number, and date. Any amendment(s) should also bear the amendment number(s) and date(s).

6.1.2   Name and address of the sponsor and monitor (if other than the sponsor).

6.1.3   Name and title of the person(s) authorized to sign the protocol and the protocol amendment(s) for the sponsor.

6.1.4   Name, title, address, and telephone number(s) of the sponsor's medical expert (or dentist when appropriate) for the trial.

6.1.5   Name and title of the investigator(s) who is (are) responsible for conducting the trial, and the address and telephone number(s) of the trial site(s).

6.1.6   Name, title, address, and telephone number(s) of the qualified physician (or dentist, if applicable), who is responsible for all trial-site related medical (or dental) decisions (if other than investigator).

6.1.7   Name(s) and address(es) of the clinical laboratory(ies) and other medical and/or technical department(s) and/or institutions involved in the trial.

6.2   Background Information

6.2.1   Name and description of the investigational product(s).

6.2.2   A summary of findings from nonclinical studies that potentially have clinical significance and from clinical trials that are relevant to the trial.

6.2.3   Summary of the known and potential risks and benefits, if any, to human subjects.

6.2.4   Description of and justification for the route of administration, dosage, dosage regimen, and treatment period(s).

6.2.5   A statement that the trial will be conducted in compliance with the protocol, the institution's policies and procedures, GCP and the applicable regulatory requirement(s).

6.2.6   Description of the population to be studied.

6.2.7   References to literature and data that are relevant to the trial, and that provide background for the trial.

6.3   Trial Objectives and Purpose

A detailed description of the objectives and the purpose of the trial.

6.4   Trial Design

The scientific integrity of the trial and the credibility of the data from the trial depend substantially on the trial design. A description of the trial design, should include:

6.4.1   A specific statement of the primary endpoints and the secondary endpoints, if any, to be measured during the trial.

6.4.2   A description of the type/design of trial to be conducted (e.g., double-blind, placebo-controlled, parallel design) and a schematic diagram of trial design, procedures, and stages.

6.4.3   A description of the measures taken to minimize/avoid bias, including:

a. Randomization

b. Blinding

6.4.4   A description of the trial treatment(s) and the dosage and dosage regimen of the investigational product(s). Also include a description of the dosage form, packaging, and labelling of the investigational product(s).

6.4.5   The expected duration of subject participation, and a description of the sequence and duration of all trial periods, including follow-up, if any.

6.4.6   A description of the "stopping rules" or "discontinuation criteria" for individual subjects, parts of trial, and entire trial.

6.4.7   Accountability procedures for the investigational product(s), including the placebo(s) and comparator(s), if any.

6.4.8   Maintenance of trial treatment randomization codes and procedures for breaking codes.

6.4.9   The identification of any data to be recorded directly on the CRFs (i.e., no prior written or electronic record of data), and to be considered to be source data.

6.5   Selection and Withdrawal of Subjects (Participants)

6.5.1   Subject inclusion criteria.

6.5.2   Subject exclusion criteria.

6.5.3   Subject withdrawal criteria (i.e., terminating investigational product treatment/trial treatment) and procedures specifying:

   a. When and how to withdraw subjects from the trial/investigational product treatment.

   b. The type and timing of the data to be collected for withdrawn subjects.

   c. Whether and how subjects are to be replaced.

   d. The follow-up for subjects withdrawn from investigational product treatment/trial treatment.

6.6   Treatment of Subjects (Participants)

6.6.1   The treatment(s) to be administered, including the name(s) of all the product(s), the dose(s), the dosing schedule(s), the route/mode(s) of administration, and the treatment period(s), including the follow-up period(s) for subjects for each investigational product treatment/trial treatment group/arm of the trial.

6.6.2   Medication(s)/treatment(s) permitted (including rescue medication) and not permitted before and/or during the trial.

6.6.3   Procedures for monitoring subject compliance.

6.7   Assessment of Efficacy

6.7.1   Specification of the efficacy parameters.

6.7.2   Methods and timing for assessing, recording, and analysing of efficacy parameters.

6.8   Assessment of Safety

6.8.1   Specification of safety parameters.

6.8.2   The methods and timing for assessing, recording, and analyzing safety parameters.

6.8.3   Procedures for eliciting reports of and for recording and reporting adverse event and intercurrent illnesses.

6.8.4   The type and duration of the follow-up of subjects after adverse events.

6.9 **Statistics**

    6.9.1   A description of the statistical methods to be employed, including timing of any planned interim analysis(ses).

    6.9.2   The number of subjects planned to be enrolled. In multicenter trials, the numbers of enrolled subjects projected for each trial site should be specified. Reason for choice of sample size, including reflections on (or calculations of) the power of the trial and clinical justification.

    6.9.3   The level of significance to be used.

    6.9.4   Criteria for the termination of the trial.

    6.9.5   Procedure for accounting for missing, unused, and spurious data.

    6.9.6   Procedures for reporting any deviation(s) from the original statistical plan (any deviation(s) from the original statistical plan should be described and justified in protocol and/or in the final report, as appropriate).

    6.9.7   The selection of subjects to be included in the analyses (e.g., all randomized subjects, all dosed subjects, all eligible subjects, evaluable subjects).

6.10 **Direct Access to Source Data/Documents**

The sponsor should ensure that it is specified in the protocol or other written agreement that the investigator(s)/institution(s) will permit trial-related monitoring, audits, IRB/IEC review, and regulatory inspection(s), providing direct access to source data/documents.

6.11 **Quality Control and Quality Assurance Procedures**

6.12 **Ethics**

Description of ethical considerations relating to the trial.

6.13 **Data Handling and Record Keeping**

6.14 **Financing and Insurance**

Financing and insurance, if not addressed in a separate agreement.

6.15 **Publication Policy**

Publication policy, if not addressed in a separate agreement.

6.16 **Supplements**

[ICH, Guideline for Good Clinical Practice, Guideline 6 (Modified)]

The Investigator's Brochure

As part of a clinical trial, a sponsor will compile clinical and nonclinical data on the investigational product that are relevant to the proposed study. This document is often referred to as an Investigator's Brochure (IB). Its purpose is to be a comprehensive reference for the investigator in understanding the protocol and being able to comply with it. The sponsor should update the IB as more information becomes available. If new information has an important impact on the study, it should be conveyed to the investigator and the IRB without waiting to update the IB. Key elements of an Investigator's Brochure, as described by GCP, are the following:

7.2   General Considerations

The IB should include:

7.2.1   Title Page

This should provide the sponsor's name, the identity of each investigational product (i.e., research number, chemical or approved generic name, and trade name(s) where legally permissible and desired by the sponsor), and the release date. It is also suggested that an edition number, and a reference to the number and date of the edition it supersedes, be provided.

7.2.2   Confidentiality Statement

The sponsor may wish to include a statement instructing the investigator/recipients to treat the IB as a confidential document for the sole information and use of the investigator's team and the IRB/IEC.

7.3   Contents of the Investigator's Brochure

The IB should contain the following sections, each with literature references where appropriate:

7.3.1   Table of Contents

7.3.2   Summary

A brief summary (preferably not exceeding two pages) should be given, highlighting the significant physical, chemical, pharmaceutical, pharmacological, toxicological, pharmacokinetic, metabolic, and clinical information available that is relevant to the stage of clinical development of the investigational product.

7.3.3   Introduction

A brief introductory statement should be provided that contains the chemical name (and generic and trade name(s) when approved) of the investigational product(s), all active ingredients, the investigational product(s') pharmacological class and its expected position within this class (e.g., advantages), the rationale for performing research with the investigational product(s), and the anticipated prophylactic, therapeutic, or diagnostic indication(s). Finally, the introductory statement should provide the general approach to be followed in evaluating the investigational product.

7.3.4   Physical, Chemical, and Pharmaceutical Properties and Formulation

A description should be provided of the investigational product substance(s) (including the chemical and/or structural formula(e)), and a brief summary should be given of the relevant physical, chemical, and pharmaceutical properties.

To permit appropriate safety measures to be taken in the course of the trial, a description of the formulation(s) to be used, including excipients, should be provided and justified if clinically relevant. Instructions for the storage and handling of the dosage form(s) should also be given.

Any structural similarities to other known compounds should be mentioned.

7.3.5 Nonclinical Studies

Introduction:

The results of all relevant nonclinical pharmacology, toxicology, pharmacokinetic, and investigational product metabolism studies should be provided in summary form. This summary should address the methodology used, the results, and a discussion of the relevance of the findings to the investigated therapeutic and the possible unfavorable and unintended effects in humans.

The information provided may include the following, as appropriate, if known/available:

Species tested

Number and sex of animals in each group

Unit dose (e.g., milligram/kilogram (mg/kg))

Dose interval

Route of administration

Duration of dosing

Information on systemic distribution

Duration of post-exposure follow-up

Results, including the following aspects:

Nature and frequency of pharmacological or toxic effects

Severity or intensity of pharmacological or toxic effects

Time to onset of effects

Reversibility of effects

Duration of effects

Dose response

Tabular format/listings should be used whenever possible to enhance the clarity of the presentation.

The following sections should discuss the most important findings from the studies, including the dose response of observed effects, the relevance to humans, and any aspects to be studied in humans. If applicable, the effective and nontoxic dose findings in the same animal species should be compared (i.e., the therapeutic index should be discussed). The relevance of this information to the proposed human dosing should be addressed. Whenever possible, comparisons should be made in terms of blood/tissue levels rather than on a mg/kg basis.

Nonclinical Pharmacology

A summary of the pharmacological aspects of the investigational product and, where appropriate, its significant metabolites studied in animals, should be included. Such a summary should incorporate studies that assess potential therapeutic activity (e.g., efficacy models, receptor binding, and specificity) as well as those that assess safety (e.g., special studies to assess pharmacological actions other than the intended therapeutic effect(s)).

Pharmacokinetics and Product Metabolism in Animals

A summary of the pharmacokinetics and biological transformation and disposition of the investigational product in all species studied should be given. The discussion of the findings should address the absorption and the local and systemic bioavailability of the investigational product and its metabolites, and their relationship to the pharmacological and toxicological findings in animal species.

Toxicology

A summary of the toxicological effects found in relevant studies conducted in different animal species should be described under the following headings where appropriate:

Single dose

Repeated dose

Carcinogenicity

Special studies (e.g., irritancy and sensitization)

Reproductive toxicity

Genotoxicity (mutagenicity)

7.3.6   *Effects in Humans*

Introduction:

A thorough discussion of the known effects of the investigational product(s) in humans should be provided, including information on pharmacokinetics, metabolism, pharmacodynamics, dose response, safety, efficacy, and other pharmacological activities. Where possible, a summary of each completed clinical trial should be provided. Information should also be provided regarding results of any use of the investigational product(s) other than from clinical trials, such as from experience during marketing.

Pharmacokinetics and Product Metabolism in Humans

A summary of information on the pharmacokinetics of the investigational product(s) should be presented, including the following, if available:

Pharmacokinetics (including metabolism, as appropriate, and absorption, plasma protein binding, distribution, and elimination)

Bioavailability of the investigational product (absolute, where possible, and relative) using a reference dosage form

Population subgroups (e.g., gender, age, and impaired organ function)

Interactions (e.g., product-product interactions and effects of food)

Other pharmacokinetic data (results of population studies performed within clinical trial(s))

Safety and Efficacy

A summary of information should be provided about the investigational product's/products' (including metabolites, where appropriate) safety, pharmacodynamics, efficacy, and dose response that were obtained from preceding trials in humans (healthy volunteers and patients). The implications of this information should be discussed. In cases where a number of clinical trials have been completed, the use of summaries of safety and efficacy across multiple trials by indications in subgroups may provide a clear presentation of the data. Tabular summaries of adverse drug reactions for all the clinical trials (including those for all the studied indications) would be useful. Important differences in adverse drug reaction patterns/incidences across indications or subgroups should be discussed.

The IB should provide a description of the possible risks and adverse drug reactions to be anticipated on the basis of prior experiences with the product under investigation and with related products. A description should also be provided of the precautions or special monitoring to be done as part of the investigational use of the product(s).

Marketing Experience

The IB should identify countries where the investigational product has been marketed or approved. Any significant information arising from the marketed use should be summarized (e.g., formulations, dosages, routes of administration, and adverse product reactions). The IB should also identify all the countries where the investigational product did not receive approval/registration for marketing or was withdrawn from marketing/registration.

7.3.7 Summary of Data and Guidance for the Investigator

This section should provide an overall discussion of the nonclinical and clinical data, and should summarize the information from various sources on different aspects of the investigational product(s), wherever possible. In this way, the investigator can be provided with the most informative interpretation of the available data and with an assessment of the implications of the information for future clinical trials.

Where appropriate, the published reports on related products should be discussed. This could help the investigator to anticipate adverse drug reactions or other problems in clinical trials.

The overall aim of this section is to provide the investigator with a clear understanding of the possible risks and adverse reactions, and of the specific tests, observations, and precautions that may be needed for a clinical trial. This understanding should be based on the available physical, chemical, pharmaceutical, pharmacological, toxicological, and clinical information on the investigational product(s). Guidance should also be provided to the clinical investigator on the recognition and treatment of possible overdose and adverse drug reactions that are based on previous human experience and on the pharmacology of the investigational product.

[ICH, *Guideline for Good Clinical Practice*]

••••••••••••

THE GENERAL ISSUES TO BE CONSIDERED BY AN IRB IN REVIEWING A PROPOSED STUDY

OHRP offers the following points for an IRB to consider in reviewing proposed protocols for various types of studies:

1. Does the study involve reviews of records, observation, surveys, or interviews? If so, does it qualify for exemption or expedited review under the federal regulations and institutional policy?

2. Is the scientific design adequate to answer the questions posed? Is the sample size (number of subjects) adequate? Is the method proposed for selecting and assigning subjects to treatment groups unbiased?

3. Does the investigator serve a dual role that may pose a conflict of interest?

4. Is any of the information to be collected sensitive (related to sexual practices, substance abuse, or illegal behavior)?

5. Are there adequate plans to protect participants from the risks of breach of confidentiality and invasion of privacy?

6. Are there plans for approaching subjects in a way that will respect their privacy and their right to refuse? If the protocol involves an epidemiologic study, will participants or their relatives be protected from learning inappropriate information?

7. Does the recruitment process protect participants from being coerced or unduly influenced to participate? Are any payments to participants reasonable in relation to the risks, discomfort, or inconvenience to which subjects will be exposed?

8. Are there adequate plans to exclude participants who are vulnerable to injury during the period of withdrawal of active and effective therapy, if that is part of the research design?

9. Have the rights and interests of vulnerable participants (for example, desperately ill persons) been adequately considered?

10. Are all appropriate elements of informed consent clearly provided for, including

    a. Do the consent documents describe the study design (including plans for randomization, use of placebos, and the probability that the subject will receive a given treatment) and conditions for breaking the code (if the study is masked)?

    b. Do the consent documents describe the risks and benefits of each of the proposed interventions and of alternative courses or actions available to the participants?

    c. Do the consent documents clearly describe the extent to which participation in the study precludes other therapeutic interventions?

    d. Are provisions made for supplying new information to participants during the course of the study and for obtaining continuing consent, where appropriate?

    e. Must investigators obtain consent before reviewing records?

11. Will the consent process take place under conditions most likely to provide potential participants an opportunity to make a decision about participation without undue pressure?

12. If the study is a clinical trial, how will the trial be monitored? What will be done with preliminary data? Should an independent data and safety monitoring board be established? How will decisions about stopping the trial be made? By whom? On what basis?

13. At what interval should the IRB perform continuing review of this project?

Review of the Underlying Science of a Proposed Study by the IRB

"Clearly, if it is not good science, it is not ethical" (OPRR, *Institutional Review Board Guidebook*). While federal regulations do not expressly demand that an IRB review the scientific validity of a proposed study, federal regulations do require that an IRB determine whether the risks are reasonable in relation to the importance of the knowledge that may be reasonably expected to be learned (45 CFR §46.111(a)(2)). If the study is fundamentally flawed, then little if any knowledge will be learned from the study. Therefore, little, if any, risk can be justified.

Most IRBs defer to the research sponsor as to the scientific validity of a proposed study. OHRP has stated "an IRB may rely on the FDA, institutions, scientific review committees, funding agencies (e.g. NIH), or others for this determination" (OPRR, *Institutional Review Board Guidebook*). Where an outside body will not be reviewing the scientific merits of a study, an IRB will need to rigorously evaluate the study. IRB members need to understand the basic features of experimental design. Outside consultants may be of value when additional expertise can be provided to the IRB members.

Considerations in Advertising for Research Participants

The FDA expects IRBs to review the advertising to ensure that it is not unduly coercive and does not promise a certainty of cure beyond what is outlined in the consent and the protocol. This is especially critical when a study may involve participants who are likely to be vulnerable to undue influence (21 CFR §50.20, 50.25, 56.111(a)(3), 56.111(b) and 812.20(b)(11)). Selection and recruitment are discussed in Chapter Four. The OIG has called for stronger guidelines on participant recruitment practices (OIG, 2000).

When direct advertising is to be used, the IRB should carefully review the information contained in the advertisement and the mode of its communication, to determine that the procedure for recruiting participants is not coercive and does not state or imply a certainty of favorable outcome or other benefits beyond what is outlined in the consent document and the protocol. The IRB should review the final copy of printed advertisements to evaluate the relative size of type used and other visual effects. When advertisements are to be taped for broadcast, the IRB should review the final audio/video tape. The IRB may wish to caution a clinical investigator to obtain IRB approval of message text prior to taping, in order to avoid retaping because of inappropriate wording. The review of the final taped message prepared from IRB-approved text may be accomplished through expedited procedures.

No claims should be made, either explicitly or implicitly, that the drug, biologic, or device is safe or effective for the purposes under investigation, or that the test article is known to be equivalent or superior to any other drug, biologic, or device. Such representation would not only be misleading to participants but would also be a violation of FDA regulations concerning the promotion of investigational drugs (21 CFR §312.7(a)) and of investigational devices (21 CFR §812.7(d)).

Advertising for recruitment into clinical trials should not use terms such as "new treatment," "new medication," or "new drug" without explaining that the test article is investigational. A phrase such as "receive new treatments" leads study participants to believe they will be receiving newly improved products of proven worth.

Advertisements should not promise "free medical treatment" when the intent is only to say participants will not be charged for taking part in the investigation. Advertisements may state that participants will be paid, but should not emphasize the payment or the amount to be paid, by such means as larger or bold type.

Generally, the FDA believes that any advertisement to recruit participants should be limited to the information the prospective participants need to determine their eligibility and interest. When appropriately worded, the following items may be included in advertisements:

1. The name and address of the clinical investigator and/or research facility
2. The condition under study and/or the purpose of the research
3. In summary form, the criteria that will be used to determine eligibility for the study
4. A brief list of participation benefits, if any (such as a no-cost health examination)
5. The time or other commitment required of the participants
6. The location of the research and the person or office to contact for further information

(However, it should be noted that the FDA does not require inclusion of all of the listed items).

Records to Be Maintained About a Study

A comprehensive agreement between a sponsor and an investigator will likely address what data is to be collected and how it is to be maintained. As a general rule, an investigator should consider the following GCP guidance (ICH, *Guidelines for Good Clinical Practice,* modified):

- The investigator should ensure the accuracy, completeness, legibility, and timeliness of the data reported to the sponsor in the Case Report Forms (CRF) and in all required reports.
- Data reported on the CRF, which are derived from source documents, should be consistent with the source documents or the discrepancies should be explained.
- Any change or correction to a CRF should be dated, initialed, and explained (if necessary) and should not obscure the original entry (an audit trail should be maintained); this applies to both written and electronic changes or corrections (see GCP 5.18.4 (n)). Sponsors should provide guidance to investigators and/or the investigators' designated representatives on making such corrections. Sponsors should have written procedures to ensure that changes or corrections in CRFs made by sponsors' designated representatives are documented, are necessary, and are endorsed by the investigator. The investigator should retain records of the changes and corrections.
- The investigator/institution should maintain the trial documents as specified in Essential Documents for the Conduct of a Clinical Trial (see GCP 8) and as required

by the applicable regulatory requirement(s). The investigator/institution should take measures to prevent accidental or premature destruction of these documents.

- Essential documents should be retained until at least two years after the last approval of a marketing application in the United States and until there are no pending or contemplated marketing applications in another country or at least two years have elapsed since the formal discontinuation of clinical development of the investigational product. These documents should be retained for a longer period if required by the applicable regulatory requirements or by an agreement with the sponsor. It is the responsibility of the sponsor to inform the investigator/institution as to when these documents no longer need to be retained (see GCP 5.5.12).

- The financial aspects of the trial should be documented in an agreement between the sponsor and the investigator/institution.

- Upon request of the monitor, auditor, IRB, or regulatory authority, the investigator/ institution should make available for direct access all requested trial-related records.

The following documents are considered to be essential documents to be maintained for a study under the Good Clinical Practice Guidelines:

—	Title of Document	Purpose	Located in Files of	
			Investigator/ Institution	Sponsor
8.2.1	**INVESTIGATOR'S BROCHURE**	To document that relevant and current scientific information about the investigational product has been provided to the investigator	X	X
8.2.2	**SIGNED PROTOCOL AND AMENDMENTS, IF ANY, AND SAMPLE CASE REPORT FORM (CRF)**	To document investigator and sponsor agreement to the protocol/ amendment(s) and CRF	X	X
8.2.3	**INFORMATION GIVEN TO TRIAL SUBJECT**			
	- INFORMED CONSENT FORM (including translations)	To document the informed consent	X	X
	- ANY OTHER WRITTEN INFORMATION	To document that subjects will be given appropriate written information (content and wording) to support their ability to give fully informed consent	X	X
	- ADVERTISEMENT FOR SUBJECT RECRUITMENT (if used)	To document that recruitment measures are appropriate and not coercive	X	
8.2.4	**FINANCIAL ASPECTS OF THE TRIAL**	To document the financial agreement between the investigator/ institution and the sponsor for the trial	X	X
8.2.5	**INSURANCE STATEMENT** (where required)	To document that compensation to subject(s) for trial-related injury will be available	X	X

(Continued)

—	Title of Document	Purpose	Located in Files of	
			Investigator/ Institution	Sponsor
8.2.6	**SIGNED AGREEMENT BETWEEN INVOLVED PARTIES**, e.g.:	To document agreements		
	- investigator/institution and sponsor		X	X
	- investigator/institution and CRO		X	X (where required)
	- sponsor and CRO X			X
	- investigator/institution and authority(ies)		X	X
8.2.7	**DATED, DOCUMENTED APPROVAL/FAVOURABLE OPINION OF INSTITUTIONAL REVIEW BOARD (IRB)/ INDEPENDENT ETHICS COMMITTEE (IEC) OF THE FOLLOWING:**	To document that the trial has been . subject to IRB/IEC review and given approval/favourable opinion. To identify the version number and date of the document(s)	X	X
	- protocol and any amendments - CRF (if applicable) - informed consent form(s) - any other written information to be provided to the subject(s) - advertisement for subject recruitment (if used) - subject compensation (if any) - any other documents given approval/favorable opinion			
8.2.8	**INSTITUTIONAL REVIEW BOARD/INDEPENDENT ETHICS COMMITTEE COMPOSITION**	To document that the IRB/IEC is constituted in agreement with GCP (where required)	X	X
8.2.9	**REGULATORY AUTHORITY(IES) AUTHORISATION/ APPROVAL/NOTIFICATION OF PROTOCOL** (where required)	To document appropriate authorization/approval/ notification by the regulatory authority(ies) has been obtained prior to initiation of (where the trial in compliance with the applicable regulatory requirement(s)	X (where required)	X (where required)
8.2.10	**CURRICULUM VITAE AND/ OR OTHER RELEVANT DOCUMENTS EVIDENCING QUALIFICATIONS OF INVESTIGATOR(S) AND SUBINVESTIGATOR(S)**	To document qualifications and eligibility to conduct trial and/or provide medical supervision of subjects	X	X
8.2.11	**NORMAL VALUE(S)/ RANGE(S) FOR MEDICAL/ LABORATORY/TECHNICAL PROCEDURE(S) AND/OR TEST(S) INCLUDED IN THE PROTOCOL**	To document normal values and/ or ranges of the tests results	X	X

—	Title of Document	Purpose	Located in Files of	
			Investigator/ Institution	Sponsor
8.2.12	**MEDICAL/LABORATORY/ TECHNICAL PROCEDURES/ TESTS** - certification or - accreditation or - established quality control and/ or external quality assessment or - other validation	To document competence of facility to perform required test(s), and support reliability of results	X (where required)	X
8.2.13	**SAMPLE OF LABEL(S) ATTACHED TO INVESTIGATIONAL PRODUCT CONTAINER(S)**	To document compliance with applicable labelling regulations and appropriateness of instructions provided to the subjects		X
8.2.14	**INSTRUCTIONS FOR HANDLING OF INVESTIGATIONAL PRODUCT(S) AND TRIAL-RELATED MATERIALS** (if not included in protocol or Investigator's Brochure)	To document instructions needed to ensure proper storage, packaging, dispensing and disposition of investigational products and trial-related materials	X	X
8.2.15	**SHIPPING RECORDS FOR INVESTIGATIONAL PRODUCT(S) AND TRIAL-RELATED MATERIALS**	To document shipment dates, batch numbers and method of shipment of investigational product(s) and trial-related materials. Allows tracking of product batch, review of shipping conditions, and accountability	X	X
8.2.16	**CERTIFICATE(S) OF ANALYSIS OF INVESTIGATIONAL PRODUCT(S) SHIPPED**	To document identity, purity, and strength of investigational product(s) to be used in the trial		X
8.2.17	**DECODING PROCEDURES FOR BLINDED TRIALS**	To document how, in case of an emergency, identity of blinded investigational product can be revealed without breaking the blind for the remaining subjects' treatment	X (third party if applicable)	X
8.2.18	**MASTER RANDOMISATION LIST**	To document method for randomisation of trial population	X	X (third party if applicable)
8.2.19	**PRE-TRIAL MONITORING REPORT**	To document that the site is suitable for the trial (may be combined with 8.2.20)		X
8.2.20	**TRIAL INITIATION MONITORING REPORT**	To document that trial procedures were reviewed with the investigator and the investigator's trial staff (may be combined with 8.2.19)	X	X

[ICH, *Guidelines for Good Clinical Practice*]

•••••••••••

TYPES OF STUDIES AND ISSUES RELATED TO EACH

Investigations can be separated into two broad categories: experimental and descriptive. In an experimental study, participants are randomly assigned to groups under carefully controlled situations manipulated by the investigator "according to a strict logic allowing causal inference about the effects of the treatments under investigation" (OPRR, *Institutional Review Board Guidebook*). In a descriptive study, the lack of rigid control through random assignment and precise manipulation of variables make causal inferences unreliable.

An Observational Study

A true observational study is one where people are solely observed in public places (shopping centers, parks, or restaurants). If the human research subjects are adults and the information recorded (1) does not identify the subjects, (2) could not reasonably place the subjects at risk for civil or criminal liability, or (3) damage the subject's social, employment, or financial situation, then IRB approval is not necessary under federal regulations (45 CFR §46.101(b)(2)). Observational research involving public observations of children is also exempt from IRB approval if, in addition to the above criteria, the investigator is not involved in the activities being observed (45 CFR §46.101(b)(2); 45 CFR §46.401(b)). However, observational research may be subject to IRB review under an institution's internal policies or its Assurance.

An observational study that involves manipulation of the subject's environment does require IRB review. For example, yelling fire in a theatre and recording the reactions of audience members would require IRB review because the audience members are exposed to risk of injury or stress. Observational studies to be conducted in settings where subjects would reasonably expect privacy are also subject to IRB approval.

Record Review or Historical Study   Many studies are conducted entirely using data contained in public or private records. If the data for a study is extracted solely from public records, IRB review is not necessary unless mandated by the institution's policies or assurance (45 CFR §46.101(b)(4)). When using medical records as the source of data, a study would be exempt from a regulatory mandate for IRB approval if the data pre-existed the start of the study and the information was assimilated in such a manner that an individual patient could not be identified (45 CFR §46.101(b)(4)). If an individual patient could be identified directly or through the use of an identifier, IRB approval is required to ensure protection of the patient's privacy and confidentiality. Any time that records are reviewed without a patient's consent, privacy issues are raised. Regulations under HIPAA are discussed in Chapter Six.

Surveys, Questionnaires, or Interviews   Social sciences such as psychology, sociology, anthropology or political science often employ surveys, questionnaires, or interviews. This type of research using adult participants is exempt from the federal regulatory mandate for IRB approval unless the information is 1) recorded in a manner that the participant could be identified, 2) could place the participant at risk for civil or criminal liability, or 3) damage the participant's social, employment, or financial situation (45 CFR §46.101(b)(2)). Surveys or interviews of children are not exempt and require IRB approval (45 CFR §46.101(b)(2); 45 CFR §401(b)). In addition, some institutions require IRB approval of all studies.

Epidemiologic Studies   Epidemiologic studies often examine and link data from a number of sources, such as medical, insurance, employment, or police records. Many researchers also combine this with surveys or interviews to expand the data available or test a hypothesis. Because of concerns about privacy and confidentiality, the better course is for epidemiologic studies to be reviewed and approved by an IRB. OHRP suggests that an IRB consider the ethical guidelines for epidemiologists when reviewing such studies (OPRR, Institutional Review Board Guidebook, Chap. IV, sec. E, suggesting Beauchamp, Tom L. et al. *Ethical Issues in Social Science Research,* Baltimore, MD: John Hopkins University Press, 1982). The validity of epidemiologic studies is directly related to the level of participation by potential subjects.

As to the role of an IRB in reviewing epidemiologic studies, OHRP cites the following list of objectives for the investigator with approval:

- Take adequate steps to preserve the confidentiality of the data that is collected;
- Specify who will have access to the data;
- State how and at what point in the research personal information will be separated from other data;
- State whether the data will be retained at the conclusion of the study;
- Thoroughly describe the interview instruments and questionnaires;
- Assure that the informed consent of participants will be obtained before interviews are conducted;
- Justify the project according to its anticipated risks and benefits

[OPRR, *Institutional Review Board Guidebook,* Chap. IV, sec. E, quoting Wallace, R. Jay. "Privacy and the Use of Data in Epidemiology" in *Ethical Issues in Social Science Research,* edited by Tom L. Beauchamp, Ruth R. Faden, R. Jay Wallace, Jr., and LeRoy Walters, pp. 274–291. Baltimore, MD: Johns Hopkins University Press, 1982]

The primary ethical challenge of an epidemiologic study is protection of the research participant's privacy (the right to determine what will be known about oneself) and confidentiality (the right to determine that information will not be disclosed without permission). Both of these rights are important components of the informed consent process. When a participant is contacted as part of the study, a potential for harm exists. At the early stage of a study, efforts to recruit potential subjects may advise patients for the first time that they either suffer or are at risk for suffering a particular disease. "In general, wherever possible, potentially eligible subjects should be contacted either by the person to whom they originally gave the information, or by a person with whom they have a trust relationship." [OPRR, *Institutional Review Board Guidebook,* Chap. IV, sec. E, quoting McCarthy, Charles R., and Porter, Joan P. "Confidentiality: The Protection of Personal Data in Epidemiological and Clinical Research Trials." *Law, Medicine and Health Care* 19 (No. 3-4, Fall/Winter 1991): 238–241]. After this stage, the investigator can obtain the consent of the research subject for participation in the study. This can be particularly stressful in studies such as of HIV or cancer.

Case-Control Study   A case-control study is a descriptive study in which people with a specific condition (the cases) and people without the condition (the controls) are recruited to participate. The frequencies of certain characteristics occurring between the cases and the controls are then compared.

An IRB should carefully consider each case-control study on an individual basis as the risk varies from study to study. Protection of privacy and confidentiality are always issues. The risk of physical injury should not be present as no intervention is being performed. However, the investigator and his IRB need to be sensitive to the risk of psychological injury—for example, in discussing a traumatic event, or legal injury—for example from the exposure to illegal drug use. Where the study is solely based on existing medical record review, expedited review or exemption from review may be appropriate in some cases (45 CFR §46.101(b)(4); 45 CFR §46.110). When interviews are an additional component of the study, full IRB review is the better course. Informed consent and the appropriate means of contacting potential participants are prominent issues to be considered.

Prospective Study   A *prospective study* is designed to observe future events (behavioral or physiological responses) that may occur after the research participants have been recruited. For example, a clinical trial is a prospective study. A *longitudinal study* follows one or more cohorts of research subjects over an extended period of time. A well-known example of such a study is the Harvard Physicians Study, where physicians have been followed for many years as they have aged. The issues of a prospective study to be considered by an IRB are discussed next in relation to a clinical trial.

Clinical Trial   A *clinical trial* (also called a randomized clinical trial, RCT) is designed to assess the safety and efficacy of a new drug, device, treatment, or preventive measure in humans by comparing two or more interventions. A clinical trial is controlled, that is, a case group receives the treatment while a control group either receives an alternative treatment or no treatment, with the participants being randomly assigned to the case group or control group. A *single-masked study* is designed to hide the identity of who is assigned to which group from either the participants or the investigators. A *double-masked study* hides the identity of who is assigned to which group from both the subjects and the investigators.

An investigator (usually a physician) conducting a clinical trial of an investigational drug agrees to conduct the study within the parameters of FDA regulations. The investigator documents this by signing an FDA form certifying that the investigator has obtained IRB review and approval prior to initiating the study.

IRB Considerations in Reviewing and Approving a Clinical Trial

An IRB evaluates the risks and benefits of a clinical trial by considering the various aspects of the study design, especially the study population, the trial phase, and mechanisms for data analysis and surveillance. Human participants must be advised that the FDA will have access to their medical records as they pertain to the study. In addition to the usual concern about informed consent, an IRB must consider two additional important ethical concerns of a clinical trial: randomization of the patients, and placebos.

Randomization of the Patients   The primary ethical concern of randomizing who will receive the experimental treatment and who will not is fairness. "If the trial therapy is known to be superior to currently available alternative therapies (prior research indicates that it is superior), it is unethical to assign subjects to the inferior treatment. Furthermore it would not be ethical to perform a clinical trial comparing two treatments when there is a third therapy that is known to be superior to either or both, unless there is some reason why that therapy is not useful for the study population" (OPRR, *Institutional Review Board Guidebook*). This leads to the necessity of a researcher being able to honestly say that there is "theoretical equipoise" (the assumption that the trial therapy and the control therapy will not lead to different outcomes) before starting a clinical trial. However, a clinical trial may be justified by the somewhat broader concept of "clinical equipoise" ("a current or likely dispute among expert members of the clinical community as to which of two or more therapy is superior in all relevant respects," OPRR, *Institutional Review Board Guidebook,* Chap. IV, sec. H, quoting Freedman, Benjamin. "Equipoise and the Ethics of Clinical Research." *New England Journal of Medicine* 317 (No. 3, July 16, 1987): 141–145). The goal of a clinical trial is to show strong enough results to resolve any debate as to the superior intervention. The control therapy must be the best accepted therapy currently available for the condition being treated (OPRR, *Institutional Review Board Guidebook*).

Placebos   No therapy (placebos) can be used as the control therapy where the research participants can tolerate no known or available alternative therapy. A placebo should not be used where a standard treatment has been shown to be superior to a placebo by convincing evidence. In contrast, some have argued that placebos must be used when experimental therapy is of "dubious efficacy" or when the side effects are known to be serious (OPRR, *Institutional Review Board Guidebook,* Chap. IV, sec. H, citing Freedman, Benjamin, "Placebo-Controlled Trials and the Logic of Clinical Purpose," *IRB* 12 (No. 6, November/December 1990):1–6). The use of placebos must be justified in a proposed protocol by a beneficial risk/benefit ratio. Further, the control participants should not be deceived into believing that they are receiving an active therapy (OPRR, *Institutional Review Board Guidebook*). They must be fully advised of the risks involved in assignment to the placebo group. Continued use of a placebo control group is unethical once good evidence shows efficacy of the trial therapy (OPRR, *Institutional Review Board Guidebook*). An investigator also needs to be concerned about the ability of participants to communicate among themselves. Patients being able to ascertain whether they are on the study drug or a placebo may bias a study (Bulkeley, 1995).

Clinical trial protocols should be stopped or modified as soon as sufficient evidence is found to support either a causal relationship of a beneficial therapeutic effect or an unacceptable adverse effect (OPRR, *Institutional Review Board Guidebook*).

A placebo washout may be conducted prior to initiation of a study. During this period all of the research participants receive a placebo to 1) terminate the effects of any drug the participant may have been taking before entering the clinical trial; 2) learn whether the participant cooperates with instructions to take drugs (compliance); and 3) learn which participants experience a high degree of placebo effect (placebo responders). Many studies attempt to weed out participants who are noncompliant or placebo responders. An IRB should carefully consider the risk to participants during a placebo washout. Participants who are vulnerable to injury due to no therapeutic treatment should be excluded from the study. Participants who do participate in the study should be told that at some point they will be receiving placebo therapy.

The Phases of Clinical Trials

Clinical trials are usually conducted in three phases under FDA regulation. In Phase 1 trials, the drug is administered to a small number of healthy volunteers to test for safety. In Phase 2 studies, the drug is tested for efficacy in a larger number of patients who have the disease that is intended to be treated. Phase 3 includes a much larger number of patients to gather further data on safety and efficacy. Phase 4 studies are performed after a drug is placed on the market. More formal definitions of each phase follow:

Phase 1 Drug Trial: Phase 1 trials include the initial introduction of an investigational new drug into humans. These studies are typically conducted with healthy volunteers; sometimes, where the drug is intended for use in patients with a particular disease, however, such patients may participate as subjects. Phase 1 trials are designed to determine the metabolic and pharmacological actions of the drug in humans, the side effects associated with increasing doses (to establish a safe dose range), and, if possible, to gain early evidence of effectiveness; they are typically closely monitored. The ultimate goal of Phase 1 trials is to obtain sufficient information about the drug's pharmacokinetics and pharmacological effects to permit the design of well-controlled, sufficiently valid Phase 2 studies. Other examples of Phase 1 studies include studies of drug metabolism, structure-activity relationships, and mechanisms of actions in humans, as well as studies in which investigational drugs are used as research tools to explore biological phenomena or disease processes. The total number of subjects involved in Phase 1 investigations is generally in the range of 20–80 (21 CFR §312.21(a)).

Phase 2 Drug Trial: Phase 2 trials include controlled clinical studies conducted to evaluate the drug's effectiveness for a particular indication in patients with the disease or condition under study, and to determine the common short-term side effects and risks associated with the drug. These studies are typically well-controlled, closely monitored, and conducted with a relatively small number of patients, usually involving no more than several hundred subjects (21 CFR §312.21(b)).

Phase 3 Drug Trial: Phase 3 trials involve the administration of a new drug to a larger number of patients in different clinical settings to determine its safety, effectiveness, and appropriate dosage. They are performed after preliminary evidence of effectiveness has been obtained and are intended to gather necessary additional information about effectiveness and safety for evaluating the overall benefit-risk relationship of the drug, and to provide an adequate basis for physician labeling. In Phase 3 studies, the drug is used the way it would be administered when marketed. When these studies are completed and the sponsor believes that the drug is safe and effective under specific conditions, the sponsor applies to FDA for approval to market the drug. Phase 3 trials usually involve several hundred to several thousand patient-subjects (21 CFR §312.21(c)).

Phase 4 Drug Trial: Concurrent with marketing approval, FDA may seek agreement from the sponsor to conduct certain postmarketing (Phase 4) studies to delineate additional information about the drug's risks, benefits, and optimal use. These studies could include, but would not be limited to, studying different doses or schedules of administration than were used in Phase 2 studies, use of the drug in other patient populations or other stages of the disease, or use of the drug over a longer period of time. [21 CFR §312.85; OPRR, *Institutional Review Board Guidebook*]

Important Considerations with the Various Phases of Clinical Trials

OPRR offered the following guidance as to the various phases of clinical trials (OPRR, *Institutional Review Board Guidebook*):

Phase 1 trials are historically safest because they usually involve administering a single dose to healthy volunteers. However, Phase 1 trials may pose the highest level of unknown risk because they involve the drug's first administration to humans. (With highly toxic drugs such as cancer chemotherapies, Phase 1 trials are usually conducted with cancer patients as subjects.) Insofar as possible, risks should be identified from previous laboratory experiments and animal trials. The FDA, which reviews Phase 1 trials submitted in the initial IND application, may have valuable information and recommendations on particular protocols.

Participants in Phase 2 trials are usually patients with the condition that the new drug is intended to detect or treat. An IRB should recognize that although Phase 2 testing is preceded by earlier clinical trials, the physiological responses of healthy volunteers to a therapeutic drug may not be reliable indicators of how safe the drug is for persons who are ill, taking other medication, or have immunodeficiencies. Since the primary purpose of a Phase 2 trial is to test the drug's effectiveness in achieving its purpose, the responses of participants receiving the drug are usually compared with those of participants who are not receiving the drug (control subjects). Whether control subjects receive some existing therapy or a placebo is a research design issue with serious ethical implications. Where an alternate safe and effective drug is available for a serious condition being studied, it should generally be given to the control subjects; however, existing therapies may be inadequate because they are of limited effectiveness against the disease, they have relatively high levels of toxicity, or because they are inconvenient to administer. When determining the acceptability of a proposed research design, IRBs must examine the risks and effectiveness of existing therapies, as well as the risks associated with providing no therapy (or a placebo).

While most drug trials involve agents that the FDA has not yet approved for marketing, some drugs may be the subject of further testing concurrent with or following FDA approval. Postmarketing investigations, also called Phase 4 trials, are conducted to develop further information about the article's safety or effectiveness. Such studies might, for example, seek to establish the safety or effectiveness of using the drug for a new indication, with a new dosage level or a new route of administration (21 CFR §312.85).

Phase 4 studies should be distinguished from use of a marketed product by a physician for an indication not in the approved labeling as part of the "practice of medicine." Investigational use of a marketed product differs from such uses by physicians in that the principal intent of the investigational use of a test article is to develop information about its safety or efficacy; the submission of an IND or IDE may therefore be required.

Charging Study Participants for Investigational Products Used in a Study

While FDA regulations allow for a sponsor to recoup its actual costs for an investigational product from research participants, the simpler path is not to do so. If a sponsor seeks to recoup its actual costs, it must advise the research participant and usually obtain prior approval from the FDA (FDA, 1998). The exceptions to this are usually mandated by state law. For example, many states require health insurance companies to pay for oncology studies approved by the National Cancer Institute. An IRB must grapple with the ethical issue of whether charging participants to enroll in a study is appropriate.

Special Concerns of Vaccine Trials

The risks and benefits of *vaccine trials* may differ from those of drug trials. A vaccine is a biological product. It is not intended to diagnose or treat a disease but to prevent its occurrence. Vaccines trigger the body's immune response. Some vaccines, those using live microorganisms, have a small but real possibility of actually causing the disease in some patients. However, most often participants transiently suffer some the symptoms of the disease while they acquire immunity. An IND is required before clinical trials can be undertaken.

Scientific terms that may be used in vaccine trials may include these (OPRR, *Institutional Review Board Guidebook*):

- **Biologic:** Any therapeutic serum, toxin, anti-toxin, or analogous microbial product applicable to the prevention, treatment, or cure of diseases or injuries.
- **Purity:** The relative absence of extraneous matter in a vaccine that may or may not be harmful to the recipient or deleterious to the product.
- **Sterility:** The absence of viable contaminating microorganisms; aseptic state.
- **Vaccine:** A biologic product generally made from an infectious agent or its components—a virus, bacterium, or other microorganism—that is killed (inactive) or live-attenuated (active, although weakened). Vaccines may also be biochemically synthesized or made through recombinant DNA techniques.

In considering the benefits to a participant in receiving a new vaccine, an IRB might consider the following:

1. The severity of the disease to be avoided
2. The likelihood that the participant will be exposed to or will contract the disease
3. The likelihood that the participant would suffer adverse consequences if he does contract the disease (children, elderly, or participants suffering other diseases)

Among the risks in most vaccine trials is the generally small risk of contracting the disease. Slight fever, headache, muscle soreness, and muscle aches are common side effects and are usually temporary inconveniences. However, the side effects may be more severe in participants who are already suffering a disease or otherwise debilitated. Anaphylactic reactions are generally unpredictable but can be potentially life-threatening.

Risks associated with vaccine trials that use vaccines produced synthetically or by using recombinant DNA techniques may be unknown at present. The participants that receive the vaccine are often those that are most at risk for coercion (children, or institutionalized patients). The most difficult balancing of benefits to risks is when the population that would most benefit from the vaccine comprises those at greatest risk of suffering the vaccine's potential adverse effects.

Vaccine trials may be difficult to monitor because they may involve thousands of participants in many locations. An IRB should confirm that the sponsor has made arrangements for monitoring data such as the progress of the research, the participants' immune status, and reported side effects. The results of the trial must be communicated to the participants. Control participants may erroneously believe that they have been immunized. Participants receiving the vaccine may need to be advised as to the duration of immunization, if the vaccine is effective.

FDA regulations specific to biological products and viral vaccines are at 21 CFR §600-800 and 21 CFR §630.

The dynamic of vaccine trials is likely to change dramatically after the events of September 11, 2001. The new federal Department of Homeland Security is anticipated to have a large budget for funding bioterrorism research, in which many vaccines may fall. The push by government and industry to bring products along rapidly will be significant. These pressures should not change the fundamental charge of the investigator or IRB to protect the participants in clinical trials.

Special Concerns of a Study Using Radioactive Materials or X Rays

Most institutions have a Radioactive Drug Research Committee (RDRC) that is responsible for evaluating the risks of medical studies involving radiation (21 CFR §361.1). However, an IRB must also approve such research. The most common types of radiation used in clinical investigations are X rays, gamma rays, and beta radiation as well as radiopharmaceuticals. OHRP (*Institutional Review Board Guidebook*) defines the following scientific terms used in such studies:

- **Radioactive Drug:** Any substance defined as a drug in §201(b)(1) of the Federal Food, Drug and Cosmetic Act that exhibits spontaneous disintegration of unstable nuclei with the emission of nuclear particles or photons (21 CFR §310.3(n)). Included are any nonradioactive reagent kit or nuclide generator that is intended to be used in the preparation of a radioactive drug and "radioactive biological products," as defined in 21 CFR §600.3(ee). Drugs such as carbon-containing compounds or potassium- containing salts containing trace quantities of naturally occurring radionuclides are not considered radioactive drugs.

- **Radioactive Drug Research Committee (RDRC):** An FDA-approved institutional committee responsible for the use of radioactive drugs in human subjects for certain research purposes (21 CFR §361.1). Research involving human subjects that proposes to use radioactive drugs must be approved by the RDRC and must meet various FDA requirements, including limitations on the pharmacological dose and the radiation dose. The research must be basic research, not intended for diagnosis or treatment of a disease. Furthermore, the exposure to radiation must be justified by the quality of the study and the importance of the information it seeks to obtain. The committee is also responsible for continuing review of the drug use to ensure that the research continues to comply with FDA requirements, including reporting obligations. The committee must include experts in nuclear medicine as well as other medical and scientific members.

- **Radiopaque Contrast Agents:** Materials that stop or attenuate radiation that is passed through the body, creating an outline on film of the organ(s) being examined. Contrast agents, sometimes called "dyes," do not contain radioisotopes. When such agents are used, exposure to radiation results only from the X-ray equipment used in the examination. The chemical structure of radiopaque contrast agents can produce a variety of adverse reactions, some of which may be severe—and possibly life-threatening—in certain individuals.

- **Radiopharmaceuticals:** Radioactive drugs that are labeled or tagged with a radioisotope. These materials are largely physiological or subpharmacological in action, and, in many cases, function much like materials found in the body. The principal risk associated with these materials is the consequent radiation exposure to the body or to specific organ systems when they are introduced into the body.

- **REM:** Acronym for Roentgen Equivalent in Man; the unit of measurement for a dose of an ionizing radiation that produces the same biological effect as a unit of absorbed dose (1 rad) of ordinary X rays. One millirem is equal to 1/1000 of a rem. [*Institutional Review Board Guidebook*]

Disagreement exists over the degree of radiation risk from medical procedures and other sources. This includes a debate about whether theoretical thresholds exist below which no harm will occur. The Nuclear Regulatory Commission (NRC) has developed occupational dose limits, which vary according to which part of the body is exposed

(10 CFR §20). The National Council for Radiation Protection and Measurement (NCRPM) has established recommended dose standards but has taken the position that there is no absolutely safe dose of radiation. The NRC regulates radioactive materials in twenty-one states (10 CFR §30, 40 & 70). The other twenty-nine states, known as Agreement States, have entered into agreements with the NRC to regulate uses in their states. The state regulations may be more restrictive than federal regulations.

The FDA requires an Investigational New Drug Application (IND) for radioactive drugs, kits, or generators that are to be used for investigational diagnostic or therapeutic purposes. Radioactive drugs that are used in certain research to study metabolism of the drug or to study human physiology, pathophysiology, or biochemistry and that are not intended for immediate therapeutic, diagnostic or similar purposes are exempt (21 CFR §361.1). To meet this exemption from submitting an IND, the radiation dose must not exceed the limits set by the regulations, the study design meets other research criteria, and the protocol is approved by an RDRC. The current radiation limits (including radiation doses from radiology procedures that would not have occurred but for the study) are these:

- For an adult research subject, radiation to the whole body, active blood-forming organs, the lens of the eye, or the gonads may not exceed a single dose of 3 rems or an annual cumulative dose of 5 rems.

- The amount of radiation to other organs may not exceed a single dose of 5 rems or an annual cumulative dose of 15 rems.

- Permissible doses for children (persons under age 18) are 10 percent of those for adults. The FDA must approve studies involving children before the study begins.

Most medical institutions have an Institutional Radiation Safety Committee (IRSC), in addition to an RDRC, that assesses the risks of radiation exposure for both patients and employees. IRSC review may be mandated by state law or by the institution's policy. It may also serve as an advisory body to an IRB.

The major risks of radiopharmaceuticals are a factor of the radioisotope's energy, its half-life, the radiosensitivity of the organ system being studied, and the radiation dosage to the target organ, adjacent organs, and the body as a whole. Radiopharmaceuticals have relatively low risks unrelated to their radioactivity (OPRR, *Institutional Review Board Guidebook*).

Although an IRB should distinguish between a study where radiation exposure is incidental as part of medical management and a study where radiation exposure is part of the research, the fundamental concern of radiation exposure is the same. Occupational dose limits give some guidance for an IRB but are not conclusive. An IRB should ensure that radiation exposure is minimized. Excessive radiation exposure can cause immediate injury such as burns. The subtler but more devastating risks are certain types of cancer and genetic damage. No radiation dose should be considered risk-free if it is directed toward, or absorbed by, the reproductive organs (OPRR, *Institutional Review Board Guidebook*). An IRB should also consider the potential risk of radiation exposure to research personnel, other healthcare providers, family, and others. For example, radioactive seeding of a tumor may create a zone of very high radiation for a short period of time. If the patient goes home, his or her spouse may have a dangerous exposure level. The informed consent process of any study where radiation exposure occurs should discuss the topic.

Intravascular contrast agents used in radiology procedures (angiograms, intravenous pylograms, and venograms) can have additional risks to some patients. For example, the type of contrast material (ionic versus nonionic) may have additional risks. An IRB should carefully consider the age and medical condition of the research participants. Patients suffering advanced age, renal disease, chronic respiratory disease, and other conditions are at increased risk. Anaphylactic reactions are a serious but rare risk.

Special Concerns in HIV-Related Research Protocols

In reviewing an HIV-related research protocol, the primary concerns for an IRB are privacy, confidentiality, and justice (fairness in distribution of the benefits and risks in research) (OPRR, *Institutional Review Board Guidebook*). An IRB should consider including people (either as members or consultants) knowledgeable about HIV and experienced in working with those suffering the disease (45 CFR §46.107 (a) and (f)). This is an important means of not only ensuring that the interests of this population are adequately considered but also of keeping the population apprised of clinical research being conducted.

As to confidentiality in HIV studies, OPRR gave the following guidance:

where identifiers are not required by the design of the study, they are not to be recorded. If identifiers are recorded, they should be separated, if possible, from data and stored securely, with linkage restored only when necessary to conduct the research. No lists should be retained identifying those who elected not to participate. Participants must be given a fair, clear explanation of how information about them will be handled.

As a general principle, information is not to be disclosed without the subject's consent. The protocol must clearly state who is entitled to see records with identifiers, both within and outside the project. This statement must take account of the possibility of review of records by the funding agency. . . . [NIH, 1984]

An IRB also must consider issues surrounding confidentiality such as:

- How much data will be recorded in the research participant's medical records.
- Informing the participant as to what data will be collected, who will have access to data, and whether state law requires reporting of HIV infection to government agencies.
- How will the investigator respond to subpoenas or court orders to divulge information about a participant and whether a participant will be notified.
- How requests for information by third parties who have the participant's permission will be handled.

An extensive set of guidelines for confidentiality in HIV research are set forth in Bayer, Levine, and Murray, "Guidelines for Confidentiality in Research on AIDS." *IRB* 6 (No. 6, November/December 1984): 1–9. and cited with approval in OPRR, *Institutional Review Board Guidebook,* Chap. V, sec. F.

Recruitment of research participants, as with any study, is a concern in HIV-related investigations. Efforts to minimize coercion of a vulnerable population should be taken. An equitable basis, not preferring one social group to another, should be chosen for recruiting participants. This may require consideration of providing adjunct services to economically or educationally disadvantaged. As part of reviewing the informed consent process, an IRB should ensure that provisions are present if consent is sought from participants suffering late stages of HIV, as dementia can be a component of this condition. Studies that screen blood for HIV serostatus should address, where applicable, state laws that require a patient to be counseled about HIV prior to testing for the disease. For example, see Va. Code 32.1-37.2(A) as well as OPRR Reports ("Dear Colleague" letters dated December 26, 1984 and June 10, 1988). Research participants also need to be advised if a risk exists that their HIV serostatus may change from negative to positive.

Major ethical issues are raised in clinical trials of HIV-related therapies or vaccines. What is the acceptable risk to participants when the disease is fatal and no effective therapy is available? Can HIV-infected patients be used as a placebo group that is not given experimental treatment? How should participants be selected for experimental treatment? Can healthy and at-risk individuals be asked to participate in vaccine trials?

Randomized clinical trials (RCTs), while anticipated to yield the most valid scientific results, create an ethical dilemma. "Ethical use of RCTs depends on the existence of both the ability to state a null hypothesis (also called "theoretical equipoise") and that there be no other therapy known to be more effective than the one being studied in the RCT" (OPRR, *Institutional Review Board Guidebook*). However, a working group of the American Foundation for AIDS Research argues that other forms of controls such as historical controls (comparisons of outcomes before the use of the investigational therapy) can be justified where there is no known effective therapy (Levine, Dubler, and Levine (1991), pp. 3, 6 cited by OPRR, *Institutional Review Board Guidebook*, Chap. V, sec. F).

The use of placebo controls in lieu of an active control where a disease is fatal is difficult to ethically justify. Levine, Dubler, and Levine (1991) argue that placebo controls can ethically only be used in two situations: 1) when there is either no known effective therapy that can be used as an active control, or participants are persons who cannot tolerate a known effective therapy; and 2) the trial therapy is "so scarce that only a limited number of patients can receive it." They contend that the only fair way to then assign participants to the active and control arms is through a lottery. The trial should be stopped or the protocol modified as soon as sufficient evidence is collected of a beneficial effect, unacceptable side effects, or a very low probability of statistically significant results being obtained.

Special Concerns in Organ Transplant Studies

An IRB should begin by organizing its thoughts about ethical concerns along the lines of risks to tissue donors and risks to recipients. Informed consent, coercion, selection of participants, risk/benefit ratio and other issues usually considered by an IRB should address both of these constituencies. The selection criteria of recipients is an ongoing issue for all organ transplantation programs.

Many candidates for experimental transplant procedures are facing imminent death, with the experiment offering the only hope of survival. This makes the population highly vulnerable, and an IRB should carefully scrutinize a proposed investigation. In addition, children, of course, are the subject of specific federal regulations (45 CFR §46.401-409). An IRB must weigh the risks and benefits carefully. What is the intended therapeutic benefit to the patient? What is the benefit to society from the knowledge gained by the research? Obviously, the latter should not be given so much weight as to overshadow the former. What is the availability of alternative therapies? What is the patient's prospect for survival and quality of life with the transplant in comparison to the available alternatives? For a detailed discussion of ethical issues in using live donors, see R. Adams, "Organ Donors & Informed Consent: A Difficult Minuet," 8 *Journal of Legal Medicine* 555 (1987).

An open question is whether cadaver donors fall within an IRB's jurisdiction. Federal regulations define a research subject as a "living individual" (45 CFR §46.102(f)). However, the President's Commission for the Study of Ethical Problems in Medicine and Biomedical and Behavioral Research (1983), p. 41, recommended that IRBs consider requiring review of studies on brain dead patients "to determine whether . . . it is consistent with 'commonly held convictions about respect for the dead.'" The better course is for an institution to require IRB approval of such studies.

The use of xenografts (transplantation of organs or tissue from an animal to a human) is a blossoming area of research. However, the lack of experience in the area heightens the need for careful evaluation of a study. Under a proposed rule, published on January 17, 2001, the FDA would provide public access to most of the study design and safety information about these types of studies. The FDA would not release confidential business information or personal information related to study participants.

COMPLIANCE ISSUES IN RESEARCH PROTOCOLS

Clinical investigations are often found to have weaknesses such as:

- Failure to report adverse events.
- Modifying either the protocol or the informed consent documents without IRB or FDA approval.
- Initiating or continuing investigational therapy on a patient that does not meet the parameters of the research protocol.
- Failure to make timely periodic reports to the IRB.

An investigator, an institution, an IRB, and a sponsor must be vigilant to ensure that these problems occur as rarely as possible. Chapter Sixteen discusses compliance in more detail.

CONCLUSION

The research protocol is the detailed plan by which an investigator will conduct his research. The investigator must simultaneously stick to his protocol and make changes to the protocol that reflect findings that become evident during the course of the study. Using good scientific methodology includes careful documentation of adjustments to the protocol to protect participants and to obtain valid results. The investigator must include the IRB and other interested parties in creating the research protocol and then closely monitoring its execution.

References

Adams, R. (1987) "Organ Donors & Informed Consent: A Difficult Minuet," 8 *Journal of Legal Medicine 555*.

Bulkeley, W. M. E-Mail Medicine: Untested Treatments, Cures Find Stronghold on On-Line Services, *Wall St. J.* Feb. 27, 1995, at A1.

Ezekiel, Wendler, & Grady. "What Makes Clinical Research Ethical?" *JAMA*. 2000; 283: 2701–2711.

FDA. Information Sheets, Guidance to IRBs, 1998.

Freedman, B. "Placebo-Controlled Trials and the Logic of Clinical Purpose," *IRB* 12 (No. 6, November/December 1990): 1–6.

Freedman, B. "Equipoise and the Ethics of Clinical Research." *New England Journal of Medicine* 317 (No. 3, July 16, 1987): 141–145.

International Conference on Harmonization, Guideline for Good Clinical Practice, Guidelines 4, 6, 7, and 8.

Levine, Dubler, & Levine. (1991), pp. 3, 6 cited by OPRR, *Institutional Review Board Guidebook,* Chap. V, sec. F.

McCarthy, R., & Porter, J. P. "Confidentiality: The Protection of Personal Data in Epidemiological and Clinical Research Trials." *Law, Medicine and Health Care* 19 (No. 3-4, Fall/Winter 1991): 238–241.

NIH. "Guidance for Institutional Review Boards for AIDS Studies" [Dear Colleague Letter]. *OPRR Reports,* December 26, 1984.

OIG. "Recruiting Subjects for Industry-Sponsored Clinical Research," OEI-01-97-00196 (June 2000), http://oig.hhs.gov/oei/reports/a458.pdf.

OPRR, *Institutional Review Board Guidebook,* 1993, Chaps. IV and V.

President's Commission for the Study of Ethical Problems in Medicine and Biomedical and Behavioral Research (1983).

Wallace, R. J. (1982) "Privacy and the Use of Data in Epidemiology." In *Ethical Issues in Social Science Research,* Tom L. Beauchamp, Ruth R. Faden, R. Jay Wallace, Jr., and LeRoy Walters, (Eds.) pp. 274–291. Baltimore, MD: Johns Hopkins University Press.

9.

The Institutional Review Board

Introduction 269
General Observations About Institutional Review Boards 270
    Defining an Institutional Review Board (IRB) 270
    The Function of an IRB 270
    An IRB by Another Name 270
    The Types of Research That Must Be Approved by an IRB 271
    The Types of Research That Are Exempt from the Requirement for IRB Approval 271
    Situations in Which IRB Review Can Be Waived 272
    Use of a Test Article by a Physician in an Emergency Without Prior IRB Review 272
    IRB Review and Approval of a Study Involving a Marketed Product 273
    Manufacturer Compliance with Federal Regulations When Conducting
    Trials Within Its Own Facility Using Employees As Participants 273
    IRB Registration with the OHRP 273
    IRB Registration with the FDA 274
    An Assurance, a Multiple Project Assurance, or a Federalwide Assurance 274
    An Assurance for FDA Regulated Products 275
    Whether an Institution Must Establish Its Own IRB 275
    The IRB in the Institution's Organizational Structure 276
    Scrutiny of an Independent IRB Used by an Institution 276
    Review and Approval of a Study by an Independent
    IRB to Be Conducted in an Institution with an IRB 277
    IRB Approval for a Physician, in Private Practice, Conducting
    Research with an FDA Regulated Product 277
    Hospital IRB Review of a Study That Will Be Conducted Outside
    of the Hospital 277
Composition of Institutional Review Board 278
    The Minimum Number and Mixture of IRB Members 278
    The Maximum Number of IRB Members 279
    Consideration of Financial Interests in Selecting IRB Members 279
    A Clinical Investigator As an IRB Member 279
    One Member Satisfying More Than One Membership Category 280
    Distinguishing Which IRB Members Are Scientists and Nonscientists 280
    The Qualities Sought in a Nonaffiliated IRB Member 280
    Meeting the Mandate That an IRB Possess Sufficient
    Knowledge of the Local Research Context 281
    Selecting the Chairperson of an IRB 283

Substitutes for IRB Members at Convened Meetings 283
Alternate Members of an IRB 284
Attendance by a Nonaffiliated Member at Every IRB Meeting 284
Use of Consultants to an IRB in Its Decision-Making 284
The Ability of an IRB to Function if a Quorum Is Lost at an IRB Meeting 284
Educational Requirements for IRB Members 285
Education Requirements for IRB Members and Others Under an FWA 285
Compensation of IRB Members for Their Services 286
Disclosure of Financial Interests by IRB Members 286
Activities of an IRB 286
Basic Policies and Procedures of an IRB 287
Frequency of IRB Meetings 289
Documents to Be Reviewed by an IRB As Part of Its Review Process 289
The "Primary Reviewer" System 289
An Investigator's Brochure As Mandatory Documentation
to Be Reviewed by an IRB of an Investigational Drug Study 290
Policy and Procedure on Financial Interests 290
Clinical Trials Being Conducted at an Institution That Has
a Financial Interest in the Product's Commercialization 291
The Format of an IRB's Decision 291
An IRB's Obligation to Review Ongoing Research 292
The Frequency of Reviewing Approved Research by an IRB 294
The Consequences if a Study Is Not Reviewed
at Least Annually by an IRB 294
Annual IRB Reviews When Studies Are Reviewed
by an IRB Each Quarter 294
Continuing IRB Review of a Project When Research Interventions
Are Completed but Investigators Are Still Collecting Follow-Up Data 294
Reporting to an IRB When a Study Has Been Completed 294
The Role of Institution Officials When an IRB Does Not Approve a Research Proposal .. 295
Notifying an IRB That Another IRB Previously Denied Approval of the Study 295
Events to Occur if an IRB Suspends or Terminates Its Approval of a Clinical Study 295
Direct Communication Between Sponsors and IRBs 296
A Sponsor's Responsibility for IRB Actions 296
Promising Approaches for IRBs 296
Decision-Making by an IRB 297
The Basic Obligations of an IRB Before Approving Research 297
The Criteria for IRB Approval of Research 297
The Risk/Benefit Analysis 298
Defining Benefit 298
Assessing Anticipated Benefits 298
Defining Risk 299
Consideration of Potential Harms When Looking at Risk 299
Defining Minimal Risk 300
IRB Determination That the Risks to Participants Are Minimized 300
IRB Determination That the Risks to the Participants
Are Reasonable in Relation to Anticipated Benefits 301
IRB Consideration of Additional Safeguards 301
IRB Determination That Selection of Participants Is Equitable 301

IRB Consideration As to Incentives for Participation 302
IRB Determination That Informed Consent Has Been Obtained and Documented 302
Review of a Standard Cooperative Research Protocol
or a Standard Informed Consent Document by a Local IRB 302
IRB Procedure When an Exception to Informed Consent Is Sought
for Emergency Research 302
IRB Waiver of Informed Consent 303
IRB Consideration During Its Prestudy Review with
Regard to Monitoring and Observation 303
IRB Determination That Data Will Be Monitored to Ensure the Participant's Safety 304
IRB Reliance on DSMB Reports 304
IRB's Role in Protecting a Participant's Privacy 304
Expedited Review 305
Conditional Approval of a Study 305
Proposed Changes to IRB Review 305
Workload 306
Record Keeping 306
Records That an IRB Must Keep 306
Information That Must Be Maintained by the IRB in Its Records About IRB Members . . . 306
IRB Minutes 307
Retention of IRB Records 307
The "Research Proposal Reviewed" Is the Same As the Formal Study Protocol
That the Investigator Receives from the Sponsor of the Research 307
IRB Records for Studies That Are Approved but Never Started 307
Sponsor Access to IRB Written Procedures, Minutes, and Membership Rosters 308
Mandatory Reports to OHRP 308
Quality Assurance 308
Common Examples of IRB Non-Compliance 308
Common Non-Compliance Problems for Institutions 309
IRB Response to Non-Compliance in a Protocol 309
IRB Reporting of Each Instance of Non-Compliance with Federal Regulations to OHRP . . 310
The Current Effectiveness of IRBs 310
Self-Evaluation of the IRB 310
FDA's Self-Evaluation Tool 311
Regulatory Oversight of IRBs 317
Federal Agencies Overseeing Local IRBs 317
FDA Inspection Procedure of an IRB 318
Sponsor Access to Whether an IRB Has Been Inspected
by the FDA, and the Results of the Inspection 318
Administrative Actions by HHS for Non-Compliance 318
Conclusion 319
References 319

· · · · · · · · · · ·

INTRODUCTION

An Institutional Review Board (IRB) is the group charged under the Common Rule with reviewing research protocols on a local level to ensure that the human participants are adequately protected. The Food & Drug Administration (FDA) since 1971 has required that any study testing new drugs or biologics on human participants within an institution be approved by an IRB. In 1976, this was expanded to include medical device studies. The mandate was further expanded in 1981 to include IRB review of any study conducted outside an institution (HHS, OIG June 2000). Long operating behind the scenes, recent federal investigations have brought IRBs into the spotlight of the media. The IRB's role has taken on new significance, and its work is under ever more scrutiny. The following questions and answers will assist an IRB and its members to carry out the IRB's functions more effectively.

....

GENERAL OBSERVATIONS ABOUT INSTITUTIONAL REVIEW BOARDS

Defining an Institutional Review Board (IRB)

According to the Office for Protection from Research Risk (OPRR), now succeeded by the Office of Human Research Protection (OHRP), "[a]n IRB is an administrative body established to protect the rights and welfare of human research participants recruited to participate in research activities conducted under the auspices of the institution with which it is affiliated" (OPRR, Institutional Review Board Guidebook, Chap. I, sec. A). An IRB has the authority to approve, require modifications in (to secure approval), or disapprove research (45 CFR §46.109(2), FDA, Information Sheets, 1998). This group review serves an important role in the protection of the rights and welfare of human research participants. To accomplish its purpose of protecting human participants, an IRB reviews research protocols and related materials (informed consent documents and investigator brochures) in advance and periodically during a study.

The Function of an IRB

An IRB is responsible for the initial review and continuing review of research involving human participants. An IRB reviews and approves a research project before the research is started (45 CFR Part 46). The review includes the research protocol, the informed consent document to be signed by research participants, any advertisements to be used to recruit research participants, and other relevant documents. The IRB must seek to ensure that any risks to which a participant is exposed are outweighed by anticipated benefits; that the participant is clearly advised of the proposed research, the risks, the benefits, and available alternatives (informed consent); that the advertising is not misleading; and that selection of participants is equitable and justified. Continuing review of a research project includes consideration of unexpected adverse events and amendments to the research protocol as well as other scrutiny of the research project to ensure that the risk/benefit ratio continues to remain favorable to the research participants.

An IRB by Another Name

IRB is a generic term used to refer to a group whose purpose is to review research to ensure the protection of human participants. Any name may be used by an organization to denote this group. For example, the Virginia statute regulating research uses the term, "human research review committee." In other countries, the group may be referred to as an Independent Ethics Committee (IEC). Regardless of the name chosen, an IRB is subject to the regulations of OHRP for most studies under the Common Rule (45 CFR Part 46). An IRB is subject to the regulations of the FDA when studies of FDA-regulated products are considered by the IRB.

The Types of Research That Must Be Approved by an IRB

Any research involving human participants "conducted, supported, or otherwise subject to regulation by any federal department or agency" requires approval by an IRB (OPRR, *Institutional Review Board Guidebook,* Chap. I, sec. A citing 45 CFR §46.101(a)). In addition, an institution is likely to have agreed in an *Assurance* with the OHRP that all research involving human participants, regardless of funding source, will be subject to approval of an IRB (45 CFR §46.103(b)(1)). *Research* is defined as "a systemic investigation, including research, development, testing and evaluation, designed to develop or contribute to generalized knowledge" (45 CFR §46.102(d)). The support of an activity by a research grant is one practical, if not artificial, reference point in determining if an activity is research (OPRR, *Institutional Review Board Guidebook*). *Human subjects* are defined as "living individuals about whom an investigator (whether professional or student) conducting research obtains (1) data through intervention or interaction with the individual, or (2) identifiable private information" (45 CFR §46.102(f)). Research involving human subjects as defined by federal regulations has been summarized in the following question: "Is there an intervention or an interaction with a living person that would not be occurring or would be occurring in some other fashion but for this research?" (OPRR, http://www.nih.gov/grants/oprr/humansubjects/guidance/decisioncharts.htm). When in doubt as to whether the research will involve human subjects, the investigator should seek assistance from the IRB in making the determination, says OHRP (OPRR, *Institutional Review Board Guidebook* 45 CFR §46.101(b)(1-6), §46.118, and §46.119). All research subject to the Common Rule or FDA regulations must be approved by the IRB (45 CFR §46.102, §46.103, §46.108(a)) (21 CFR §56.103).

The Protection of Human Subjects Assurance Identification/IRB Certification/Declaration of Exemption form appears on page 322.

The Types of Research That Are Exempt from the Requirement for IRB Approval

Not all research requires consideration by an IRB under the Common Rule. Research that is exempted from IRB approval (45 CFR §101(b)) under the Common Rule includes:

1. Educational testing and educational research.

2. Survey or interview techniques where the human subject remains anonymous.

3. Public observation where the human subject remains anonymous.

4. The collection or study of existing data, documents, records, pathological specimens, or diagnostic specimens, if these sources are publicly available or if the information is recorded so that the human subjects remain anonymous.

5. Research and demonstration projects of the Social Security program.

"Existing data, documents, records, pathological specimens, or diagnostic specimens" refer to these items that "are on the shelf" before the protocol begins (45 CFR §101(b)(4)). For example, testing blood for a purpose other than that for which it is drawn would not be exempt from IRB review. Conversely, testing of blood samples in a reference bank that are not identifiable to an individual is exempt. "Masked studies" are not exempt from IRB review (OPRR, *Institutional Review Board Guidebook*). Research records will reflect the identity of subjects, either directly or through identifiers (codes) that can be linked to individuals.

The government agency overseeing the program retains final authority to determine whether a particular activity is covered by federal regulations (45 CFR §101(c)). A further determinant is the institution's Assurance. The institution may have pledged to have all research reviewed and approved by its IRB. The form for notifying a federal agency of an exempt study appears at the end of this chapter.

An institution's policies or a state's regulations may require IRB approval of any type of study despite federal exemptions.

Situations in Which IRB Review Can Be Waived

An IRB does not have the authority to waive its review of a proposed study. However, FDA regulations allow the FDA to waive any of the requirements pertaining to IRBs, including the requirement for IRB review, for specific research activities or for classes of research activities. Sponsors or investigators must request such a waiver directly from the FDA (21 CFR §56.105). Requests for waiver are submitted to the Center for Drug Evaluation and Research (CDER) or the Center for Biologic Evaluation and Research (CBER) division responsible for reviewing the IND. If the responsible division is unknown, the request can be sent to the Bioresearch Monitoring Staff, Office of the Associate Commissioner of Regulatory Affairs (HFC-30). Even if FDA waiver of IRB review is obtained, other federal agencies or the institution may still require IRB review of the study. Other federal agencies also have the authority to waive applicability of the regulations to specific research activities or classes of research activity (45 CFR §101(e)).

Use of a Test Article by a Physician in an Emergency Without Prior IRB Review

FDA regulations (21 CFR §56.104(c)) allow for one emergency use of a test article in an institution without prospective IRB review, provided that such emergency use is reported to the IRB within five working days after such use. *Emergency* is defined as a life-threatening situation in which no standard acceptable treatment is available and in which there is not sufficient time to obtain IRB approval (21 CFR §56.102(d)). An *emergency use* is defined as a single use (or single course of treatment, such as multiple doses of antibiotic) with one patient. *Subsequent use* is defined as a second use with that patient or the use with another patient.

In its review of an emergency use, if use of the test article in the future is anticipated, an IRB should request that a protocol and informed consent process be developed so that an approved protocol will be in place when the next need arises. The FDA recognizes that, in spite of the best efforts of a clinical investigator and an IRB, a situation may occur where a second emergency use needs to be considered. The FDA has stated that it believes denial of emergency treatment to an individual is inappropriate when the only obstacle is lack of time for the IRB to convene, review the use, and give approval (FDA, Information Sheets, 1998).

A physician retains the authority to provide emergency medical care to his patients (45 CFR §46.116(f)). On May 15, 1991, OPRR issued the following statement clarifying emergency treatment of a patient by a physician when that patient is also a research subject:

> Whenever emergency care is initiated without prior IRB review and approval, the patient may not be considered to be a research subject. Such emergency care may not be claimed as research, nor may the outcome of such care be included in any report of a research activity. Simply stated: [D]HHS regulations for the protection of human subjects do not permit research activities to be started, even in [an] emergency, without prior IRB review and approval.
>
> If the emergency care involves drugs, devices, or biologics that are considered to be investigational by the Food and Drug Administration (FDA), then it may be necessary to meet FDA requirements to use the investigational article for emergency purposes.

> Thus, the distinction under HHS regulations is that while a physician may, without prior IRB approval, treat a patient using a test article (if the situation meets the FDA requirements), the patient may not be considered a research participant, and data derived from use of the test article may not be used in the study (OPRR, *Institutional Review Board Guidebook*).

IRB Review and Approval of a Study Involving a Marketed Product

> If an investigation involves human participants, then IRB review and approval is required (21 CFR §56.101, §56.102(c), §312.2(b)(1), §361.1, 601.2, and §812.2). This is true even of studies involving products that have previously been approved for marketing by the FDA. For example, *off-label* use requires IRB approval if clinical research is being conducted (FDA, Information Sheets, 1998). Also, see the FDA information sheet entitled "'Off-label' and Investigational Use of Marketed Drugs and Biologics" for more information. IRB approval is not required if "off-label" is strictly part of practicing medicine (FDA, Information Sheets, 1998). *Investigational* is a term applied by the FDA as to availability of a product for distribution, and the term does not address regulatory oversight of clinical studies (21 CFR §510(k)).

Manufacturer Compliance with Federal Regulations When Conducting Trials Within Its Own Facility Using Employees As Participants

> A manufacturer must comply with federal, and even state, regulations relating to clinical research when conducting studies involving human participants. No exception is made for either conducting the study entirely within the sponsor's facility or using solely its own employees. In fact, just the opposite is true. This situation represents a prime example of a vulnerable subject population (FDA, Information Sheets, 1998). When a vulnerable subject population is being used for a study, special precautions need to be put into place. These are discussed in earlier chapters.

IRB Registration with the OHRP

> Registration of an IRB with OHRP is not mandatory. However, OHRP does maintain a voluntary registry, and any organization that applies for a Federalwide Assurance (FWA) must register its IRB or IEC. IRBs already designated under a Multiple Project Assurance or FWA will be automatically registered. This permits OHRP to quickly disseminate

information to the IRB. Information on registering an IRB with OHRP can be found at http://ohrp.osophs.dhhs.gov/irbasur.htm. An IRB can be registered by (i) going to OHRP's IRB Registration and Assurance Web site (http://ohrp.osophs.dhhs.gov/irbasur. htm); (ii) downloading, completing, and forwarding to OHRP the three-page IRB registration form (http://ohrp.osophs.dhhs.gov/humansubjects/Assurance/regirbi.htm); and (iii) in three to five days, checking OHRP's IRB registration listings to verify that processing has been completed (http://ohrp.osophs.dhhs.gov/polasur.htm#LST). In most instances, the IRB will be known to OHRP through an institution's Assurance.

IRB Registration with the FDA

An IRB is not required to register with the FDA prior to approving research protocols. The FDA becomes aware of an IRB when an investigator identifies it. The Form FDA-1572 "Statement of Investigator" for a study conducted under an IND requires the name and address of the IRB that will be responsible for review of the study. The OIG has complained that the lack of federal registration is a major impediment to federal oversight. The FDA is currently studying an IRB registration system (OIG, April 2000).

An Assurance, a Multiple Project Assurance, or a Federalwide Assurance

An Assurance is an agreement negotiated between an institution and the Department of Health and Human Services (HHS) in accordance with HHS regulations (45 CFR §46.103). Federal regulations require a written Assurance from an institution proposing to host research that the institution will comply with the HHS protection of human subjects regulations (45 CFR part 46). "An institution involved in biomedical or behavioral research should have in place a set of principles and guidelines that govern the institution, its faculty, and staff, in the discharge of its responsibilities for protecting the rights and welfare of human participants taking part in research conducted at, or sponsored by, the institution, regardless of the source of funding" (45 CFR §46.103(b)(1)). At a minimum, an Assurance must contain a statement of principles, which may include an appropriate existing code, declaration, and a statement of ethical principles formulated by the institution (45 CFR §46.103(b)(1)). The *Belmont Report* or *Declaration of Helsinki* is frequently cited. "This set of principles should be in the form of a document that is readily available to all staff or faculty personnel who have need of it and can be a part of the staff or faculty manual. It should be written in clear, concise, unambiguous language, understandable to its intended audience" (OPRR, *Institutional Review Board Guidebook*).

The Assurance mechanism is described in 45 CFR §46.103. (See also Chapters Two and Thirteen.) Once HHS has approved an institution's Assurance, a number is assigned to the Assurance. In the past, the Assurance may have been for a single grant or contract (a Single Project Assurance); for multiple grants (Multiple Project Assurances— formerly called General Assurances); or for certain types of studies such as oncology group studies and AIDS research group studies (Cooperative Project Assurances). Currently, a simplified process for filing Institutional Assurances of Protection for Human Subjects is being introduced by OHRP. Assurances approved under this process will cover all of the institution's federally supported human subject research. Each legally separate institution will need its own Federalwide Assurance (FWA). OHRP no longer routinely accepts Assurances that are limited to HHS-supported research, to special categories of research, or to individual research projects. However, all existing Assurances will remain in effect through the earlier of either their expiration date or December 31, 2003.

An Assurance for FDA Regulated Products

Currently, FDA regulations do not require an Assurance. However, when research studies involving products regulated by the FDA are funded or supported by a federal agency, the research institution must comply with both the federal agency's regulations (usually the Common Rule) as well as FDA regulations (FDA, Information Sheets, 1998). Most institutions will have entered into an Assurance with OHRP that includes research that will also be regulated by the FDA.

Whether an Institution Must Establish Its Own IRB

An institution engaged in research involving human subjects will usually have its own IRB to oversee research conducted within the institution or by the staff of the institution. An institution without an IRB can arrange for an outside IRB to be responsible for initial and continuing review of studies conducted at the non-IRB institution. Such arrangements should be documented in writing. Individuals conducting research in a noninstitutional setting often use established IRBs (independent or institutional) rather than form their own IRBs (45 CFR §46.114).

OHRP has cautioned against institutions relying on outside IRBs and recommends that institutions not enter into such arrangements unless prior approval by OHRP is granted (OPRR, *Institutional Review Board Guidebook*). "Local laws, institutional policies and constraints, professional and community standards, and population differences are examples of pertinent local factors that can influence the setting of research." (45 CFR §46.103(d), §107(a), and §111(a)(3)). For example, the considered opinion of an IRB of one institution may be blind to information that would alter its decision for another where:

- Institutions draw from culturally dissimilar patient populations.
- Institutions are located in different states or other geographical subdivisions with varied legal or regulatory constraints.
- Institutions are not accustomed to each other's operational policies, constraints, procedures, or commitments.
- There is uncertain satisfaction of drug control responsibilities, or other FDA requirements (OPRR, 1991).

However, where these concerns are appropriately addressed, OHRP has said that it will approve the use of an outside IRB (OPRR, 1991). OHRP may require that the institution have a representative serve as a consultant to the outside IRB (OPRR, *Institutional Review Board Guidebook*).

In contrast, the Office of Inspector General has criticized low-volume IRBs (defined as IRBs that conduct less than 125 initial reviews annually), which are particularly susceptible to problems because they are often hospital-based and isolated from other IRBs and research cultures. Occasionally this gives the opportunity for "IRB shopping" by sponsors (OIG, 1998). Also see a Canadian government report on low-volume IRBs: National Council on Bioethics in Human Research (1995). (This report concluded that low-volume IRBs lacked adequate breadth and depth to adequately conduct reviews. It recommended that IRBs that review less than fifty proposals per year should merge with another IRB.)

The IRB in the Institution's Organizational Structure

OHRP has stated, "It is vital that IRB members, department heads, and other officials with responsibility for oversight of research have open and ready access to the highest levels of authority within the institution" (OPRR, *Institutional Review Board Guidebook*). An IRB chairman must have the rank and authority to ensure effectiveness of the IRB. Investigators, faculty, and staff must have open communication with an IRB in addition to having confidence and respect for an IRB's decisions. Oversight of research and the IRB must be in the hands of an official at the institution who has the legal authority to act and speak for the institution. "If the CEO does not function as the Authorized Institutional Official, that person should be the equivalent of the director of research and development, a dean or assistant dean, or hospital administrator" (OPRR, *Institutional Review Board Guidebook*). Examples of who should not be appointed to be the Authorized Institutional Official include a department chair, a research coordinator, or director of a service. The IRB should not report to a unit of the institution responsible for bringing in research funds (OIG, 2000). HHS regulations require that an institution provide meeting space and adequate staff to support the IRB's review and recordkeeping duties (45 CFR §46.103(b)(2)).

Scrutiny of an Independent IRB Used by an Institution

OPRR, now known as OHRP, has set forth the following considerations that it will use to determine if an independent IRB meets the institution's obligation for research oversight:

- Prior to approval of an Assurance, OPRR must review and approve any contract between: (1) an institution that assures OPRR of compliance with 45 CFR §46 and (2) an independent IRB that agrees to provide IRB services in compliance with procedural requirements of 45 CFR §46 as related, for example, to IRB membership, functions, review responsibilities, criteria for approval, and recordkeeping. The contract or other clarifying documentation must explicitly state how the institution's responsibilities under 45 CFR §46 will be carried out and enable the institution to fulfill its obligation as specified in its Assurance to OPRR (e.g., procedures for prompt delivery of minutes and other records for retention by an institution not otherwise affiliated with the IRB).

- No arrangement between an institution and an independent IRB may contain disincentives, impediments, or conflicts of interest which may hamper the exercise of an IRB's function or objectivity throughout the duration of a research activity involving human subjects by or under the direction of the institution which the IRB serves (e.g., fee, employment or other arrangements that discourage prompt, continuing, flexible, or objective response to the need for even unforeseeable IRB action).

- Any IRB, independent or not, must possess and maintain the diversity of membership and/or consultant input to ensure its ability to objectively account, amongst other things, for local institutional, population, legal, and cultural influences on risk to subjects, to compare those risks to anticipated benefits, and make decisions about the equitable selection of subjects. In order to avoid a conflict of interest, no "unaffiliated" IRB member may have an equity interest (e.g., partnership, stocks, or profit-sharing) in the organization providing IRB review nor may any member be paid more than reasonable compensation for IRB services.

[OPRR Memorandum, 1997]

Contracts or other documents (OPRR Memorandum, 1997) submitted by an institution are considered deficient if:

1. They merely allude to 45 CFR §46;
2. They discourage the objectivity or continuing use of the IRB through the nature of fee arrangements or otherwise; or
3. They do not employ effective local representation in convened meetings.

Review and Approval of a Study by an Independent IRB to Be Conducted in an Institution with an IRB

Most institutional IRBs have jurisdiction over all studies conducted within that institution. An independent IRB may become the IRB of record for such studies only upon written agreement with the administration of the institution or the in-house IRB (FDA, Information Sheets, 1998). Government overseers are likely to question why a study was approved and monitored by an outside IRB. However, an institution may have a study in which this is the best means of ensuring human participant safety. Federal regulations permit an institution in multisite studies to use joint review, reliance on the review of another qualified IRB, or similar arrangements intended to avoid duplication of effort (45 CFR §46.114).

IRB Approval for a Physician, in Private Practice, Conducting Research with an FDA Regulated Product

FDA regulations require IRB review and approval of regulated clinical investigations, whether or not the study uses participants that are admitted to an institution. "FDA has included non-institutionalized subjects because it is inappropriate to apply a double standard for the protection of research subjects based on whether or not they are institutionalized" (FDA, Information Sheets, 1998). In addition, several states require an investigator to have IRB approval of any human subject research regardless of funding source. An investigator may be able to obtain IRB review by submitting his research proposal to an IRB at a community hospital, a university/medical school, or an independent IRB. If IRB review cannot be accomplished by one of these means, the FDA has invited investigators to contact the FDA for assistance (Health Assessment Policy Staff at 301-827-1685) (FDA, Information Sheets, 1998).

Hospital IRB Review of a Study That Will Be Conducted Outside of the Hospital

A hospital IRB may agree to review research from affiliated or unaffiliated investigators. If an IRB routinely conducts these reviews, the IRB's policies should authorize such reviews, and the process should be described in the IRB's written procedures. A hospital IRB may review outside studies on an individual basis when the minutes clearly show that the members are aware of where the study is to be conducted and when the IRB possesses appropriate knowledge about the study site(s) (FDA, Information Sheets, 1998).

∙∙∙∙∙∙∙∙∙∙∙∙

COMPOSITION OF INSTITUTIONAL REVIEW BOARD

An IRB should be organized to address the scope of the institution's research activities, the types of participant populations likely to be involved and the size and complexity of the institution. "An IRB must be 1) sufficiently qualified through . . . the diversity of the members, including consideration of race, gender, and cultural backgrounds and sensitivity to such issues as community attitudes, to promote respect for its advice and counsel; and 2) able to ascertain the acceptability of proposed research in terms of institutional commitments and regulations, applicable law, and standards of professional conduct and practice" (45 CFR §46.107(a)).

An IRB must also be capable of ensuring that (1) selection of participants is equitable; (2) privacy of participants is protected; (3) confidentiality of data is maintained; (4) informed consent is sought in language understandable to the participant and under conditions that minimize the possibility of coercion or undue influence; and (5) appropriate safeguards are in place to protect the rights and welfare of vulnerable participants (45 CFR §46.111 and §46.116).

The requirements for IRB composition apply equally to all functions of the IRB. For example, an IRB dedicated to conducting continuing review must meet the IRB membership requirements (OHRP, 2002).

The Minimum Number and Mixture of IRB Members

An IRB must have at least five members. The board must include people representative of various backgrounds and professions to capture the prevailing values of the communities in which it operates. Experience, expertise, and diversity of the IRB members must be adequate "to promote respect for its advice and counsel in safeguarding the rights and welfare of human subjects" (45 CFR §46.107(a)). OPRR recommended that to achieve this, members should be selected with consideration of "their racial and cultural heritage and their sensitivity to issues such as community attitudes" (OPRR, *Institutional Review Board Guidebook*). At least one member must have primarily scientific interests, one must have primarily nonscientific interests, and one must be otherwise unaffiliated with the institution (45 CFR §46.107(c)). The IRB must make every nondiscriminatory effort to ensure that it does not consist entirely of men or entirely of women. Selections must not, however, be made on the basis of gender. The members must not be entirely of one profession (45 CFR §46.107(b)). A quorum, with at least one nonscientific member present, is needed for voting. "[T]he independent ethical review of research trials should involve individuals with training in science, statistics, ethics, and law, as well as reflective citizens who understand social values, priorities, and the vulnerability and concerns of potential subjects" (Ezekiel, Wendler, and Grady, 2000).

The OIG has complained that IRBs need more nonscientific and noninstitutional members. "At present just one IRB member can wear both of these hats and satisfy the requirement. We found that to be an untenable situation, one that can deprive IRBs of a valuable counterbalance to internal, institutional pressures that can threaten their independence" (OIG, 2000). The OIG was also critical of many institutions that do not make the IRB adequately independent.

When an IRB regularly reviews research proposals where vulnerable populations are involved, such as children, prisoners, pregnant women, or the handicapped, the IRB must consider having one or more members that are knowledgeable about and experienced in working with these groups (45 CFR §46.107(a)). Department of Education regulations require that when an IRB reviews research for one of its programs that purposefully includes handicapped children or mentally disabled persons, the IRB must include at least one member who is primarily concerned with the welfare of these individuals (34 CFR §350.3(d)2; 34 CFR §356.3(c)(2)).

The Maximum Number of IRB Members

"An IRB can have as many members as necessary for it to perform its duties effectively" (OPRR, *Institutional Review Board Guidebook*). Federal guidelines do not set forth any maximum number of members for an IRB. However, the institution should be cognizant of what size group is efficient in decision-making. Many institutions have opted to create more than one IRB in lieu of increasing the size of a committee to an unworkable number. An institution may divide oversight of particular categories of studies between its multiple IRBs (OPRR, *Institutional Review Board Guidebook*).

Consideration of Financial Interests in Selecting IRB Members

The institution should be very conscious of conflicting interests as well as the appearance of conflicting interests when selecting IRB members. The board and its members should not only be independent, they should also avoid any appearance of not being independent. As the HHS has pointed out,

> Institutions engaged in human research should take great care to ensure that the composition of the membership of an affiliated IRB and its positioning within or relative to the administrative structure of the institution ensures that the review board is free to make its decisions and conduct its oversight activities in an autonomous manner, free from institutional pressures to follow a preferred course of action. Broad participation of members from outside the institution, who will have no interest in the outcome of the research or the business interests of the institution, is considered to be one of the most effective means of protecting the integrity of the IRB process. [HHS, 2000.]

Financial relationships and other potentials for conflict of interest among IRB members are a growing concern. For example, a sponsor of a study under review may also fund research for several IRB members. This raises the concern that the IRB members may be under pressure to approve the sponsor's studies. However, if anyone who is doing research for a sponsor of the current study is excluded, the IRB may suffer from the loss of his or her expertise.

A Clinical Investigator As an IRB Member

A clinical investigator can be a member of an IRB. However, FDA regulations (21 CFR §56.107(e)) and the Common Rule (45 CFR §46.107(e)) prohibit any IRB member from participating in an IRB's initial or continuing review of any study in which the member has a conflicting interest, except to provide information requested by the IRB. The selection process of IRB members should consider how often conflicting interests would be of concern. When members frequently have conflicts and must recuse themselves from deliberation and abstain from voting, their contributions to the group review process may be diminished and could hinder the review procedure. This is of utmost concern if the investigator is chairperson of the IRB (FDA, Information Sheets, 1998). The IRB minutes should explicitly reflect that when a member had a conflict of interest, he or she left the room during the discussion and voting phases of the review and approval process (OPRR, *Institutional Review Board Guidebook*).

One Member Satisfying More Than One Membership Category

One IRB member may fulfill more than one membership category. For example, one member could be otherwise unaffiliated with the institution and have a primary concern in a nonscientific area. This individual would satisfy two of the membership requirements of the regulations. However, an IRB should strive for a membership that is thoroughly diverse in representative capacities and disciplines. In fact, federal regulations require that, as part of being qualified as an IRB, the IRB must have ". . . diversity of members, including consideration of race, gender, cultural backgrounds and sensitivity to such issues as community attitudes. . . ." (45 CFR §46.107).

The OIG has complained that the present situation in which one IRB member can wear both the nonscientific and noninstitutional hats is untenable, "one that can deprive IRBs of a valuable counterbalance to internal, institutional pressures that can threaten their independence." The OIG continues "to regard this as a significant area warranting attention. In this increasingly commercialized research environment, the potential for conflicts within research institutions loom larger than ever" (OIG, 2000).

Distinguishing Which IRB Members Are Scientists and Nonscientists

At least one member of the IRB must have primary concerns in the scientific area and at least one must have primary concerns in the nonscientific area (45 CFR §46.107(c)). Physicians and Ph.D. level physical or biological scientists satisfy the requirement for at least one scientist. The members of an IRB must understand the fundamental aspects of experimental design. When an IRB encounters studies involving science beyond the expertise of the members, the IRB may use a consultant to assist in the review (45 CFR §46.107(f)).

The FDA believes the intent of the requirement for diversity of disciplines was to include members who had little or no scientific or medical training or experience. Therefore, the FDA cautions that nurses, pharmacists, and other biomedical health professionals should not be regarded to have "primary concerns in the nonscientific area." In the past, lawyers, clergy, and ethicists have been utilized as persons whose primary concerns would be in nonscientific areas. Some individuals may have training in both scientific and nonscientific disciplines, such as a nurse/lawyer. While such members are of great value to an IRB, the FDA has cautioned that other members who are unambiguously nonscientific should be appointed to satisfy the nonscientist requirement (FDA, Information Sheets, 1998).

The Qualities Sought in a Nonaffiliated IRB Member

"The person selected should be knowledgeable about the local community and be willing to discuss issues and research from that perspective. Consideration should be given to the type of community from which the institution will draw its research subjects" (OPRR, *Institutional Review Board Guidebook*). Nonaffiliated members should be drawn from the community-at-large. Possible candidates include ministers, teachers, attorneys, business people, or community volunteers. "The nonaffiliated member(s) should not be vulnerable to intimidation by the professionals on the IRB, and their services should be fully utilized by the IRB" (OPRR, *Institutional Review Board Guidebook*).

Meeting the Mandate That an IRB Possess Sufficient Knowledge of the Local Research Context

OPRR, now succeeded by OHRP, has pointed out that institutions have a profound responsibility to ensure that IRBs possess sufficient knowledge of the local research context to satisfy the regulatory mandates (OPRR Memorandum, 1998). This obligation is present even if an institution uses an independent IRB and is amplified where research involves more than minimal risk to research subjects. OPRR has said that it will use the following criteria to evaluate the adequacy of an IRB meeting its obligation for possessing sufficient knowledge of the local research context:

(A) OPRR considers the following standards when evaluating the adequacy of IRBs designated under an institutional Assurance, particularly when the IRBs are geographically removed from the local research context. These standards reflect minimum levels of adequacy. More stringent standards may be required, depending upon the nature of the proposed research or the relevant research context.

(1) Where the research involves minimal risk to subjects, the IRB should demonstrate that it has obtained necessary information about the local research context through written materials or discussions with appropriate consultants.

(2) Where the research involves greater than minimal risk to subjects *but* (i) the local research context involves no intervention or interaction with subjects *and* (ii) the principal risk associated with the local research context is limited to the potential harm resulting from a breach of confidentiality, the IRB should (i) demonstrate that it has obtained necessary information[1] about the local research context through written materials or discussions with appropriate consultants; and (ii) determine and specifically document that provisions to protect the privacy of subjects and maintain the confidentiality of data are adequate.

(3) Where the research involves greater than minimal risk to subjects *and* item (A)(2) does not apply, the IRB should demonstrate that it has obtained necessary information[1] about the local research context through one or more of the following mechanisms, or through other mechanisms deemed appropriate by OPRR for the proposed research and the local research context.

---

[1]Necessary information under DHHS regulations includes all of the following:
- The anticipated scope of the institution's research activities;
- The types of subject populations likely to be involved;
- The size and complexity of the institution;
- Institutional commitments and regulations;
- Applicable law;
- Standards of professional conduct and practice;
- Method for equitable selection of subjects;
- Method for protection of privacy of subjects;
- Method for maintenance of confidentiality of data;
- Language(s) understood by prospective subjects;
- Method for minimizing the possibility of coercion or undue influence in seeking consent; and
- Safeguards to protect the rights and welfare of vulnerable subjects.

(a) Personal knowledge of the local research context on the part of one or more IRB members, such knowledge having been obtained through extended, direct experience with the research institution, its subject populations, and its surrounding community.

(b) Participation (either physically or through audiovisual or telephone conference) by one or more appropriate consultants in convened meetings of the IRB. Such consultant(s) should have personal knowledge of the local research context, such knowledge having been obtained through extended, direct experience with the research institution, its subject populations, and its surrounding community.

(c) Prior written review of the proposed research by one or more appropriate consultants (see (b) above), in conjunction with participation (either physically or through audiovisual or telephone conference) by the consultant(s) in convened meetings of the IRB, *when such participation is deemed warranted* either by the consultant(s) or by any member of the IRB.

(d) Systematic, reciprocal, and documented interchange between the IRB and elements of the local research context. Such interchange should include (i) periodic visits to the research site, occurring several times per year, by one or more IRB members in order to obtain and maintain knowledge of the local research context, including the research institution, its subject populations, and its surrounding community; (ii) periodic discussion with appropriate consultants knowledgeable about the local research context; (iii) regular interaction with one or more designated institutional liaisons; and (iv) review of relevant written materials.

(B) The following standards apply where an institution holding an OPRR-approved Assurance wishes to avoid duplication of effort, in accordance with DHHS regulations at *45 CFR §46.114,* by relying upon the IRB review of another Assurance-holding institution:

(1) The review arrangement must be approved in writing by OPRR and by appropriate officials of the institutions involved.

(2) The institution relying upon another institution's IRB has a responsibility to ensure that the particular characteristics of its local research context are considered, either (i) through knowledge of its local research context by the reviewing IRB (see (A) above); or (ii) through subsequent review by appropriate designated institutional officials, such as the Chairperson and/or other members of its local IRB.

(C) Regardless of the IRB's geographic location, each institution holding an OPRR-approved Assurance is expected to maintain a unified system of protections applicable to all human subjects research covered under the Assurance.

(1) Each institution remains responsible for safeguarding the rights and welfare of human subjects within its local research context.

(2) Each institution remains responsible for educating the members of its research community in order to establish and maintain a culture of compliance with Federal regulations and institutional policies relevant to the protection of human subjects.

(3) Each institution remains responsible for implementation, within its local research context, of appropriate oversight mechanisms in order to ensure compliance with the determinations of the reviewing IRB.

(4) Where institutions holding an OPRR-approved Assurance engage a separate entity to perform human subject protection activities, OPRR must review and approve those portions of the contract and/or other clarifying documentation detailing responsibilities and implementation mechanisms relevant to such activities.

   (a) Such documentation must specify mechanisms to ensure that all institutional responsibilities under the Assurance are fulfilled (e.g., procedures for retention and accessibility of records in accordance with DHHS regulations at *45 §CFR 46.115;* procedures for prompt reporting to the IRB of proposed changes in approved research and for prompt reporting to OPRR of unanticipated problems in accordance with DHHS regulations at *45 CFR §46.103*(b)(4), (5)).

   (b) No arrangement may contain disincentives, impediments, or conflicts of interest that may hamper the exercise of the IRB's function or objectivity (e.g., procedures or fee schedules that could discourage prompt reporting to the IRB of proposed changes or unanticipated problems or that could impede the IRB's flexibility to take prompt, objective action where necessary to protect human subjects).

   (c) In order to avoid real or perceived conflicts of interest, (i) no IRB member may hold an equity interest (e.g., partnership, stock, or profit-sharing) in the organization providing IRB review; (ii) no IRB member may be paid more than reasonable compensation or receive more than reasonable benefits for IRB-related activities; and (iii) no IRB member may receive compensation or benefits under arrangements that could impede or discourage objective decision-making on behalf of human subjects.

[OPRR Memorandum, 1998]

Selecting the Chairperson of an IRB

Federal regulations do not articulate any specific criteria for the person to serve as the chairperson of an IRB. Therefore, the chairperson may be a scientist or a nonscientist, affiliated or nonaffiliated. The key to success of an IRB is choosing a chairperson who is highly respected, fully capable of managing the IRB, and fair. "The task of making the IRB a respected part of the institutional community will fall primarily on the shoulders of this individual" (OPRR, *Institutional Review Board Guidebook*).

Substitutes for IRB Members at Convened Meetings

An IRB member cannot unilaterally send a personal representative to fill in for him at a convened IRB meeting that he is unable to attend. Alternates who are formally appointed and listed in the membership roster may substitute, but ad hoc substitutes are not permissible as members of an IRB. In addition, a member who is unable to be present at the convened meeting may participate by videoconference or conference telephone call when the member has received a copy of the documents that are to be reviewed at the meeting. Such members may vote and be counted as part of the quorum. If allowed by

IRB procedures, ad hoc substitutes may attend as consultants and gather information for the absent member, but they may not be counted toward the quorum or participate in either deliberation or voting with the board. The IRB may, of course, ask questions of this representative just as they could of any nonmember consultant. Opinions of the absent members that are transmitted by mail, telephone, fax, or e-mail may be considered by the attending IRB members but may not be counted as votes or toward the quorum for convened meetings (FDA, Information Sheets, 1998).

Alternate Members of an IRB

The use of formally appointed alternate IRB members is acceptable, provided that the IRB's written procedures describe the appointment and function of alternate members. The IRB roster should identify the primary member(s) for whom each alternate member may substitute. To ensure maintaining an appropriate quorum, the alternate's qualifications should be comparable to the primary member to be replaced. The IRB minutes should document when an alternate member replaces a primary member. When an alternate substitutes for a primary member, the alternate member should have received and reviewed the same material that the primary member received or would have received (FDA, Information Sheets, 1998).

Attendance by a Nonaffiliated Member at Every IRB Meeting

A nonaffiliated member is not required to attend every IRB meeting. A word of caution, however. Although FDA regulations (21 CFR §56.108(c)) do not specifically require the presence of a member not otherwise affiliated with the institution to constitute a quorum, the FDA considers the presence of such members an important element of the IRB's diversity. Therefore, frequent absence of all nonaffiliated members is not acceptable to the FDA. Acknowledging their important role, many IRBs have appointed more than one member who is not otherwise affiliated with the institution. The FDA encourages IRBs to appoint members in accordance with 21 CFR §56.107(a) who will be able to participate fully in the IRB process (FDA, Information Sheets, 1998).

Use of Consultants to an IRB in Its Decision-Making

An IRB can ask individuals with special competence to assist in the review of issues that are beyond the expertise of the members. However, these individuals are not allowed to vote (21 CFR §56.107(f) and 45 CFR §46.107(f)).

The Ability of an IRB to Function if a Quorum Is Lost at an IRB Meeting

If a quorum fails during an IRB meeting for whatever reason, recusal, early departure, absence of nonscientist member, the IRB can take no further actions or votes until the quorum is restored (OHRP, 2002).

An IRB loses its quorum whenever during a meeting less than a majority of its members are present. "The quorum is the count of the number of members present. If the number present falls below a majority, the quorum fails. The regulations only require that a member who is conflicted not participate in the deliberations and voting on a study on which he or she is conflicted. Under FDA guidelines, the IRB may decide whether an individual should remain in the room" (FDA, Information Sheets, 1998). This is in contrary to OHPR guidance that forbids a conflicted member to remain in the room (OPRR, *Institutional Review Board Guidebook,* Chap. I, sec. B). The minutes should reflect when this situation occurred.

Educational Requirements for IRB Members

Until recently no educational requirements existed for IRB members. This is quickly changing following a scathing report by the OIG. The OIG believed that minimum standards should exist, and it expressed frustration that federal agencies had not enacted guidelines (OIG, 2000). "Such a requirement exits for research involving animal subjects. We found the case for education requirements no less compelling for research involving humans. The mandatory education we called for could be provided through media such as seminars, individual instruction, videos, or on-line tutorials" (OIG, 2000). The OIG believed that each IRB member must be educated in both applicable federal regulations and ethical principles (OIG, 2000). As discussed next, OHRP is now requiring certain basic educational standards as part of an FWA.

The National Institute of Health (NIH) has created a Web site that lists bioethics resources as an aid to educating IRB members [www.nih.gov/sigs/bioethics/]. Other resources are available through Public Responsibility in Medicine and Research (PRIM&R) [http://www.primr.org/] and its subsidiary, the Applied Research Ethics National Association (ARENA) [http://www.primr.org/arena.html] as well as MCWIRB, an online discussion forum.

Education Requirements for IRB Members and Others Under an FWA

The Institutional Signatory Official, the Human Protections Administrator (e.g., Human Subjects Administrator or Human Subjects Contact Person), and the IRB Chairperson(s) must complete the OHRP basic educational modules (or training certified to OHRP by the institution as equivalent to the OHRP modules) prior to submitting a Federalwide Assurance (see Chapters Two and Thirteen). If an institution wishes to use an alternative educational program, the institution must certify via an appropriate person taking the OHRP program and the alternative program that the alternative equivalently covers the following topics contained in the OHRP program:

1. The responsibilities of the institutional signatory official

2. Institutional responsibilities

3. The responsibilities of the IRB chair

4. IRB responsibilities

5. The administrative responsibilities of a human research protections program

6. Investigator responsibilities

OHRP requires that "members and staff of the IRBs must complete relevant training before reviewing human subject research. Research investigators must complete appropriate institutional training before conducting human subject research" [http://ohrp. osophs.dhhs.gov/humansubjects/Assurance/faq.htm]. OHRP offers Internet-based training modules [http://137.187.172.201/cbttng_ohrp/default.asp?CBTID=2] as a means of educating IRB members and investigators but adds, "OHRP expects that many institutions will decide that other types of training are more appropriate for these individuals. OHRP will expect institutions to be able to provide details about their training upon request" [http://ohrp.osophs.dhhs.gov/humansubjects/Assurance/faq.htm]. "IRB members and others charged with responsibility for reviewing and approving research should receive detailed training in the regulations, guidelines, and policies applicable to human subjects research. Attending workshops and other educational opportunities focused on IRB functions should be encouraged and supported to the extent possible" (OPRR, *Institutional Review Board Guidebook*). OHRP has stated that the PRIM&R 101 program is a comprehensive program and the equivalent of the OHRP program (OHRP, 2001).

The Public Health Service recently announced a new policy that requires certain core areas of education for research staff (ORI, 2000). The text of the policy and frequently asked questions can be found at http://ori.hhs.gov. This includes conflict of interest issues and commitment. HHS has proposed regulations that would require institutions to establish education programs on conflicts of interest (HHS, 2000). IRB members should participate (HHS, 2000).

Compensation of IRB Members for Their Services

IRB members, though frequently volunteers, can be paid for their services. The federal regulations do not preclude a member from being compensated for services rendered. However, payment to IRB members should not be in any way connected to a favorable decision. Expenses, such as travel costs, may also be reimbursed (FDA, Information Sheets, 1998).

Disclosure of Financial Interests by IRB Members

HHS has proposed regulations that require an institution to collect and review information from IRB members and staff on their financial interests with commercial sponsors at least annually (HHS, 2000). HHS also has proposed regulations that require institutions to have policies and procedures that include specific guidance for investigators, IRB members, and others involved in clinical research regarding "potential and actual financial conflicts and their management" (HHS, 2000).

HHS's proposed regulations require an IRB to have clear procedures for disclosure by IRB members of any potential conflict of interest related to a protocol under consideration and for recusal of any IRB member who does have a potential conflict (HHS, 2000). The IRB minutes should specifically reflect that the IRB members were reminded of these policies at the beginning of the meeting and the recusal of any member from a vote.

············

ACTIVITIES OF AN IRB

The institution is responsible for seeing that the IRB has written policies and procedures when conducting its initial and continuing review of research, as well as for reporting its findings and actions to the investigator and the institution's administration (OPRR, *Institutional Review Board Guidebook*). These are usually required as part of the institution's Assurance.

Basic Policies and Procedures of an IRB

An IRB should have policies and procedures (45 CFR §46.103(b)(4) and (5), 21 CFR §56.108; also see ICH, *Guideline for Good Clinical Practice*, 3.3) that address at least:

- Determining its composition (names and qualifications of the members) and the authority under which it is established.
- Scheduling, notifying its members of, and conducting its meetings.
- Conducting initial and continuing review of research.
- Reporting findings to the investigator and the institution's administration in a timely manner.
- Determining which projects require review more often than annually.
- Providing, according to the applicable regulatory requirements, expedited review and approval of minor change(s) in ongoing trials that have the approval of the IRB.
- Specifying that no participant should be admitted to a trial before the IRB issues its written approval of the trial.
- Identifying which projects require verification from sources other than the investigator that no material changes have occurred since the last IRB review.
- Ensuring that proposed changes in approved research activity may not be initiated without IRB review and approval except when necessary to eliminate apparent immediate hazards to the human participant(s).
- Specifying that the investigator promptly report to the IRB, appropriate institutional officials, and, when appropriate, federal agencies:
  (1) Proposed changes in the research protocol.
  (2) Any unanticipated problems involving risks to participants or others.
  (3) All adverse drug reactions that are both serious and unexpected.
  (4) Any serious or continuing non-compliance with federal regulations, IRB directives, or the research protocol.
  (5) Any suspension or termination of IRB approval.

OHRP has recently gone further to state that written IRB procedures "should provide sufficient step-by-step operational details so that an independent observer can understand how an IRB operates and conducts its major functions" (OHRP, 2002). While declining the opportunity to set forth a model set of written procedures with the admonition that one size will not fit all, OHRP stated that the written procedures should include the following:

1. A description of any primary reviewer system used for initial review, continuing review, review of protocol changes, and/or review of reports of unanticipated problems involving risks to subjects or others or of serious or continuing non-compliance.

2. Lists of specific documents distributed to primary reviewers (if applicable) and to all other IRB members for initial review, continuing review, review of protocol changes, and review of reports of unanticipated problems involving risks to subjects or others or of serious or continuing non-compliance.

3. Details of any process (e.g., a subcommittee procedure) that may be used to supplement the IRB's initial review, continuing review, review of protocol changes,

and/or review of reports of unanticipated problems involving risks to subjects or others or of serious or continuing non-compliance.

4. The timing of document distribution prior to IRB meetings.

5. The range of possible actions taken by the IRB for protocols undergoing initial or continuing review and protocol changes undergoing review.

6. A description of how expedited review is conducted and how expedited approval actions are communicated to all IRB members.

7. A description of the procedures for (a) communicating to investigators IRB action regarding proposed research and any modifications or clarifications required by the IRB as a condition for IRB approval of proposed research; and (b) reviewing and acting upon investigators' responses.

8. A description of which institutional office(s) and official(s) are notified of IRB findings and actions and how notification to each is accomplished.

9. A description, if applicable, of which institutional office(s) or official(s) is responsible for further review and approval or disapproval of research that is approved by the IRB. Please note that, in accordance with HHS regulations at 45 CFR §46.112, no other institutional office or official may approve research that has not been approved by the IRB.

10. A specific procedure for how the IRB determines which protocols require review more often than annually, including specific criteria used to make these determinations (e.g., an IRB may set a shorter approval period for high-risk protocols or protocols with a high risk: potential benefit ratio).

11. A specific procedure for how the IRB determines which projects need verification from sources other than the investigators that no material changes have occurred since previous IRB review, including specific criteria used to make these determinations (e.g., such criteria could include some or all of the following: (i) randomly selected projects; (ii) complex projects involving unusual levels or types of risk to subjects; (iii) projects conducted by investigators who previously have failed to comply with the requirements of the HHS regulations or the requirements or determinations of the IRB; and (iv) projects where concern about possible material changes occurring without IRB approval have been raised based upon information provided in continuing review reports or from other sources).

12. A description of what steps are taken to ensure that investigators do not implement any protocol changes without prior IRB review and approval, except when necessary to eliminate apparent immediate hazards to subjects (e.g., this might be addressed through training programs and materials for investigators, specific directives included in approval letters to investigators, and random audits of research records).

13. A description of which office(s) or institutional official(s) is responsible for promptly reporting to the IRB, appropriate institutional officials, any supporting Agency or Department heads, and OHRP any (i) unanticipated problems involving risks to subjects or others; (ii) any serious or continuing non-compliance with 45 CFR Part 46 or the requirements or determinations of the IRB; and (iii) any suspension or termination of IRB approval.

14. A description of the required time frame for accomplishing the reporting requirements in the preceding paragraph.

15. The range of possible actions taken by the IRB in response to reports of unanticipated problems involving risks to subjects or others or of serious or continuing non-compliance.

Frequency of IRB Meetings

An IRB should meet on a regular basis, depending on its workload. One of the basic written procedures of an IRB should be delineating a schedule for meetings. IRB decisions should be made only at announced meetings when at least a quorum of members is present (ICH, *Guideline for Good Clinical Practice*).

Documents to Be Reviewed by an IRB As Part of Its Review Process

ICH, *Good Clinical Practice Guidelines* recommend that an IRB should review the following documents as part of reviewing a research protocol:

- Trial protocol(s)/amendment(s).
- Written informed consent form(s) and consent form updates that the investigator proposes for use in the trial.
- Participant recruitment procedures (advertisements).
- Written information to be provided to participants.
- Investigator's Brochure (IB).
- Available safety information.
- Information about payments and compensation available to participants.
- The investigator's current curriculum vitae and/or other documentation evidencing qualifications.
- Any other documents that the IRB may need to fulfill its responsibilities.

The "Primary Reviewer" System

The IRB system was designed to foster open discussion and debate at convened meetings of the full IRB membership. Although it is preferable for every IRB member to have personal copies of all study materials, each member must be provided with sufficient information to be able to actively and constructively participate. Some institutions have developed a primary reviewer system to promote a thorough review. Under this system, studies are assigned to one or more IRB members for a full review of all materials. Then, at the convened IRB meeting the study is presented by the primary reviewer(s) and, after discussion by IRB members, a vote for an action is taken.

The primary reviewer procedure is acceptable to the FDA and OHRP if each member receives, at a minimum, a copy of consent documents and a summary of the protocol in sufficient detail to determine the appropriateness of the study-specific statements in the consent documents. In addition, the complete documentation should be available to all members for their review, both before and at the meeting. The materials for review should be received by the membership sufficiently in advance of the meeting to allow for adequate review of the materials. If a primary review system is not used by the IRB, then full documentation should be provided to each member (OHRP, 2002).

Some IRBs are also exploring the use of electronic submissions and computer access for IRB members. Whatever system the IRB develops and uses, it must ensure that each study receives an adequate review and that the rights and welfare of the participants are protected (FDA, Information Sheets, 1998).

An Investigator's Brochure As Mandatory Documentation to Be Reviewed by an IRB of an Investigational Drug Study

For studies conducted under an investigational new drug application, the FDA usually requires an investigator's brochure (21 CFR §312.23(a)(5) and §312.55). Even though FDA regulations do not mention the investigator's brochure by name, much of the information contained in such brochures is clearly required to be reviewed by the IRB. An IRB must ensure that risks to the participants are minimized and that the risks to participants are reasonable in relation to the anticipated benefits (21 CFR §56.111(a)). These risks cannot be adequately evaluated without review of the results of previous animal and human studies, which are summarized in the investigator's brochure. An investigator's brochure is commonly submitted to the IRB, and the IRB may establish written procedures that require its submission (FDA, Information Sheets, 1998). OHRP has taken the position that an investigator's brochure, if one exists, should be provided to the IRB (OHRP, 2002).

Policy and Procedure on Financial Interests

The better course is for an IRB to have a policy and procedure on financial interests. HHS has proposed regulations that would require an IRB to have a policy on institutional/IRB financial conflict of interest and financial relationship (HHS, 2000). HHS also suggests that an IRB's policy and procedure manual contain references to medical literature on conflict of interest as well as the HHS August 2000 conference materials (HHS, 2000). The HHS conference materials on conflict of interest issues can be found at http://ohrp. osophs.dhhs.gov/coi/index.htm.

An IRB, under HHS's proposed regulation, should consider the financial relationship of an institution and/or investigator to a sponsor and determine whether a clinical trial should be allowed to be carried out at the institution. If so, the IRB must consider how the study, particularly the protocol and informed consent process, can be best managed (HHS, 2000). The IRB also should be aware of the funding for each protocol that it reviews as well as the funding source for the IRB's review of the protocol (HHS, 2000).

HHS has proposed the following questions for an IRB to consider in its review of a proposed clinical study:

Who is the sponsor?

Who designed the clinical trial?

Who will analyze the safety and efficacy data?

Is there a Data Safety Monitoring Board (DSMB)?

What are the financial relationships between the clinical investigator and the commercial sponsor?

Is there any compensation that is affected by the study outcome?

Does the investigator have any proprietary interests in the product including patents, trademarks, copyrights, and licensing agreements?

Does the investigator have equity interest in the company—publicly held company or non–publicly held company?

Does the investigator receive significant payments of other sorts (grants, compensation in the form of equipment, retainers for ongoing consultation, and honoraria)?

What are the specific arrangements for payment?

Where does the payment go? To the institution? To the investigator?

What is the payment per participant? Are there other arrangements? (HHS, 2000).

Under HHS's proposed regulations, an IRB should consider the specific mechanisms proposed "to minimize the potential adverse consequences of the conflict in an effort to optimally protect the interests of the research subjects" (HHS, 2000). An investigator with a conflict of interest should not be permitted to directly be engaged in parts of the study where the conflict of interest could have a detrimental effect on human participants, such as design of the trial, monitoring of the trial, obtaining the informed consent, adverse event reporting, or analyzing data (HHS, 2000).

An IRB should consider including funding arrangements for the study and for the IRB's review of the protocol in the consent document (HHS, 2000). This is particularly true whenever that information is material to the potential participant's decision-making process (HHS, 2000). If the financial conflict of interest has not or cannot be eliminated, the existence of the conflict and how it is being managed should be disclosed in the consent document (HHS, 2000).

In this era of fraud and abuse suspicion, an IRB must also be cognizant as to funding of research in the context of the Anti-Kickback Statute and Stark regulations (OIG, Advisory Opinion No. 02-11). Similar concerns may be raised as to gifts and other inducements to Medicare and Medicaid patients (see OIG, Special Advisory Bulletin, 2002).

The Association of American Medical Colleges has taken the issue a step further with proposed standards for dealing with conflicts of interest. Principal investigators, IRBs, and institutions are presumed to have conflicts of interest in human studies research when they have actual or potential significant financial interests in the project. This includes funding of the study, licensure of technology, or future income. While it is still possible to approve such endeavors under the AAMC approach, there are several factors that must be navigated before such a study can receive IRB approval. In practical terms, this may mean a significant change to present policies and procedures as well as definitions, such as conducting research and management of financial relationships (AAMC, 2002).

Clinical Trials Being Conducted at an Institution That Has a Financial Interest in the Product's Commercialization

HHS has suggested that an institution should avoid conducting clinical investigations of medical devices in which the institution has a financial interest in the success of the product. If the clinical investigation is carried out at the institution, then it should be conducted "with special safeguards to maximally protect the scientific integrity of the study and the research participants" (HHS, 2000). The institution is also advised to consider establishing an independent conflicts of interest committee to determine if conflicts do exist and, if so, how to manage those conflicts.

The Format of an IRB's Decision

An IRB (45 CFR §46.109(d); 21 CFR §56.109(e); ICH, *Guideline for Good Clinical Practice*, 3.1.2) should review a proposed clinical trial within a reasonable time and document its determinations in writing, clearly identifying the trial, the documents reviewed, reasons for the determination, and the dates for the following:

- Approval/favorable opinion.
- Modifications required prior to its approval/favorable opinion.
- Disapproval/negative opinion.
- Termination/suspension of any prior approval/favorable opinion.

The FDA has stated that it does not specify the procedure that IRBs must use regarding the signature of an IRB-approval letter. The written operating procedures for an IRB should outline the procedure that is followed (FDA, Information Sheets, 1998).

An IRB's Obligation to Review Ongoing Research

The ongoing review of research by an IRB is a very hot topic. OHRP and OIG have recently become quite vocal that this may be the weakest link in the protection of research participants. To the contrary, the FDA stated earlier that it does not expect IRBs to routinely observe consent interviews, observe the conduct of the study, or review study records even though FDA regulations (21 CFR §56.109(f)) give an IRB the authority to observe, or have a third party observe, the consent process and the research. When and if the IRB is concerned about the conduct of the study or the process for obtaining consent, the IRB may consider whether, as part of providing adequate oversight of the study, an active audit is warranted (FDA, Information Sheets, 1998).

Per the OHRP, *review* is defined as "the concurrent oversight of research on a periodic basis by an IRB" (OIG, *Institutional Review Board Guidebook,* Chap. III, sec. E). An IRB is obligated to perform at least annual reviews of research studies. Where appropriate, an IRB also must conduct continuous or periodic review (45 CFR §46.108(e)). However, the OIG has been very vocal that it believes IRBs are guilty of doing minimal substantive review of continuing research projects:

> The IRBs' limited efforts in conducting continuing review of active research is a serious national issue because it compromises their protection of human participants. It inhibits their capacity to identify and address situations where unacceptable risks emerge, or research results prove to be too favorable to continue, or protocols stray beyond approved limits. It also inhibits their capacity to ensure that the participants have sufficient understanding of the risks they may incur in the research process.
>
> [OIG, 1998].

"[T]heir reviews of the annual reports, adverse-event reports, and protocol amendments submitted by research sponsors are often hurried and superficial" (OIG, 1998). Almost all of an IRB's work is limited to paperwork reviews, complained the OIG: "They rarely visit the research site to determine how the consent process is actually working or to review the records of active protocols" (OIG, 1998). The OIG (1998) attributes this situation to:

- Heightened workload pressures.
- Limited useful feedback on multisite trials by DSMBs or clinical audit teams.
- Limited feedback on FDA actions against investigators.
- Limited IRB expertise.

- Limited nonscientific and noninstitutional input.
- The "Trust Factor."

Changes to a previously approved protocol that are minor do not require review by the IRB. However, the challenge is to determine what is minor and what is not. "Any change that would materially affect the assessment of risks and benefits should not be considered minor" (OPRR, *Institutional Review Board Guidebook*).

OHRP has stated that, "Under normal circumstances, it is neither necessary nor desirable for the IRB itself to undertake data monitoring" (OPRR, *Institutional Review Board Guidebook*). However, an independent person should be responsible for monitoring a clinical trial. "It is the IRB's responsibility to ensure that these functions are carried out by an appropriate group. The review group should be required to report its findings to the IRB on an appropriate schedule" (OPRR, *Institutional Review Board Guidebook*). "The IRB should not delegate the monitoring of the informed consent process to others" (OPRR, *Institutional Review Board Guidebook*).

OHRP has recently stated the following position on what should be considered during continued review:

> In conducting continuing review of research not eligible for expedited review, all IRB members should at least receive and review a protocol summary and a status report on the progress of the research, including:
>
> - The number of subjects accrued.
> - A summary of adverse events and any unanticipated problems involving risks to subjects or others and any withdrawal of subjects from the research or complaints about the research since the last IRB review.
> - A summary of any relevant recent literature, interim findings, and amendments or modifications to the research since the last review.
> - Any relevant multicenter trial reports.
> - Any other relevant information, especially information about risks associated with the research.
> - A copy of the current informed consent document and any newly proposed consent document.
>
> At least one member of the IRB (a primary reviewer) also should receive a copy of the complete protocol including any modifications previously approved by the IRB. Furthermore, upon request, any IRB member also should have access to the complete IRB protocol file and relevant IRB minutes prior to or during the convened IRB meeting.
>
> When reviewing the current informed consent documents, the IRB should ensure the following:
>
> - The currently approved or proposed consent document is still accurate and complete
> - Any significant new findings that may relate to the subject's willingness to continue participation are provided to the subject in accordance with HHS regulations at 45 CFR §46.116(b)(5).
> - Review of currently approved or newly proposed consent documents must occur during the scheduled continuing review of research by the IRB, but informed

consent documents should be reviewed whenever new information becomes available that would require modification of information in the informed consent document.

Furthermore, the minutes of IRB meetings should document separate deliberations, actions, and votes for each protocol undergoing continuing review by the convened IRB. [OHRP, 2002a; OHRP, 2002b]

The Frequency of Reviewing Approved Research by an IRB

An IRB is required to review approved research at intervals appropriate to the degree of risk but at least once annually (45 CFR §46.109(e) & 21 CFR §56.109(f)). The frequency of continuing review should be focused on ensuring the continued protection of research participants. To this end, the IRB should consider:

- Whether the risk/benefit ratio has shifted.
- Whether there are unanticipated findings involving risks to research participants.
- Whether any new information regarding the risks and benefits should be provided to the research participants.

Recent reports and position statements by federal agencies have argued for more frequent scrutiny. For example, see OIG's report on the IRB's role in reviewing approved research, [http://oig.hhs.gov/oei/summaries/b273.pdf]. Between reviews, the investigator is primarily responsible for keeping the IRB informed of significant findings. In larger studies, a DSMB may be responsible for keeping the IRB updated.

The Consequences if a Study Is Not Reviewed at Least Annually by an IRB

OHRP has taken the position that IRB approval for a study lapses if continuing review does not occur at least annually and the investigation must stop unless the IRB determines that it is in the best interests of the participants to continue the research activities. Enrollment of new participants after expiration of IRB approval is forbidden. Lapse of approval does not need to be reported to OHRP as a suspension (OHRP, 2002a).

Annual IRB Reviews When Studies Are Reviewed by an IRB Each Quarter

An IRB may decide to review all studies under its supervision on a quarterly basis. If every quarterly report contains sufficient information for an adequate continuing review and is reviewed by the IRB under procedures that meet the requirements for continuing review, an additional "annual" review is not mandated (FDA, Information Sheets, 1998).

Continuing IRB Review of a Project When Research Interventions Are Completed but Investigators Are Still Collecting Follow-Up Data

An IRB is obligated to continue reviewing a study even after the completion of interventions as long as investigators continue to collect follow-up data. "So long as data are being collected for an organized research project, the IRB must continue to review the status of the protocols and the details of the continuing data gathering activity. If the continuing research meets the requirements for expedited review, the expedited review process may be used, if desired by the IRB" (OHRP, *Institutional Review Board Guidebook*).

Reporting to an IRB When a Study Has Been Completed

An investigator must report to his IRB when a study is completed. An investigator is required to report to the IRB when a change in research activity occurs (21 CFR §56.108(a)(3)). The completion of a study is a change in activity and should be reported to the IRB. "Although subjects will no longer be 'at risk' under the study, a final report/notice to the IRB allows it to close its files as well as providing information that may be used by the IRB in the evaluation and approval of related studies" (FDA, Information Sheets, 1998).

The Role of Institution Officials When an IRB Does Not Approve a Research Proposal

If an IRB refuses to approve a research protocol, other officials at an institution are not allowed to override that decision. An IRB is the final arbiter of whether a research proposal should be approved for the reasons under the IRB's mandate. However, institutional officials may refuse to allow a research project to go forward for other reasons, even though the IRB has approved. For example, the officials may feel that the study would be too costly, that staffing would be too burdensome, or that the subject matter was inappropriate for the institution (45 CFR §46.112).

Notifiying an IRB That Another IRB Previously Denied Approval of the Study

An investigator is obligated to notify an IRB that another IRB has denied approval of his study. When an IRB disapproves a study, it must provide a written statement of the reasons for its decision to the investigator and the institution (21 CFR §56.109(e)). If the study is submitted to a second IRB, a copy of this written statement should be included with the study documentation so that the second IRB can make an informed decision about the study. An IRB would be well served to require that review decisions of similar protocols by other IRBs be submitted for consideration along with the other study documents. For example, FDA regulations require an IRB to ". . . review . . . all research activities [emphasis added] . . ." (21 CFR §56.109(a)).

FDA regulations do not prohibit submission of a study to another IRB following disapproval. However, all pertinent information about the study should be provided to the second IRB. (FDA, Information Sheets, 1998). The FDA is considering an amendment to its regulations explicitly requiring that IRBs be advised of what other IRBs have concluded in reviewing similar protocols (FDA 2002a).

Events to Occur if an IRB Suspends or Terminates Its Approval of a Clinical Study

An IRB is authorized by the Common Rule and FDA regulations to suspend or terminate its approval of a study that fails to comply with the IRB's directives or when a research participant suffers serious harm. An IRB should report its decision immediately to the investigator, the appropriate institutional officials, and OHRP (or other federal agency with oversight of the study such as the FDA) (21 CFR §56.113). The IRB's written decision must include a statement of the reasons for the IRB's decision (45 CFR §46.113). A federal agency may not continue funding a project from which IRB approval has been withdrawn (45 CFR §46.122).

Direct Communication Between Sponsors and IRBs

Sponsors and IRBs are permitted to directly communicate. It is important that a formal line of communication be established between the clinical investigator and the IRB. Clinical investigators should report adverse events directly to the responsible IRB and should send progress reports directly to that IRB. The investigator often acts as the conduit between the sponsor and an IRB. However, the FDA does not prohibit direct communication between the sponsor and the IRB, and recognizes that direct communication could result in more efficient resolution of some problems. The investigator should be kept abreast of such discussions.

The FDA requires direct communication between a sponsor and the IRB for certain studies of medical devices and when the informed consent waiver has been invoked. A sponsor and the IRB are required to communicate directly for medical device studies under 21 CFR §812.2, §812.66 and §812.150(b). For informed consent waiver studies, direct communication between a sponsor and the IRB is mandated under 21 CFR §50.24(e), §56.109(e), §56.109(g), §312.54(b), §312.130(d), §812.38(b)(4), and §812.47(b) (FDA, Information Sheets, 1998).

A Sponsor's Responsibility for IRB Actions

FDA regulations (21 CFR §312.23(a)(1)(iv)) require that a sponsor assure the FDA that a study will be conducted in compliance with the informed consent and IRB regulations (21 CFR parts 50 and 56). However, it is not a sponsor's obligation to determine IRB compliance with the regulations. Sponsors should rely on the clinical investigator, who assures the sponsor on Form FDA-1572 for drugs and biologics or the investigator agreement for devices that the study will be reviewed by an IRB. Because clinical investigators work directly with IRBs, it is appropriate that they assure the sponsor that the IRB is functioning in compliance with the regulations.

Conversely, a sponsor should be vigilante for any indications that an IRB is not functioning appropriately. The FDA may disallow the use of data generated from a study where adequate IRB oversight did not occur (21 CFR §56.121(d)).

Promising Approaches for IRBs

A committee of the Institute of Medicine recently recommended sweeping changes to the current IRB system in its report, "Responsible Research: A Systems Approach to Protecting Research Participants" (2002). One of the major recommendations was to delegate the broad duties of the IRB to at least two other entities that would address (1) scientific validity of the research; and (2) potential conflicts of interest. The IRB's remaining responsibility would be to address the ethics of the proposed research. To this end, the IRB would be renamed the Ethics Review Board (ERB). An independent body would conduct data and safety monitoring. The OIG has published a collection of innovative practices in its report *Institutional Review Boards: Promising Approaches* (OEI-01-97-00191).

....
DECISION-MAKING BY AN IRB

The Basic Obligations of an IRB Before Approving Research

An IRB must consider the following in reviewing and approving research protocols (OPRR, *Institutional Review Board Guidebook*):

- Risk/benefit analysis
- Informed consent
- Selection of participants
- Privacy and confidentiality
- Monitoring and observation
- Additional safeguards
- Incentives for participation
- Continuing review

An IRB must determine that the risks to human participants are minimized, the risks to the participants are reasonable in relation to anticipated benefits, selection of participants is equitable, informed consent has been obtained and documented, data will be monitored to ensure that the participant's safety and privacy are respected, and other human rights of the participants are protected (21 CFR §56.111).

Maintaining quality standards is also a function of the IRB. "Insistence upon well-conceived and well-conducted research should be evident both in written polices and in actions of institutional officials. Research that is conducted so poorly as to be invalid exposes participants and the institution to unnecessary risk. Approval procedures should be devised such that the institution supports only well-designed and properly executed research" (OPRR, *Institutional Review Board Guidebook*).

The Criteria for IRB Approval of Research

The Common Rule sets forth the criteria that an IRB must use in determining whether a research proposal should be approved. All of the following requirements must be satisfied:

(a) In order to approve research covered by this policy the IRB shall determine that all of the following requirements are satisfied:

(1) Risks to subjects are minimized: (i) by using procedures which are consistent with sound research design and which do not unnecessarily expose subjects to risk, and (ii) whenever appropriate, by using procedures already being performed on the subjects for diagnostic or treatment purposes.

(2) Risks to subjects are reasonable in relation to anticipated benefits, if any, to subjects, and the importance of the knowledge that may reasonably be expected to result. In evaluating risks and benefits, the IRB should consider only those risks and benefits that may result from the research (as distinguished from risks and benefits of therapies subjects would receive even if not participating in the research). The IRB should not consider possible long-range effects of applying knowledge gained in the research (for example, the possible effects of the research on public policy) as among those research risks that fall within the purview of its responsibility.

(3) Selection of subjects is equitable. In making this assessment the IRB should take into account the purposes of the research and the setting in which the research will be conducted and should be particularly cognizant of the special problems of research involving vulnerable populations, such as children, prisoners, pregnant women, mentally disable persons, or economically or educationally disadvantaged persons.

(4) Informed consent will be sought from each prospective subject or the subject's legally authorized representative, in accordance with, and to the extent required by §46.116.

(5) Informed consent will be appropriately documented, in accordance with, and to the extent required by §46.117.

(6) When appropriate, the research plan makes adequate provision for monitoring the data collected to ensure the safety of subjects.

(7) When appropriate, there are adequate provisions to protect the privacy of subjects and to maintain the confidentiality of data.

(b) When some or all of the subjects are likely to be vulnerable to coercion or undue influence, such as children, prisoners, pregnant women, mentally disabled persons, or economically or educationally disadvantaged persons, additional safeguards have been included in the study to protect the rights and welfare of these subjects.

[45 CFR §46.111]

The Risk/Benefit Analysis

The IRB must determine whether an anticipated benefit, such as new knowledge or improved health of a participant, justifies asking a person to undertake the risks of a study. The IRB must:

1. Identify the risks associated with the research, as distinguished from the risks of therapies the participants would receive even if not participating.
2. Determine that the risks will be minimized to the extent possible.
3. Identify the probable benefits to be derived from the research.
4. Determine that the risks are reasonable in relation to be benefits to participants, if any, and the importance of the knowledge to be gained.
5. Assure that potential participants will be provided with an accurate and fair description of the risks or discomforts and the anticipated benefits (informed consent).
6. Determine intervals of periodic review, and, where appropriate, determine that adequate provisions are in place for monitoring the data collected.

Defining Benefit

Benefit is defined as a valued or desired outcome; an advantage. A benefit may be to the individual human participant, to others similarly situated as the human participant, or to society as a whole.

Assessing Anticipated Benefits

An IRB should distinguish between benefits to the research participant and benefits to society. Research that has no immediate therapeutic benefit to the participant may benefit society in general by increasing our understanding of a disease, improve safety, advance technology, or improve public health.

Incentives or rewards in the form of cash or other remuneration should not be considered a benefit. Personal satisfaction from participating in a personally rewarding activity or humanitarian effort should not be part of the IRB's assessment of anticipated benefits. The IRB should carefully identify what benefits are anticipated (OPRR, *Institutional Review Board Guidebook*).

Defining Risk

Risk is the probability of harm or injury (physical, psychological, social, or economic) occurring as a result of participation in a research study. Both the probability and magnitude of possible harm may vary from minimal to significant. Only *Minimal Risk* is used in the Common Rule.

Risk, in an IRB's consideration, should be that which is a result of the research and not that routinely associated with therapy that a participant would undergo even if not in a clinical trial. For example, a protocol's risk may be minimal even though a patient routinely has significant risk associated with a therapy. However, an IRB needs to be vigilant in identifying what is research and what is therapy.

Potential risk faced by a research participant may be due to design features of the protocol. For example, a participant in a randomly assigned treatment group may suffer from a less efficacious treatment than another. Risk may also involve the potential for violation of privacy and confidentiality.

A risk less often considered is the potential application of knowledge obtained from a study. For example, would research on the effect of subliminal messages have a long-range impact on society? However, federal regulations specifically articulate that an IRB is not to consider this risk "as among those risks that fall within the purview of its responsibilities" (45 CFR §46.111(a)(2)).

Consideration of Potential Harms When Looking at Risk

Research participants may be exposed to the following risks:

- Physical Harms: An IRB should consider a human participant's exposure to minor pain, discomfort, or injury from invasive medical procedures, or possible harmful side effects of drugs. Some adverse events can be permanent, even though most are transient.

- Psychological Harms: An IRB should consider whether participation in a research protocol might result in undesired changes in thought processes and emotion (depression, hallucination, stress, or other psychological problems). These adverse states may be temporary, recurrent, or permanent. Psychological harm (stress or feelings of guilt) may occur where the research participant is given false feedback about his own performance. An IRB should also consider the effect of any invasion of the research participant's privacy or a breach of confidentiality.

- Social and Economic Harm: Invasion of privacy or breach of confidentiality in some research protocols may cause embarrassment, loss of employment, or criminal prosecution. A research participant may be "labeled" or "stigmatized." Safeguards to protect the research participant's privacy and confidentiality should be vigorously reviewed by an IRB. Plans for follow-up contact should carefully be considered.

Defining *Minimal Risk*

Minimal Risk is where the probability and magnitude of harm or discomfort anticipated in the proposed research are not greater, in and of themselves, than those ordinarily encountered in daily life or during the performance of routine physical or psychological examinations or tests (45 CFR §46.102(i)). The definition for minimal risk involving prisoners is more restrictive (45 CFR §303(d)).

Determination of whether the risks are minimal in a research protocol is very important. For example, if an IRB determines that minimal risk exists, then an IRB may be allowed to perform an expedited review (45 CFR §46.110 and 21 CFR §56.110) or waiver or modification of informed consent requirements may be permitted (45 CFR §46.116(d)). These variations in routine IRB approval and monitoring are discussed in more detail elsewhere in this book.

If a research protocol presents more than minimal risk, the potential research participants must be informed of the availability of medical treatment and compensation for protocol-related injury, including who will pay for the treatment (45 CFR §46.116(a)(6); 21 CFR §50.25(a)(6)). (An institution is not required to provide medical treatment or compensation, but many do.)

Minimal risk must also be considered in the context of the research population. For example, geriatric men may have a higher potential for injury from an investigational drug than young men.

IRB Determination That the Risks to Participants Are Minimized

An IRB is responsible for ensuring that risks are minimized to the extent possible. This requires careful scrutiny of precautions, safeguards, and alternatives that can be incorporated into a research protocol. An IRB needs to consider:

- The underlying scientific basis (including previous animal and human studies).
- The anticipated beneficial and harmful effects.
- The potential harmful effects can be adequately detected, prevented, or treated.
- The risks and complications of any underlying disease that may be present.
- Whether the investigator is competent to conduct the study.
- Whether the investigator serves dual roles (treating physician, teacher, counselor in addition to researcher).
- What useful data will be obtained from the study design (sufficient sample size; well-articulated hypothesis).
- If adequate safeguards are incorporated into the research design, such as frequent monitoring, sufficient personnel who can respond to emergencies, adequate treatment facilities, or proper coding of data to protect confidentiality. Data monitoring is important to ensure that a study does not continue after reliable data has been obtained.
- A mechanism for another professional to break the code of a masked study so that a patient suffering medical problems can be properly treated.
- Obtaining data from diagnostic or treatment situations in lieu of using risky procedures, such as spinal tap or cardiac catheterization.
- Where deception or incomplete disclosure occurs and psychological stress, guilt, or embarrassment may occur, the research participant is adequately debriefed.

IRB Determination That the Risks to the Participants Are Reasonable in Relation to Anticipated Benefits

This is the major ethical judgment made by an IRB in reviewing research proposals. It is often a determination based on local community standards and subjective assessments of risk and benefit. Consequently, different IRBs may reach differing conclusions as to the risk/benefit ratio.

The risk/benefit ratio should be analyzed in light of whether the research (1) involves the use of interventions that have the intent and high likelihood of providing benefit to the research participant; or (2) only involves procedures performed for research purposes. The amount of risk can be justified at a higher level where the research participant is likely to benefit from the intervention. However, the risk/benefit ratio in a new or not-yet-validated treatment evaluation should be similar to that of available therapy (OPRR, *Institutional Review Board Guidebook*).

Where the study will have no anticipated benefit to the research participant, an IRB must weigh whether the risks are ethically acceptable. "There should be a limit to the risks society (through the government and research institutions) asks individuals to accept for the benefit of others, but IRBs should not be overprotective. While the IRB must consider the importance of the knowledge that may result from the research, the IRB's appreciation of that importance may, at times, be limited. If only minimal risks are involved IRBs do not need to protect competent adult participants from participating in research considered unlikely to yield any benefit" (OPRR, *Institutional Review Board Guidebook*).

IRB Consideration of Additional Safeguards

Where "some or all of the participants are likely to be vulnerable to coercion or undue influence," federal regulations 45 CFR §46.111(b), require that additional safeguards be used to protect the participants' rights and welfare. A participant's vulnerability may be subtle, and the IRB should be attentive in ensuring that due consideration is given to this in a proposed research protocol. Examples of vulnerable populations include children, prisoners, pregnant women, mentally ill or disabled people, employees, students, and people who are economically or educationally disadvantaged. A research protocol must minimize the possibility of coercion or undue influence to give consent. OHRP (Institutional Review Board Guidebook) suggests that an IRB consider the following points with regard to safeguards for vulnerable populations:

1. Are recruitment procedures designed to ensure that informed consent is freely given?

2. What special safeguards are included to protect the rights and welfare of participants who are likely to be vulnerable to coercion or undue influence (children, prisoners, pregnant women, persons with physical or mental illness, and persons who are economically or educationally disadvantaged)?

3. Does the nature of the disease or behavioral issue to be studied permit free consent?

4. Are any incentives offered for participation likely to unduly influence a prospective participant's (or surrogate's) decision to participate?

5. Is there an adequate procedure for monitoring the consent process, and should the IRB or its representative observe the process?

IRB Determination That Selection of Participants Is Equitable

The topic of participant recruitment and selection is discussed in Chapter Four.

IRB Consideration As to Incentives for Participation

While federal regulations do not specifically address how an IRB should weigh incentives for participation of research participants, an IRB must ensure that a participant's consent is truly voluntary and that it was obtained under conditions that minimized coercion or undue influence (45 CFR §46.116; 21 CFR §50.20). An IRB should consider who the participants will be, what incentives will be offered, and the conditions under which consent will be sought.

In looking at the appropriateness of incentives, an IRB must become familiar with the accepted rates in the community and the complexity, discomforts, and inconveniences of the particular protocol. Payments may be based on time incurred, per tissue or fluid sample collected, additional inconveniences, and other factors.

A very difficult decision by an IRB is at what amount of money or type of reward undue influence occurs. This can be effected by the pool of volunteers from which recruiting will occur. IRB members may split as to the level of personal autonomy that can be exercised by a potential volunteer.

IRB Determination That Informed Consent Has Been Obtained and Documented

IRBs are entrusted with ensuring that informed consent is adequate (45 CFR §46.103). The topic of informed consent is discussed at length in Chapter Five. By way of illustration, the OPRR (1993) offered the following guidelines for IRBs specific to genetic research. These guidelines suggest that patients should be informed about specific issues, including:

1. Confidentiality Assurances that are in place.
2. Unreimbursed costs, including for counseling.
3. The possibility of disclosure of information to the donor and the donor's relatives.
4. The consequences of withdrawing from the study.

Review of a Standard Cooperative Research Protocol or a Standard Informed Consent Document by a Local IRB

The local IRB must review even a standard cooperative research protocol or a standard informed consent document. While a cooperative research protocol or an informed consent document may be standard, the research setting is not always standard across the nation or even across an institution. The IRB also needs to be cognizant that a standard protocol or informed consent document may not conform to state law, local regulations, or institutional policies and procedures. (See 45 CFR §46.103(d), §46.107(a), and §46.111(a)(3)).

IRB Procedure When an Exception to Informed Consent Is Sought for Emergency Research

The FDA (2000) has given the following guidance for IRBs in the situation where an exception to informed consent is sought for emergency research:

> The IRB must have the concurrence of a licensed physician, both initially and at the time of continuing review, that the criteria of 21 CFR §50.24 are met. The licensed physician must be 'a member of or consultant to the IRB and . . . not otherwise participating in the clinical investigation' [21 CFR §50.24(a)]. A licensed physician

consultant would be necessary in cases where the licensed physician member(s) cannot participate in the deliberation and voting due to conflict(s) of interest. Because the documented concurrence of the licensed physician member or licensed physician consultant is required for the IRB to allow these studies to proceed, IRBs should ensure that meeting minutes specifically record the licensed physician member's affirmative vote or the licensed physician consultant's concurrence.

In contrast, Common Rule regulations permit waiver of informed consent requirements only in the case of research that has no more than minimal risk (45 CFR §46.116). If emergency use of a test article occurs without informed consent, the patient cannot be considered a research participant and no data derived from the emergency use of the test article can be used in the study (OPRR, *Institutional Review Board Guidebook*).

IRB Waiver of Informed Consent

When a researcher seeks to have the requirement of informed consent waived, IRB members must be alert to the distinction between the Common Rule and FDA regulations allowing such a waiver. HHS allows the IRB to waive informed consent where the research "poses minimal risk" (45 CFR §46.116(d)). The FDA exception is at the other end of the spectrum: where the therapy is for a life-threatening condition, no alternative exists, and the patient or his representative is not able to consent in a timely manner (21 CFR §50.23(a), 21 CFR §50.24). A third consideration is state law. Informed consent, and whether it can be waived, is almost always a matter of state statute, regulation, or common law.

IRB Consideration During Its Prestudy Review with Regard to Monitoring and Observation

Proposed research should be reviewed for the researcher's plan to collect, store, and analyze data. Monitoring is important because preliminary data may alert the researcher, sponsor, and IRB to the need for change in the research design, information given to subjects, or even to terminate the project. *Monitoring* is defined as "the collection and analysis of data as the project progresses to assure the appropriateness of the research, its design, and subject protections" (OPRR, *Institutional Review Board Guidebook*). Federal regulations (45 CFR §46.111(a)(6)) require that, where appropriate, the researcher's monitoring plan must be included in the proposed protocol for the IRB's approval. The level of monitoring should be directly related to the degree of risk in the study. An IRB should be assured that, as a study progresses, adequate monitoring will occur to determine that information generated will:

- Be conveyed to the research participants.
- Affect recruitment of participants.
- Change the risk/benefit ratio.
- Lead to modification or discontinuation of the protocol.

OHRP (*Institutional Review Board Guidebook*) has suggested the following points for an IRB to consider with respect to reviewing a protocol for adequate monitoring:

1. How will the research data be recorded and maintained?
2. Considering the degree of risk, is the plan for monitoring the research adequate in terms of timeliness and thoroughness?

3. If the principal investigator is other than full-time on the project, is the oversight and monitoring time sufficient?

4. Is there a mechanism for providing information to the IRB in the event that unexpected results are discovered? (Unexpected results may raise the possibility of unanticipated risks to participants.)

5. Does the institution have a data and safety monitoring board? If so, should it be asked to monitor the project under review? If the institution does not have a data and safety monitoring board, should the IRB request or recommend that one be appointed, either by the institution or the sponsor, for this project?

IRB Determination That Data Will Be Monitored to Ensure the Participant's Safety

A well-developed research protocol should include constant monitoring, evaluation, and evolving methodology that is responsive to the data gathered as the study progresses. The OIG has expressed frustration that most IRBs view continuing review as a low priority. "IRBs know little of what actually occurs during the consent and research processes (OIG, 2000). The OIG has highlighted the requirement that "call for IRBs to conduct full, annual reviews of approved protocols and that call for complete reviews of Federal funding applications prior to funding decisions" (OIG, 2000).

The OIG has recommended that IRBs "move beyond their focus on the informed consent document and periodically check for themselves how the actual consent process is working" (OIG, 2000). This sentiment has been echoed by the Chairman of the President's National Bioethics Advisory Commission: "One problem we have heard again and again is that, once an experiment is approved, there is a failure to follow what's going on with the patients. I think there is a growing consensus that something must be done" (Hilts, 2000). The topic of participant safety is discussed at length in Chapter Ten.

IRB Reliance on DSMB Reports

In many multisite trials and other major studies, a Data and Safety Monitoring Board (DSMB) will often be used to review adverse events, interim findings, and relevant literature. Often the DSMB is in a better position than a local IRB to spot trends and emerging issues because the DSMB is drawing its information from broader sources. OHRP has stated that an IRB can rely on current statements from the DSMB or the sponsor as to the state of adverse events, interim findings, and recent literature. The local IRB does not have to review the raw data. However, the local IRB is still responsible for reviewing adverse events or unanticipated problems that occur within its jurisdiction. The IRB may request additional information from the sponsor, DSMB, or investigator as necessary to conduct a "substantive and meaningful" review (OHRP, 2002a).

IRB's Role in Protecting a Participant's Privacy

Personal privacy has become a very important issue in society. Human research depends on access to personal data. Yet, the research participant has a right of privacy. Balancing this interest is increasingly falling to the IRB.

Private information is defined as "information about behavior that occurs in a context in which an individual can reasonably expect that no observation or recording is taking place, and information which has been provided for specific purposes by an individual and which the individual can reasonably expect will not be made public (a medical record)" (45 CFR §46.102(f)).

OPRR gave the following guidance:

> Privacy can be defined in terms of having control over the extent, timing, and circumstances of sharing oneself (physically, behaviorally, or intellectually) with others. Confidentiality pertains to the treatment of information that an individual has disclosed in a relationship of trust and with the expectation that it will not be divulged to others in ways that are inconsistent with the understanding of the original disclosure without permission. [OPRR Guidebook, 1993]

The IRB's role of protecting a participant's privacy under HIPAA is discussed extensively in Chapter Six.

Expedited Review

Expedited review is a procedure through which certain kinds of research may be reviewed and approved without convening a meeting of the full IRB. The OHRP and the FDA agency's IRB regulations permit, but do not require, an IRB to review certain categories of research through an expedited procedure if the research involves no more than minimal risk (45 CFR §110 and 21 CFR §56.110). A list of minimal risk categories was last published in the *Federal Register* on November 9, 1998 (63 FR 60364-60367).

The IRB may also use the expedited review procedure to review minor changes in previously approved research during the period covered by the original approval. Under an expedited review procedure, review of research may be carried out by the IRB chairperson or by one or more experienced members of the IRB designated by the chairperson. The reviewer(s) may exercise all the authorities of the IRB, *except* disapproval. Research may only be disapproved following review by the full committee. An IRB is required to adopt a method of keeping all members advised of research studies that have been approved by expedited review.

Expedited review procedures may be used for continuing review of a study if it continues to meet the criteria for expedited review. This usually falls under the category of minimal risk. OHPR has added in a recent statement that expedited review may be used when a study may be ongoing at other sites but has closed to new human research, interventions have ceased within the IRB's jurisdiction, and the remainder of the study is long-term follow-up of participants and data analysis (OHPR, 2002a).

Conditional Approval of a Study

IRBs, in an effort to be efficient, have fallen into the custom of giving conditional approval of research protocols where an issue is outstanding. OHRP has taken the position that IRB approval should be deferred if substantive clarifications or modifications of a protocol or informed consent documents are requested by the IRB. Where only simple matters that merely require the investigator's concurrence may be stated specifically by the IRB, subsequent approval under an expedited review procedure may be appropriate (OHRP, 2002b).

Proposed Changes to IRB Review

The NIH's Regulatory Burden Advisory Group has recommended that a change be made to the requirement that IRBs review all protocols before funding decisions are made.

OPRR and the National Cancer Institute are developing a pilot project that establishes a central IRB for certain trials that would take on the review functions previously carried out by separate IRBs and streamline the process (OIG, 2000).

· · · · · · · · · · · ·

WORKLOAD

An IRB's institution must provide sufficient meeting space, support staff, and other resources for an IRB to function effectively (45 CFR §46.103(b)(2)). The OIG has pointed out that this includes not only staff and board members but also space, computers, and other essential elements. The OIG has called on OPRR (now OHRP) to hold institutions accountable for their representations of resource commitment in Assurances. The OIG has also called on the FDA to modify its site visit protocol so that it could more readily identify situations where resource shortages jeopardize IRB oversight of research. While the OIG lauded OPRR's enforcement efforts that have heightened awareness of the need for IRB resources, the OIG complained that no "indicators of adequate resource levels or to enable greater investments to support IRB functions" have been forthcoming. The NIH is considering giving an additional increment of grant funds to institutions to provide necessary resources for IRBs (OIG, 2000). However, the OIG has warned that "IRBs alone can not do the job and that in various subtle ways IRBs are expected to carry too much of the burden. We ought not to allow the reform agenda to focus strictly on what can be done to buttress IRBs" (OIG, 2000). The OIG also has expressed frustration at the heavy workloads of IRBs (OIG, 2000).

· · · · · · · · · · · ·

RECORD KEEPING

Records That an IRB Must Keep

An IRB must keep research proposals, evaluations, statements of significant new findings provided to participants (as provided by 45 CFR §46.116(b)(5)), progress reports, minutes of IRB meetings, records of continuing review of activities, correspondence, a list of board members, board policies and procedures, and other records (45 CFR §46.115; 21 CFR §56.115).

Information That Must Be Maintained by the IRB in Its Records About IRB Members

An IRB must maintain the following information about its members (45 CFR §46.103(b) (3) and 45 CFR §46.115(a)(5)):

- Name
- Earned degrees
- Representative capacity
- Indications of experience (such as board certifications and licenses) sufficient to describe each member's chief anticipated contributions to IRB deliberations
- Any employment or other relationship between the member and the institution (such as full-time employee, stockholder, unpaid consultant, or board member)

This information is usually submitted to OHRP as part of the Assurance process. Any changes in IRB membership must be reported to OHRP (45 CFR §46.103(b)(3) and 45 CFR §46.115(a)(5)).

IRB Minutes

IRB minutes must have sufficient detail to reflect (45 CFR §46.115(a)(2)):

- Attendance at each meeting
- Actions taken by the IRB
- The vote on actions taken (including the number of members voting for, against, and abstaining)
- The basis for requiring changes in or disapproving research
- A written summary of the discussion of controverted issues and their resolution

Retention of IRB Records

All of the records described should be kept for at least three years pursuant to federal regulations (45 CFR §46.115(b); 21 CFR §56.115). Records pertaining to research that is conducted must be retained for three years after completion of the research. Facilities may wish to retain records longer. All records must be accessible for inspection and copying by federal representatives at reasonable times and in a reasonable manner (45 CFR §46.115(b)).

The "Research Proposal Reviewed" Is the Same as the Formal Study Protocol That the Investigator Receives from the Sponsor of the Research

The IRB should receive and review all research activities (21 CFR §56.109(a)). The documents reviewed should include the complete documents received from the clinical investigator, such as the protocol, the investigator's brochure, a sample consent document, and any advertising intended to be seen or heard by prospective study participants. Some IRBs also require the investigator to submit an institutionally developed protocol summary form. A copy of all documentation reviewed is to be maintained for at least three years after completion of the research at that institution (21 CFR §56.115(b)). However, when the IRB makes changes, such as in the wording of the informed consent document, only the finally approved copy needs to be retained in the IRB records (FDA, Information Sheets, 1998).

IRB Records for Studies That Are Approved but Never Started

When an IRB approves a study, continuing review should be performed at least annually. All of the records listed in 21 CFR §56.115(a)(1)-(4) are required to be maintained. The clock starts on the date of approval, whether or not participants have been enrolled. Written progress reports should be received from the clinical investigator for all studies that are in approved status prior to the date of expiration of IRB approval. If participants were never enrolled, the clinical investigator's progress report would be brief. Such studies may receive continuing IRB review using expedited procedures. If the study is finally canceled without participant enrollment, records should be maintained for at least three years after cancellation (FDA, Information Sheets, 1998).

Sponsor Access to IRB Written Procedures, Minutes, and Membership Rosters

FDA regulations do not require public or sponsor access to IRB records. However, the FDA does not prohibit the sponsor from requesting IRB records. The IRB and the institution may establish a policy on whether minutes or a pertinent portion of the minutes are provided to sponsors. Because of variability, each IRB also needs to be aware of state and local laws regarding access to IRB records (FDA, Information Sheets, 1998). The confidentiality of the peer-review privilege may apply.

Mandatory Reports to OHRP

An institution must report to OHRP whatever information it has agreed to report in its Assurance. At a minimum, this would be (45 CFR §46.103(b)(5)(ii) and §46.113):

- IRB membership changes
- Serious or continuing non-compliance (45 CFR §46.103(b)(5)(i))
- Any unanticipated problems involving risks to participants or others (45 CFR §46.103(b)(5)(i))
- Any suspension or termination of IRB approval of a project

....

QUALITY ASSURANCE

The topic of quality assurance and compliance are discussed in detail in Chapters Fifteen and Sixteen. Issues peculiar to IRBs are discussed below.

Common Examples of IRB Non-Compliance

IRB non-compliance occurs when it fails to fulfill its duties imposed by federal regulations: "A demonstrated inability to carry out IRB responsibilities in accordance with DHHS regulations can be cause for the suspension or withdrawal of an institution's Assurance" (OPRR, *Institutional Review Board Guidebook*) identified the following as common problems:

- Inadequate review of research protocols by failing to ensure that the consent document and process provide sufficient information to allow prospective participants to make an informed decision.
- Failing to ensure that the research design included adequate monitoring of the data and any additional safeguards necessary to protect the welfare of particularly vulnerable participants.
- Failing to conduct continuing review of research at intervals appropriate to the degree of risk.
- Failing to maintain adequate records of IRB business.
- Failing to hold IRB meetings with a majority of members present, including a non-scientific member.

The FDA has issued Warning Letters to several IRBs for the following, among other, deficiencies:

- Failing to have adequate written procedures as required by 21 CFR §56.108, in:
  - Conducting initial and continuing review of studies.
  - Performing expedited review according to 21 CFR §56.110.
  - Determining which projects require review more often then annually.
  - Ensuring prompt reporting to the IRB of changes in research protocols.
  - Ensuring that changes in approved research are not initiated prior to IRB approval.
  - Ensuring prompt reporting to the IRB and FDA of unanticipated adverse events.
  - Ensuring that investigator non-compliance is addressed.
  - Suspending or terminating research.
  - Requiring that a majority of members are present at convened meetings and that at least one member has nonscientific interests.
  - Ensuring that a majority of members approve a research proposal.
- Failing to follow written procedures as required by 21 CFR §56.108, §56.109, and §50.25.
- Failing to implement expedited review procedures in accordance with 21 CFR §56.110(b) and (c).
- Failing to ensure adequate initial and continuing review of research as required by 21 CFR §56.108, §56.109, and §56.111.
- Failing to maintain adequate records of IRB activities and operations as required by 21 CFR §56.115.
- Failing to ensure compliance with informed consent requirements as required by 21 CFR §56.109 and §50.25.
- Failing to meet IRB membership requirements as set forth in 21 CFR §56.107.
- Failing to provide written notification of IRB decisions and perform continuing review at the required frequency as required by 21 CFR §56.109(e) and (f).

Common Non-Compliance Problems for Institutions

In addition to being responsible for the actions of individual investigators and the IRB, an institution can be in non-compliance by failing to implement practices and procedures contained in the institution's Assurance. For example, if the IRB is not properly constituted or does not function in accordance with regulations; the IRB does not receive appropriate institutional support and staffing; or investigators do not meet their obligations to the IRB. "While recognizing both individual and institutional responsibility for compliance with the regulations, OPRR [now OHRP] generally negotiates Assurances only with institutions, which are ultimately responsible for ensuring that the regulatory requirements are met. Investigators and IRBs, however, also retain responsibility for complying with the regulations" (OPRR, *Institutional Review Board Guidebook*).

IRB Response to Non-Compliance in a Protocol

An IRB is required to take immediate and effective steps to ensure compliance when the IRB discovers that research is being conducted outside of the approved protocol. The IRB must report non-compliance to any federal agency that is funding the research and take appropriate follow-up measures (OPRR, *Institutional Review Board Guidebook*). The FDA requires that the IRB itself notify FDA of instances of non-compliance if such reporting would not otherwise occur (FDA, 1991).

IRB Reporting of Each Instance of Non-Compliance with Federal Regulations to OHRP

An IRB does not necessarily need to report each instance of non-compliance to OHRP (OPRR, *Institutional Review Board Guidebook*). An institution must have written procedures that ensure that instances of serious or continuing non-compliance will be reported to the IRB, appropriate institutional officials, and the head of the federal department or agency supporting the research (45 CFR §46.103(b)(5)). "The IRB is only responsible for doing the reporting if it is required to do so under the institution's written procedures [NOTE: FDA requires that the IRB report to FDA if such reporting would not otherwise occur (*Federal Register* 56 (June 18, 1991): 28026).]" (OPRR, *Institutional Review Board Guidebook*).

The Current Effectiveness of IRBs

The OIG has frequently voiced its concern that IRBs are functioning at a subpar level. The OIG (2000) has identified the following factors that put the effectiveness of IRBs in jeopardy:

- They face major changes in the research environment
- They review too much, too quickly, with too little expertise
- They conduct minimal continuing review of approved research
- They face conflicts that threaten their independence
- They provide little training for investigators and board members
- Neither IRBs nor the HHS devote much attention to evaluating IRB effectiveness

OHRP has found many problems in the functioning of IRBs [http://ohrp.osophs.dhhs.gov/references/findings.pdf].

Self-Evaluation of the IRB

An IRB needs to continually evaluate itself. The major weaknesses often found include

- Sloppy record keeping
- Shortage of review staff
- Lack of oversight and ongoing monitoring for research projects
- Insufficient procedures for informing patients about and obtaining consent
- Questionable safety and ethics standards

Examples of these problems found by OPRR include well-publicized actions against West Los Angeles VA Healthcare Center, Duke University, University of Pennsylvania, University of Oklahoma, and many other institutions.

The OIG has complained that it was "struck by how little attention federal oversight bodies and IRBs themselves gave to evaluating how successful IRBs were in protecting human subjects. It is time, we concluded, for the federal government to mandate self-evaluations or, better yet, evaluations conducted by independent, outside parties. We also urged that the results of such evaluations be made public" (OIG, 2000).

FDA's Self-Evaluation Tool

The FDA has proposed the following self-evaluation tool checklist;

> Three "response" columns are provided—"Yes," "No," and "N/A." A "Yes" means that the institution has a written policy/procedure and that it is current. A "No" may mean that a policy/procedure is lacking or needs to be updated. The "N/A" column indicates that a topic is not applicable or a procedure is not needed by the IRB.
>
> The columns may be completed by checking the appropriate box. Instead of a check mark, some IRBs record the date of issuance or revision date. Others have found it useful to record the policy/procedure number on the form. Any "No" responses indicate a need to write/revise policies and/or procedures.
>
> Footnoted items are referenced in the FDA regulations. Asterisked items are those for which written procedures are specifically required by the FDA regulations.

FDA Self-Evaluation Tool for IRBs

YES	NO	N/A		DOES THE INSTITUTION HAVE WRITTEN POLICIES OR PROCEDURES THAT DESCRIBE:
____	____	____	I.	THE INSTITUTIONAL AUTHORITY UNDER WHICH THE IRB IS ESTABLISHED AND EMPOWERED.¾
____	____	____	II.	THE DEFINITION OF THE PURPOSE OF THE IRB, i.e., THE PROTECTION OF HUMAN SUBJECTS OF RESEARCH.
____	____	____	III	THE PRINCIPLES WHICH GOVERN THE IRB IN ASSURING THAT THE RIGHTS AND WELFARE OF SUBJECTS ARE PROTECTED.
			IV.	THE AUTHORITY OF THE IRB.
____	____	____		A. The scope of authority is defined, i.e., what types of studies must be reviewed.
____	____	____		B. Authority to disapprove, modify or approve studies based upon consideration of human subject protection aspects.[4]
____	____	____		* C. Authority to require progress reports from the investigators and oversee the conduct of the study.[5]
____	____	____		* D. Authority to suspend or terminate approval of a study.[6]
____	____	____		* E. Authority to place restrictions on a study.[7]
			V.	THE IRB'S RELATIONSHIP TO
____	____	____		A. The top administration of the institution.
____	____	____		B. The other committees and department chairpersons within the institution.
____	____	____		C. The research investigators.
____	____	____		D. Other institutions.
____	____	____		E. Regulatory agencies.
			VI.	THE MEMBERSHIP OF THE IRB.
____	____	____		A. Number of members.[8]
____	____	____		B. Qualification of members.[9]

(Continued)

FDA Self-Evaluation Tool for IRBs (Continued)

YES	NO	N/A	DOES THE INSTITUTION HAVE WRITTEN POLICIES OR PROCEDURES THAT DESCRIBE:
			C. Diversity of members[10] (for example, representation from the community, and minority groups), including representation by:
____	____	____	— both men and women[11]
____	____	____	— multiple professions[12]
____	____	____	— scientific and nonscientific member(s)[13]
____	____	____	— not otherwise affiliated member(s)[14]
____	____	____	D. Alternate members (if used).
			VII. MANAGEMENT OF THE IRB.
			A. The Chairperson
____	____	____	— selection and appointment
____	____	____	— length of term/service
____	____	____	— duties
____	____	____	— removal
			B. The IRB Members.
____	____	____	— selection and appointment
____	____	____	— length of term/service and description of staggered rotation or overlapping of terms, if used
____	____	____	— duties
____	____	____	— attendance requirements
____	____	____	— removal
____	____	____	C. Training of IRB Chair and members
____	____	____	— orientation
____	____	____	— continuing education
____	____	____	— reference materials (IRB library)
____	____	____	D. Compensation of IRB members.
____	____	____	E. Liability coverage for IRB members.
____	____	____	F. Use of consultants.[15]
____	____	____	G. Secretarial/administrative support staff (duties).
____	____	____	H. Resources (for example, meeting area, filing space, reproduction equipment, computers).
			I. Conflict of interest policy
____	____	____	— no selection of IRB members by investigators
____	____	____	— prohibition of participation in IRB deliberations and voting by investigators.[16]
			VIII. FUNCTIONS OF THE IRB.
____	____	____	* A. Conducting initial and continuing review.[17]
____	____	____	* B. Reporting, in writing, findings and actions of the IRB to the investigator and the institution.[18]
____	____	____	* C. Determining which studies require review more often than annually.[19]
____	____	____	* D. Determining which studies need verification from sources other than the investigators that no material changes have occurred since previous IRB review.[20]

FDA Self-Evaluation Tool for IRBs (Continued)

YES	NO	N/A	DOES THE INSTITUTION HAVE WRITTEN POLICIES OR PROCEDURES THAT DESCRIBE:
____	____	____	E. Ensuring prompt reporting to the IRB of changes in research activities.[21]
____	____	____	* F. Ensuring that changes in approved research are not initiated without IRB review and approval except where necessary to eliminate apparent immediate hazards.[22]
			G. Ensuring prompt reporting to the IRB, appropriate institutional officials, and the FDA of:
____	____	____	* — unanticipated problems involving risks to subjects or others[23]
____	____	____	* — serious or continuing non-compliance with 21 CFR parts 50 and 56 or the requirements of the IRB[24]
____	____	____	* — suspension or termination of IRB approval[25]
____	____	____	H. Determining which device studies pose significant or nonsignificant risk.
		IX.	OPERATIONS OF THE IRB.
____	____	____	* A. Scheduling of meetings.[26]
____	____	____	B. Pre-meeting distribution to members, of, for example, place and time of meeting, agenda, and study material to be reviewed.
			C. The review process
			* — description of the process ensuring that[27]
____	____	____	1) all members receive complete study documentation for review (see XI.B);
			or
____	____	____	2) one or more "primary reviewers"/"secondary reviewers" receives the complete study documentation for review, reports to IRB and leads discussion; if other members review summary information only, these members must have access to complete study documentation
____	____	____	— role of any subcommittees of the IRB
____	____	____	* — emergency use notification and reporting procedures[28]
____	____	____	* — expedited review procedure[29]
____	____	____	— for approval of studies that are both minimal risk <u>and</u> on the FDA approved list (see Appendix A)
____	____	____	— for approval of modifications to ongoing studies involving no more than minimal risk
____	____	____	D. Criteria for IRB approval contain all requirements of 21 CFR §56.111.
			E. Voting requirements[30]
____	____	____	— quorum required to transact business
____	____	____	— diversity requirements of quorum (for example requiring at least one physician member when reviewing studies of FDA regulated articles)
____	____	____	— percent needed to approve or disapprove a study
____	____	____	— full voting rights of all reviewing members
____	____	____	— no proxy votes (written or telephone)
____	____	____	— prohibition against conflict-of-interest voting

(Continued)

FDA Self-Evaluation Tool for IRBs (Continued)

YES	NO	N/A	DOES THE INSTITUTION HAVE WRITTEN POLICIES OR PROCEDURES THAT DESCRIBE:
____	____	____	F. Further review/approval of IRB actions by others within the institution. (Override of disapprovals is prohibited.)[31]
			G. Communication from the IRB.
____	____	____	* — to the investigator for additional information[32]
____	____	____	* — to the investigator conveying IRB decision[33]
____	____	____	* — to institution administration conveying IRB decision[34]
____	____	____	— to sponsor of research conveying IRB decision
			H. Appeal of IRB decisions.
____	____	____	— criteria for appeal
____	____	____	— to whom appeal is addressed
____	____	____	— how appeal is resolved (Override of IRB disapprovals by external body/official is prohibited.)[35]
		X.	IRB RECORD REQUIREMENTS.
____	____	____	A. IRB membership roster showing qualifications[36]
____	____	____	* B. Written procedures and guidelines.[37]
			C. Minutes of meetings.[38]
____	____	____	— members present (any consultants/guests/others shown separately)
____	____	____	— summary of discussion on debated issues—record of IRB decisions
____	____	____	— record of voting (showing votes for, against and abstentions)
____	____	____	D. Retention of protocols reviewed and approved consent documents[39]
____	____	____	E. Communications to and from the IRB.[40]
____	____	____	* F. 1) Adverse reactions reports, and[41]
____	____	____	2) documentation that the IRB reviews such reports.
____	____	____	H. Records of continuing review.[42]
			I. Record retention requirements. (at least 3 years after completion for FDA studies)[43]
			J. Budget and accounting records.
____	____	____	K. Emergency use reports.[44]
____	____	____	L. Statements of significant new findings provided to subjects.[45]
		XI.	INFORMATION THE INVESTIGATOR PROVIDES TO THE IRB.
____	____	____	A. Professional qualifications to do the research (including a description of necessary support services and facilities).
			B. Study protocol which includes/addresses[46]
____	____	____	— title of the study
____	____	____	— purpose of the study (including the expected benefits obtained by doing the study)
____	____	____	— sponsor of the study
____	____	____	— results of previous related research
____	____	____	— subject inclusion/exclusion criteria
____	____	____	— justification for use of any special/vulnerable subject populations (for example, the decisionally impaired, children)
____	____	____	— study design (including as needed, a discussion of the appropriateness of research methods)

FDA Self-Evaluation Tool for IRBs (Continued)

YES	NO	N/A	DOES THE INSTITUTION HAVE WRITTEN POLICIES OR PROCEDURES THAT DESCRIBE:
____	____	____	— description of procedures to be performed
____	____	____	— provisions for managing adverse reactions
____	____	____	— the circumstances surrounding consent procedure, including setting, subject autonomy concerns, language difficulties, vulnerable populations
____	____	____	— the procedures for documentation of informed consent, including any procedures for obtaining assent from minors, using witnesses, translators and document storage
____	____	____	— compensation to subjects for their participation
____	____	____	— any compensation for injured research subjects
____	____	____	— provisions for protection of subject's privacy
____	____	____	— extra costs to subjects for their participation in the study
____	____	____	— extra costs to third party payers because of subject's participation
____	____	____	C. Investigator's Brochure (when one exists).[47]
____	____	____	D. The case report form (when one exists).
			E. The proposed informed consent document.[48]
____	____	____	— containing all requirements of 21 CFR §50.25(a)
____	____	____	— containing requirements of 21 CFR §50.25(b) that are appropriate to the study
____	____	____	— meeting all requirements of 21 CFR §50.20
____	____	____	— translated consent documents, as necessary, considering likely subject population(s)
____	____	____	* F. Requests for changes in study after initiation.[49]
____	____	____	* G. Reports of unexpected adverse events.[50]
____	____	____	* H. Progress reports.[51]
____	____	____	I. Final report.
____	____	____	J. Institutional forms/reports.
		XII.	EXEMPTION FROM PROSPECTIVE IRB REVIEW[52]
____	____	____	* A. Notify IRB within 5 working days.[53]
____	____	____	B. Emergency use.[54]
____	____	____	C. Review protocol and consent when subsequent use is anticipated.[55]
		XIII.	EMERGENCY RESEARCH CONSENT EXCEPTION[56]
____	____	____	A. The IRB may find that the 50.24 requirements are met.[57]
____	____	____	B. The IRB shall promptly notify in writing the investigator and the sponsor when it determines it cannot approve a 50.24 study.[58]
____	____	____	C. The IRB shall provide in writing to the sponsor a copy of the information that has been publicly disclosed under 50.24(a)(7)(ii) and (a)(7)(iii).[59]
____	____	____	D. In order to approve an emergency research consent waiver study, the IRB must find and document:
____	____	____	(1) subjects are in a life-threatening situation, available treatments unproven or unsatisfactory and collection of scientific evidence is necessary[60]

(Continued)

FDA Self-Evaluation Tool for IRBs (Continued)

YES	NO	N/A	DOES THE INSTITUTION HAVE WRITTEN POLICIES OR PROCEDURES THAT DESCRIBE:
			(2) Obtaining informed consent is not feasible because:[61]
____	____	____	— medical condition precludes consent[62]
____	____	____	— no time to get consent from legally authorized representative[63]
____	____	____	— prospective identity of likely subjects not reasonable[64]
			(3) Prospect of direct benefits to study subjects because:[65]
____	____	____	— life-threatening situation that necessitates treatment
____	____	____	— data support potential for direct benefit to individual subjects
____	____	____	— risk/benefit of both standard and proposed treatments reasonable
____	____	____	(4) waiver needed to carry out study
____	____	____	(5) plan defines therapeutic window, during which investigator will seek consent rather than starting without consent. Summary of efforts will be given to IRB at time of continuing review.
____	____	____	(6) IRB reviews and approves consent procedures and document. IRB reviews and approves family member objection procedures
			(7) Additional protections, including at least:
____	____	____	— consultation with community representatives
____	____	____	— public disclosure of plans, risks and expected benefits
____	____	____	— public disclosure of study results
____	____	____	— assure an independent Data Monitoring Committee established
____	____	____	— objection of family member summarized for continuing review
____	____	____	(8) Ensure procedures in place to inform at earliest feasible opportunity of subject's inclusion in the study, participation may be discontinued. Procedures to inform family the subject was in the study if subject dies.
____	____	____	(9) Separate IND or IDE required, even for marketed products.
____	____	____	(10) IRB disapproval must be documented in writing and sent to the clinical investigator and the sponsor of the clinical investigation. Sponsor must promptly disclose to FDA, other investigators and other IRBs.

[3] 21 CFR §56.109(a)

[?] 21 CFR §56.101(a)

[4] 21 CFR §56.109(a)

[5] 21 CFR §56.108(a)(1) and §56.109(f)

[6] 21 CFR §56.108(b)(3) and §56.113

[7] 21 CFR §56.108(a)(1), 56.109(a) and §56.113

[8] 21 CFR §56.107(a)

[9] 21 CFR §56.107(a)

[10] 21 CFR §56.107(a)

[11,12] 21 CFR §56.107(b) Only requires every nondiscriminatory effort

[13] 21 CFR §56.107(a)

[?] 21 CFR §56.107(c)

[14] 21 CFR §56.107(d)

[15] 21 CFR §56.107(f) Consultant use not required by FDA regulation.

[16] 21 CFR §56.107(e)

[17] 21 CFR §56.108(a)(1) and §56.109(a–f)

[18] 21 CFR §56.108(a)(1) and §56.109(e)

[19] 21 CFR §56.108(a)(2) and §56.109(f)

[20] 21 CFR §56.108(a)(2)

[21] 21 CFR §56.108(a)(3)

[22] 21 CFR §56.108(a)(4) and §56.115(a)(1)

[23] 21 CFR §56.108(b)(1) and §56.115(a)(1)

[24] 21 CFR §56.108(b)(2)

[25] 21 CFR §56.108(b)(3) and §56.113

[26] 21 CFR §56.108(a)(1)

[27] 21 CFR §56.108(a)(1)

[28] 21 CFR §56.104(c), 56.108(a)(1) and §108(b)(1)

[29] 21 CFR §56.108(a)(1) and §56.110(a–c) not required if IRB does not use expedited procedures

[30] 21 CFR §56.108(c) and §56.107(e–f)

[31] 21 CFR §56.112

[32] 21 CFR §56.108(a)(1), §56.109(a) and §56.115(a)(4)

[33] 21 CFR §56.108(a)(1) and §56.109(e)

[34] 21 CFR §56.108(a)(1) and §56.109(e)

[35] 21 CFR §56.112

[36]21 CFR §56.115(a)(5)

[37]21 CFR §56.108(a–b) and §56.115(a)(6)

[38]21 CFR §56.115(a)(2)

[39]21 CFR §56.115(a)(1)

[40]21 CFR §56.115(a)(4)

[41]21 CFR §56.108(a) and §56.115(a)(1 and 4)

[42]21 CFR §56.115(a)(3)

[43]21 CFR §56.115(b)

[44]21 CFR §56.115(a)(4) and §56.104(c)

[45]21 CFR §56.115(a)(7)

[46]21 CFR §56.103(a) and §56.115(a)(1)

[47]21 CFR §56.111 (a)(2), §56.115(a)(1) and 21 CFR §312.55

[48]21 CFR §56.111(a)(4–5) and §56.111(a)(1)

[49]21 CFR §56.108(a)(4) and §56.115(a)(3–4)

[50]21 CFR §56.108(b)(1), §56.115(a)(3–4), §56.115(b)(1) and §56.113

[51]21 CFR §56.108(a)(1) and §56.115(a)(1, 3 and 4)

[52]Not required when the scope of studies reviewed by the IRB does not include serious and life-threatening diseases or conditions.

[53]21 CFR §56.104(c) and §56.108(a)(3)

[54]21 CFR §56.102(d) and §56.108(a)(3)

[55]21 CFR §56.104(c) and §56.108(a)(3) The IRB may determine that a rapid means of approval is preferable to a preapproved protocol and consent. Also see information sheet: "Emergency Use of a Drug or Biologic."

[56]21 CFR §50.24 The IRB/institution may determine that research in emergent settings will not be conducted or supported. When that is the case,

written procedures for this section need not be prepared.

[57]21 CFR §56.109(c)(2)

[58]21 CFR §56.109(e) The written statement shall include a statement of the reasons for the IRB's determination.

[59]21 CFR §56.109(g)

[60]21 CFR §50.24(a)(1)

[61]21 CFR §50.24(a)(2)

[62]21 CFR §50.24(a)(2)(i)

[63]21 CFR §50.24(a)(2)(ii)

[64]21 CFR §50.24(a)(2)(iii)

[65]21 CFR §50.24(a)(3)

[66]21 CFR §50.24(a)(3)(i)

[67]21 CFR §50.24(a)(3)(ii)

[68]21 CFR §50.24(a)(3)(iii)

[69]21 CFR §50.24(a)(4)

[70]21 CFR §50.24(a)(5)

[71]21 CFR §50.24(a)(6) Family member objection procedures at 50.24 (a)(7)(v)

[72]21 CFR §50.24(a)(7)

[73]21 CFR §50.24(a)(7)(i)

[74]21 CFR §50.24(a)(7)(ii)

[75]21 CFR §50.24(a)(7)(iii)

[76]21 CFR §50.24(a)(7)(iv)

[77]21 CFR §50.24(a)(7)(v)

[78]21 CFR §50.24(b)

[79]21 CFR §50.24(d) The study may not begin until FDA approves the separate IND/IDE.

[80]21 CFR §50.24(e)

REGULATORY OVERSIGHT OF IRBS

Federal Agencies Overseeing Local IRBs

Historically, the Office for Protection from Research (OPRR) had focused its oversight of IRBs at the Assurance stage. However, OPRR conducted ten on-site investigations at institutions in Fiscal Year 1999. It also conducted more than 140 document reviews off-site in 1998 and 1999. OPRR has now been replaced by the Office of Human Research Protection (OHRP). The FDA's primary mode of IRB oversight is through the inspection process. The FDA performed 336 routine on-site investigations in Fiscal Year 1999. The FDA's Center for Drug Evaluation and Research took administrative action against eight IRBs during FY 1998 and 1999 (OIG, 2000).

The primary mechanism for oversight by OHRP is the Assurance process. The Assurance is a document filed by an institution that states the institution's commitment to uphold human-subject protection regulations and its policies and procedures for meeting the regulations. After an initial three-year period, the Assurance is renewed every five years. OPRR conducts a limited number of IRB inspections. These are primarily in response to complaints or concerns about compliance. The OIG reports that spontaneous reviews have been rare (OIG, 2000). However, this is anticipated to change as OHRP's resources are increased. The clear indication is that government scrutiny will continue to heighten for the foreseeable future.

The FDA also inspects IRBs. Investigator inspection is primarily through the FDA's bioresearch monitoring program when the investigator's research is associated with a product approval application. However, for-cause inspections are also conducted (OIG, 2000). Study sponsors, who frequently conduct their own auditing programs of research sites, may bring compliance concerns to the attention of the FDA and OHRP (OPRR, *Institutional Review Board Guidebook*). Both the OIG and the Government Accounting Office have criticized the FDA for its focus on verifying data and ensuring researchers' adherence to study protocols with little attention to protection of human participants (OIG, 2000). The OIG has complained that the OPRR oversight process has been concentrated on the up-front Assurance process: "We found the Assurance process to be paperwork-laden with little effect on IRB functioning." The OIG has called on the OPRR to devote more of its resources to periodic performance-based reviews.

The OIG (2000) has called on the FDA to expand its on-site inspections from primarily compliance to a more results-oriented focus. For example, how are potential research participants being approached? How are IRBs making assessments of risk/benefit ratios?

FDA Inspection Procedure of an IRB

FDA field investigators interview institutional officials and examine the IRB records to determine compliance with the FDA regulations. The FDA is anticipated to become more comprehensive in the inspection process. This may, for example, include interviews of staff and participants (FDA, Information Sheets, 1998).

Sponsor Access to Whether an IRB Has Been Inspected by the FDA, and the Results of the Inspection

The FDA's Division of Scientific Investigations, Center for Drug Evaluation and Research, maintains a list of the IRBs that have been inspected, including dates of inspection and classification. The Division recently began including the results of inspections assigned by the Center for Biologics Evaluation and Research and the Center for Devices and Radiological Health. This information is available through the Freedom of Information Act (FOIA) procedures. Once an investigational file has been closed, the correspondence between FDA and the IRB and the narrative inspectional report are also available under FOIA (FDA, Information Sheets, 1998).

Administrative Actions by HHS for Non-Compliance

HHS regulations do not specify administrative actions for non-compliance "except to state that material failure to comply with the regulations can result in termination or suspension of support for department or agency projects, and that HHS will take terminations or suspensions of funding due to non-compliance into consideration when making future funding decisions" (OPRR, *Institutional Review Board Guidebook*). One or more of the following outcomes can occur:

1. OHRP may determine that protections under an institution's Assurance of Compliance are in compliance with the HHS Regulations or the PHS Policy.

2. OHRP may determine that protections under an institution's Assurance of Compliance are in compliance with the HHS Regulations or the PHS Policy but that recommended improvements to those protections have been identified.

3. OHRP may restrict its approval of an institution's Assurance of Compliance. HHS cannot support affected research projects until the terms of the restriction have been

satisfied. Examples of such restrictions include, but are not limited to:

    a. Suspending the Assurance's applicability relative to some or all research projects until specified protections have been implemented.

    b. Requiring prior OHRP review of some or all research projects to be conducted under the Assurance.

    c. Requiring that some or all investigators conducting research under the Assurance receive appropriate human subject or animal welfare education.

    d. Requiring special reporting to OHRP.

4. OHRP may withdraw its approval of an institution's Assurance of Compliance. Affected research projects cannot be supported by any HHS component until an appropriate Assurance is approved by OHRP.

5. OHRP may recommend to appropriate HHS officials or PHS agency heads:

    a. That an institution or an investigator be temporarily suspended or permanently removed from participating in specific projects.

    b. That peer review groups be notified of an institution's or an investigator's past non-compliance prior to review of new projects.

6. OHRP may recommend to HHS that institutions or investigators be declared ineligible to participate in HHS-supported research (Debarment). If OHRP makes this recommendation, the Debarment process will be initiated in accordance with the procedures specified at 45 CFR §76 and discussed in Chapter Eight.

....
CONCLUSION

The Institutional Review Board has the fundamental responsibility of protecting the well being of study participants. That responsibility has many facets ranging from considering financial conflicts of interest to gauging the amount of risk for significant harm a study may pose. This mandate includes the practical application of ethics and scientific analysis. Thoughtful discussion and detailed documentation of the deliberative process are required of the IRB.

References

Applied Research Ethics National Association (ARENA) [http://www.primr.org/arena.html].

Case Study, Letter from Michael Carome, Chief, Compliance Oversight Branch, March 4, 1999.

Association of American Medical Medical Colleges, Protecting Subjects, Preserving Trust, Promoting Progress II: Principles and Recommendations for Oversight of an Institution's Financial Interests in Human Subjects Research, October 2002.

Ezekiel, Wendler, and Grady. "What Makes Clinical Research Ethical?," *JAMA.* 2000; 283:2701–2711.

FDA. "Institutional Review Boards: Requiring Sponsors and Investigators to Inform IRBs of Any Prior IRB Reviews." Federal Register 10115-10116, March 6, 2002a.

FDA. Federal Register 10115-10116, March 6, 2002b.

FDA. Federal Register 56 (June 18, 1991): 28026 (FDA interpretation of 21 CFR §56.108(b).

FDA. Guidance for Institutional Review Boards, Clinical Investigators, and Sponsors: Exception from Informed Consent Requirements for Emergency Research (Draft). FDA, Office of Regulatory Affairs, 30 March 2000.

FDA. Information Sheets, Guidance for Institutional Review Boards and Clinical Investigators, 1998 Update, FAQS, http://www.fda.gov/oc/oha/IRB/toc2.html#IRBOrg.

FDA. Minimal risk clinical trials, Federal Register, November 9, 1998 [63 FR 60364-60367].

FDA. Warning Letters to several IRBs.

HHS. Financial Relationships in Clinical Research: Issues for Institutions, Clinical Investigators, and IRBs to Consider when Dealing with Issues of Financial Interests and Human Subject Protection. Draft Interim Guidance, Jan. 2000.

HHS. Financial Relationships in Clinical Research: Issues for Institutions, Clinical Investigators, and IRBs to Consider when Dealing with Issues of Financial Interests and Human Subject Protection. Draft Interim Guidance, Jan. 2000.

HHS. OIG, "FDA Oversight of Clinical Investigators," June 2000, OEI-05-99-00350, p. 11.

Hilts, P. "Panel Seeks Better Monitoring of Experiments Using People," *New York Times,* March 2, 2000.

ICH. *Guideline for Good Clinical Practice,* 1996.

Institute of Medicine, Committee on Assessing the System for Protecting Human Research Participants. *Responsible Research: A Systems Approach to Protecting Research Participants.* Washington, DC: The National Academics Press, 2002.

National Council (Canada) on Bioethics in Human Research. "Protecting and Promoting the Human Research Subject: A Review of the Function of Research Ethics boards in Canadian Faculties of Medicine." NCBHR Communique CNBRH, Vol. 6 (1995) No. 1.

NIH. Bioethics Resources Web site, www.nih.gov/sigs/bioethics/.

Office for Protection from Research Risk. Institutional Review Board Guidebook (available at http://ohrp.osophs.dhhs.gov/irb/irb_guidebook_t.htm).

OHRP. March 9, 2001 Newsflash.

OHRP. "Open Letter to the Human Research Community [OHRP quality assurance program], April 17, 2002.

OHRP. Assurance Web site [http://ohrp.osophs.dhhs.gov/humansubjects/Assurance/faq.htm].

OHRP. Guidance on Continuing Review, July 11, 2002a.

OHRP. Guidance on Written IRB Procedures, July 11, 2002b.

OHRP. http://ohrp.osophs.dhhs.gov/references/findings.pdf.

OHRP. Training Modules, http://137.187.172.201/cbttng_ohrp/default.asp?CBTID=2.

OIG, Advisory Opinion No. 02-11.

OIG, Advisory Opinion No. 02-11, University grant for funding research in medical school, issued December 8, 2002. [http://www.oig.hhs.gov/fraud/advisoryopinions/opinions.html]

OIG. "FDA Oversight of Clinical Investigators" (OEI-05-99-00350), June 2000.

OIG, Final Report on Low-Volume Institutional Review Boards (OEI-01-97-00194), October 23, 1998.

OIG, Institutional Review Boards: Promising Approaches (OEI-01-97-00191).

OIG. "Institutional Review Boards: Their Role in Reviewing Approved Research." (OEI-01-97-00190), June 1998.

OIG, Protecting Human Research Subjects: Status of Recommendations, April 2000, OEI-01-97-00197.

OIG, Special Advisory Bulletin, August 29, 2002.

OIG, Special Advisory Bulletin, Gifts and Inducements, issued August 29, 2002, published in Federal Register August 30, 2002. [http://oig.hhs.gov/fraud/docs/alertsandbulletins/SABGiftsandInducements.pdf]

OIG's report re: IRB's role in reviewing approved research, [http://oig.hhs.gov/oei/summaries/b273.pdf]

OPRR, Institutional Review Board Guidebook, 1993.

OPRR Memorandum: IRB Knowledge of Local Research Context, August 27, 1998.

OPRR Memorandum: Update – Suitability of a Designated Institutional Review Board (IRB), February 4, 1997.

OPRR, General Guidance on the Use of Another Institution's IRB (July 7, 1991).

OPRR, [http://www.nih.gov/grants/oprr/humansubjects/guidance/decisioncharts.htm]

ORI, "PHS Policy on Instruction in the Responsible Conduct of Research (RCR)," January 7, 2000, [http://ori.hhs.gov]

Public Responsibility in Medicine and Research (PRIM&R) [http://www.primr.org/]

OMB No. 0990-0263
Approved for use through 07/31/2005

Protection of Human Subjects
Assurance Identification/IRB Certification/Declaration of Exemption
(Common Rule)

Policy: Research activities involving human subjects may not be conducted or supported by the Departments and Agencies adopting the Common Rule (56FR28003, June 18, 1991) unless the activities are exempt from or approved in accordance with the Common Rule. See section 101(b) of the Common Rule for exemptions. Institutions submitting applications or proposals for support must submit certification of appropriate Institutional Review Board (IRB) review and approval to the Department or Agency in accordance with the Common Rule.

Institutions must have an assurance of compliance that applies to the research to be conducted and should submit certification of IRB review and approval with each application or proposal unless otherwise advised by the Department or Agency.

1. Request Type [ ] ORIGINAL [ ] CONTINUATION [ ] EXEMPTION	2. Type of Mechanism [ ] GRANT [ ] CONTRACT [ ] FELLOWSHIP [ ] COOPERATIVE AGREEMENT [ ] OTHER:_____	3. Name of Federal Department or Agency and, if known, Application or Proposal Identification No.
4. Title of Application or Activity		5. Name of Principal Investigator, Program Director, Fellow, or Other

6. Assurance Status of this Project (*Respond to one of the following*)

[ ] This Assurance, on file with Department of Health and Human Services, covers this activity:

Assurance Identification No. _____, the expiration date _____ IRB Registration No. _____

[ ] This Assurance, on file with (*agency/dept*) _____, covers this activity.

Assurance No. _____, the expiration date _____ IRB Registration/ Identification No. _____ (if applicable)

[ ] No assurance has been filed for this institution. This institution declares that it will provide an Assurance and Certification of IRB review and approval upon request.

[ ] Exemption Status: Human subjects are involved, but this activity qualifies for exemption under Section 101(b), paragraph_____.

7. Certification of IRB Review (Respond to one of the following IF you have an Assurance on file)

[ ] This activity has been reviewed and approved by the IRB in accordance with the Common Rule and any other governing regulations. by:
   [ ] Full IRB Review on (date of IRB meeting) _____ or [ ] Expedited Review on (date) _____
   [ ] If less than one year approval, provide expiration date _____

[ ] This activity contains multiple projects, some of which have not been reviewed. The IRB has granted approval on condition that all projects covered by the Common Rule will be reviewed and approved before they are initiated and that appropriate further certification will be submitted.

8. Comments

9. The official signing below certifies that the information provided above is correct and that, as required, future reviews will be performed until study closure and certification will be provided.	10. Name and Address of Institution	
11. Phone No. (*with area code*)		
12. Fax No. (*with area code*)		
13. Email:		
14. Name of Official	15. Title	
16. Signature		17. Date

Authorized for local Reproduction   Sponsored by HHS

10

Patient Safety in Clinical Trials Research

Overview 326
Data Safety Monitoring Board 327
   Purpose and Function of a Data Safety Monitoring Board (DSMB) 327
   Indications for Use of a DSMB 328
   Composition of a DSMB 329
   The Relationship of a DSMB to an IRB 329
   Activities of a DSMB 330
   NIH Requirements for Data and Safety Monitoring 330
Specific Steps That Can Be Taken to Create a Patient
Safety Style Environment for Clinical Trials 330
   Screening Tools 330
   Consent Tools 331
   Checklists 331
   Signage 332
   Research Bracelets 332
   On-Call and Interactive Web Sites 333
   Clinical Contingency Plan for Adverse Events 334
   Education 334
Adverse Event Reporting 334
   A Systematic Approach to Managing Adverse Events 335
      Investigation 335
      Sequestration of Documentation 335
      Sequestration of Ancillary Record Information 335
      Sequestration of Equipment 336
      Interviews 336
      Process Indicators 336
      Develop a Visual Algorithm for Adverse Event Investigations 336
      Determination: Does the Adverse Event Require Reporting 336
   Determining to Whom to Report Adverse Events 338
   Multiple Adverse Event Reporting Obligations 339
   Disclosure of Adverse Event Information to Research Subjects 339
   Directions for Adverse Event Reporting by Research Subjects 340
   The Duty to Warn Research Subjects About Emergency Treatment for Adverse Events . . . 340
Conclusion 341
References 341

....

OVERVIEW

In fall 1999 the Institute of Medicine issued a remarkable report, *To Err is Human,* describing the pitfalls in the American healthcare system that lead to as many as 98,000 deaths per year from medical error. The report sparked a call for new legislation at both the federal and state levels and quality-based initiatives among a number of federal agencies to rectify the problem.

The problems described in *To Err is Human* were not restricted to conventional medical therapy. Indeed, some well-publicized events occurred in Boston, Philadelphia, and elsewhere in the country that pointed out error and safety were of serious concern for subjects of clinical trials. As much as a year prior to the IOM Report the Deputy Inspector-General of HHS testified before Congress in essence challenging IRBs to do a better job to ensure the rights and safety of clinical trial participants. The testimony was encapsulated in an OIG report in June 1998, *Institutional Review Boards: A Time for Reform* (OEI-01-97-00193). In that report, the OIG called for Data Safety Monitoring Boards (DSMBs) that would provide summary assessments of adverse event reports to IRBs so that the ongoing safety of a research trials could be accomplished by IRBs. Further, it recommended elimination of a type of "forum shopping" done when sponsors unhappy with the reviews done by one IRB took their business to another IRB without telling the second body about the earlier one's involvement or determinations. This was seen by the OIG as denying the second IRB important information and short-circuiting the opportunity for subject protection.

In keeping with the theme of subject protection, the OIG recommended that IRBs become more involved in terms of what transpired during research trials. It was suggested that for particularly risk-prone trials this might involve the use of intermediaries, counselors, or observers to observe the consent process or IRB members might conduct random unannounced visits to review relevant documents and to oversee the consent process.

In an April 2000 report (*Protecting Human Research Subjects—Status of Recommendations,* OEI-01-97-00197), the OIG found that a number of changes had been made but many recommendations remained unheeded. Some of these recommendations included those involving research subject safety.

During this time frame, major structural changes were initiated involving the Office of Protection from Research Risks, a part of the National Institutes of Health (NIH) with authority over NIH-funded research. In June 2000, the Secretary of Health and Human Services replaced OPRR with the Office of Human Research Protection (OHPR), situating it in the Department of Health and Human Services. Positioned at the departmental level, the new agency was designed to provide leadership for the seventeen federal agencies funding human research. Since its inception, OHPR has moved to develop strategies for education of IRB and clinical trial investigators and to improve regulatory compliance.

The Institute of Medicine (IOM) has also weighed in on the subject of research subject safety and protection. In one report, the IOM accreditation was recommended as a means of improving the protection of research subjects (*Preserving Public Trust: Accreditation and Human Research Protection Programs,* 2001). In another, the IOM went further, emphasizing the need to refocus the mission of the IRB, enhancing consent to participate in clinical research, and a compensation program for participants who experience harm in clinical trials (*Responsible Research: A Systems Approach to Protecting Research Participants* [October 3, 2002]).

As a backdrop to all these changes is a set of federal regulations that set out a process for addressing adverse events affecting human research subjects (45 CFR §46.103(5); and 21 CFR §312.32). Under the HHS rules, the IRB must have a *written process* in place for prompt reporting of *unanticipated problems* involving risks to research subjects. Under the FDA Investigational New Drug (IND) requirements the sponsor of the IND has to notify the FDA and participating investigators in a written safety report of those adverse experiences associated with the use of the drug that are both serious and unexpected. The FDA may also request that the sponsor telephone or fax reports of unexpected fatal or life-threatening experience associated with the use of the drug as soon as possible. The requirement must be completed no later than seven calendar days after the time that the sponsor received the information. This means that the IRB and clinical investigators must be cognizant of the different reporting triggers for research conducting under HHS style regulations and those funded as IND protocols by the FDA.

Sometimes the line is blurred between patient and research subject. A patient who is also a research subject may be unhappy with the outcome or the care received while at a teaching hospital. Under the Conditions of Participation for Medicare and Medicaid in Hospitals, the patient is entitled to file a grievance under the patients rights standards. This will trigger a detailed probe and report. It may be quite a challenge to sort out the conventional treatment-related events from those that took place under the aegis of the clinical research protocol in which the individual is enrolled as a subject. This multiplicity of investigations and fact-finding, all done in the name of creating a safe environment, could prove expensive, time-consuming, and possibly generate contradictory results since there are differences in the enabling laws. An outcome may generate a confirmation that the patient had a genuine point of grievance, but on the research side there may not be a basis for considering the occurrence as an adverse event. In the accreditation area the situation may constitute an "unanticipated outcome" triggering a different type of reporting to the patient as described in the patient safety standards published by the Joint Commission on Accreditation of Healthcare Organizations. This is an important consideration when trying to put in place the infrastructure for a patient-research subject safety-oriented protocol.

This chapter describes the role of the Data Safety Monitoring Board (DSMBs) and a practical approach to reporting, responding to, and documenting adverse events. It addresses reports to and the work of DSMBs. Effective patient safety-style research strategies are also described to lessen the risk of adverse events or unanticipated outcomes. Management of concurrent situations, incident reporting, and sentinel event reporting are discussed in the context of clinical trials.

....

DATA SAFETY MONITORING BOARD

Purpose and Function of a Data Safety Monitoring Board (DSMB)

When constructing a research protocol, an investigator must ensure ongoing evaluation of data as it is accumulated. In an FDA-regulated study, data monitoring is also the responsibility of the sponsor. An IRB must ensure that this critical element is part of a research protocol. The Office of Human Research Protections (OHRP) suggests an independent group, often called a Data Safety Monitoring Board (DSMB), is an excellent way to achieve objective analysis of information from a study. A DSMB is occasionally referred to as a Data Monitoring Committee (DMC), particularly in FDA publications.

A DSMB provides an important service of being able to analyze interim data, often from multiple sites, as well as external data from other studies and reports. A DSMB should be looking for efficacy of the therapy under study, its relative merit compared with other treatment (including no treatment), and any adverse events causally related to the therapy. A DSMB often is the first to be in a position to make a sound judgment that a study should be terminated because the investigational therapy is clearly superior or inferior to the control therapy or patient safety is clearly in jeopardy. More often, a DSMB will recommend that a study continue as this conclusion cannot yet be statistically supported. A DSMB may also recommend alterations to the protocol, populations enrolled, or information that should be supplied to participants.

The OIG believes that an IRB alone cannot provide a sufficient degree of protection to research participants, and that DSMBs can play a vital role for trials that pose significant risks to patients (OIG, 2000), especially for certain high-risk and multisite trials. The OIG believes that "DSMBs are independent assessment bodies that provide medical, scientific and other expertise that is not typically available on IRBs, thereby serving an invaluable function in protecting human subjects" (OIG, 2000). However, an IRB does not absolve itself of responsibility for protecting research participants. A DSMB is merely a useful tool for an IRB to fulfill its responsibility.

DSMBs should provide their summary assessments of adverse event reports to IRBs. "IRBs are swamped with individual adverse event reports from multi-site trials, but these reports lack the essential context to confer meaning about the relative safety of the trial. DSMBs can provide this context and thereby enhance the IRB's capacity to assess the ongoing safety of a trial" (OIG, 2000). In addition, the DSMB decides how missing or suspect data are to be assessed in overall analyses of a study.

Indications for Use of a DSMB

DSMBs have gained favor in large, randomized multisite studies that evaluate interventions intended to prolong life or reduce risk of a major adverse health outcome such as a cardiac event or recurrence of cancer (FDA, 2001). They are not practical generally in short-term studies where a DSMB would not have the opportunity to analyze the data in a timely fashion. The FDA has suggested the following should be considered in determining if a DSMB should be utilized for a study:

1. Risk to study participants.
2. Practicality of DSMB review.
3. Assurance of scientific validity.

A study sponsor, especially in pharmaceutical and medical device studies, often considers whether a DSMB is indicated when the sponsor designs the study. A DSMB can be one component of a sponsor meeting its obligation to monitor studies evaluating new drugs, biologics, and devices and report adverse events to the FDA (21 CFR §312.50 and 312.56 for drugs and biologics; 21 CFR §812.40 and 812.46 for devices). Many sponsors now routinely use a DSMB as part of clinical trials, and prudence would counsel that a DSMB be used in any study where the ability to monitor data is beyond the resources of a local IRB. However, FDA regulations do not require the use of a DSMB, except for studies in emergency settings under 21 CFR §50.24(a)(7)(iv) where informed consent may be waived.

An IRB should determine at the time of its initial assessment whether a DSMB is required. What is the complexity of the study? Is mortality or major morbidity a primary or secondary end point? What is the size and duration of the study? What is the degree of risk? Is a fragile population, such as children or elderly, being utilized? A DSMB is intended to review unblended interim data. A DSMB usually does not monitor a single test site for points including protocol compliance, and appropriate data entry.

NIH guidance gives an excellent example of when DSMBs are indicated. NIH funded or conducted Phase 3 trials are generally required to have DSMBs and most involve site monitoring as part of the quality assurance program of the funding institute or center (NIH, 1998). NIH has also recommended the use of a DSMB or similar arrangement for Phase 1 and Phase 2 studies, especially when large numbers of participants are enrolled or multiple sites are used (NIH, 2000). DSMBs associated with NIH trials are expected to forward summary reports of adverse events to IRBs (NIH, 1999).

Composition of a DSMB

Unfortunately, federal regulations and policy statements give little guidance as to what the quantity or attributes of individuals serving on a DSMB should be. The FDA has noted that as few as three members may compose a DSMB, but it encourages a broader group than this (FDA, 2001). The better course would be to weight the composition with members who have scientific backgrounds useful in evaluating the data being collected from an investigation. A biostatistician needs to undertake the analysis of the data. Whether the biostatistician should be a member of the DSMB is debated. Specialists in pharmacokinetics, toxicology, epidemiology, and cardiology may be needed. The FDA has also suggested that factors of gender, ethnic, and representation of the disease process under study are important (FDA, 2001). Equally important is the independence and influence of the DSMB. Thus, the members must have standing in the scientific community sufficient to be effective in persuading an investigator, an IRB, and the sponsor to modify or terminate a study when indicated by data analysis.

Some sponsors create a DSMB from its upper scientific management team. This approach has the benefits of being easily organized, efficient in gathering the members for a meeting, and usually persuasive in its recommendations. However, this approach may suffer from being pressured explicitly or implicitly to minimize the significance of adverse events or dubious clinical effectiveness of the investigational drug. The FDA points out that independence of a DSMB protects the sponsor from pressure toward premature disclosure of results due to SEC reporting requirements, fiduciary responsibilities, and other business considerations (FDA, 2001). A better approach is to include a sufficient number of independent members on the DSMB to assure that data is critically analyzed and appropriate responses are made. Clearly, an investigator or a participant in the study should not be a member of its DSMB. Scientists who have outspoken views on the merits of the therapy under investigation also should not be on the DSMB.

The Relationship of a DSMB to an IRB

A DSMB will collect and interpret data from all of the clinical sites of a study. Often an IRB will approve and give continued approval to only one research site. Therefore, the DSMB may be able to spot significant data earlier by seeing it from more than one location and from a larger population. "IRBs conducting continuing review of research may rely on a current statement from the DSMB indicating that it has reviewed study-wide adverse events, interim findings, and any recent literature that may be relevant to the research, in lieu of requiring that this information be submitted directly to the IRB. Of course, the IRB must still receive and review reports of local, on-site unanticipated problems involving risks to subjects or others and any other information needed to ensure that its continuing review is substantive and meaningful" (OHRP, 2002). The IRB always maintains the responsibility of protecting patients at its site. It may rely on reports from the DSMB, but it has the responsibility to take whatever actions are necessary to protect the participants.

Activities of a DSMB

The activities of a DSMB should be structured in a manner similar to an IRB. Participant safety, public relations, and scientific validity require that the DSMB operate in a logical and predictable manner. Policies and procedures should be written and followed. These should include a schedule of meetings and the format for each meeting, the format for presentation of data to the DSMB, the format for reporting of interim findings, and the statistical methods to be utilized. Minutes of every meeting should be written in detail and filed. The Board's recommendations should be clearly communicated to the sponsor. A DSMB usually does not report directly to the FDA unless this was part of the study's design. However, the sponsor has an obligation to report the DSMB's recommendations in a timely manner to the FDA and the responsible IRB. The DSMB's activities will be reviewed as part of the FDA's consideration of data.

NIH Requirements for Data and Safety Monitoring

The National Institute of Health (NIH) requires data and safety monitoring, generally in the form of DSMBs, for Phase III clinical trials sponsored by NIH. It also recommends that a DSMB may be appropriate for Phase I and Phase II clinical trials if the studies (1) have multiple clinical sites; (2) are blinded (masked); or (3) employ particularly high-risk interventions or vulnerable populations. Conversely, an independent DSMB may not be necessary or appropriate if the proposed intervention is low risk. Monitoring by the investigator or by an independent individual may be sufficient. When a DSMB is employed, an IRB can rely on the summary reports of adverse events from the DSMB (NIH, 2000).

· · · · · · · · · · · ·

SPECIFIC STEPS THAT CAN BE TAKEN TO CREATE A PATIENT SAFETY STYLE ENVIRONMENT FOR CLINICAL TRIALS

There are a number of practical steps that can be implemented to create a safe environment for clinical trials. These include effective screening tools to use with subjects who are at risk of experiencing an adverse event, consent procedures, training, signage, checklists, and Medic-Alert style bracelets. Even with so much attention focused on individually identifiable information, it is possible to create an HIPAA compliant, "fire wall" protected Web site for posting important clinical trial information needed for the treatment of a research subject who becomes ill miles away from the clinical trial location. A related concept is a contingency plan for adverse events. Each of these categories is explained below.

Screening Tools

Critical to successful management of a clinical trial is the proper selection of research subjects. Not only must the subject population include those who meet the study design, they must also present with a reasonable constellation of risk factors. These risk factors may have nothing to do with the clinical study, yet the mere presence of these attributes could deter the individual from being selected for inclusion in the investigation. For example, a trial might involve investigation of a new diabetic medication. From screening information obtained from the individual it is clear that the person is eligible for the study. However, additional questions reveal a history of non-compliance with structured medication schedules. There is no familial caregiver or friend who might assist the individual with staying on the required regimen. Since it is critical to stay within the rigid parameters of the study, this is a person "at risk" who might be rejected from enrollment.

Consent Tools

As discussed in Chapter Five, consent is a pivotal component in clinical trials. It is equally important in terms of subject safety. Consent is more than securing a written authorization for inclusion in a study; it is a communications tool that enables the principal investigator and study personnel to impart important information for safe participation in a clinical trial. Disclosure of possible anticipated side effects should always be part of the discussion. However, from a safety perspective what is equally important is to use the consent process as a forum for schooling subjects on what steps to take if such side effects occur. Additionally, research consent procedures usually include some discussion about unforeseeable risk factors. Subjects may have unusual or unanticipated responses to a study intervention or a investigational drug. Rather than dismissing it as "nothing to worry about," subjects should be encouraged to report it promptly. Although considered somewhat radical, another useful approach is to involve a family member of the research subject in the consent process. This *must* be done with the permission of the research subject. The rationale is that the family member may have a different perspective than the subject on key issues such as predisposing risk factors, ability to adhere to the protocol, and early detection of adverse events. At the same time, the family member can school others about what to look for in terms of reactions or adverse events and the appropriate response to such situations. For example, a subject may be enrolled in a study that involves an implanted investigational device. He collapses at home on the living room floor and 911 is called. The EMS response team has no idea that the individual is enrolled in a clinical trial. No one in the immediate family is aware of the individual's role in a study and so they are unable to shed light on what might have caused the person to experience such an event. The upshot is a therapeutic intervention that is incompatible with the study, resulting in harm to the subject-patient. The chance of avoiding such real-life risk situations is increased if one or more family members are involved from the outset in the communication process called consent. As a communications tool the consent process can be used to reinforce the importance of alerting study personnel to risk-prone situations and aid those assisting a subject-patient who requires a therapeutic intervention.

Checklists

A practical approach to maintaining research subject safety involves the use of checklists. When used as guidelines or pathways, these tools do not become "cookbook" clinical research. Instead, the documents serve as reminders or helpful algorithms for reducing unwanted or risk-prone variations in the proper management of a clinical trial. Some of the checklists will be for the use of clinical trials staff personnel. Others will be useful guides for in-patient, emergency department, and urgent care personnel who encounter research subjects as patients. Finally, other checklists will provide important reminders to research subjects and their family members regarding what to do when reactions or adverse effects occur. Sample checklists are found in the Appendix.

Signage

Another research subject safety tool involves well-displayed notices in languages used by members of the community in which the facility is situated. This is particularly important for hospitals, free-standing urgent care units, ambulatory patient care units, and retail pharmacies. The message is quite simple:

> **Are You Taking Part in a Clinical Trial or Research?**
> **If so, please tell us when you register for treatment.**

The signage serves as a friendly reminder, a prompt to disclose an important consideration for caregivers to take into account when evaluating a patient's needs, performing therapeutic interventions, or prescribing medication. Why the same type of signage at multiple locations? The rationale is simple: a communications safety net to "catch" research subjects who might otherwise miss an opportunity to provide salient information about participation in a clinical trial that has or could have an adverse impact on proposed treatment. For example, a research subject-patient might have missed the prompt in a free-standing urgent care center. However, upon seeing it at the retail pharmacy, the subject says to the pharmacy technician, "Yes, I am in a study. Why is that important? After all, the doctor only prescribed some antibiotics and over-the-counter pain medication." It *is important* since this may be the last opportunity to prevent an untoward synergistic effect between an investigational drug and "accepted" medical treatment. When told about the participation in the study, the pharmacy technician should inform the pharmacist. In turn, the pharmacist would contact the prescribing doctor and discussion should follow with a study investigator or coordinator. This conversation may be the first early warning of an adverse effect or it may be a routine infection that has nothing to do with the study. At the very least, the communication provides peace of mind for the prescribing physician and professionals involved in the research study. Once a decision is made about next steps, the outcome may be to clear the proposed prescription or suggest an alternative. The root of this safety process was the signage in the retail pharmacy that prompted the research subject to notify staff about involvement in a clinical trial.

Research Bracelets

Many individuals wear decorative bracelets or necklaces emblazoned with medical warnings or alerts, which may include information about allergies, underlying medical conditions, medication requirements, or organ donor status. Still others provide instructions on resuscitation requests. The information is designed to alert first responders, EMS, and emergency personnel of what to do when assisting the person wearing these bracelets and necklaces. It is a very practical idea in terms of safety for clinical trial participants. Study subjects often travel miles away from the investigation location in which they participate. If they require any treatment there is no way in which caregivers might know that these individuals are enrolled in a study. The need for treatment might be the result of an adverse reaction to a study drug or injuries sustained in an unrelated event. Without the benefit of knowing that the patient is taking part in a clinical trial, misdiagnosis or inappropriate treatment based upon the medications or devices involved in the clinical study could occur. Providing subjects with warning bracelets or necklaces can greatly reduce this risk to subject safety. In practical terms the information should include the following:

→ The name of the *protocol.*

→ The patient's clinical research *identification number.*

→ A toll-free *number or e-mail address* to contact for urgent information.

In addition, the information should include a warning statement as follows:

> ### Warning!
> **I am enrolled in a clinical research. Please contact the study coordinator before performing treatment!**

Taking this additional step helps to ensure the safety of clinical trial participants. It may also help in terms of maintaining the integrity of the study so that subjects are not lost to follow-up as a result of an unfortunate response to a need for treatment.

On-Call and Interactive Web Sites

Related measures should be considered to complete the loop on safety communication for clinical research trials. One involves an on-call protocol so that when research subjects call with questions or to report what they believe is an adverse event, someone can respond quickly. This is especially important with high-risk trials and also in those protocols in which the consent document "assures" participants that if they call, *someone will get back to them promptly.* An on-call system may involve forwarding calls to someone carrying a cell phone or a pager. In practical terms, this means that there must be follow through in a timely manner. Another technique may be to provide participants with address information for a secure Web site. This presupposes that research subjects have access to the Internet. Using their protocol identification number or a similar code process, research subjects could visit a Web site that includes Frequently Asked Questions (FAQs) and answers to common concerns stemming from involvement in the research trial. It might also have a monitored chat room or "e-mail us" function through which participants could receive prompt answers to questions such as, "Am I experiencing an adverse reaction to the study drug?" or "I missed two of my medications yesterday and this morning. What should I do?" From the perspective of the principal investigator, it is important that someone on the study staff *monitor* the web and e-mail traffic and that a response is made in a timely manner. The Internet provides a powerful tool for overseeing the concerns or questions of participants and for preventing possible harm to subjects or their dropping out of the investigation. In this way the Web site information might contribute to enhancements in the study design.

Clinical Contingency Plan for Adverse Events

Along with the use of properly trained personnel to field questions and the use of warning bracelets and necklaces, there should be in place a clinical plan to manage the care of subjects who experience an adverse event. Such a plan would include:

→ Clinical management algorithms for differentiating what is an adverse reaction to a device or drug under investigation in the study and what might be the result of drug-drug, or drug-food interaction or other factors.

→ Notification of clinical care team of related reported adverse events and successful treatment plans in other cases.

→ Instruction sheets for subjects provided to them at the time of enrollment in the study reminding them to alert their primary care provider, family, and urgent care or ED staff that they are involved in a clinical trial of an investigational drug or device.

→ Instruction sheets for on-call personnel or those monitoring e-mail traffic on how to manage a subject believed to be experiencing an adverse event.

→ Follow-up once care is completed to determine what worked and what did not work in terms of managing the person who experiences an adverse event related to the drug or device under investigation.

Education

Everyone involved in clinical research trials can benefit from safety education. Providing staff with practical training on safety practices prevents harmful experiences. In managing research subjects, the same is quite true: knowing what to look for in terms of early warning signs of adverse effects, how to talk with subjects and their families to provide calm responses that channel appropriate responses, and how to interact with clinical treatment facilities can all contribute to positive outcomes. By the same token, education is important for research subjects and their family members. They need a firm understanding of how to detect when there is evidence of adverse effect, who to call, and how to respond. Taking this approach provides a useful way of addressing what can potentially become a life or health-threatening event. Rather than letting situations evolve into a crisis, the prudent approach is to anticipate possible adverse events through cogent education that develops success strategies for managing such problems.

These measures are illustrative of the steps to take in creating a culture of safety in studies involving the use of human subjects. Other steps may be added, consistent with ongoing patient safety strategies in a healthcare organization or Contract Research Organization.

············

ADVERSE EVENT REPORTING

It is imperative that IRBs receive prompt notification about adverse events stemming from research studies. This would include situations in which subjects experience serious harm and unforeseen accidents or problems. When an adverse event such as a serious injury to or the death of a subject occurs, a thorough review is warranted. A failure analysis or root cause analysis is warranted to ascertain why the situation occurred. The results may be surprising, too.

Many observers may be ready to ascribe the outcome to the investigational device or drug, but the event may prove to be the culmination of a series of failures that came to cause the subject's injury or death. Delving into the issue could make the difference between suspending a valid research protocol and correcting system failures that led to the untoward event. Models exist for this type of investigation, including those with which accredited hospitals are familiar (Sentinel Event—Root Cause Analysis from the Joint Commission on Accreditation of Healthcare Organizations) and others with which many manufacturing industries are conversant (PROACT from the Reliability Center).

Other considerations include the possibility of litigation stemming from injury or death to a subject, investigations by a coroner or medical examiner, criminal probes by law enforcement, and compliance oversight investigations by pertinent federal regulatory bodies such as the FDA or the Office of Human Research Protections (OHRP).

A Systematic Approach to Managing Adverse Events

With such an array of possible regulatory investigations, it is important that healthcare facilities or CROs have in place a systematic approach to investigating, managing, and eventually reporting the finding on adverse events. Such an approach would include the following considerations.

Investigation   Once an adverse event occurs, steps should be taken to determine what gave rise to it. Care should be taken not to jump to conclusions but rather to look at processes that should have occurred and compare this information with what did occur. For example, a research subject may have received ten times the dose of radiation expected in the research protocol. The investigation would not jump to the conclusion that somebody did something wrong. Rather, it would look at documentation, communication, and equipment calibration processes as well as staff education. Taking this approach, it may turn out that several processes or procedures failed and coalesced into a systems failure. Alternatively, it may be a human factors issue, in which a staffer perhaps took it for granted that the radiation machine was always set at the right setting and did not bother to double-check the calibrations per study protocol. In such a situation, the event involves a human failure as well as a systems failure, implicating the lack of fail-safes to prevent such an adverse event. An Investigation Checklist is provided in the Appendix to use as a sample for purposes of thoroughly studying the causes of adverse outcomes in clinical trials.

Sequestration of Documentation   As part of an investigation, all pertinent documentation should be obtained and copies kept for safe-keeping, pending the disposition of the matter. This does not mean, however, that the original documents must be sequestered; rather, verified copies can be maintained. These copies should be date- and time-stamped to indicate when the photocopies were prepared along with the name and position of the person doing it. Most qualified health information specialists are conversant with applicable state laws that address the issue of usual and customary business practices that may be used to prepare a credible, authenticated copy of such records. Taking these measures does not impede the use of the original record for purposes of on-going clinical trials work or the treatment of the research subject.

Sequestration of Ancillary Record Information   Paper documentation alone is not sufficient for purposes of an adverse event investigation. As with hard copy information, verified copies should be made of electronic record data. This can be preserved in a format that is timed and dated and impenetrable to modification. It also should include the name and title of the individual who makes the reproduction. A recognized process should be used so that the reproduction will be considered authentic.

Sequestration of Equipment   It is important to secure any devices involved in an adverse event. This includes investigational devices. Care should be taken in the handling of such equipment, too. Specific procedures should be in place to address who can examine the device and whether the equipment is removed from the premises for this purpose. Manufacturer's warranty language often carries warnings that any tampering with or removal of the factory seal on a device breaches the warranty. However, when the manufacturer's representative and a biomedical engineer from a reputable third party examine the device, this does not void the warranty. The idea of a third party viewing investigational devices can prove very sensitive. Confidentiality agreements may be necessary to allay fears of potential theft of intellectual property information. The representative from the third-party biomedical engineering firm may examine the device and document or testify about the findings, but he or she is precluded for sharing or using the information for any other purpose.

Interviews   An important part of the adverse event investigation is to get information from first-hand observers. The interviews should be carefully constructed to avoid bias or presuppositions about what transpired. The interview process should include those involved in the event, from those who prepared the trial, test article, or equipment to the person carrying out the trial. Interviews with the study subject are equally important. Documentation of the interviews should include the following:

→ Name of the subject of the interview

→ Interviewer's name and title

→ Time, date, and location

→ List of questions posed

→ Responses to questions

Process Indicators   An adverse event investigation can be time-consuming and expensive. Since the results may mean suspension of a trial or a regulatory investigation for subject safety non-compliance, it is important that there be a consistent, meticulous approach to examining adverse events. A series of process indicators can be used to ensure a consistent approach to adverse event investigations. These indicators are essentially a series of prompts to thoroughly aid those conducting the investigation. Figure 10.1 delineates some suggested adverse event indicators.

Develop a Visual Algorithm for Adverse Event Investigations   For those who must manage an adverse event, a flowchart can be very useful. It would depict the steps to take in identifying, managing, and reporting an adverse event involving clinical trials.

Determination: Does the Adverse Event Require Reporting   One of the important aspects of the investigation is determining the types of reports that must be

FIGURE 10.1.   Identified opportunities for process improvement

---

Identify processes involved in the event:
- Consent
- Confidentiality
- Medication
- Surgery
- Radiation
- Chemotherapy
- Physical therapy
- Psychotherapy
- Behavioral Management/Modification
- Investigational device
- Investigational new drug
- Clinical Trial Staff education and training
- Education and training for research subjects or family members
- Combination investigational device and conventional treatment (describe treatment)
- Combination investigational drug and conventional treatment (describe treatment)
- Identification of onset of adverse event
- Communication linked to identification of onset of adverse event
- Reporting of adverse event
- Treatment for adverse event

Authenticated copies of relevant documentation obtained?
Authenticated copies of electronic files obtained?
Equipment sequestered?
Interviews completed

Name   Title (if applicable)   Date of Interview   Interviewer

For each process identified
- Was there a process variance?
- No
- If yes: describe variance

---

made subsequent to an adverse event. The threshold consideration, however, is determining if the outcome constitutes an adverse event. Once a determination has been made there could be a host of reporting obligations. It is useful to remember too, that what constitutes a reportable event for one purpose may not meet the requirements for another constituency. For example, an end-user device-related serious injury may trigger reporting under the Safe Medical Device Act and its accompanying regulations. If an individual is receiving both accepted treatment (patient) and an experimental protocol (research subject), there may be no obligation to report the situation to the IRB. In practical terms, however, it may be prudent to notify the IRB that a nonresearch aspect of the subject's treatment led to an adverse outcome. Moreover, even if federal regulations do not trigger a reporting obligation in such situations, a contract with a private sponsor may do so. Hence the sponsor of an experimental drug under investigation for treatment of cancer might want to know that the serious injury to a study subject came about *not* as a result of the study but for totally different reasons. An investigation should yield sufficient information to make a reporting determination.

Determining to Whom to Report Adverse Events

An adverse event may trigger reporting obligations under several federal, state, and contractual requirements. Questions asked in making determinations can include the following:

- Did the event stem from a clinical protocol or was the individual a participant in a clinical trial *and* a patient receiving accepted treatment?

- Did the event involve an approved or an investigational device?

- Did the event involve an approved drug or drug under investigation?

- Did the event involve an approved drug that was being tested for a new use?

- Did the adverse event result in the unexpected death of the subject?

- Did the adverse event occur in a JCAHO accredited facility? If so, did it constitute a reviewable event?

- Did the adverse event trigger a mandatory reporting obligation under applicable state law?

- Under the terms of a sponsor's agreement, does the adverse event require a mandatory report?

- Under the policies and procedures of the IRB, do the facts require reporting of an adverse event?

- Under the terms of the protocol, the policies and procedures of the IRB, or the sponsor's agreement, does the adverse event necessitate a notification to other facilities carrying out the same or similar studies?

- Under the policies and procedures of the healthcare facility or Contract Research Organization, is there a requirement to notify either the quality or risk management officer about the adverse event?

- If the facility in which the adverse event took place is obliged to follow the Conditions of Participation for Hospitals under Medicare or Medicaid, is there a requirement to notify senior management of subject complaints or grievances linked to a research-related adverse event?

- If the healthcare organization has a corporate compliance plan, is there a responsibility to notify the compliance officer about a research-related adverse event?

- Is there a responsibility to notify liability insurance carriers about a research-related adverse event? If the healthcare organization has an insurance captive, is there an obligation to report to the captive manager?

- If the adverse event is related to competency, misrepresentation, fraud, deceit, or unprofessional conduct, is there an obligation to report to state licensing bodies or the Federal Office of Research Integrity?

Depending on the circumstances of a specific case, the answer may be that there are *multiple* reporting obligations. Some reporting obligations may compete with or conflict with one another in terms of order of priority and the amount of detail to be provided in each instance.

To be certain that all the necessary reports are made, it is suggested that the IRB and research office personnel work together to develop a reporting matrix tool. A sample is provided on page 22. Developed by a team of key stakeholders, the tool would provide a common ground for determining when reports should be made, to whom, and in what priority. Any concerns about adverse event reporting would be referred to the risk   management department or legal counsel. The multidisciplinary approach is important to capture information about the need to report. Thus, the design team may include representatives from the IRB, legal counsel, research office staff, compliance, risk management, and accreditation. As both state and federal laws are changed with respect to reporting, the tool should be updated accordingly. To be certain that adverse events do not go unreported, the matrix should be provided to principal investigators and their key administrative staff. Protocol approval should be contingent upon meeting the IRB's policy on adverse event reporting. Training on the importance of reporting should also be included in the process.

Multiple Adverse Event Reporting Obligations

There is always the chance that one adverse event report may appear contradictory to another about the same adverse event. Remember what is required for meeting the reporting obligations for a specific purpose. For example, a sponsor's agreement may oblige the principal investigator to report the deaths of all study subjects. It may go on to specify, however, to provide a detailed report only if the subject's death was known to be or believed to be related to the investigational device. The result would be that the sponsor would never know that a medication was involved in the subject's demise. This detailed information may be part of a root cause analysis completed by the JCAHO accredited hospital in which the person was a participant in the research trial. These reports might appear contradictory. However, on further review, each report is made for a *specific purpose* and in each instance the information supplied met the reporting requirements.

Difficulties can arise, when those required to receive essentially the same information end up with contradictory reports. This is not acceptable, and all reports should be reviewed carefully to be certain that the information is accurate and complete. Inconsistencies should trigger a further review of the situation.

Disclosure of Adverse Event Information to Research Subjects

Subjects should be told when it is determined that they have experienced a research-related adverse event. Doing so is part of the ongoing communication that is so important in restoring public confidence in the safety of human clinical trials. That an adverse event has occurred *does not* mean, however, that there must be an admission of liability or culpability. In fact, it may be some time before an investigation determines the cause or causes of the adverse event. What subjects want to know is quite understandable:

- What does this mean to me?
- Will I recover?
- How long will it take?
- Does this episode mean I am out of the study?
- Who pays for my continued care?
- I want to complain about what happened. Who do I contact?

A related issue is what should be disclosed to the subject's family or the legally authorized representative. If the subject has authorized the involvement of family members or surrogates, there should be no difficulty in disclosing information about the adverse event. However, if a subject specifically asked that information not be revealed to family members or a legally authorized representative, that request should be respected. Some exception may be permitted under the terms of state law or the impending HIPAA regulations dealing with health information.

What may be more problematic for some investigators is revealing to unaffected research subjects that other participants have experienced adverse events. Some would argue that by disclosing this information, investigators could bias the study by planting the suggestion of possibly experiencing similar adverse events. Others would argue that it is important to be open and honest with subjects and to let them know when adverse events have become a documented part of the study. In between these viewpoints is a third perspective. This middle stance looks to the facts and circumstances of the adverse event. If it is one that is likely to be experienced throughout the study population, it is information that subjects should receive so that they can pinpoint it and take appropriate action. However, if it is a rare event, the IRB may not require the investigator to disclose this finding if it were to jeopardize the integrity of the study, if the research could not carry on if the information were revealed, and if the risk of harm to other subjects is minimal. At the very least, once the adverse event is known to occur, the IRB and sponsor should be notified so that an ethical and legal decision can be made upon disseminating information to the study population.

Directions for Adverse Event Reporting by Research Subjects

Research subjects need clear, understandable information regarding what is considered an adverse event. Some reactions to test drugs may not be adverse events. Instead, the outcomes may be anticipated reactions. To be certain that subjects understand what is an adverse event and what they should do when such an event occurs, research coordinators should do the following:

- Develop some standard information to be provided to all research subjects.
- Test the required comprehension level of the tool by using it among a sample of individuals who would be research subjects and those who would act as their legally authorized representatives.
- Adjust the language to meet the reading level of the would-be study population.
- Develop in-service training for investigators and their staff regarding practical ways to teach subjects to identify and report adverse events.
- Obtain input from and the approval of the IRB for the standard format.

The Duty to Warn Research Subjects About Emergency Treatment for Adverse Events

Because many research studies are based in hospitals or near such facilities, subjects are often encouraged to seek assistance at the hospital emergency department. Some research consent documents or instruction sheets may state, "Should you experience a problem and you are unable to contact us, please proceed to *our* [or the named] emergency department and *they* will be able to assist you." This type of language often alarms healthcare attorneys and risk managers, as it creates the impression that there is a legal relationship between the study and the hospital emergency department.

Moreover, it is seen as creating a false sense of security in the emergency department based on the phrase "they will take care of you." The emergency department personnel may not have any idea that the individual is enrolled in a study, and even if that information was known, they may not know what is involved and if in fact it relates to the presenting ailment.

A related concern is the notation in the instruction sheet that directs subjects to "call or e-mail our office night or day if you have an adverse event or problem." Unless the phone line or e-mail system *is* manned around the clock, a research subject could be waiting hours for a response. What might have been a manageable adverse event at the outset may become impossible to control. The false expectation of a manned phone line or e-mail system could create an unwanted liability risk exposure.

There are several practical options for researchers to explore to avoid needless delay in responding to an adverse event:

- Provide a phone "roll over" service through which calls that are not picked up after five or six rings are forwarded to a manned call center.

- Make certain the call center can get a research staff member to respond to the subject within a defined time period.

- Use a pager system that can be manned twenty-four hours every day.

- Have the e-mail message system linked to a pager, cell phone, or personal data assistant (PDA) to alert the on-call research staff member to respond to the subject.

- Perform quality audits to be certain that voice and e-mail messages are answered within a designated time period.

If a decision is made to encourage subjects to seek emergency services at a designated facility, or to telephone an on-call medical group, it is important that the facility or group have sufficient background information on the study with which to plan appropriate treatment. This is why there is merit in providing subjects with a MedicAlert style bracelet or necklace. With pertinent information such as the study number, subject identifier, a manned toll-free number to call or Internet Web address to contact, the MedicAlert style notification provides caregivers with important details needed in treating a subject who presents with an adverse event.

············

CONCLUSION

Research subject safety will remain a core issue for regulators and subjects. Steps can be taken to minimize needless risk exposure to research subjects. Communications, documentation practices, training, and managing adverse events are important considerations in developing a culture of safety for clinical trials. Strong investigatory tools, methodologies, and reporting practices help to develop the necessary infrastructure for a safe environment of research for clinical trials subjects. Knowing to whom to report and when are also factors to consider in developing a culture of safety in human research.

References

FDA. Guidance for Clinical Trial Sponsors On the Establishment and Operation of Clinical Trial Data Monitoring Committees (Draft Guidance). November 2001.

Institutional Review Boards: A Time for Reform. OEI-01-97-00193, June, 1998.

Institute of Medicine, *Preserving Public Trust: Accreditation and Human Research Protection Programs,* 2001.

Institute of Medicine, *Responsible Research: A Systems Approach to Protecting Research Participants.,* October 3, 2002.

Joint Commission on Accreditation of Healthcare Organizations, Sentinel Event Policy And Procedures, Revised: July 2002.

NIH. Further Guidance on Data and Safety Monitoring for Phase I and Phase II Trials (OD-00-038), June 5, 2000.

NIH. Guidance on Reporting Adverse Events to Institutional Review Boards for NIH-supported Multicenter Clinical Trials. June 11, 1999. [http://grants.nih.gov/grants/guide/notice-files/not99-107.html].

NIH. Policy for Data and Safety Monitoring, June 10, 1998. [http://www.nih.gov/grants/guide/notice-files/not98-084.html].

OHRP. *Guidance on Continuing Review.* July 11, 2002.

OIG. *Protecting Human Research Subjects: Status of Recommendations.* (OEI-01-97-00197) April 2000.

OPRR. *Institutional Review Board Guidebook,* Chap. III, sec. E.

Protecting Human Research Subjects–Status of Recommendations, OEI-01-97-00197, April 2000.

To Err is Human, Institute of Medicine, November, 1999.

45 CFR Part §46.103(5) (2001).

21 CFR §312.32 (2001).

The PROACT Patient Safety Suite,™ The Reliability Center, Hopewell, Virginia, www.reliability.com

Woods, J. and Rozovsky, F. *How Do I Say It?* San Francisco: Jossey-Bass, 2003.

11

Human Research Under the Food, Drug & Cosmetic Act

The Steps of Scientific Research for Drug or Medical Device Approval 344
Investigational New Drug Application (IND) 344
Investigational Device Exemption (IDE) 345
The Definition of a Medical Device. 345
Offices at the FDA That an IRB May Contact to Determine
Whether an IND or IDE Is Required 345
The Common Rule and FDA Regulations. 345
The *Significant* Differences Between FDA and the Common
Rule Regulations for Clinical Research 346
A 510(k) Device 347
The Difference Between Marketing Approval
Under a 510(k) and Under a PMA 347
IRB Review of a Clinical Investigation Being Done
After Submission of a 510(k). 348
The Distinction Between Significant Risk and Nonsignificant
Risk in Medical Device Studies. 348
The Significance of the Distinction Between SR and NSR Device Studies 348
Sponsor Determination of Whether a Study Is SR or NSR. 349
The Information That a Sponsor Should Provide to an IRB
for an Investigational Device Protocol to Determine SR/NSR 349
IRB Determination of Whether a Study Is SR or NSR 349
IRB and Sponsor Responsibilities Following SR/NSR Determination 350
The Methodology for an IRB to Decide Whether a Device is SR or NSR 350
Defining Class I, II, and III Devices 351
General Controls. 352
Distinguishing Postamendments Devices and Preamendments Devices 352
FDA Regulations on IRB Review and Approval of
the Off-Label Use of a Marketed Drug or Device 352
Clinical Trials for Approval of Generic Drugs. 353
Defining an *Open* Label Protocol or an *Open* Protocol IND 353
Gender Issues That Should Be Considered by an IRB
in Clinical Trials for FDA Studies 353
Defining Compassionate Use 354

Defining a Treatment IND/IDE 354
IRB Approval of a Treatment IND/IDE 355
Local IRB Review: FDA Waiver Versus HHS Regulations 355
The Role of an IRB in Reviewing a Treatment IND 355
The Requirements for the Emergency Use Exception 355
A Physician's Responsibilities After Emergency Use
of a Nonapproved Medical Device 356
Informed Consent in the Emergency Use Setting 357
A Group C Drug. 357
Defining a Single Patient Use 357
The Parallel Track. 358
An IRB's Role in Reviewing a Parallel Track Protocol 358
The Protections of Patients in a Parallel Track 358
A Pharmacist's Special Duties in Dispensing an Investigational Drug 358
References 358

The Food and Drug Administration (FDA) established a set of regulations for clinical research involving human subjects in 1981. The FDA regulations pertaining to human subject research are codified in 21 CFR Part 50 (Protection of Human Subjects) and 21 CFR Part 56 (Institutional Review Boards). These apply to all clinical investigations regulated by the FDA, as well as clinical investigations that support applications for research or marketing permits for products regulated by the FDA (21 CFR Part 312). The FDA regulations were harmonized as much as possible to conform to the Common Rule (45 CFR Part 46) in 1991. However, these regulations have some *significant* variations from the Common Rule. This chapter will help the institution, researcher, and IRB to understand FDA regulation.

The Steps of Scientific Research for Drug or Medical Device Approval

The steps of research toward FDA approval are well defined by statute and regulation. New products are tested in vitro, followed by administration to laboratory animals. The product's sponsor submits an Investigational New Drug Application (IND) containing the test results to the FDA. If the FDA approves further research, additional studies will be conducted in a series of trials, commonly referred to as phases. At the conclusion of the trials, the sponsor submits a New Drug Application (NDA) containing complete reports of all investigations conducted. The FDA then determines whether to approve or deny the application after granting the sponsor an opportunity to be heard.

Investigational New Drug Application (IND)

A sponsor (for example, a drug manufacturer) will submit an Investigational New Drug Application (IND) to the FDA. The IND must include the complete composition of the drug, its source, how it is made, and all animal study data that support the drug's potential usefulness in humans and that define its toxicity; an investigational plan; detailed protocols for the trials; chemistry, manufacturing, and control information; pharmacology and toxicology information; previous human experience with the drug;

and dependence and abuse potential (21 CFR §312.23). The data should support the sponsor's representation that no human subject will be exposed to unreasonable risk. A protocol for testing in humans must be submitted. The sponsor must wait thirty days after submitting the IND to the FDA before commencing the clinical investigation protocol. The sponsor may begin testing at the end of the thirty-day period unless the FDA asks for additional time because of potential safety problems.

Investigational Device Exemption (IDE)

An investigational device is a medical device that is the subject of clinical research to determine its safety and efficacy. Clinical investigations are required to support a request for premarket approval. Such investigations that involve human subjects must be conducted according to the Investigational Device Exemption (IDE) regulations (21 CFR §812) or Investigational Exemptions for Intraocular Lenses (21 CFR §813).

The Definition of a Medical Device

The FDA defines a *medical device* as any instrument, apparatus, or other similar or related article, including component, part, or accessory, which is (a) recognized in the official National Formulary, or the United States Pharmacopeia, or any supplement to them; (b) intended for use in the diagnosis of disease or other conditions, or in the cure, mitigation, treatment, or prevention of disease, in humans or other animals; or (c) intended to affect the structure or any function of the human body or in animals; and does not achieve any of its principal intended purposes through chemical action within or on the human body or in animals and is not dependent upon being metabolized for the achievement of its principal intended purposes.

Offices at the FDA That an IRB May Contact to Determine Whether an IND or IDE Is Required

For drugs, an IRB may contact the Drug Information Branch, Center for Drug Evaluation and Research (CDER), at (301) 827-4573.

For a biological blood product, an IRB may contact the Office of Blood Research and Review, Center for Biologics Evaluation and Research (CBER), at (301) 827-3518. For a biological vaccine product, an IRB may contact the Office of Vaccines Research and Review at (301) 827-0648. For a biological therapeutic product, an IRB may contact the Office of Therapeutics Research and Review, CBER, at (301) 594-2860.

For a medical device, an IRB may contact the Program Operation Staff, Office of Device Evaluation, Center for Devices and Radiological Health (CDRH), at (301) 594-1190.

If an IRB is unsure about whether a test article is a drug, a biologic or a device, an IRB may contact the Health Assessment Policy Staff, Office of Health Affairs, at (301) 827-1685 (FDA, Information Sheets, 1998).

The Common Rule and FDA Regulations

On many occasions a study will be subject to the Common Rule, either because of funding sources or because of an institution's assurance. If the study involves a medication or device, FDA regulations are also likely to apply. Each federal agency that has jurisdiction over a study requires compliance with its regulations. For example, FDA regulations may permit the waiver of informed consent. However, the HHS regulations require informed consent. The IRB should require that the researcher obtain informed consent.

The *Significant* Differences Between FDA and the Common Rule Regulations for Clinical Research

The Department of Health and Human Services (HHS) regulations apply to research involving human subjects conducted by the HHS or funded in whole or in part by the HHS (45 CFR Part 46). The Food and Drug Administration (FDA) regulations apply to research involving products regulated by the FDA (21 CFR parts 50 and 56). Federal support is not necessary for the FDA regulations to be applicable. For research involving products regulated by the FDA that is funded, supported, or conducted by FDA and HHS, both the HHS and FDA regulations apply. The FDA has given the following guidance as to *significant* differences between FDA and HHS regulations:

<u>IRB Regulations</u>

§56.102 (FDA) §46.102 (HHS)	FDA definitions are included for terms specific to the type of research covered by the FDA regulations (test article, application for research or marketing permit, clinical investigation). A definition for emergency use is provided in the FDA regulations.
§56.104 (FDA) §46.116 (HHS)	FDA provides exemption from the prospective IRB review requirement for "emergency use" of test article in specific situations. HHS regulations state that they are not intended to limit the provision of emergency medical care.
§56.105 (FDA) §46.101 (HHS)	FDA provides for sponsors and sponsor-investigators to request a waiver of IRB review requirements (but not informed consent requirements). HHS exempts certain categories of research and provides for a Secretarial waiver.
§56.109 (FDA) §46.109 (HHS) §46.117(c) (HHS)	Unlike HHS, FDA does <u>not</u> provide that an IRB may waive the requirement for signed consent when the <u>principal</u> risk is a breach of confidentiality because FDA does not regulate studies which would fall into that category of research. (Both regulations allow for IRB waiver of <u>documentation</u> of informed consent in instances of minimal risk.)
§56.110 (FDA) §46.110 (HHS)	The FDA list of investigations eligible for expedited review (published in the Federal Register) does not include the studies described in category 9 of the HHS list because these types of studies are not regulated by FDA
§56.114 (FDA) §46.114 (HHS)	FDA does not discuss administrative matters dealing with grants and contracts because they are irrelevant to the scope of the Agency's regulation. (Both regulations make allowances for review of multi-institutional studies.)
§56.115 (FDA) §46.115 (HHS)	FDA has neither an assurance mechanism nor files of IRB membership. Therefore, FDA does not require the IRB or institution to report changes in membership whereas HHS does require such notification.

| §56.115(c) (FDA) | FDA may refuse to consider a study in support of a research or marketing permit if the IRB or the institution refuses to allow FDA to inspect IRB records. HHS has no such provision because it does not issue research or marketing permits. |
| §56.120 — §56.124 (FDA) | FDA regulations provide sanctions for non-compliance with regulations. |

Informed Consent Regulations

§50.23 (FDA)	FDA, but not HHS, provides for an exception from the informed consent requirements in emergency situations. The provision is based on the Medical Device Amendments of 1976, but may be used in investigations involving drugs, devices, and other FDA regulated products in situations described in §50.23.
§46.116(c) & (d) (HHS)	HHS provides for waiving or altering elements of informed consent under certain conditions. FDA has no such provision because the types of studies which would qualify for such waivers are either not regulated by FDA or are covered by the emergency treatment provisions (§50.23).
§50.25(a)(5) (FDA) §46.116(a)(5) (HHS)	FDA explicitly requires that subjects be informed that FDA may inspect the records of the study because FDA may occasionally examine a subject's medical records when they pertain to the study. While HHS has the right to inspect records of studies it funds, it does not impose that same informed consent requirement.
§50.27(a)	FDA explicitly requires that consent forms be dated as well as signed by the subject or the subject's legally authorized representative. The HHS regulations do not explicitly require consent forms to be dated.

A 510(k) Device

A medical device that is substantially equivalent to a device that was or is being legally marketed is covered by section 510(k) of the Food, Drug & Cosmetic Act. The legally marketed device is referred to as a *predicate device*. A sponsor planning to market a substantially equivalent device must submit notification to the FDA ninety days in advance of placing the device on the market. If the FDA agrees with the sponsor, the device may then be marketed.

The Difference Between Marketing Approval Under a 510(k) and Under a PMA

A 510(k) application by a sponsor demonstrates that a new device is substantially equivalent to another device that is legally on the market without a Premarket Approval (PMA). If the FDA agrees that the new device is substantially equivalent, it can be marketed. Clinical data are not required in most 510(k) applications; however if clinical data are necessary to demonstrate substantial equivalence, the clinical studies need to be conducted in compliance with the requirements of the IDE regulations, IRB review, and informed consent (21 CFR parts 812, 56, and 50, respectively) (FDA, Frequently Asked Questions About IRB Review of Medical Devices, #2).

IRB Review of a Clinical Investigation Being Done After Submission of a 510(k)

An IRB must review any clinical study, even of a 510(k) device. If it's research related to a drug or medical device, then FDA regulations apply and an IRB should review it (21 CFR Part 50 and Part 56). A 510(k) allows commercial distribution but does not address research use. A 510(k) application can take time to process, during which it remains an investigational product. It cannot be distributed except for investigational use until the FDA approves the 510(k) application (FDA, Frequently Asked Questions About IRB Review of Medical Devices, #9).

The Distinction Between Significant Risk and Nonsignificant Risk in Medical Device Studies

FDA regulations for Investigational Device Exemption (IDE) (21 CFR part 812) describe two types of device studies, significant risk (SR) and nonsignificant risk (NSR). An SR device study is defined as a study of a device that presents a potential for serious risk to the health, safety, or welfare of a participant and (1) is intended as an implant; or (2) is used in supporting or sustaining human life; or (3) is of substantial importance in diagnosing, curing, mitigating, or treating disease, or otherwise prevents impairment of human health; or (4) otherwise presents a potential for serious risk to the health, safety, or welfare of a participant (21 CFR §812.3(m)). An NSR device investigation is one that does not meet the definition for a significant risk study. NSR device studies, however, should not be confused with the concept of minimal risk, a term utilized in the FDA's IRB regulations (21 CFR part 56) to identify certain studies that may be approved through an expedited review procedure. For both SR and NSR device studies, IRB review and approval prior to conducting clinical trials and continuing review are required (21 CFR part 50).

The Significance of the Distinction Between SR and NSR Device Studies

The effect of the SR/NSR decision is very important to research sponsors and investigators. SR device studies are governed by the IDE regulations (21 CFR Part 812). NSR device studies have fewer regulatory controls than SR studies and are governed by the abbreviated requirements (21 CFR §812.2(b)). The major differences are in the FDA approval process and in the record keeping and reporting requirements. The SR/NSR decision is also important to the FDA because the IRB serves, in a sense, as the FDA's surrogate with respect to review and approval of NSR studies. FDA is usually not apprised of the existence of approved NSR studies because sponsors and IRBs are not required to report NSR device study approvals to the FDA. If an investigator or a sponsor proposes the initiation of a claimed NSR investigation to an IRB, and if the IRB agrees that the device study is NSR and approves the study, the investigation may begin at that institution immediately, without submission of an IDE application to the FDA.

If an IRB believes that a device study is SR, the investigation may not begin until both the IRB and FDA approve the investigation. To help in the determination of the risk status of the device, an IRB should review information such as reports of prior investigations conducted with the device, the proposed investigational plan, a description of participant selection criteria, and monitoring procedures. The sponsor should provide the IRB with a risk assessment and the rationale used in making its risk determination (21 CFR §812.150(b)(10)).

Sponsor Determination of Whether a Study Is SR or NSR

The assessment of whether or not a device study is NSR is initially made by the sponsor. If the sponsor considers that a study is NSR, the sponsor provides the reviewing IRB an explanation of its determination and any other information that may assist the IRB in evaluating the risk of the study including determinations by other IRBs. The sponsor must inform the IRB of the FDA's assessment of the device's risk if such an assessment has been made. The IRB may also seek the FDA's opinion.

The IRB may agree or disagree with the sponsor's initial NSR assessment. If the IRB agrees with the sponsor's initial NSR assessment and approves the study, the study may begin without submission of an IDE application to the FDA. If the IRB disagrees, the sponsor must notify the FDA that an SR determination has been made regardless of whether the study is ultimately conducted at the institution. The study can be conducted as an SR investigation following FDA approval of an IDE application.

The FDA makes the ultimate decision in determining if a device study is SR or NSR. If the Agency does not agree with an IRB's decision that a device study presents an NSR, an IDE application must be submitted to FDA. On the other hand, if a sponsor files an IDE with the FDA because it is presumed to be an SR study, but the FDA classifies the device study as NSR, the Agency will return the IDE application to the sponsor and the study would be presented to IRBs as an NSR investigation.

The Information That a Sponsor Should Provide to an IRB for an Investigational Device Protocol to Determine SR/NSR

In presenting an investigational device protocol for consideration by an IRB to determine SR versus NSR, a sponsor should provide the following to the IRB:

- A description of the device
- The study proposal/protocol
- An explanation of why the device study presents a *nonsignificant* risk
- Any other supporting information, such as reports of prior investigations
- A statement of whether the FDA or any other IRB has made a risk assessment and what the results of that assessment were

IRB Determination of Whether a Study Is SR or NSR

Full IRB review is required for determination of either SR or NSR medical device studies. If a NSR study is considered to be a minimal risk study, then an IRB's expedited review procedure can be used. Otherwise, IRB review of an investigational device study is the same as review of other studies.

The risk determination should be based on the proposed use of a device in an investigation, and not on the device alone. In deciding if a study poses an SR, an IRB must consider the nature of the harm that may result from use of the device. Studies where the potential harm to participants could be life-threatening, could result in permanent impairment of a body function or permanent damage to body structure, or could necessitate medical or surgical intervention to preclude permanent impairment of a body function or permanent damage to body structure should be considered SR. Also, if the participant must undergo a procedure as part of the investigational study, e.g., a surgical procedure, the IRB must consider the potential harm that could be caused by the procedure in addition to the potential harm caused by the device.

In the usual IRB review process, the IRB considers whether the risks to the participant are reasonable in relation to the anticipated benefits. The risks and benefits of the investigation are compared with the risks and benefits of alternative devices or procedures. This differs from the judgment about whether a study poses an SR or NSR, which is based solely upon the seriousness of the harm that may result from the use of the device.

The FDA gives the following examples in addition to extensive lists of products:

1. The study of a pacemaker that is a modification of a commercially available pacemaker poses an SR because the use of any pacemaker presents a potential for serious harm to the participants. This is true even though the modified pacemaker may pose less risk, or only slightly greater risk, in comparison with the commercially available model. The amount of potential reduced or increased risk associated with the investigational pacemaker should only be considered (in relation to possible decreased or increased benefits) when assessing whether the study can be approved.

2. The study of an extended-wear contact lens is considered SR because wearing the lens continuously overnight while sleeping presents a potential for injuries not normally seen with daily wear lenses, which are considered NSR.

IRB and Sponsor Responsibilities Following SR/NSR Determination

If the IRB decides that a study is Significant Risk (SR), the IRB must notify the sponsor and investigator of the decision.

After the sponsor obtains an IDE, the IRB can proceed to review the study applying the usual criteria (21 CFR §56.111). If the IRB determines that the study is Not Significant Risk (NSR), then it may proceed with its usual review of the study for approval. The FDA considers studies of all SR devices to present more than minimal risk. Therefore, full IRB review for all studies involving SR devices is necessary. Usually, similar review of NSR studies is required. However, some NSR studies may qualify as minimal risk, and the IRB may elect to review those studies under its expedited review procedures.

The sponsor has the responsibility to submit an IDE to the FDA or, if deciding not to proceed with the study, notify the FDA of the SR determination. The study may not begin until the FDA has approved the IDE and the IRB has approved the study. If the study is NSR, then the sponsor and investigator must follow the abbreviated IDE requirements (21 CFR §812.2(b)).

The Methodology for an IRB to Decide Whether a Device Is SR or NSR

The FDA advises that an IRB should use its best abilities, the information in the regulations and the guidelines, and the risk evaluation provided by the applicant. An IRB can, as always, seek outside assistance. An IRB should have written policies and procedures regarding device review (FDA, Frequently Asked Questions About IRB Review of Medical Devices, #5).

Like other activities, an IRB that reviews study protocols to determine whether a device is SR or NSR must have written procedures in how it will conduct its deliberations on the topic. Regulation 21 CFR §56.108(a)(1) requires an IRB to follow written procedures for conducting its initial review of research and for reporting its findings and actions to the investigator. The procedures followed in determining whether a study is SR or NSR should be included among those written procedures. When an IRB determines that an investigation presented for approval as involving an NSR device actually involves an SR device, 21 CFR §812.66 requires the IRB to notify the investigator and, where appropriate, the sponsor (FDA, Frequently Asked Questions About IRB Review of Medical Devices, #6).

Defining Class I, II, and III Devices

Medical devices are classified as Class I, Class II, or Class III, depending on the following criteria:

- Class I medical devices are those such that their safety and efficacy can be ensured by the general controls of the 1976 Medical Device Amendments to the Food, Drug & Cosmetic Act.

- Class II medical devices must comply with the general controls. In addition the sponsor must provide enough information about the device to establish special controls that are sufficient to provide assurance. Examples of special controls are promulgation of performance standards, postmarket surveillance, and patient registries.

- Class III devices are those that (1) their safety and effectiveness cannot be reasonably ensured through either general or special controls; and (2) they are life-sustaining, life-supporting, implanted in the body, or of substantial importance in preventing impairment to health.

When a manufacturer develops a new device that it contends is the substantial equivalent of a currently marketed device (predicate device), the manufacturer must notify the FDA of its intent to market the device. If the FDA concurs with the manufacturer, the device can be marketed without further approval. If the FDA does not concur, the device will be automatically classified as a Class III device, and premarket approval from the FDA is required. The sponsor can petition the FDA to reclassify the device to Class I or Class II.

The distinctions among Class I, II, and III are made primarily on the level of risk to patients and, therefore, the level of FDA oversight needed to ensure that the device is safe and effective as labeled. Generally, but not always, this corresponds to logical risk evaluations (FDA, Frequently Asked Questions About IRB Review of Medical Devices, #1). A few examples follow:

Class I:	General controls	crutches, Band-Aids
Class II:	Special controls	wheelchairs, tampons
Class III:	Premarket Approval	heart valves (known to present hazards requiring clinical demonstration of safety and effectiveness)—OR—not enough known about safety or effectiveness to assign to Class I or II

General Controls

General Controls are certain FDA statutory provisions designed to control the safety of marketed drugs and devices. These include provisions on adulteration, misbranding, banned devices, good manufacturing practices, notification and record keeping, and other sections of the 1976 Medical Device Amendments to the Food, Drug & Cosmetic Act (21 U.S.C. §360(c) and §513).

Distinguishing Postamendments Devices and Preamendments Devices

Medical devices marketed after enactment of the 1976 Medical Device Amendments are referred to as *postamendments devices*. Medical devices marketed before the enactment of the 1976 Medical Device Amendments are called *preamendments devices*.

FDA Regulations on IRB Review and Approval of the Off-Label Use of a Marketed Drug or Device

The FDA requires that an IRB approve off-label use of a marketed drug or device if the off-label use is part of a research project involving human subjects. IRB approval is not required if the off-label use is intended to be solely the practice of medicine, such as for a physician treating a patient and no research is being done (FDA, Frequently Asked Questions About IRB Review of Medical Devices, #7). The FDA has given the following guidance.

Off-Label Use of Marketed Drugs, Biologics, and Medical Devices

Good medical practice and the best interests of the patient require that physicians use legally available drugs, biologics, and devices according to their best knowledge and judgment. If physicians use a product for an indication not in the approved labeling, they have the responsibility to be well informed about the product, to base its use on firm scientific rationale and on sound medical evidence, and to maintain records of the product's use and effects. Use of a marketed product in this manner when the intent is the practice of medicine does not require the submission of an Investigational New Drug Application (IND), Investigational Device Exemption (IDE), or review by an IRB. However, the institution at which the product will be used may, under its own authority, require IRB review or other institutional oversight.

Investigational Use of Marketed Drugs, Biologics, and Medical Devices

The investigational use of approved, marketed products differs from the situation just described. "Investigational use" suggests the use of an approved product in the context of a clinical study protocol (21 CFR §312.3(b)). When the principal intent of the investigational use of a test article is to develop information about the product's safety or efficacy, submission of an IND or IDE may be required. However, according to 21 CFR §312.2(b)(1), the clinical investigation of a marketed drug or biologic does not require submission of an IND if all six of the following conditions are met:

1. It is not intended to be reported to FDA in support of a new indication for use or to support any other *significant* change in the labeling for the drug.

2. It is not intended to support a *significant* change in the advertising for the product.

3. It does not involve a route of administration or dosage level, use in a subject population, or other factor that significantly increases the risks (or decreases the acceptability of the risks) associated with the use of the drug product.

4. It is conducted in compliance with the requirements for IRB review and informed consent (21 CFR parts 56 and 50).

5. It is conducted in compliance with the requirements concerning the promotion and sale of drugs (21 CFR §312.7).

6. It does not intend to invoke 21 CFR §50.24.

Clinical Trials for Approval of Generic Drugs

A sponsor does not need to conduct clinical trials if it files an Abbreviated New Drug Application (ANDA) stating that the new generic drug is the bioequivalent of a drug that has been previously approved. However, the sponsor must also certify that the new generic drug will not infringe on any valid patent (21 USC §355(j)).

Defining an *Open* Label Protocol or an *Open* Protocol IND

An open label protocol and an open protocol IND are usually uncontrolled studies, carried out to obtain additional safety data (Phase 3 studies). They are typically undertaken when the controlled trials have ended and treatment is continued so that the case participants and the control participants may continue to receive the benefits of the investigational drug until marketing approval is obtained. Like other studies, an open label protocol or an open protocol IND requires prospective IRB approval and other customary safeguards for participants (e.g. informed consent).

Gender Issues That Should Be Considered by an IRB in Clinical Trials for FDA Studies

Historically, most clinical trials used men as research subjects. Not only does this call into question the safety and efficacy of a medication, but the paternalistic approach of not letting women choose treatments for themselves has fallen out of favor. On July 22, 1993, the FDA published the Guideline for the Study and Evaluation of Gender Differences in the Clinical Evaluation of Drugs (58 FR 39406). Therein the FDA encourages the enrollment of women in clinical investigations to study any differences between genders as well as to let women decide for themselves. An IRB should consider the Guideline as part of its initial deliberations about protocols and ongoing surveillance of research for not only the cited drug and biologic testing but medical device studies also.

The Guideline has the following important changes in policy by the FDA:

1. The restriction on participation by most women with childbearing potential from entering Phase 1 and early Phase 2 trials is lifted, and their participation is now encouraged. Protocol designs should include monitoring for pregnancy as well as measures to prevent pregnancy during exposure to investigational agents. Pregnancy testing is recommended, and women must be counseled about the reliable use of contraception or abstinence from intercourse while participating in the clinical trial. Assistance of gynecology consultants is important to ensure appropriate steps in the protocol.

2. Sponsors should collect gender-related data during research and development and should analyze the data for gender effects in addition to other variables such as age

and race. FDA requires sponsors to include a fair representation of both genders as participants in clinical trials so that clinically *significant* gender-related differences in response can be detected. Collecting pharmacokinetics data on demographic differences beginning in the Phase 1 and 2 studies is important, so that relevant study designs are developed for later trials.

3. Three specific pharmacokinetics issues should be considered when feasible: (1) effect of the stages of the menstrual cycle; (2) effect of exogenous hormonal therapy including oral contraceptives; and (3) effect of the drug or biologic on the pharmacokinetics of oral contraceptives.

Defining Compassionate Use

The term compassionate use refers to allowing the use of investigational drugs outside of an ongoing clinical trial to a limited number of patients that are desperately ill and for whom no accepted alternative therapy is available. However, compassionate use does not appear in either FDA or HHS regulations. Therefore, using the term adds more confusion than assistance (OPRR, *Institutional Review Board Guidebook*). Communication is easier using the names of the specific programs, such as emergency use or Treatment IND, that allow access to investigational drugs outside of clinical trials.

Defining a Treatment IND/IDE

A *Treatment IND/IDE* is a procedure whereby the FDA allows investigational drugs or devices to be administered to very ill patients earlier in the development process. A Treatment IND may be approved by the FDA (21 CFR §312.34) where

- The drug is used to treat an immediately life-threatening or serious condition
- No satisfactory alternative drugs are available
- The drug is under investigation in a controlled clinical trial
- The sponsor of the clinical trial is actively seeking approval

A Treatment IND is a treatment protocol that is added to an existing investigational new drug application (IND). It allows physicians to treat qualifying patients according to the protocol. "The purpose of the *Treatment IND* exemption is to facilitate the availability of promising new drugs to desperately ill patients as early in the drug development process as possible (before marketing begins) and to obtain additional data on the drug's safety and effectiveness" (OPRR, *Institutional Review Board Guidebook*). A Treatment IND may be granted after sufficient data have been collected to show that the drug may be effective and does not have unreasonable risks. Because data related to safety and side effects are collected, Treatment INDs also serve to expand the body of knowledge about the drug.

Treatment IND studies require prospective IRB approval and the other usual safeguards for participants. A sponsor may apply to the FDA for a waiver of local IRB approval under a Treatment IND if it can be shown to be in the best interest of the participants, and if a satisfactory alternative mechanism for ensuring the protection of human participants is available (review by a central IRB). Such a waiver does not apply to the informed consent requirement. A local IRB may still opt to review a study even if the FDA has granted a waiver, pursuant to the institution's policy or state law.

IRB Approval of a Treatment IND/IDE

Test articles given to human subjects under a Treatment IND/IDE require prior IRB approval, with two exceptions. If a life-threatening emergency exists, as defined by 21 CFR §56.102(d), the procedures described in 56.104(c) ("Exemptions from IRB Requirement") may be followed. In addition, the FDA may grant the sponsor or sponsor/investigator a waiver of the IRB requirement in accord with 21 CFR §56.105. An IRB may still choose to review a study even if the FDA has granted a waiver of local IRB approval (FDA, Frequently Asked Questions About IRB Review of Medical Devices, #58).

Local IRB Review: FDA Waiver Versus HHS Regulations

Local IRB review may be required under HHS regulations even though the FDA has waived local IRB approval if the research is subject to regulation by both the FDA and HHS. In addition, the institution's Assurance is likely to require local IRB review despite FDA waiver. However, HHS may grant a waiver of its regulations. For example, HHS may waive some of its regulations for *Parallel Track* protocols (OPRR, *Institutional Review Board Guidebook*).

The Role of an IRB in Reviewing a Treatment IND

An IRB's role in reviewing a Treatment IND is the same as it is for reviewing any proposed protocol: "to determine whether the proposed use exposes the subjects to unreasonable or unnecessary risk, to review the informed consent forms and process, and to monitor the progress of the *Treatment IND*" (OPRR, *Institutional Review Board Guidebook*). An IRB must be very vigilant in reviewing a Treatment IND in which a patient is being charged for the cost of the investigational drug. "The question here is one of equitable selection and the involvement in research of vulnerable populations, particularly economically disadvantaged persons" (OPRR, *Institutional Review Board Guidebook*). An IRB must also be sensitive to the idea that the availability of a Treatment IND may create difficulty for an investigator to attract patients to Phase 3 clinical trials. To control this problem, the FDA may place a clinical hold on a Treatment IND (OPRR, *Institutional Review Board Guidebook*).

The Requirements for the Emergency Use Exception

Each of the following conditions must exist to justify *emergency use* without prior FDA and IRB approval of an investigational drug or device:

1. The patient is in a life-threatening condition that needs immediate treatment.

2. No generally acceptable alternative for treating the patient is available.

3. Because of the immediate need to use the device, there is no time to use existing procedures to get FDA approval for the use.

The FDA expects the physician to determine whether these criteria have been met, to assess the potential for benefits from the unapproved use of the device, and to have substantial reason to believe that benefits will exist. The physician may not conclude that an emergency exists in advance of the time when treatment may be needed based solely on the expectation that IDE approval procedures may require more time than is available. The FDA expects physicians to exercise reasonable foresight with respect to potential emergencies and to make appropriate arrangements under the IDE procedures far enough in advance to avoid creating a situation in which IDE procedures are impracticable.

The FDA recognizes that emergencies arise when an unapproved device may offer the only possible life-saving alternative, but an IDE for the device does not exist, or the proposed use is not approved under an existing IDE, or the physician or institution is not approved under the IDE. Using its enforcement discretion, FDA has not objected if a physician chooses to use an unapproved device in such an emergency, provided that the physician later justifies to the FDA that an emergency actually existed.

In the event that an investigational device is to be used in an emergency, the device developer must notify the Center for Devices and Radiological Health (CDRH), Program Operation Staff by telephone, (301) 594-1190, immediately after shipment is made. During nights and weekends, the device developer can contact the Division of Emergency and Epidemiological Operations, (202) 857-8400. The FDA makes a point of noting that an unapproved device may not be shipped in anticipation of an emergency.

The FDA expects the treating physician to follow as many human subject protection procedures as possible during emergency use of an investigational drug or device. These include

- Obtaining an independent assessment by an uninvolved physician
- Obtaining informed consent from the patient or a legal representative
- Notifying institutional officials as specified by institutional policies
- Notifying the Institutional Review Board (IRB)
- Obtaining authorization from the IDE holder, if an approved IDE for the device exists

A Physician's Responsibilities After Emergency Use of a Nonapproved Medical Device

After an unapproved device is used in an emergency, the physician should

1. Report to the IRB within five days (21 CFR §56.104(c)) and otherwise comply with provisions of the IRB regulations (21 CFR part 56)
2. Evaluate the likelihood of a similar need for the device occurring again, and if future use is likely, immediately initiate efforts to obtain IRB approval and an approved IDE for the device's subsequent use
3. If an IDE for the use does exist, notify the sponsor of the emergency use, or if an IDE does not exist, notify the FDA of the emergency use (CDRH Program Operation Staff, (301) 594-1190) and provide the FDA with a written summary of the conditions constituting the emergency, human subject protection measures, and results

Subsequent emergency use of an investigational device may not occur unless the treating physician or another person obtains approval of an IDE for the device and its use as well as IRB approval (21 CFR §56.102(d)). If an IDE application for subsequent use has been filed with the FDA and the FDA disapproves the IDE application, the device may not be used even if the circumstances constituting an emergency exist. The FDA has advised that developers of devices that could be used in emergencies should anticipate the likelihood of emergency use and should obtain an approved IDE for such uses.

Informed Consent in the Emergency Use Setting

Emergency use does not nullify the requirement for informed consent. Even for an emergency use, the investigator is required by the FDA to obtain informed consent of the patient or the patient's legally authorized representative unless both the investigator and a physician who is not otherwise participating in the clinical investigation certify in writing all of the following (21 CFR §50.23(a)):

1. The patient is confronted by a life-threatening situation necessitating the use of the test article.

2. Informed consent cannot be obtained because of an inability to communicate with, or obtain legally effective consent from, the patient.

3. Time is not sufficient to obtain consent from the patient's legal representative.

4. No alternative method of approved or generally recognized therapy is available that provides an equal or greater likelihood of saving the patient's life.

   If, in the investigator's opinion, immediate use of the test article is required to preserve the patient's life, and if time is not sufficient to obtain an independent physician's determination that the required four conditions apply, the clinical investigator should make the determination and, within five working days after the use of the article, have the determination reviewed and evaluated in writing by a physician who is not participating in the clinical investigation. The investigator must notify the IRB within five working days after the use of the test article (21 CFR §50.23(c)). The foregoing discussion is of the FDA regulations. State law may have more strict requirements for informed consent. See Chapter Five.

A Group C Drug

Investigational drugs are made available to cancer patients under a procedure similar to the Treatment IND. This is called *Group C*. A primary difference between a Treatment IND and a Group C protocol is that the latter is administered by the National Cancer Institute (NCI), not the FDA.

The Group C program is a means for the distribution of investigational agents to oncologists for the treatment of cancer under protocols outside controlled clinical trials. Group C drugs are generally Phase 3 study drugs that have shown evidence of relative and reproducible efficacy in a specific tumor type. Properly trained physicians can generally administer Group C drugs without the need for specialized supportive care facilities. Group C drugs are distributed only by the National Institutes of Health under NCI protocols. Although treatment is the primary objective and patients treated under Group C guidelines are not part of a clinical trial, safety and effectiveness data are collected. Because administration of Group C drugs is not done with research intent, the FDA has generally granted a waiver from IRB review requirements (21 CFR §56.105). However, an IRB may still choose to conduct a review under its policies and state regulations. The Group C Guideline Protocol contains an FDA-approved informed consent document that must be used if there is no local IRB review.

Defining a Single Patient Use

A *Single Patient Use* permits a physician to obtain access to an investigational drug for treatment of a single patient. This usually occurs when the patient is in a desperate situation and is unresponsive to other drugs or therapy, or when no approved or generally recognized treatment is available. The proposed therapy must be theoretically or anecdotally plausible even if little objective supportive data exists (21 CFR §312.35).

The Parallel Track

The Parallel Track program is intended to make promising investigational agents available as quickly as possible to patients with AIDS and other HIV-related diseases (*Federal Register* 57 (April 15, 1992): 13250–13259). The FDA permits access to promising investigational drugs for such patients who are not able to take standard therapy or for whom standard therapy is no longer effective, and who are not able to participate in ongoing clinical trials. Requests under the Parallel Track must be submitted to the FDA as amendments to an existing IND. This should be thought of as a subset of the Treatment IND.

In a Parallel Track to a traditional Phase 2 study, patients are enrolled that are not eligible for a clinical trial, are too ill to participate, or do not live in an area where a study is being conducted. The Parallel Track is open only to patients who cannot take an approved treatment because either it is contraindicated or it is not effective.

An IRB's Role in Reviewing a Parallel Track Protocol

While FDA and HHS regulations apply to *Parallel Track* protocols, local IRB review may be unworkable. However, local IRBs retain the option of reviewing the expanded availability side of a Parallel Track protocol. HHS and FDA will consider waiving local IRB review on a protocol-by-protocol basis. In reviewing the noncontrolled side of a Parallel Track protocol, an IRB should be very concerned with the informed consent process and patient recruitment as well as the usual concerns for participant safety.

The Protections of Patients in a Parallel Track

The usual protections of an IND are extended to patients in a Parallel Track. However, the FDA may waive local IRB approval and use a national human subject protection review panel to review protocols and provide ongoing oversight. The FDA may terminate a Parallel Track if the FDA determines that patients are being exposed to significant unreasonable risks, the Parallel Track is interfering with the controlled clinical trials, clinical trial results indicate that the drug is not effective, or a different drug has a better risk-benefit profile (Final Policy Notice, 57 Fed. Reg. 13,250 (1992)).

A Pharmacist's Special Duties in Dispensing an Investigational Drug

A pharmacist must be aware that investigational drugs must be labeled as such (21 CFR §312.6). Dispensing must be limited to the procedures set forth in the research protocol. The pharmacist is responsible for the security, record keeping, and disposal of the investigational drug.

References

21 CFR Part 312.23

21 CFR Part 50

21 CFR Part 51

21 CFR Part 56

21 CFR §312

21 CFR §360

45 CFR Part 46

45 CFR §812

45 CFR §813

21 USC §355(j)

57 FR 13250. Final Policy Notice. (1992).

58 FR 39406.

FDA. Frequently Asked Questions About IRB Review of Medical Devices.

Office for Protection from Research Risk. *Institutional Review Board Guidebook.*

12

Behavior Research

Classic Behavior Research Techniques 361
Behavior Research That Is Exempt from Federal Regulations
for Protection of Human Subjects 362
Considerations for an IRB in Reviewing Behavior Research Protocols 362
The Extent to Which Information Must Be Disclosed if It Would
Affect the Validity of the Research Findings 363
Unique Issues of Fieldwork for an IRB to Consider 363
Considerations in Reviewing and Approving Research Involving Depressed
or Suicidal Patients 363
Unique Issues of Behavioral Research on HIV. 364
References 364

The distinction between biomedical research and behavioral research is often blurred. Biomedical research is classically thought of as that which measures a physiologic condition, such as the quantity of red blood cells. In contrast, behavior research is classically thought of as that which measures social or psychological responses. Often, however, a study may have components of both biomedical and behavioral research. For example, a study may measure the vital sign (pulse, blood pressure, respiration) response of a study participant who is watching a violent movie. Trying to categorize this as either biomedical or behavior research is a futile exercise. The more important issue is to ensure that the protocol is designed appropriately to produce scientifically valuable results and protect the human participants. This chapter will focus on issues more often present in behavior research.

Classic Behavior Research Techniques

Questionnaires, observation, studies of existing records, and experimental design involving exposure to some type of stimulus or intervention are the traditional techniques used in behavior research. Endless variations are used within these four categories. For example, questionnaires may be conducted by in-person interviews, mail, telephone, Internet, or other media.

Behavior Research That Is Exempt from Federal Regulations for Protection of Human Subjects

Review of anonymous data, such as census data, observations in public places, and other studies that do not directly identify an individual or directly affect an individual are generally exempt from federal regulations for protection of human subjects. See 45 CFR §46.101. However, an institution may still require IRB approval of such studies pursuant to its policies or state law.

Considerations for an IRB in Reviewing Behavior Research Protocols

Most behavior research does not expose participants to physical intervention or physical harm. However, participants may be exposed to social harm, as in harm to reputation, embarrassment, or financial injury. As with all research protocols, confidentiality is important in behavioral research. This is especially important to avoid any social harm to the participants. Participants may also be exposed to psychological harm, such as unwelcome revelations about themselves or deception as to whether events occurred. Deception should be kept to a minimum. If deception is necessary, then safeguards (such as debriefing) should be considered.

An IRB needs to be conscious whether the proposed study is morally wrong. This is a challenging dilemma for any group to ponder. Deceiving the participants and invading their privacy are two common examples of potential moral wrongs. How far is the potential moral wrong allowed to go in the pursuit of scientific knowledge? The proposed study should be able to justify the use of deception or invasion of privacy. A more controversial challenge is whether the social morals of the IRB members should be considered in the review and approval of research protocols. For example, the study of sexual activity among street people might be repugnant to some while others may find it scientifically important.

An IRB should be careful to avoid any social class distinction as to what studies are permissible. For example, would the proposed study of Medicaid recipients be as acceptable if the same questions were asked of college professors? The ethics of behavioral research among racial or ethnic groups is very controversial. In the past, for example, such studies have been used, or abused, to argue racial superiority. Interestingly, the former OPRR stated, "The possible use—or misuse—of research findings, however, should not be a matter for IRB review, despite the importance of this question." The government agency goes on to add:

> IRBs should resist placing restrictions on research because of its subject matter; IRBs should instead be concerned about research methods and the rights and welfare of research subjects. IRBs must differentiate disapproving a research proposal because of qualms about the subject being explored or its possible findings, such as genetic differences in intelligence, from disapproving research involving the performance of illegal or unethical acts. The former raises serious issues of academic freedom; the latter is quite different and appropriate. Whatever the propriety of institutional administrators prohibiting research to protect the institution from being associated with controversial or sensitive subjects, it is generally agreed that this is not an appropriate concern for an IRB, whose function is to protect human subjects.

[OPRR, *Institutional Review Board Guidebook,* Chap. V, sec. A]

The Extent to Which Information Must Be Disclosed if It Would Affect the Validity of the Research Findings

The Belmont Report states that:

> In many cases, it is sufficient to indicate to subjects that they are being invited to participate in research of which some features will not be revealed until the research is concluded. In all cases of research involving incomplete disclosure, such research is justified only if it is clear that (1) incomplete disclosure is truly necessary to accomplish the goals of the research, (2) there are no undisclosed risks to subjects that are more than minimal, and (3) there is an adequate plan for debriefing subjects, when appropriate, and for dissemination of research results to them. Information about risks should never be withheld for the purpose of eliciting the cooperation of subjects, and truthful answers should always be given to direct questions about the research. Care should be taken to distinguish cases in which disclosure would destroy or invalidate the research from cases in which disclosure would simply inconvenience the investigator.

> [*The Belmont Report: Ethical Principles and Guidelines,* 1979]

Unique Issues of Fieldwork for an IRB to Consider

Fieldwork, or ethnographic research, is the observation of and interaction with people or groups being studied in their native environment. This research may continue for long periods of time. The process is difficult, if not impossible, to fully capture in a study proposal as the full parameters and goals evolve during the research.

Because fieldwork involves continuing complex interaction between the researcher and the subject people, the use of an informed consent form is problematic. OPRR has suggested, "while the idea of consent is not inapplicable to fieldwork, IRBs and researchers need to adapt prevailing notions of acceptable protocols and consent procedures to the realities of fieldwork. IRBs should keep in mind the possibility of granting a waiver of informed consent" (OPRR, *Institutional Review Board Guidebook*).

Considerations in Reviewing and Approving Research Involving Depressed or Suicidal Patients

Some studies of depression may be considered low risk, but studies focused on reducing suicidality are considered high risk. No study to date has been able to adequately predict who will complete suicide. Researchers, IRB members, and DSMB members need to be aware of the risk and ways to minimize it through consent, monitoring of participants, and risk management. Assessment of risk for suicidality must be an ongoing process. A research protocol should estimate, plan to treat, and inform study participants of the perceived risk and procedures to address. In studies where suicidality is not the focus of the study but can be anticipated to occur, such as substance abuse treatment, a risk management protocol should be utilized for the expected frequency of suicidality. What are the signs, symptoms, or conditions indicative of significant change in risk? How will a suicide attempt be managed? Criteria for withdrawal from the study should be explicit and provide for additional or alternative treatment for patients (NIMH, 2001).

Unique Issues of Behavioral Research on HIV

Behavior research studying HIV has focused on three areas:

1. The social, psychological, and behavioral conditions of the disease transmission and prevention

2. The effects of psychological state on immunosuppression

3. The role of psychology in alleviating the distress experienced by persons affected by HIV, including patients, family, friends, and people at risk

Concerns of privacy, confidentiality, and justice are the primary issues to be addressed by an IRB in reviewing HIV-related research. A protocol should not cause harm to a patient or others in his community.

References

National Commission for the Protection of Human Subjects of Biomedical Research (1979). *The Belmont Report: Ethical Principles and Guidelines for the Protection of Human Subjects of Research.*

National Institutes of Mental Health Issues to Consider in Intervention Research with Person at High Risk for Suicidality, January 2001.

OPRR. Institutional Review Board Guidebook, Chap. V, sec. A.

13

Multisite and Collaborative Studies

Overview 366
The Regulatory Framework for an Assurance 366
  The Federal Assurance 366
    The Common Rule and Federal Assurances 366
    Traditional Types of Assurances 367
    The Distinction Between an Assurance and an Agreement 368
  The New Federalwide Assurance (FWA) 368
Expectations Under an FWA for Domestic Institutions 368
  The Domestic FWA 369
    Written Procedures 369
    IRB Responsibilities and Scope of Duties 369
    Requirements for Informed Consent 369
    Responsibility for Collaborating Institutions/Investigators ... 370
    Requirements for Nonaffiliated Investigators 370
    The FWA Insists Upon Institutional Support for IRB(s) ... 370
    Compliance with the Assurance 370
    Assurance and Regulatory Training 370
    Assurance Renewal 371
  Terms of the FWA for Non-U.S. Institutions 371
Practical Considerations in Obtaining and Complying with FWAs 371
  TIPS: Avoiding Regulatory, Contractual, and Tort Risks 372
    Identify All Compliance Criteria 372
    Design a Monitoring Tool 372
    Reinforce Communication Systems for Reporting Adverse Events 372
    Develop a Non-Compliance Mitigation Plan 372
    Insist on Key Contract Terms 372
Conclusion 373
References 373
Terms of the Federalwide Assurance (FWA) for
International (NON-U.S.) Institutions 374
Forms.. 378

············

OVERVIEW

Clinical trials often involve participation by research centers in many states and sometimes in other countries. Sometimes the research entails multiple projects. Whether a single project, a multicenter trial, or an international research protocol, each research entity is obliged to safeguard the rights and welfare of research subjects. In recognition of this obligation and the duty to adhere to federal standards, each institution engaged in federally supported human subject research must submit an Assurance. Based on section 103(a) of the Federal Policy known as the Common Rule, the Assurance formalizes the institution's commitment to protect human subjects. The requirement to submit an Assurance applies to awardees *and* institutions.

As seen in this chapter, the Assurance is more than a document of lofty goals or aspirations. It is a contract binding upon those who file such a document with regard to federally supported research. Seen in another light, the Assurance may be evidence of a standard of care in terms of negligence litigation. (For a discussion of liability see Chapter Fourteen.) Moreover, it can be used as evidence of either regulatory compliance or non-compliance. This is an important consideration should a federal prosecutor see non-compliance as the basis for a civil or criminal action under the False Claims Act. The prosecutor could claim that providing inaccurate information, such as false cost reports or status reports, or the failure to report adverse events constitutes a false submission and non-compliance with the terms of the Assurance. Such information could set the wheels in motion for a federal prosecutor. (See Chapter Sixteen, on compliance.)

Practical measures are available to deal with Assurances. As discussed in this chapter, these measures involve careful evaluation of the assurance requirements and ongoing monitoring and surveillance to achieve compliance.

············

THE REGULATORY FRAMEWORK FOR AN ASSURANCE

Government-sponsored or funded research is subject to a detailed regulatory schematic. Part of the mosaic of rules and regulations involves the use of Assurances that delineate the duties or obligations of the research and institutions where research will be conducted.

The Federal Assurance

An Assurance is a written, legally binding contract that obliges either a public or a private entity to adhere to the minimum federal standards for protecting clinical trials research subjects. Such a contract must be executed *before* embarking upon research either conducted or supported by a federal department or agency. There are different types of Assurances that reflect the varying types of research trials conducted or funded by federal departments and agencies.

The Common Rule and Federal Assurances   The Assurance requirement is based on Section 103(a) of the Common Rule, which requires every institution *engaged* in federally supported clinical trials to file such a document. The requirement applies to awardees and to the performance site and to each collaborating institution. If an entity *does not* meet the criteria for engaging in clinical trials, there is no need to submit an

Assurance. Traditionally, the need for an Assurance was triggered when awardees and their collaborating institutions become "engaged" in human subject research whenever their employees or agents (i) intervene or interact with living individuals for research purposes; or (ii) obtain, release, or access individually identifiable private information for research purposes. ("IRB Registration and Assurance Filing Procedures General Information" (OHRP, 2000b)). In documentation accompanying the new FWA described later in this chapter, there is a slightly different statement of applicability of a Federalwide Assurance. The Office for Human Research Protections has published guidance on the subject, delineating examples of when an entity is considered to be engaged in clinical trials (See, *Engagement of Institutions in Research* (OHRP, 2000a)). At the very least, an awardee entity is involved in human subject research whenever it receives a *direct award* from the U.S. Department of Health and Human Services to support such endeavors. The result is the same even when all research activities are performed by either a subcontractor or collaborator.

Traditional Types of Assurances   Until recently, there were several types of Assurances used to formalize an entity's commitment to protect human research subjects. The traditional Assurances are slotted to be phased out and replaced with a new system. The Multiple Project Assurances (MPAs) and Cooperative Project Assurances (CPAs) remain valid until the stated expiration date or December 2003, whichever comes first. Single Project Assurances (SPAs) remain valid through the expiration date for contract awards, grants, or any non-competitive continuation ("IRB Registration and Assurance Filing Procedures, General, Information" (OHRP, 2002b)). As explained in a later subsection, a new set of Assurances is seen as offering a more streamlined system under the title of a Federalwide Assurance (FWA).

The four traditional Assurance documents can be distinguished. A *Multiple Project Assurance* (MPA) was designed for those entities involved in a significant amount of health-oriented research. Most entities in this category have numerous federally funded projects under way at the same time. A *Single Project Assurance* (SPA) was used for a single research project involving the participation of human research subjects. Typically, facilities involved in such studies did not have an MPA on file. A *Modified Single Project Assurance* was also recognized for those instances in which an entity planned to utilize another facility's IRB to review its human subject research. To do so, the reviewing entity had to have an MPA on file or it had to file an SPA for this project. The *Cooperative Project Assurance* (CPA) was crafted to meet the needs of the Cooperative Research Protocol Programs (CRPPs) involving multiprotocol, multisite research. In these studies data from standardized protocols is collected across all the participating organizations. Such protocols were approved and monitored by Department of Health and Human Services Protocol Review Committees for purposes of human subject protection in clinical trials. When approval was obtained the CPA was valid for all recognized Cooperative Research Protocol Programs.

The traditional Assurance process recognized some variation through an amendment process. Thus an *InterInstitutional Amendment* (IIA) was created to ensure compliance by an MPA-affiliated performance site without an IRB. In such situations the employees of the MPA usually carried out HHS-funded research at the test center. By allowing the amendment, the need for a separate SPA was obviated for each project carried out at the performance center.

Under the new Federalwide Assurance (FWA), in which each legally separate facility involved in federally sponsored human subject research must have its own Assurance, the IIA and so-called Joint Assurances have been eliminated. Under this new approach entities can designate IRBs under their Assurances that are operated by other facilities ("IRB Registration and Assurance Filing Procedures, General, Information" (OHRP, 2002b)).

The Distinction Between an Assurance and an Agreement   Terminology is important in this area. An Agreement was a document approved by the Office for Protection from Research Risks (OPRR) that was submitted either by a prospective awardee or other noninstitutional performance center. An Assurance was a document approved by the Office for Protection from Research Risks (OPRR) that was submitted either by a prospective awardee or other institutional performance center. In each instance, the approved document ensured institutional compliance with human research protection regulations with research to HHS-conducted or supported research.

The New Federalwide Assurance (FWA)

The Federalwide Assurance (FWA) applies to federally supported human research, defined as "the U.S. Government providing any funding or other support (including, but not limited to, providing supplies, products, drugs, and identifiable private information collected for research purposes) and/or the conduct of the research involves U.S. Government Employees" ("Federalwide Assurance of Protection for Human Subjects" (OHRP, 2002a)).

The FWA is applicable to an institution when

(a) the Institution's employees or agents intervene or interact with human subjects for purposes of federally-supported research;
(b) the Institution's employees or agents obtain individually identifiable private information about human subjects for purposes of federally-supported research; or
(c) the Institution receives a direct federal award to conduct human subject research even where all activities involving human subjects are carried out by a subcontractor or collaborator.

["Federalwide Assurance of Protection for Human Subjects" (OHRP, 2002a)]

Under an FWA such institutions and the IRBs designated under the entity's Assurance must comply with the Common Rule and any other regulations or policies set forth by the supporting federal department or agency. For research conducted or supported by the HHS, compliance is expected with all the subparts enumerated under Title 45 Part 46 of the Code of Federal Regulations.

············

EXPECTATIONS UNDER AN FWA FOR DOMESTIC INSTITUTIONS

The Federalwide Assurance has two sets of expectations for U.S. and international institutions. Although quite similar, there are some distinctions made with regard to international entities. While recognizing these distinctions a compliant entity must meet a number of requirements under the terms and conditions for a Federalwide Assurance (FWA).

The Domestic FWA

For U.S.-based entities, the FWA focuses on a number of key areas, including written procedures, informed consent, and educational requirements. These requirements should be met before applying for an FWA. The model forms can be found at the end of this chapter.

Written Procedures   Under the terms of the FWA, an institution is expected to establish written procedures for a number of aspects of the research review process. These include

1. Prompt reporting mechanisms about unanticipated risks to subjects and other individuals, serious or continuing non-compliance with respect to the federal regulations or IRB requirements, and a decision to suspend or terminate IRB approval for a study. Those to whom reports might be made include the IRB and appropriate officials within the institution, the head of a federal department or agency, an applicable regulatory body, and the OHRP.
2. A verification process to determine when research qualifies for exemption from the Common Rule. Such a process should be completed by a qualified individual, and in practical terms, this means someone other than the investigator or research team.
3. IRB written polices for initial and continuing review.
4. IRB written policies for determining which projects require review more than once annually and those that require verification from someone other than the principal investigator, and that there have been no changes since the last review.
5. IRB written policies that provide a mechanism for prompt reporting of changes in approved research protocols and that such changes are not put into effect without previous IRB review and approval. Exception is made for those changes that eliminate immediate hazards to research subjects.

It is also expected that with respect to written procedures, when OHRP requests a copy, the institution will provide it to the Office of Human Research Protection ("Federalwide Assurance for Protection for Human Subjects," March 20, 2002).

IRB Responsibilities and Scope of Duties   The FWA requires prospective review and approval of all human subject research. An exception is made for those projects for which there is an exemption or a waiver under Sections 101(b) or 101(i) of the Common Rule. Those that have been approved remain subject to not only continuing oversight by the IRB, but at a minimum, an annual review. All human subject research will be reviewed, prospectively approved, and subject to continuing oversight and review at least annually by the designated IRBs. The IRBs will have authority to approve, require modifications in, or disapprove the covered human subject research ("Federalwide Assurance for Protection for Human Subjects," March 20, 2002).

Requirements for Informed Consent   Under the terms of the FWA, there is a requirement to seek the informed consent of would-be research subjects. The consent should meet the specifications of the Common Rule, unless it is a situation in which either an exemption or a waiver would apply. Consent may also be sought from a legally authorized representative in appropriate circumstances. Further, the consent must be documented in accordance with the Common Rule. With respect to consent, the FWA follows sections 116 and 117 of the Common Rule.

Responsibility for Collaborating Institutions/Investigators   Under the terms of the FWA, the institution is held responsible for making certain that all entities and investigators participating in its federally supported research operate under an appropriate OHRP or other federally approved Assurance for the protection of human subjects. The FWA policy recognizes that in some instances institutions may operate under an Assurance that has been issued to another institution. In order to do so, there must be approval from the supporting department or agency and the institution with the Assurance.

Requirements for Nonaffiliated Investigators   A formal written agreement must be in place to permit a nonaffiliated investigator to participate in human research projects. Here, the term "nonaffiliated" refers to those who are employees or agents of the institution. They may be covered under the FWA as long as there is in place a written commitment to pertinent human subject protection policies and the oversight of the IRB. At the end of this chapter is an OHRP-prepared sample, "Unaffiliated Investigator Agreement," that may be used or modified for this purpose. If it wishes to do so, the institution may develop its own agreement. Copies of executed agreements should be maintained on file. Upon request, OHRP should receive copies of such agreements.

The FWA Insists Upon Institutional Support for IRB(s)   It is incumbent upon the institution to furnish the IRBs it operates with adequate resources to fulfill their responsibilities. The term resources here means both professional and support staff. The institution must provide the IRBs that it operates with resources and professional and support staff sufficient to carry out their responsibilities under the Assurance effectively.

Compliance with the Assurance   The institution must accept all the requisite elements of the FWA. In addition, the institution is held accountable for making certain that any IRB designated under the Assurance agrees to comply with its terms. It is also the responsibility of the institution to make certain that the IRBs have appropriate knowledge of the "local research context for all research covered under the Assurance" ("Federalwide Assurance for Protection for Human Subjects" (OHRP, 2002a)).

When a designation is made of an independent or another entity's IRB under the institution's Assurance, it must be captured in written agreement between the institution and the IRB organization. The document should set out the relationship and a commitment that the designated IRB will comply with the requirements of this Assurance. At the end of this chapter is an OHRP-prepared sample "IRB Authorization Agreement." However, there is no requirement to use this format, and some may design their own agreements. Copies of the executed agreements should be retained at both organizations and, upon request, made available to the OHRP.

Assurance and Regulatory Training   The OHRP has developed Assurance Training Modules that provide information on the key duties of the Institutional Signatory Official, the Human Protection Administrator, and the IRB Chairs that must be met under the Assurance. OHRP encourages these individuals to complete the Assurance Training Modules or some form of similar training prior to submitting the Assurance. In fact, as noted in the introduction to the on-line training program, OHRP will not approve an Assurance without these individuals completing this type of course.

For IRB members and staff, the OHRP believes that they should receive training on applicable ethical principles and Federal Regulations, guidance published by OHRP guidance, state and local laws, as well as institutional policies on the protection of human research subjects. Such training should be completed before reviewing human subject research studies. In addition, prior to initiating human research trials, research investigators should complete relevant training.

Oversight is important in making certain that training is provided and completed. Maintaining ongoing currency of knowledge in this area is important to safeguard human subjects. To facilitate educational training, the OHRP has developed a basic on-line course for Human Subject Assurance Training. It covers the Federal Regulations and the responsibilities of both the institution and investigator. It also addresses informed consent and human research protections. The course also addresses the responsibilities of the IRB. The course can be found at the OHRP Web site.

Assurance Renewal   To maintain an active Assurance, it must be updated at the very least every three years, even if there have been no changes in this time period. Lack of compliance with this requirement can have serious consequences. This includes restriction, suspension, or termination of the Institution's FWA.

Terms of the FWA for Non-U.S. Institutions

The terms for an international institution are quite similar to those described earlier for a U.S.-based institution, but there are some major differences. For example, the FWA references the role of an IRB *and* an IEC (Independent Ethics Committee), a term used in many countries to describe an IRB.

The FWA requires compliance with the specifications of the federal department or agency supporting the research as well as the Common Rule or a recognized international policy. The FWA permits the head of a U.S. department or agency to approve the substitution of foreign procedures for the federal procedural requirements as long as these requirements are consistent with Section 101(h) of the U.S. Federal Policy under the Common Rule (OHRP, 2002a). The specific requirements for international institutions are set forth at the end of this chapter.

············

PRACTICAL CONSIDERATIONS IN OBTAINING AND COMPLYING WITH FWAs

The FWA is not an administrative document that should be taken for granted. It is a legal instrument with a number of ramifications. It is a document that promises that the covered institution will be compliant with federal requirements. Failure to follow the terms of the Assurance can be seen as regulatory non-compliance. In serious cases, this could lead to the shut-down of federally funded research projects or the elimination of the institution from the list of approved research locations. If research subjects have been injured as the result of non-compliance, such information may be used as evidence of a breach of a standard of care in a negligence claim. Where private or international sponsors base contracts on adherence to the FWA, non-compliance may be seen as a material breach of the contract.

TIPS: Avoiding Regulatory, Contractual, and Tort Risks

Given the serious consequence of non-compliance with an FWA, institutions should develop practical strategies to avoid such risk exposure. The OHRP has provided a basic course for training key stakeholders in their responsibilities. But it is just a threshold course. More can be done to augment training and to foster compliance oversight. This includes the following:

Identify **All *Compliance Criteria***   Prepare a list of what is encompassed in the Assurance for meeting federal standards. Add to this list the requirements delineated in any contract.

Design a Monitoring Tool   Use a checklist that encompasses all the compliance criteria, responsibilities, completion dates, and, where applicable, required follow-up measures. For example:

Compliance Criteria	Responsibility	Completion Date	Follow-Up
IRB Staff Education	Human Protections Administrator	June 1, 2004	Six staff members still require training. F/o by 6/15/04.

Reinforce Communication Systems for Reporting Adverse Events
Test systems in place for notification of adverse events. Any deficiencies should be rectified.

Develop a Non-Compliance Mitigation Plan   Make certain that a practical method is in place to rapidly implement to deal with FWA non-compliance. Design it to be practical. For example, if in a mock verification survey 60 percent of the research investigators report that they do not understand what an FWA is, the response plan should be immediate educational programming. This can be done in a classroom or seminar setting or interactively via on-line training. That they have now completed the training is important. Equally important is some metric to demonstrate that they understood the content and how to implement it.

Insist on Key Contract Terms   Make certain that contracts include important terms relating to regulatory compliance with respect to a subcontractor or collaborating facility. Discuss core terms with legal counsel, including

- Hold harmless and indemnification terms
- Insurance coverages (see Chapter Fifteen)
- Reimbursement for cost of defense of any regulatory or administrative proceeding
- Nonassignment of the contract without prior approval
- Noninvolvement of other subcontractors without prior approval
- Quality monitoring
- Compliance surveillance
- Adverse event reporting mechanisms

- Duty to report regulatory inquiries, professional liability claims, or debarment or sanction by a state or federal agency
- Substance performance and duty to correct deficiencies
- Triggering events for termination of the agreement and
- Continued access to records during and after term of contract

CONCLUSION

The Assurance requirements involve more than the administrative task of completing a set of papers. It is a legal obligation made by the entity filing the paperwork that it will meet the requirements for federally supported human subject research protections. It encompasses the need for education of those involved at various levels of the entity. It also requires ongoing monitoring and maintenance of compliance with the federal requirements. With contracts imposing additional obligations, it is an area ripe for the introduction of practical strategies to achieve and maintain compliance.

References

OHRP. *Engagement of Institutions in Research.* June 23, 2000a.

OHRP. "Federalwide Assurance of Protection for Human Subjects." March 20, 2002a.

OHRP. "IRB Registration and Assurance Filing Procedures General Information." 2000b.

OHRP. "IRB Registration and Assurance Filing Procedures, General Information." March 20, 2002b.

TERMS OF THE FEDERALWIDE ASSURANCE (FWA) FOR INTERNATIONAL (NON-U.S.) INSTITUTIONS

1. **Human Subject Research Must Be Guided by Ethical Principles**

   All of the Institution's human subject activities and all activities of the Institutional Review Boards (IRBs) or independent ethics committees (IECs) designated under the Assurance, regardless of funding source, will be guided by one of the following statements of ethical principles: (a) The World Medical Association's Declaration of Helsinki (as adopted in 1996 or 2000); (b) The Belmont Report: Ethical Principles and Guidelines for the Protection of Human Subjects of Research of the U.S. National Commission for the Protection of Human Subjects of Biomedical and Behavioral Research; or (c) other appropriate international ethical standards recognized by Federal Departments and Agencies that have adopted the U.S. Federal Policy for the Protection of Human Subjects.

2. **Applicability**

   These terms apply whenever the Institution becomes engaged in U.S. federally-supported* (i.e., conducted or supported) human subject research, which is not otherwise exempt from the U.S. Federal Policy for the Protection of Human Subjects. The Institution becomes engaged whenever (a) the Institution's employees or agents intervene or interact with human subjects for purposes of U.S. federally-supported research; (b) the Institution's employees or agents obtain individually identifiable private information about human subjects for purposes of U.S. federally-supported research; or (c) the Institution receives a direct award to conduct U.S. federally-supported human subject research, even where all activities involving human subjects are carried out by a subcontractor or collaborator.

   If a U.S. Department or Agency Head determines that the procedures prescribed by the institution afford protections that are at least equivalent to those provided by the U.S. Federal Policy, the Department or Agency Head may approve the substitution of the foreign procedures in lieu of the procedural requirements provided above consistent with the requirements of 101(h) of the U.S. Federal Policy.

   [*Federally-supported is defined throughout the Assurance document and the Terms of Assurance as the U.S. Government providing any funding or other support (including, but not limited to, providing supplies, products, drugs, and identifiable private information collected for research purposes) and/or the conduct of the research involves U.S. Government employees.]

3. **Compliance with Regulations, Policies, or Guidelines**

   All U.S. federally-supported human subject research will comply with the requirements of any applicable U.S. Federal regulatory agency as well as one or more of the following:

   a) The U.S. Federal Policy for the Protection of Human Subjects, known as the Common Rule (e.g., Subpart A) or the U.S. Department of Health and Human Services (DHHS) regulations at 45 CFR 46 and its Subparts A, B, C, and D;

   b) The May 1, 1996, International Conference on Harmonization E-6 Guidelines for Good Clinical Practice (ICH-GCP-E6), Sections 1 through 4;

   c) The 1993 Council for International Organizations of Medical Sciences (CIOMS) International Ethical Guidelines for Biomedical Research Involving Human Subjects;

d) The 1998 Medical Research Council of Canada Tri-Council Policy Statement on Ethical Conduct for Research Involving Humans;

e) The 2000 Indian Council of Medical Research Ethical Guidelines for Biomedical Research on Human Subjects; or

f) Other standard(s) for the protection of human subjects recognized by U.S. Federal Departments and Agencies which have adopted the U.S. Federal Policy for the Protection of Human Subjects.

4. **IRB/IEC Written Procedures**

a) The Institution should establish, and should provide a copy to OHRP upon request, written procedures for:

1) ensuring prompt reporting to the IRB/IEC, appropriate institutional officials, the relevant Department or Agency Head, any applicable regulatory body, and OHRP of any: (i) unanticipated problems involving risks to subjects or others, (ii) serious or continuing non-compliance with the Federal Regulations or IRB requirements, and (iii) suspension or termination of IRB approval.

2) Verifying, by a qualified person or persons other than the investigator or research team, whether proposed human subject research activities qualify for exemption from the requirements of the U.S. Common Rule;

b) The designated IRB(s)/IEC(s) should establish, and should provide a copy to OHRP upon request, written procedures for:

1) Conducting IRB/IEC initial and continuing review (not less than once per year), approving research, and reporting IRB/IEC findings to the investigator and the Institution;

2) Determining which projects require review more often than annually and which projects need verification from sources other than the investigator that no material changes have occurred since the previous IRB/IEC review;

3) Ensuring that changes in approved research protocols are reported promptly and are not initiated without IRB/IEC review and approval, except when necessary to eliminate apparent immediate hazards to the subject.

5. **Responsibilities and Scope of IRB(s)/IEC(s)**

Except for research exempted or waived in accordance with sections 101(b) or 101(i) of the U.S. Common Rule, U.S. federally-supported research should be reviewed, prospectively approved, and subject to continuing oversight and review at least annually by the designated IRB(s)/IEC(s). The IRB(s)/IEC(s) should have authority to approve, require modifications in, or disapprove the covered human subject research.

6. **Informed Consent Requirements**

Except for research exempted or waived in accordance with Sections 101(b) or 101(i) of the U.S. Common Rule, informed consent should be:

a) sought from each prospective subject or the subject's legally authorized representative, in accordance with, and to the extent required by Section 116 of the U.S. Common Rule;

b) appropriately documented, in accordance with, and to the extent required by Section 117 of the U.S. Common Rule.

7. **Considerations for Special Class of Subjects**

   For DHHS-supported human subject research, this Institution will comply with 45 CFR 46 Subparts B, C, and D prior to the involvement of pregnant women or fetuses, prisoners, or children, respectively. For non-DHHS U.S. federally-supported human subject research, the Institution will comply with any human subject regulations and/or policies of the supporting Department or Agency for these classes of subjects.

8. **Requirement for Assurances for Collaborating Institutions/Investigators**

   The Institution is responsible for ensuring that all institutions and investigators engaged in its U.S. federally-supported human subject research operate under an appropriate OHRP or other federally-approved Assurance for the protection of human subjects. In some cases, one institution may operate under an Assurance issued to another institution with the approval of the supporting Department or Agency and the institution holding the Assurance.

9. **Written Agreements with Non-Affiliated Investigators**

   The engagement in human research activities of each independent investigator who is not an employee or agent of the Institution may be covered under the FWA only in accordance with a formal, written agreement of commitment to relevant human subject protection policies and IRB oversight. OHRP's sample Unaffiliated Investigator Agreement may be used or adapted for this purpose, or the Institution may develop its own commitment agreement. Institutions must maintain commitment agreements on file and provide copies to OHRP upon request.

10. **Institutional Support for the IRB(s)/IEC(s)**

    The Institution should provide the IRB(s)/IEC(s) that it operates with resources and professional and support staff sufficient to carry out their responsibilities under the Assurance effectively.

11. **IRB(s)/IEC(s) Compliance with the Terms of Assurance**

    The Institution accepts and will follow items 1-10 above and is responsible for ensuring that (a) the IRB(s)/IEC(s) designated under the Assurance agree to comply with these terms, and (b) the IRB(s)/IEC(s) possesses appropriate knowledge of the local research context for all research covered under the Assurance (please refer to the OHRP posted guidance on IRB Knowledge of Local Research Context).

    Any designation under this Assurance of another Institution's IRB or an independent IRB must be documented by a written agreement between the Institution and the IRB organization outlining their relationship and include a commitment that the designated IRB will adhere to the requirements of this Assurance. OHRP's sample IRB Authorization Agreement may be used for such purpose or the two organizations may develop their own agreement. This agreement should be kept on file at both organizations and made available to OHRP upon request.

12. **Assurance Training**

    The OHRP Assurance Training Modules describe the major responsibilities of the Institutional Signatory Official, the Human Protection Administrator and the IRB Chair(s) that must be fulfilled under the Assurance. OHRP strongly recommends that the Institutional Signatory Official, the Human Protections Administrator (e.g., Human Subjects Administrator or Human Subjects Contact Person), and the IRB/IEC Chair(s) personally complete the relevant OHRP Assurance Training Modules, or comparable training that includes the content of these Modules, prior to submitting the Assurance.

13. **Educational Training**

OHRP strongly recommends that the Institution and the designated IRB(s)/IEC(s) establish educational training and oversight mechanisms (appropriate to the nature and volume of its research) to ensure that research investigators, IRB/IEC members and staff, and other appropriate personnel maintain continuing knowledge of, and comply with, relevant ethical principles, relevant U.S. regulations; procedural standards under the Assurance; OHRP guidance; other applicable guidance; national, state and local laws; and institutional policies for the protection of human subjects. Furthermore, OHRP recommends that a) IRB/IEC members and staff complete relevant educational training before reviewing human subject research; and b) research investigators complete appropriate institutional educational training before conducting human subject research.

14. **Renewal of Assurance**

All information provided under this Assurance should be updated every 36 months (3 years), even if no changes have occurred, in order to maintain an active Assurance. Failure to update this information may result in restriction, suspension, or termination of the Institution's Federalwide Assurance for the protection of human subjects.

FORMS

☐ **New Filing**   ☐ **Update or Renewal for FWA Number:** _____

U.S. Department of Health and Human Services (DHHS) Federalwide Assurance (FWA) for the Protection of Human Subjects For Domestic (U.S.) Institutions

1. Institution Filing Assurance

Legal Name:

City: State:

DHHS Institution Profile File (IPF) code, if known:

Federal Entity Identification Number (EIN), if known:

If this Assurance replaces an MPA or CPA, please provide the "M" or "T" number:

2. Institutional Components

List below all components over which the Institution has legal authority <u>that operate under a different name</u>. Also list with an asterisk (*) any <u>alternate names</u> under which the Institution operates. The Institution should have available for review by the Office for Human Research Protections (OHRP) upon request a brief description and line diagram explaining the interrelationships among the Assurance Signatory Official, the Institutional Review Board (IRB), IRB support staff, and investigators in these various components.

NOTE: The Signatory Official signing this Assurance must be legally authorized to represent the Institution providing this Assurance and all components listed below. Entities that the Signatory Official is not legally authorized to represent may <u>not</u> be listed here without the prior approval of OHRP.

Γ Please check here if there are no additional components or alternate names.

Name of Component or Alternate Names Used	City	State (or Country if Outside U.S.)

3. Statement of Principles

This Institution assures that all of its activities related to human subject research, regardless of funding source, will be guided by the ethical principles in the following document(s). (*indicate below*)

         ☐ *The Belmont Report*
         ☐ *Other* (*please submit copy to OHRP with this Assurance*)

4. Applicability

(a) This Institution assures that all of its activities related to federally-conducted or -supported human subject research will comply with the **Terms of Assurance for Protection of Human Subjects for Institutions Within the United States.** NOTE: The Terms of Assurance are contained in a separate document on the OHRP website.

(b) *Optional:* This Institution elects to apply the following to all of its human subject research regardless of source of support:

> ☐ *45 CFR 46 and all of its subparts (A,B,C,D)*
> ☐ *Common Rule (e.g., 45 CFR 46, subpart A)*

5. Designation of Institutional Review Boards (IRBs)

This Institution designates the following IRB(s) for review of research under this Assurance *(if the IRB is not previously registered with DHHS or has not provided a membership roster to DHHS, please attach the appropriate IRB registration materials available on the OHRP website).*

NOTE: Reliance on another institution's IRB or an independent IRB must be documented by a written agreement that is available for review by OHRP upon request. OHRP's sample IRB Authorization Agreement may be used for this purpose, or the institutions involved may develop their own agreement. Future designation of other IRBs requires update of the FWA.

DHHS IRB Registration Number	Name of IRB As Registered with DHHS

6. Human Protections Administrator (e.g., Human Subjects Administrator or Human Subjects Contact Person)

First Name: Middle Initial: Last Name:

Degrees or Suffix (e.g., MD, PhD):   Institutional Title:

Institution:

Telephone: FAX: E-Mail:

Address:

City: State: Zip Code:

7. <u>Signatory Official (i.e., Official Legally Authorized to Represent the Institution — cannot be IRB Chairperson or IRB member)</u>

I understand that the Assurance Training Modules on the OHRP website describe the responsibilities of the Signatory Official, the IRB Chair(s), and the Human Protections Administrator under this Assurance. Additionally, I recognize that providing all research investigators, IRB members and staff, and other relevant personnel with appropriate initial and continuing education about human subject protections will help ensure that the requirements of this Assurance are satisfied.

Acting officially in an authorized capacity on behalf of this Institution and with an understanding of the Institution's responsibilities under this Assurance, I assure protections for human subjects as specified above. The IRB(s) designated above are to provide oversight for all research conducted under this Assurance. These IRB(s) will comply with the **Terms of Assurance** and possess appropriate knowledge of the local context in which this Institution's research will be conducted. I understand that all collaborating institutions engaged in federally-conducted or -supported human subject research must submit their own Assurance.

All information provided with this Assurance is up to date and accurate. *I am aware that false statements could be cause for invalidating this Assurance and may lead to other administrative or legal action.*

Signature: _____   Date: _____

First Name: _____   Middle Initial: _____   Last Name: _____

Degrees or Suffix (e.g., MD, PhD): _____   Institutional Title: _____

Telephone: _____   FAX: _____   E-Mail: _____

Address: _____

City: _____   State: _____   Zip Code: _____

NOTE: Facilities operated by the U.S. Government may require Department or Agency clearance. Please contact the relevant Department or Agency Human Protections Officer before forwarding this Assurance to OHRP.

8. <u>DHHS Approval</u>

The Federalwide Assurance of Protection for Human Subjects submitted to DHHS by the above Institution is hereby approved.

Assurance Number: _____   Expiration Date: _____

Signature of DHHS Approving Official: _____   Date: _____

Department of Health and Human Services
Federalwide Assurance of Protection for Human Subjects

ADDITIONAL PAGE REQUIRED FOR
DEPARTMENT OF VETERANS AFFAIRS
VETERANS HEALTH ADMINISTRATION FACILITIES

Insert Institution Name
assures that all of its pertinent activities related to human subject research will comply with all requirements of Department of Veterans Affairs regulations at Title 38 Code of Federal Regulations Part 16 (38 CFR 16), and all other pertinent Department of Veterans Affairs policies and procedures, including policies and procedures of the Office of Research Compliance and Assurance (ORCA) and the Office of Research & Development (ORD), issued in Manuals, Handbooks and other relevant authorized Directives.

(7a.) Official Legally Authorized to Represent the Institution (VA Medical Center Director):

Signature: _____   Date: _____

First Name: Middle Initial: Last Name:

Degree or Suffix (e.g., MD, PhD)   Institutional Title:

Human subject protection training last taken on: (date)

Address:

City: State: Zip Code:

Telephone: FAX: E-Mail:

(7b.) Official Legally Authorized to Concur in the Institution's Approval (VHA VISN Director):

Signature: _____   Date: _____

First Name   Middle Initial: Last Name:

Degree or Suffix (e.g., MD, PhD)   Institutional Title: Director, VISN #

Human subject protection training last taken on: (date)

Address:

City: State: Zip Code:

Telephone: FAX: E-Mail:

(7c.) Department of Veterans Affairs Approval

(Section Below to be completed by the Office of Research Compliance and Assurance)

This Federal-wide Assurance of Protection for Human Subjects is hereby approved for submission to the Department of Health and Human Services (HHS).

VHA Recommending Official

Signature of VA Recommending Official:

Name: Priscilla A. Craig   Date:

Title: Health Science Specialist, Federal Wide Assurances
                 Office of Research Compliance and Assurance

Signature of VA Approving Official:

Name: John H. Mather M.D.   Date:

Title: Chief Officer,
                 Office of Research Compliance and Assurance

Any Additional Comments:

Office for Research Compliance and Assurance (10R)
811 Vermont Avenue, NW, Suite 574
Washington, DC 20420

Phone: (202) 565-8162
FAX: (202) 565-9194

E-mail: priscilla.craig@hq.med.va.gov

☐ **New Filing** ☐ **Update or Renewal for FWA Number:** _____

U.S. Department of Health and Human Services (DHHS) Federalwide Assurance (FWA) for the Protection of Human Subjects For International (Non-U.S.) Institutions

1. Institution Filing Assurance

Legal Name:

City: State/Province: Country:

DHHS Institution Profile File (IPF) code, if known:

Federal Entity Identification Number (EIN), if known:

If this Assurance replaces an MPA or CPA, please provide the "M" or "T" number:

2. Institutional Components

List below all components over which the Institution has legal authority that operate under a different name. Also list with an asterisk (*) any alternate names under which the Institution operates. The Institution should have available for review by the Office for Human Research Protections (OHRP) upon request a brief description and line diagram explaining the interrelationships among the Assurance Signatory Official, the Institutional Review Board (IRB) or the Independent Ethics Committee (IEC), IRB/IEC support staff, and investigators in these various components.

NOTE: The Signatory Official signing this Assurance must be legally authorized to represent the Institution providing this Assurance and all components listed below. Entities that the Signatory Official is not legally authorized to represent may not be listed here without the prior approval of OHRP.

Γ Please check here if there are no additional components or alternate names.

Name of Component or Alternate Names Used	City	State or Country

3. Statement of Principles

This Institution assures that all of its activities related to human subject research, regardless of funding source, will be guided by the ethical principles in the following document(s). (*indicate below*)

      ☐ *The Declaration of Helsinki*
      ☐ *The Belmont Report*
      ☐ *Other (please submit copy to OHRP with this Assurance)*

4. Applicability

This Institution assures that all of its activities related to United States (U.S.) federally-conducted or -supported human subject research will comply with a) the **Terms of Assurance for Protection of Human Subjects for Institutions Outside the U.S.** (NOTE: The Terms of Assurance are contained in a separate document on the OHRP website) and b) the following procedural standards:

(please check one or more of the following)

- ☐ *45 CFR 46 and all of its subparts (A,B,C,D)*   ☐ *45 CFR 46, subpart A (Common Rule)*
- ☐ *21 CFR 50 and 21 CFR 56*   ☐ *ICH-GCP-E6 Sections 1 through 4*
- ☐ *CIOMS International Ethical Guidelines*
- ☐ *Canadian Tri-Council Policy*   ☐ *Indian Council of Medical Research*
- ☐ *Other (please submit copy to OHRP with this Assurance)*

5. Designation of Institutional Review Boards (IRBs) or Independent Ethics Committees (IECs)

This Institution designates the following IRB(s)/IEC(s) for review of research under this Assurance [*if the IRB(s)/IEC(s) is not previously registered with DHHS or has not provided a membership roster to DHHS, please attach the appropriate IRB registration materials available on the OHRP website*].

NOTE: Reliance on another institution's IRB/IEC or an independent IRB/IEC must be documented by a written agreement that is available for review by OHRP upon request. OHRP's sample IRB Authorization Agreement may be used for this purpose, or the institutions involved may develop their own agreement. Future designation of other IRB(s)/IEC(s) requires update of the FWA.

DHHS IRB Registration Number	**Name of IRB/IEC As Registered with DHHS**

6. Human Protections Administrator (e.g., Human Subjects Administrator or Human Subjects Contact Person)

First Name: Middle Initial: Last Name:

Degrees or Suffix (e.g., MD, PhD):   Institutional Title:

Institution:

Telephone: FAX: E-Mail:

Address:

City: State/Province: Country:

7. <u>Signatory Official (i.e., Official Legally Authorized to Represent the Institution —</u> <u>cannot be IRB/IEC Chairperson or IRB/IEC member)</u>

I understand that the Assurance Training Modules on the OHRP website describe the responsibilities of the Signatory Official, the IRB/IEC Chair(s), and the Human Protections Administrator under this Assurance. Additionally, I recognize that providing all research investigators, IRB/IEC members and staff, and other relevant personnel with appropriate initial and continuing education about human subject protections will help ensure that the requirements of this Assurance are satisfied.

Acting officially in an authorized capacity on behalf of this Institution and with an understanding of the Institution's responsibilities under this Assurance, I assure protections for human subjects as specified above. The IRB(s)/IEC(s) designated above are to provide oversight for all research conducted under this Assurance. These IRB(s)/IEC(s) will comply with the **Terms of Assurance** and possess appropriate knowledge of the local context in which this Institution's research will be conducted. I understand that all collaborating institutions engaged in U.S. federally-conducted or -supported human subject research must submit their own Assurance.

All information provided with this Assurance is up to date and accurate. *I am aware that false statements could be cause for invalidating this Assurance and may lead to other administrative or legal action.*

Signature: _____ Date: _____

First Name: Middle Initial: Last Name:

Degrees or Suffix (e.g., MD, PhD):   Institutional Title:

Telephone: FAX: E-Mail:

Address:

City: State/Province: Country:

8. <u>DHHS Approval</u>

The Federalwide Assurance of Protection for Human Subjects submitted to DHHS by the above Institution is hereby approved.

Assurance Number: Expiration Date:

Signature of DHHS Approving Official: _____ Date: _____

Division of Assurances and Quality Improvement
Office for Human Research Protections (OHRP)
1101 Wootton Parkway
The Tower Building, Suite 200
Rockville, MD 20852

U.S. Department of Health and Human Services (DHHS) Office for Human Research Protections (OHRP)

Step-by-Step Instructions for Filing a Federalwide Assurance for International (Non-U.S.) Institutions

---

Version Date 03/20/2002

Each institution that is engaged (see definition of "engaged" at http://ohrp.osophs.dhhs.gov/humansubjects/assurance/engage.htm) in Department of Health and Human Services (DHHS) supported or conducted human subject research must submit a Federalwide Assurance (FWA) to the Office for Human Research Protections (OHRP). The FWA Signatory Official must be authorized to represent and commit the entire institution and all of its components to a legally-binding agreement.

Follow the instructions below for each item on the application. You should also review the Questions and Answers material found at http://ohrp.osophs.dhhs.gov/humansubjects/assurance/afaq.htm. If you have further questions **after reading these instructions and reviewing the Questions and Answers,** please go to the staffing guide at http://ohrp.osophs.dhhs.gov/dpa-staff.htm#Table2, to determine the name and phone number of the staff member assigned to your region and contact them.

TOP RIGHT-HAND CORNER - "New Filing" versus "Update or Renewal"

Indicate by an [x] whether this is either: 1) a "New Filing," or 2) an "Update or Renewal" of an **already existing** FWA. Your application is a "New Filing" if this is your institution's initial filing for a FWA. If your institution already has an approved FWA, the form should be appropriately marked as an "Update or Renewal" and include your institution's FWA number. (See Update and Renewal instructions at http://ohrp.osophs.dhhs.gov/humansubjects/assurance/renwfwa.htm)

ITEM #1 - Institution Filing Assurance

a. Type or print the legal name of the institution (or the name the institution uses in doing business) that is providing the Assurance. Please **do not provide both names in this section**. Any alternate name(s) or components of the institution filing the FWA or separate legal entities that will be covered by the FWA should be listed under Item #2 of the FWA application.

Institutions that are affiliated solely through professional or collaborative arrangements must submit their own FWA application, unless a special exception is requested and described in a cover letter submitted with the FWA application, and approved by OHRP. An exception may be made by OHRP as described in the following example.

Separate legal entities may be covered under one FWA, if there is one human subjects protection program that oversees the review and conduct of human subjects research at each entity or institution. In such cases, the Signatory Official who signs the FWA must have authority over the entire human subjects protection program and be ultimately responsible for the review and conduct of human subjects research at each component and separate legal entity covered under the FWA. A formal agreement between each separate legal entity should be prepared to outline the relationship between the institutions and document the authority granted to the Signatory Official with regard to the oversight of human subjects research at each institution. A copy of the agreement should be kept on file at each institution and made available to OHRP upon request.

Do not hesitate to contact OHRP if consultation is needed on this issue.

Any component that does business in its own name (e.g., applies for federal research funding in its own name and/or has its own IPF/EIN identifiers, described below in paragraph c) may file its own FWA application, if the organization's administrative structure permits the component to make legally binding commitments to the Terms of Assurance, independent of the "parent" institution. Such a decision may be appropriate if the component has its own human subjects protection program that is separate or distinct from the "parent" institution.

b. Type or print the city, country and mail code where the institution is located.

c. Type or print the DHHS Institution Profile File (IPF) code and the Federal Entity Identification Number (EIN; tax number), if known. OHRP does not assign these numbers; they are assigned by other federal departments or agencies for certain tracking purposes. OHRP requests these numbers to distinguish between similar institutions and to try to avoid approval of multiple assurances for a given institution. If your are not aware of your institution's IPF code or EIN, you may leave these items blank. The numbers are not required for FWA processing.

Indicate whether your FWA will replace a Multiple Project Assurance (MPA; "M" number) or a Cooperative Project Assurance (CPA; "T" number), by providing the respective number of your current Assurance.

ITEM #2 - Institutional Components

Type or print the names of all components of the institution identified in item #1 that will be covered by the FWA, including any alternate names used by your institution or components. Components are generally defined as parts of your institution that may be viewed as separate organizations, but remain part of the legal entity or institution.

For example, a ABC University can list its XYZ University Hospital, KLM School of Public Health, and EFG Institute for International Studies as components. In order to keep the listing of components manageable, only list the major components of your institution that are likely to be represented as either the applicant organization or as a research performance site. Please do not list all departments of your institution, as their participation in a study is likely to be represented by the name of the institution or one of the major components.

ITEM #3 - Statement of Principles

Indicate by an [x] the statement of ethical principles that govern your institution in fulfilling its responsibilities for the protection of the rights and welfare of human subjects in research. OHRP recognizes The Belmont Report as an acceptable statement of ethical principles for the protection of human subjects in research. International institutions may elect the Declaration of Helsinki as their statement of ethical principles for the protection of human subjects in research. If "Other" principles are named, as required by the human subjects protection regulations, a copy of those principles must be submitted with the FWA application.

ITEM #4 - Applicability

a. Review the Terms of the Federalwide Assurance (FWA) for International (non-U.S.) Institutions on the OHRP website at http://ohrp.osophs.dhhs.gov/humansubjects/assurance/filasurt.htm to obtain an understanding of the regulatory requirement that will be applied to federally-supported or -conducted human subjects research.

b. This section asks about the regulatory standards that your institution applies to human subjects research. Indicate with an [x] the alternative regulatory standards available on the FWA application for International Institutions (non-U.S.) that your institution elects to apply for U.S. federally-supported or -conducted human subjects research.

Please note that the listed alternative regulatory standards are considered to be generally consistent to the U.S. Common Rule (i.e., U.S. Federal Policy for the protection of human subjects in research). However, for DHHS-supported or -conducted human subjects research item 7 of the Terms of the FWA for International (non-U.S.) Institutions may require additional protections for the involvement of pregnant women or fetuses, prisoners, or children.

If "Other" procedural standards are named, a copy of those standards must be submitted with the FWA application.

ITEM #5 - Designation of Institutional Review Boards(s)/Independent Ethics Committee(s)

Designate the Institutional Review Boards (IRBs)/Independent Ethics Committees (IECs) of record for this assurance. You must still indicate at least one IRB/IEC in this section. Please ensure that all designated IRBs/IECs are registered, or are in the process of registering, with OHRP prior to submitting the FWA application. OHRP does not take action on a FWA application until all designated IRBs/IECs are registered and assigned IRB Registration numbers. If the registration of the IRB/IEC was in process when you submitted your FWA, OHRP will insert the IRB Registration number.

To determine if an IRB/IEC is registered with OHRP, you should go to the OHRP website at http://ohrp.cit.nih.gov/search/asearch.asp#IORG and search for it. If an IRB(s) needs to be registered, go to the instructions on the OHRP website at http://ohrp.osophs.dhhs.gov/humansubjects/assurance/regirbi.htm - with links to sample registrations in Rich Text and HTML Formats.

List the IRB Registration number(s) [not the IRB Organization number (IORG number)] and the name of the IRB(s) as registered on this website.

If your institution relies on another institution's IRB/IEC, this arrangement must be documented in writing between the two institutions. OHRP has a sample IRB Authorization Agreement on its website at http://ohrp.osophs.dhhs.gov/humansubjects/assurance/iprotsup.rtf that may be used for this purpose, or the institutions may develop their own agreement. The agreement must be kept on file at the institutions and available for review by OHRP upon request, but it should not be submitted with the FWA application.

If at any time your institution relies on an IRB/IEC not listed on your FWA, you must update your FWA and list the additional IRB(s)/IEC(s). (See Update and Renewal instructions on the OHRP website at http://ohrp.osophs.dhhs.gov/humansubjects/assurance/renwfwa.htm)

ITEM #6 - Human Protections Administrator

Designate the individual who will serve as the Human Protections Administrator (HPA) (i.e., the primary contact person for human subjects protection issues) for your institution. The HPA whould exercise operational responsibility for your institution's program for protecting human subjects in research. The HPA should have comprehensive knowledge of all aspects of your institution's system of protections for human subjects, as well as be familiar with the institution's commitments under the FWA and play a key role in ensuring that the institution fulfills its responsibilities under the FWA.

When considering who should be appointed as HPA, it is important to remember that the duration of an FWA is 3 years and that, at the institution's option, a FWA may cover all human subjects research at the filing institution, not just federally-supported or -conducted human subjects research. The HPA should be familiar with the institution's commitments under the FWA and that the HPA is responsible for assisting the institution in ensuring that it fulfills its responsibilities.

Type or print the full name, degree(s), institutional (e.g., administrative) title, institution, telephone and fax numbers, e-mail address, and full mailing address for the HPA. The e-mail address is very important, as this will provide the means for effective communication from OHRP (e.g., sending of new information regarding the FWA). If any of these fields are not available, please indicate accordingly rather than leaving the field blank. NOTE, you may also obtain news items and new guidance from OHRP by signing up on the OHRP-L LISTSERV (instructions are found on the OHRP website at http://ohrp.osophs.dhhs.gov/list.htm)

ITEM #7 - Signatory Official

The Signatory Official must be a senior institutional official who has the authority to commit the entire institution named in the FWA application, as well as all of the institutional components listed under Item #2, to a legally binding agreement. Entities that the Signatory Official is not legally authorized to represent may not be covered under the FWA. This individual must also have the authority to assure compliance of the institution and all of its components to the Terms of the Assurance. Generally, this is someone at the level of President or Chief Executive Officer (CEO) of a company or Provost or Chancellor of an academic institution, unless another official has been specifically delegated with this authority. **Thus, the IRB Chair and IRB members are not appropriate personnel to serve as the Signatory Official.**

The signature of the Signatory Official and the date of the signature must be provided on the FWA. The FWA with the original signature must be submitted to OHRP.

Type or print the full name, degree(s), institutional (e.g., administrative) title, institution, telephone and fax numbers, e-mail address, and full mailing address for the Signatory Official. The e-mail address is very important, as this will provide the means for effective communication from OHRP (e.g., sending of new information regarding the FWA). If any of these fields are not available, please indicate accordingly rather than leaving the field blank. NOTE, you may also obtain news items and new guidance from OHRP by signing up on the OHRP-L LISTSERV (instructions are found on the OHRP website at http://ohrp.osophs.dhhs.gov/list.htm)

ITEM #8 - DHHS Approval

Leave this item blank. This section is for use by OHRP for approval of the FWA.

Submitting an FWA Application to OHRP -

Please review and proofread all materials to be submitted and ensure that all parts of the FWA application are complete and accurate. **Applications that are complete will facilitate quicker review and approval by OHRP. Incomplete documents may delay processing and approval of the FWA.**

Please submit the FWA application single-sided and with the original signature of the Signatory Official by regular mail, express mail, or hand delivery to OHRP at:

FWA Submission
Division of Assurances and Quality Improvement
Office for Human Research Protections
The Tower Building
1101 Wootton Parkway, Suite 200
Rockville, MD 20852

FWA applications may be submitted by fax to 011-301-402-0527, as long as the FWA with the original signature(s) follows by mail. (Note, IRB registrations are also acceptable via fax at the above number.)

Notification of Approval of a FWA -

Notice of approval of a FWA will be sent by e-mail to the Signatory Official and the Human Protections Administrator if e-mail addresses were provided for them on the FWA application. A copy of the approved FWA will be sent by regular mail to the Signatory Official.

[**SAMPLE DOCUMENT- Rich Text Format (RTF)**]

[**SAMPLE DOCUMENT- HyperText Markup Language Format (HTML)**]

If you have any questions, please do not hesitate to contact the Division of Assurances and Quality Improvement, OHRP, at 011-301-496-7005.

If you have questions about human subject research, click **ohrp@osophs.dhhs.gov**
If you have questions/suggestions about this web page, click **Webmaster**
Updated August 7, 2002

14

Medical Malpractice Liability in Human Research

Introduction 392
Theories of Law That May Arise in Lawsuits by Research Participants 392
   Theories That a Research Participant May Use to Recover Damages 392
   Potential Liability of IRB Members 393
   The Food, Drug & Cosmetic Act as Creating a Private Cause of Action 394
   The Venues in Which a Research Participant May File a Lawsuit 394
   Defenses That an Investigator, an Institution, or a Sponsor May Raise 394
   Government Liability for Injury to Military Personnel 395
   The Time Period in Which a Research Participant Can File a Lawsuit 396
General Concepts of Professional Negligence 396
   The Basic Elements of a Negligence Lawsuit 396
   Negligence 397
   Damages 397
   Punitive Damages 397
   Proximate Cause 397
   Expert Testimony in a Research Negligence Lawsuit 397
   Proving the Standard of Care in a Research Protocol 397
   Proving a Lack of Informed Consent 398
Limiting Liability 399
   Use of a Waiver or Release in an Effort to Limit Liability 399
   Compensation of Participants for Injury Occurring as
   a Result of Participation in a Research Study 399
   Sponsor Indemnification of the Investigator
   and Others Involved in a Clinical Study 399
   NIH Certificate of Confidentiality 340
   Insurance Issues for Clinical Research 340
References 340

············

INTRODUCTION

In addition to the plethora of statutes and regulations, human research in America is influenced by medical malpractice litigation. The fear of such litigation may be a larger influence than the actual litigation. Unfortunately, much of American medical practice is conducted with this fear in mind. The following discussion is intended to explain the theories and process of medical malpractice litigation when focused on human research.

············

THEORIES OF LAW THAT MAY ARISE
IN LAWSUITS BY RESEARCH PARTICIPANTS

Theories That a Research Participant May Use to Recover Damages

The most common allegation against an investigator, an institution, or a sponsor is one of negligence. Negligence in a medical malpractice action is defined as a deviation from the standard of care for a reasonable physician in the same or similar circumstances. The law does not apply a scientific formula to this definition, and in some areas of research, the denominator of such an equation would be extremely small. However, a study participant who claims to have been injured by a study also may raise many other theories. Examples include

- **Lack of informed consent:** A participant may contend that he was not told of a risk of injury that materialized. The specifics of what constitutes informed consent in the research setting is discussed at length in Chapter Five. The burden is on the investigator to obtain informed consent. An institution may also be held liable. In contrast, one federal court of appeals has held that a sponsor cannot be held liable for failure of an investigator to obtain informed consent. *Anderson v. Lanier Memorial Hospital.*

- **Battery:** If a person does not consent to a touching, the defendant is liable for battery. The interesting feature of this tort is that a battery requires that the defendant act intentionally but the plaintiff does not have to prove a physical injury or offer expert testimony as to what a reasonable physician would do. *Woodbury v. Courtney.* Most courts disfavor this cause of action in looking at medical care because a patient usually consents to some touching and the true issue is the nature of the touching. Did the physician act negligently in performing the surgery or was he negligent in failing to disclose a risk that eventually materialized?

- **Breach of confidentiality:** A participant may seek damages for unauthorized disclosure of medical or other personal information collected during a study. The mere disclosure that a participant is in a study may be the basis for such a lawsuit.

- **Infliction of emotional distress:** A researcher may be accused of causing emotional distress to a participant, either negligently or intentionally. This claim, for example, could arise in behavioral studies where a researcher is examining the response of participants to horrific, but false, information. Participants, or even their family members, may also seek damages for events during a biomedical study that cause emotional distress.

- **Fraud:** A disgruntled participant often alleges fraud by an investigator in that the participant contends he was not aware that he was enrolled in a study or did not know the extent of the study. This was intentionally hidden from him. The allegation of fraud extends the statute of limitations (discussed below) to some period after the true nature of the events was discovered.

- **Breach of contract:** Though usually not successful, a participant may contend that the relationship between the investigator and the participant was one of contract and the researcher failed to keep his end of the bargain. Most courts do not favor categorizing the physician-patient relationship in this manner, but the detailed documents related to informed consent for a research study may sway a court to allow a breach of contract claim to go forward.

- **Product liability:** Though a common cause of action in lawsuits stemming from the use of medications or medical devices that are being marketed, product liability is not frequently seen in lawsuits arising from research studies. However, such allegations can be alleged against the sponsor, the institution, the investigator, or all of them. The strong interest in pursuing a claim under product liability in most states is that the tort is one of strict liability. This is a higher standard of care for the defendant than just simple negligence.

- **Violations of civil rights:** Research participants have also tried to recover under theories of civil rights violations. Violations of constitutional rights by government employees may give rise to a cause of action (*Bivens v. Six Unknown Fed. Narcotics*). For example, plaintiffs have alleged that research sponsored by government entities violated their right to privacy and right to be free from state-sponsored invasion of a person's bodily integrity under the right to due process. The key elements of a claim under a constitutional violation are "that (1) a government actor, (2) without obtaining informed consent and utilizing false pretenses to obtain participation, (3) conducted medical experiments known to have no therapeutic value and indeed known to be possibly harmful to the participants" (*Heinrich v. Sweet*). Exposure to government-sponsored radiation experiments that had no therapeutic value and were not disclosed to the participants have been held to be violations of the right to bodily integrity (*Bibeau v. Pacific Northwest Research Foundation*); *Stadt v. Univ. of Rochester, In re Cincinnati Radiation Litigation*.

- **Vicarious liability:** An institution, a sponsor, or even another researcher may be held liable for the acts of another because the negligent party was the employee or agent of the defendant. Many states have also endorsed the concept of *apparent agency*, which means that a defendant can be held liable for the acts of another where the injured party reasonably believed that the negligent party was the employee or agent of the defendant. This allegation, for example, frequently is raised in cases arising from emergency department care in a hospital. The patient assumed that an ED physician was the employee of the hospital, and the patient contends that he came to the defendant hospital because he believed it employed good physicians. The same allegation might be raised where an independent contract research organization (CRO) operates on a medical facility's campus.

Potential Liability of IRB Members

The IRB members and vicariously the institution may be liable for negligence in performing their responsibilities in reviewing, approving, and monitoring studies. For example, the university's chief bioethicist and the members of IRB were sued in *Robertson v. McGee et al.* However, to date, the authors have not been able to find a verdict against an IRB or its members. Immunity provided under state peer review statutes may provide a defense.

In one of the few judicial opinions examining the role of an IRB, the failure of a facility's review committee to consider the ramifications of the interinstitutional transfer of cryopreserved human prezygotes did not vitiate the contract between parties nor did it usurp the court's jurisdiction to settle contractual disputes between the parties (*York v. Jones,* interpreting former Virginia statute on human research).

The Food, Drug & Cosmetic Act as Creating a Private Cause of Action

The Food, Drug & Cosmetic Act (FDCA) does not create a private cause of action. The U.S. Court of Appeals, Sixth Circuit has held that the estate of a patient who died from a toxic reaction when he took a medication refilled without a prescription could not use the FDCA as a basis for a civil lawsuit. Only the federal government can enforce the FDCA (*Bailey v. Johnson*). Likewise, a violation of the FDCA during clinical trials should not give rise to a separate cause of action. However, violation of a statute or regulation may be admissible as evidence of negligence.

The Venues in Which a Research Participant May File a Lawsuit

Where a lawsuit can be filed varies from state to state. Some states have a very expansive view of who can be sued in its courts. For example, New York very liberally construes what is sufficient contact with the state to give its state court's jurisdiction over a defendant (*Stadt v. Univ. of Rochester*). Other states are more conservative in allowing a defendant to be sued in its courts. Most states follow a "minimum contacts" analysis looking at whether the defendant could "reasonably anticipate being hauled into court there" (*Stadt* citing *World-Wide Volkswagen Corp. v. Woodson*).

To be sued in federal district court, not more than one party can be from the state in which the district court sits. This is referred to as complete diversity. Plaintiff may also gain access to the federal district court by alleging a federal cause of action.

Defenses That an Investigator, an Institution, or a Sponsor May Raise

Depending on the facts of a case, a defendant may be able to argue that he was not negligent, the participant was not injured, and the alleged injury was not proximately caused by any action or inaction of the defendant. In addition, the defendant may be able to raise one or more affirmative defenses such as the following:

- **Statute of Limitations:** Procedural law of each state mandates the time limit in which a research participant has to file a lawsuit. This ranges from one year to many years. Further confounding the calculation of a time limit are various exceptions to the statute of limitations. For example, some jurisdictions do not start the clock until the patient discovers the injury regardless of how long ago the medical care was. Many jurisdictions toll the statute of limitations until a child reaches the age of majority or for as long as an incompetent patient remains incompetent. Some states have imposed limits on these long-tails of exposure.

- **Consent:** A researcher may raise the affirmative defense that the participant consented to the touching (the study protocol). Consent is a complete defense to an allegation of battery.

- **Assumption of the risk:** Similar to the defense of consent, a researcher may allege that the participant was aware of the risk and agreed to assume the risk. The informed consent process is very useful in this defense. The more explicit and well documented that the process was, the stronger the defense (assuming the risk that is at issue was appropriately disclosed). Assumption of the risk should not be confused with a pre-injury release. Pre-injury releases of liability by a participant are prohibited in federally regulated research studies. Likewise most state court decisions and statutes either severely restrict or prohibit such agreements on the rationale that the injured person cannot agree to release the defendant from liability before he knows what the negligence will be or what his injury will be.

- **Contributory negligence:** A jury can consider whether a participant was also negligent. In a few states, any negligence by the plaintiff is a complete bar to recovery. In other states, negligence merely reduces the amount that the plaintiff can recover. This is often referred to as *comparative negligence.*

- **Learned intermediary:** Some states have adopted the defense of the learned intermediary. A product manufacturer can use this as a shield where its product must be prescribed or dispensed by a physician or other licensed professional. A physician, for example, is the one who has the superior knowledge of whether an investigational drug is appropriate for a particular patient. To illustrate the point, the Illinois Supreme Court held that a drug manufacturer could not be held liable for a patient who took a medication shortly before wrecking his car and injuring his passenger. The physician, not the manufacturer, had the responsibility to determine whether the drug was appropriate for the patient and to advise the patient of the risks (*Kirk v. Michael Reese Hospital*).

- **Sovereign immunity:** Governmental entities, whether federal, state, or local, enjoy immunity from civil liability. This extends to its employees when they are acting in their official capacities. By statute and court decisions, a multitude of exceptions have been created to this broad doctrine. For example, in Virginia, resident physicians but not faculty physicians are entitled to sovereign immunity (*James v. Jane*). The federal government permits itself to be sued under the conditions set forth in the Federal Tort Claims Act, 28 USC §2671 et seq. Employees of the federal government enjoy *qualified immunity* for their actions.

Government Liability for Injury to Military Personnel

The *Feres* doctrine holds that active duty military personnel cannot sue the government or other soldiers for alleged negligence (*Feres v. United States*). For example, soldiers are not allowed to sue a government hospital or physicians for negligent medical care. This doctrine extends even to situations where the soldier discovers that he was an unwitting human participant in a secret military experiment (*United States v. Stanley*). Some justices of the U.S. Supreme Court, in a dissenting opinion, pointed out the egregiousness of the *Feres* doctrine in this circumstance:

> Having invoked national security to conceal its actions, the Government now argues that the preservation of military discipline requires that Government officials remain free to violate the constitutional rights of soldiers without fear of money damages. What this case and others like it demonstrate, however, is that Government officials (military or civilian) must not be left with such freedom. See, e.g., Jaffee v.

United States, 663 F.2d 1226 (CA3 1981) (en banc) (exposure of soldiers to nuclear radiation during atomic weapons testing); Schnurman v. United States, 490 F. Supp. 429 (ED Va. 1980) (exposure of unknowing soldier to mustard gas); Thornwell v. United States, 471 F. Supp. 344 (D.C. 1979) (soldiers used to test the effects of LSD without their knowledge); cf. Barrett v. United States, No. 76 Civ. 381 (SDNY, May 5, 1987) (death of mental hospital patient used as the unconsenting participant of an Army experiment to test mescaline derivative). [483 U.S. 669, 690].

The Time Period in Which a Research Participant Can File a Lawsuit

The statute of limitations, as discussed above, varies from state to state. For example, Virginia has a two-year limit on filing actions alleging medical malpractice. Tennessee has a one-year limitation (*Hughes v. Vanderbilt University*).

Another state-dependent issue is when the statute of limitations period begins to run. Some states hold that the period begins to run from the date that the cause of action accrued. This is usually the date on which the negligence occurred. However, it may also be construed to be the date that the injury occurred (when the cancer developed) or the date that the injury was discovered (when the patient discovers that he had cancer). For example, a plaintiff was not barred from filing a lawsuit in 1995 stemming from a 1945 experiment where school children were given radioactive lemonade. The press did not cover the story until 1994. However, a suit filed in 1997 was untimely in light of the 1994 press coverage (*Hughes v. Vanderbilt University*). As to when a plaintiff first has or reasonably should have knowledge of the critical facts of his injury, which are that he has been hurt and who has inflicted the injury, is a question of fact generally to be decided by a jury (*Bibeau v. Pacific Northwest Research Foundation*). In the *Bibeau* case, for example, the U.S. Court of Appeals held that the key question was "whether, had Bibeau seen a doctor about his symptoms [severe testicular pain, rash, enlarged lymph nodes, etc.], the doctor would have discovered Bibeau's participation in the experiments [testicular radiation of state prison inmates] and then made a connection between the two" (*Id.* at 11).

The limitations period for allegations of fraudulent concealment does not usually begin to run until the fraud is discovered (*Heinrich v. Sweet et al.*). The date of discovery by a plaintiff is a question of fact to be determined by a jury when fraud is alleged (*Anderson v. Lanier Memorial Hospital*) (interpreting the tolling of Alabama's statutes of limitation). The judge should decide this issue as a matter of law only when a plaintiff actually knew of the facts that would put a reasonable person on notice of fraud (*Id.* quoting *Green v. Wedowee Hospital*).

· · · · · · · · · · ·

GENERAL CONCEPTS OF PROFESSIONAL NEGLIGENCE

The Basic Elements of a Negligence Lawsuit

A plaintiff must allege and prove that the defendant was negligent, that the plaintiff was injured, and that the plaintiff's injury was proximately caused by the defendant's negligence.

In a negligence action stemming from human research, a research participant must prove the standard of care for a reasonable clinical investigator, the defendant investigator deviated from the standard of care (negligence) and the participant was injured by the deviation from the standard of care (damages and proximate cause). Other causes of action may require different elements of proof.

Negligence

Negligence when applied to a medical malpractice case is usually defined as a deviation from the standard of care. Standard of care means what a reasonable physician or clinical investigator would do in the same or similar circumstances. This is not a scientific formula and is determined by the testimony of expert witnesses.

Damages

Damages are often obvious (blindness or other physical impairment, medical bills, lost income, etc.). However, a plaintiff may also seek to recover for psychological injuries, embarrassment, loss of companionship, and other hard-to-quantify damages. The challenging task for a jury is to attach a dollar figure to any damages that the plaintiff has proved that he suffered.

Punitive Damages

Also called *exemplary damages,* punitive damages are intended to punish the defendant for willful or wanton misconduct. This requires more than simple negligence by a defendant. The conduct must have been egregious.

Proximate Cause

Proximate cause is the legal requirement that a defendant's negligence must have caused or contributed to the plaintiff's injuries. In other words, the plaintiff would not have suffered the alleged injury (or the extent of injury) but for the defendant's negligence. This is often a challenging task when the plaintiff's condition before the alleged negligence was likely to lead to some physical impairment. The task for the jury to determine was what amount of a plaintiff's condition was caused or contributed to by the defendant's negligence.

Expert Testimony in a Research Negligence Lawsuit

Usually the testimony of an expert witness is required on the issue of what a reasonable investigator would have done. Plaintiff, because he has the burden of proof, usually must have an expert witness who will state to a reasonable degree of certainty that the defendant deviated from the standard of care for a reasonable investigator. Plaintiff, using the same expert witness or another, is usually also required to present evidence that the plaintiff's injury was proximately caused by defendant's negligence. If the plaintiff's alleged damages are not obvious, he may also need an expert witness to describe the kind and extent of injury suffered (For a more in-depth discussion, see Morin (1998)).

Proving the Standard of Care in a Research Protocol

In order to prove *the standard of care* for an investigator in a clinical trial, plaintiff will usually be required to call an expert witness. The expert witness must have expertise in the same or similar field as the defendant investigator. The expert witness must show through education, training, or experience that he knows what the standard of care for a reasonable investigator in similar circumstances is. He then must testify that the defendant deviated from the standard of care for a reasonable investigator. Obviously, the precision of matching clinical experience to that of the defendant can be difficult where the defendant is on the cutting edge of a field. The trial court may give leeway in qualifying an expert witness in this area. The decision is left to the jury as to the credibility of an expert witness.

Another means of trying to establish the standard of care is by proving that an investigator violated a federal or state regulation. State courts have interpreted the significance of violating a statute or regulation differently. Many states have held that the violation of a statute is some evidence of negligence. Others, such as Maryland, have held that violating a federal research regulation is negligence per se (*Grimes v. Kennedy Krieger Institute, Inc.*).

A research agreement between an investigator and a participant can, as a matter of law, create a special relationship giving rise to duties of the investigator to the participant. A breach of those duties may constitute negligence (Restatement of Torts, 2nd; *Grimes v. Kennedy Krieger Institute, Inc.; Moore v. Regents of University of California*).

Proving a Lack of Informed Consent

Traditionally, a plaintiff must prove what a reasonable physician would tell a patient (standard of care), a deviation from that by the defendant, plaintiff was injured, and that but for the defendant's deviation from the standard of care the plaintiff would not have been injured (proximate cause). Plaintiff usually must offer expert testimony on these elements. The state courts have split as to whether the standard for determining proximate cause is one of an objective nature or subjective nature. The objective test is whether a reasonable patient would have refused the intervention if he had been told of the risk that materialized. The plaintiff's testimony, while relevant, is not determinative (*Pardy v. U.S., Dessi v. U.S.*). In contrast, the subjective test is whether the plaintiff, based on whatever was important to him, would have refused the intervention if he had been advised of the risk that materialized (*Canterbury v. Spence*). Although not often considered by courts in the clinical research setting, the subjective standard, which has been rejected in most jurisdictions for medical malpractice actions, may be accepted as the rule for informing patients in purely elective studies. The amount of information that must be disclosed to a patient is usually inversely related to the immediacy of needing treatment. For example, emergency repair of a ruptured aortic aneurysm does not have to be preceded by the degree of detailed discussion on risks and benefits as compared with an elective breast augmentation.

Some states require in a medical malpractice trial that an expert witness testify as to what a reasonable patient would do when a plaintiff alleges that informed consent was not obtained. That is, a plaintiff must elicit from an expert witness that a reasonable patient would not have agreed to undergo the experimental therapy. Other states do not require, and some do not permit, an expert witness to testify as to what a reasonable patient would do. This is left to the jury to determine. Due to the elective nature of participation in a research project, few states are likely to require expert testimony as to what a reasonable participant would do if he had been informed of a risk that materialized.

············

LIMITING LIABILITY

Use of a Waiver or Release in an Effort to Limit Liability

Federal regulations expressly prohibit a clinical investigator from attempting to limit his liability through the use of a waiver or release signed by the participant prior to enrolling in the study (21 CFR §50.20). Several states have similar statutes. The law frowns on a person being asked to waive his right to be compensated for the negligence of another before the negligence occurs and before the extent of the injury is known. This is particularly true where a study participant is at a disadvantage to the better-informed investigator about the potential risks of a study.

The Supreme Court of Washington, for example, has held that a pre-injury release of negligence by a medical investigator is void as a matter of public policy. However, it made a point of saying that a patient or research participant remains free to waive the right to recover for injury in other situations. The courts in Washington will enforce a pre-injury release of liability for recreational activities. It apparently would also recognize a patient's right to give informed consent (as distinguished from a release) in a clinical study setting: "With proper informed consent, an ill patient may wish to consent to a highly experimental treatment which might otherwise not be generally accepted" (*Vodopest v. MacGregor*). A well-crafted informed consent document will advise the participant of risks, benefits, and alternatives. This is important from the perspective of reducing allegations that the participant was not adequately warned of potential adverse outcomes before agreeing to enroll in the study. Though not usually well received by a jury, an investigator may raise the defense that the participant assumed the risk of injury after being fully advised.

Compensation of Participants for Injury Occurring as a Result of Participation in a Research Study

Institutional policy, not federal regulation, determines whether compensation and medical treatment(s) will be offered and the conditions that might be placed on participant eligibility for compensation or treatment(s). The FDA informed consent regulation on compensation (21 CFR §50.25(a)(6)) requires that, for research involving more than minimal risk, the participant must be told *whether* any compensation and any medical treatment(s) are available if injury occurs and, if so, what they are, or where further information may be obtained (FDA, Information Sheets, 1998). Many commentators contend that the sponsor of a clinical trial should be responsible for providing medical care and compensation for study-induced illness or injury, regardless of the cost and strength of the proximate cause relationship.

Sponsor Indemnification of the Investigator and Others Involved in a Clinical Study

Federal regulations do not prohibit a sponsor from agreeing to indemnify an investigator for any expenses related to defending claims for compensation for injuries suffered in a clinical trial. The investigator would be well advised to carefully review the contract with a sponsor to ascertain the scope of such an indemnity agreement: Does it include attorney's fees and other costs related to defending a claim or lawsuit? Does it include allegations of willful misconduct by the investigator? Does the investigator have the right to determine whether or not the sponsor settles a claim? Does the investigator have the right to choose what lawyer will defend him? Likewise, an institution would be well advised to consider these issues before hosting a research study.

NIH Certificate of Confidentiality

The National Institutes of Health (NIH) has the authority under federal law to issue a Certificate of Confidentiality. The certificate protects an investigator and institution from being compelled by a subpoena or court order to divulge information that would identify research participants in civil, criminal, or administrative tribunals (42 USC §241(d)). The certificates can be granted for studies collecting information that if disclosed could have adverse consequences on the research participants or damage their financial standing, employability, insurability, or reputation. The federal government need not fund a study in order to grant a certificate. Additional information on this recent federal initiative can be found at http://grants1.nih.gov/grants/policy/coc/.

Insurance Issues for Clinical Research

Investigators, institutions need to confirm that existing insurance coverage extends to research activities. As soon as an institution, investigator, or sponsor becomes aware of potential liability claims, their insurance company needs to be notified. Failure to do so in a timely manner may be a breach of the insurance contract, resulting in the defendant having no insurance coverage (*United States Fire Ins. Co. v. Vanderbilt University*).

References

Anderson v. Lanier Memorial Hospital. 982 F.2d 1513 (Eleventh Cir., 1993).

Bailey v. Johnson, 48 F.3d 965 (Sixth Cir., 1995).

Bibeau v. Pacific Northwest Research Foundation. Case No. 95-06410 (D. Ore. September 27, 1996), dismissed on other grounds, 980 F. Supp. 349 (1998)

Bivens v. Six Unknown Fed. Narcotics Agents, 403 US §388 (1971).

Canterbury v. Spence

Cincinnati Radiation Litigation, 874 F. Supp. 796. 810-11 (S.D. Ohio 1995).

Dessi v. United States, 489 F. Supp. 722, 728 (ED Va. 1980).

FDA. Information Sheets, Guidance for Institutional Review Boards and Clinical Investigations. Frequently Asked Question #11. 1998.

Federal Tort Claims Act. 28 USC §2671 et. seq.

Feres v. United States, 340 US §135 (1950).

42 USC §241(d).

Green v. Wedowee Hospital, 584 So. 2d 1309, 1312 (Ala. 1991).

Grimes v. Kennedy Krieger Institute, Inc. 782 A.2d 807 (Md. 2001).

Heinrich v. Sweet, 62 F. Supp. 2d 282 (D. Mass. 1999).

Hughes v. Vanderbilt University, 2000 Fed. App. 0193P (Sixth Cir., 2000).

James v. Jane, 221 Va. 43 (1980).

Kirk v. Michael Reese Hospital, 117 Ill. 2D 507 (1987).

Moore v. Regents of University of California, 793 P.2d 479 (Cal. 1990).

Morin, K. The Standard of Disclosure in Human Participant Experimentation. 19 J. Legal Med. 157, 202 (1998).

Pardy v. United States, 783 F.2d 710, 715 (Seventh Circ., 1986).

Robertson v. McGee et al., Case No. 01CV00G0H(M). U.S. District Court, Oklahoma.

Stadt v. Univ. of Rochester, 921 F. Supp. 1023, 1027–28 (WDNY, 1996). 21 CFR §50.20.

United States Fire Ins. Co. v. Vanderbilt University, 267 F.3d 465 (2001).

United States v. Stanley, 483 US §669 (1987).

Vodopest v. MacGregor, 128 Wn. 2d 840, 861; 913 P.2d 779, 789 (1996).

Woodbury v. Courtney, 239 Va. 651, 654 (1990).

World-Wide Volkswagen Corp. v. Woodson, 444 US §286, 297 (1980).

York v. Jones, 717 F. Supp. 421 (ED Va. 1989).

15

Quality Improvement, Accreditation, and Risk Management in Clinical Trials

Overview 404
Quality Improvement 404
    The OHRP Approach to Quality Improvement in Clinical Trials 405
    Confidentiality and QI Activities 406
    The OHRP Tool 406
Accreditation 407
    The VAHRPAP Approach to Accreditation 407
    The AAHRPP Approach to Accreditation 408
    Comparison of Accreditation Programs 409
Risk Management 409
    Risk Management in Clinical Trials 410
    Risk Identifiers for a Clinical Trials Risk Management Program 410
    Practical Examples of Risk Management in Clinical Trials 412
        Research Subject Risk Elimination Example 412
        Regulatory Compliance Risk Prevention Example 412
        Risk Reduction Example 412
        Risk Minimization Example 412
    The Role of the Risk Manager in Clinical Trials 413
    Practical Risk Management Strategies to Follow in Terms
    of Developing Policies and Procedures for Clinical Trials Administration 414
    Credentialing Principal Investigators and IRB Members:
    A Risk Management Perspective 416
    Criteria for a Research Credentialing Program 418
    Insurance Coverages and Solutions for Clinical Trials 419
Record Management and Reporting 421
    Record Retention and Clinical Trials 421
    Documenting and Managing Clinical Trial-Related Adverse Events 422
    The Risk Management Challenges in Reporting Adverse Events 423
    The Claims Management Process for a Clinical Trial Adverse Event 424
Conclusion 425
References 426
Forms 427

· · · · · · · · · · · ·

OVERVIEW

Clinical trials research is now the focal point of a myriad of interventions from quality improvement, to accreditation, and risk management. On the basis of concerns about research subject safety and regulatory compliance, the OHRP has embarked on a quality improvement campaign to help institutions assess and enhance the quality of human research protection programs.

Accreditation models have emerged for human research protection programs. One, developed by the National Committee on Accreditation (NCQA) and the Department of Veterans Affairs, accredits VA medical centers through its mandatory Veterans Affairs Human Research Protection Accreditation Program (VAHRPAP). In December 2002, NCQA published draft standards for a human research accreditation program that will go beyond VA facilities ("NCQA Releases Draft Standards for Human Research Protection Accreditation Program," NCQA, December 3, 2002). In January 2003, NCQA announced that it had formed a partnership with the Joint Commission on Accreditation of Healthcare Organizations (JCAHO) to accredit human research protection programs in the United States and abroad ("NCQA, JCAHO Form Partnership," January 16, 2003). Called the "Partnership for Human Research, Inc." PHRP Accreditation expect to publish their final accreditation standards in 2003. The accreditation field has another participant, the Association for the Accreditation of Human Research Protection Programs, Inc. (AAHRPP). The AAHRPP is applicable to academic institutions, hospitals, government agencies, private corporations, independent review boards, and eligible international entities.

Beyond quality improvement and accreditation, many human research protection programs are developing concrete loss prevention and loss control programs. Built on the model of healthcare risk management, these programs recognize that conducting clinical trials research is an activity fraught with all types of risk exposure. Noncompliance with federal and state legal requirements, breach of sponsor contracts, failure to follow IRB rules, and injury-producing adverse events all create risk exposures. As discussed in this chapter, the activities involved in the clinical trials risk management program include education, development of cogent policies, and procedures for clinical trials administration, and practical measures for managing adverse events. Also discussed is documentation management, claims management, and insurance coverages for clinical trials.

· · · · · · · · · · · ·

QUALITY IMPROVEMENT

Quality improvement is a process for identifying and enhancing activities ripe for change. It is a process found in industry and it has been an integral part of the healthcare field for two decades. Through quality improvement wasteful practices can be eliminated and efficiencies can be implemented. Needless process variation once removed from the system can lead to greater job and customer satisfaction. This is as true for an automobile assembly plant as it is in the activities surrounding review and oversight of clinical trials research.

Described in this section is a quality improvement initiative launched by the Office for Human Research Protections (OHRP). Included in the discussion is a review of the methods used by OHRP and the tool specially designed for use in the quality improvement initiative.

The OHRP Approach to Quality Improvement in Clinical Trials

According to the OHRP (2002) there are three objectives to its Quality Improvement (QI) Program:

1. To increase quality, performance, and efficiency of institutional human subjects protection programs
2. To ensure compliance with federal regulations regarding the protection of human research subjects
3. To help prepare institutions to achieve accreditation of their programs through private-sector accrediting organizations

Through the auspices of the Division of Assurances and Quality Improvement (DAQI), OHRP offers both consultative services and support to those with institutional human subjects protection programs. It addresses the needs of institutions that conduct biomedical, behavioral, and social research. It also encompasses the activities of independent IRBs (OHRP, 2002).

As described by OHRP, the program has three components. The first is a self-assessment that is designed to evaluate institutional compliance with the regulations governing human research protection. The DAQI will help guide the self-assessment process, and it may review the operating procedures of the human research protection program.

DAQI will evaluate the self-assessment and communicate with the institution. This may be done through written correspondence, teleconference, videoconference, or on-site consultation (OHRP, 2002). DAQI will then provide guidance and recommendations for quality improvement. The interactions between DAQI and the institution "will include mechanisms to protect the confidentiality of information voluntarily provided by the institution" (OHRP, 2002).

With the baseline information in hand, DAQI will work with the institution on the second stage of the process. This second component is the actual Quality Improvement component. It will include consultations on improvements and posting on the OHRP Web site of best practices and tools designed to enhance quality and performance. OHRP will also facilitate networking or sharing of best practices information among willing participant institutions.

The third component will focus on continuous quality improvement (CQI) at the institutional level. On a voluntary basis, DAQI wants to share successful strategies among willing participant organizations (OHRP, 2002).

To "incentivize" human protection programs to participate in the QI Program, OHRP has implemented a new strategy. OHRP has announced the expansion of its not-for-cause evaluations (NFC) carried out by the Division of Compliance Oversight. Institutions will be selected for NFC evaluations on the basis of criteria that is designed to result in a representative sampling on a regular basis. The evaluations will focus on IRB documentation and policies and procedures. On some occasions the NFC evaluations will include a site visit (Koski, 2002).

An effort will be made to avoid NFC evaluations for those institutions with a QI Program. Indeed, OHRP has indicated that if an institution within the past two years has participated in the QI Program or is in the process of doing so, it will defer doing an NFC evaluation on the entity. If, however, the institution that is in process cannot complete the QI Program in a mutually agreed upon time period, it will be put back in the pool of entities subject to an NFC evaluation. Hence, the prospect of an NFC serves as an incentive to participate in the QI Program.

Of the two approaches, the QI Program is the more preferable approach. It is voluntary, and it puts the institution on the road to preparing for accreditation. Having a QI program in place can also lead to efficiencies and lessen the prospect of process variation. Because process variation can lead to subject injury, quality improvement is a positive development.

Confidentiality and QI Activities

As noted, confidentiality in the QI Program will be addressed through a determination made under Exemption 4 of the Freedom of Information Act (FOIA). As OHRP suggested, Exemption 4 enables it to withhold information submitted on a voluntary basis to the QI Program that is confidential or privileged. Prior to submitting information, an institution can identify data that it believes is within the scope of Exemption 4. Should a request be submitted under the Freedom of Information Act, OHRP FOIA officials will review the data to see if the exemption is applicable. If the information is subject to release, the institution supplying it will be notified prior to disclosing it.

This confidentiality mechanism is not air tight. One can envision situations in which disputes can arise over the applicability of Exemption 4. A better approach would be to develop a legislative solution that recognizes a quality improvement protection for such voluntary reporting. Until that step is taken, however, care should be exercised in providing sensitive data under the QI Program.

There is another reason to be cautious on the issue of disclosure of confidential information. In the ordinary course of its work, DAQI does not convey information about its QI activity to the Division of Compliance Oversight (DCO) of OHRP. However, this may not be the case when during a QI consultation DAQI learns about serious systemic noncompliance or serious problems that have resulted in or may cause a threat to research subject safety. In such instances, DAQI will notify institutional officials. They will be expected to take prompt action to rectify the problem, and these institutional officials will be expected to submit to OHRP a corrective action plan. For its part, OHRP is committed to working in a collegial manner to help the institution develop and implement such an action plan.

The situation is not encompassed in any form of rigid evidentiary protection. Input is imperative from legal counsel on practical measures to take in such instances. The intent is not to hide or cover up improper conduct; rather, it is not to develop action plans or documentation that lead to needless liability exposure at the expense of quality improvement.

The OHRP Tool

As noted earlier, OHRP has created a self-assessment tool for use in its QI Program. The purpose is to help human subjects protection programs determine if they comply with relevant federal requirements. Some of the questions in the tool go beyond regulatory compliance, focusing on IRB work volume and resources available to the human protection program.

The tool was designed for ease of completion, with most answers requiring a yes, no, or not applicable response. Once the tool has been completed, the human research protection program and OHRP can identify institutional compliance with the federal requirements. OHRP believes that the answers will also identify areas of strength and weakness. The need for education may also be identified as a result of the answers provided in the self-assessment process. OHRP also believes that with the answers provided it can help an institution enhance its performance, efficiency, and the quality of its human research program.

A copy of the OHRP *QA Self-Assessment Tool* is found at the end of this chapter. The answers gleaned from the tool track general administration of the IRB functions, management of non-compliance and conflict of interest, IRB workload and staffing issues, education and training, and IRB policies and procedures. The submission process is also evaluated in the QA Self-Assessment Tool. This is for both new protocols and those under continuing review. The tool also examines the actual review process utilized by the IRB. Several questions address the content of the minutes of the IRB and communication with investigators.

From a practical standpoint, the QA Self-Assessment Tool is a useful review for any human subjects protection program. For IRBs, investigators, and institutions it is a blueprint of what OHRP sees as key elements of the human subjects protection program. Honest answers are imperative. If the responses indicate strong adherence to the regulations, it is a good indicator of a quality program. However, if there is little compliance, it is a warning that steps should be taken to rectify identified problems.

Once completed, the Tool serves as notice that a facility knows or ought to know where it is having difficulties in terms of regulatory compliance. Failure to take corrective action when there is an awareness of non-compliance resulting in foreseeable harm to a research subject may serve as grounds in a claim of negligence. Regulatory compliance is not the only incentive for adhering to the regulations in this arena.

···········

ACCREDITATION

The VAHRPAP Approach to Accreditation

The National Committee for Quality Assurance (NCQA), long known for managed care accreditation, joined forces with the Department of Veterans Affairs (VA) to launch an accreditation program to protect human subjects in research projects (NCQA, 2001). The VAHRPAP reviews the systems in place to protect research subjects in studies at Veterans Affairs Medical Centers (VAMC).

The VAHRPAP program addresses six key areas:

- Institutional accountability for the protection of human research subjects
- Organization and process of the IRB
- The way in which the IRB evaluates risks and benefits
- The way in which the IRB evaluates research subject recruitment and selection
- IRB evaluation of risks to privacy and confidentiality in research
- IRB evaluation of informed consent practices for research participants

Changes have been proposed to the initial set of accreditation standards ("VA Human Research Protection Accreditation Program Accreditation Standards," Version 2.0, September 5, 2002). If adopted, the revised standards will reflect changes in scoring and an attempt to streamline the accreditation process. The revised standards would also require institutions to seek input from current and potential subjects regarding improvements in research and human subject protection programs.

In December 2002, NCQA released a draft set of standards for a *new* Human Research Protection Accreditation Program (HRPAP) for public comment. Based on the VAHRPAP model, the new program was to target hospitals, medical schools, and pharmaceutical firms, as well as independent IRBs that *review but do not undertake* research. The focus on the proposed standards was to be on organizational responsibilities, the structure and operations of an IRB, consideration of risks and benefits, and informed consent ("NCQA Releases Draft Standards for Human Research Protection Accreditation Program," NCQA, December 3, 2002).

In January 2003 NCQA and the Joint Commission on Accreditation of Healthcare Organization announced the creation of the Partnership for Human Research Protection, Inc. (PHRP) Accreditation Program. A separate corporate entity, the Partnership subsumed the draft accreditation standards announced by NCQA in December 2002. The PHRP accreditation program will place heavy reliance on a Web-based review. For this purpose, the entity that wants to go through the accreditation process will use a Standards Guideline and Assessment Tool (SGAT). It will provide a framework for determining accreditation review readiness status and areas in need of improvement. Provision is made for a site review by surveyors who will validate actual performance with the accreditation standards. Through the SGAT, the organization will receive detailed performance reports to help advance quality improvement initiatives.

The PHRP Accreditation Program focuses on a continuous quality improvement approach. It is not focused on compliance with minimum standards. The PHRP program will be looking for best practices as well.

The new accreditation process is expected to be finalized in 2003 ("NCQA Releases Draft Standards for Human Research Protection Accreditation Program," NCQA, December 3, 2002). Once implemented it is expected that accreditation status will serve as a differentiator for accredited human research protection programs. In essence the PHRP accredited programs will be seen as the "go to" organizations for research activities premised on quality, safety, and subjects' rights.

Hospitals with human research protection programs that are currently accredited by JCAHO will not be expected to undergo PHRP accreditation. This is a choice that hospitals must make as it is a voluntary process offered by a separate corporate entity.

The AAHRPP Approach to Accreditation

The Association for the Accreditation of Human Research Protection Programs, Inc. (AAHRPP) provides another opportunity for accreditation of human subject protection programs. The AAHRPP is a voluntary accreditation process that is focused on education and developing "a culture of conscience and responsibility" ("Accreditation Step-by-Step," AAHRPP). It was founded by well-respected organizations, including the Association of American Medical Colleges (AAMC), the Association of American Universities (AAU), the Federation of American Societies for Experimental Biology, the National Associate of State Universities and Land Grant Colleges, and Public Research in Medicine and Research (PRIM&R).

The accreditation process includes a self-assessment, completion of a detailed outline, and submission of a complete description of the human subjects protection program. Thereafter, a team of experts conducts an on-site review. The AAHRPP Council on Accreditation reviews the findings of the site survey team and makes a determination of accreditation status.

AAHRPP has divided its standards into what it calls five domains. These domains focus on organization, the research review unit, the investigator, the sponsor, and the participant (AAHRPP, 2002).

Comparison of Accreditation Programs

Both the VAHRPAP and the AAHRPP accreditation programs embrace a series of standards. The same is true of the newly announced accreditation process, PHRP. The idea is to set a foundation or benchmark for clinical trials programs. In doing so the goal has been to set standards to safeguard the health and welfare of research subjects.

By becoming an accredited program, the IRB or institution agrees to abide by the accreditation standards. The failure to abide by these standards can have serious consequences. These include breach of contract with a funding entity or sponsor and regulatory non-compliance. In a situation in which a subject has experienced injury, accreditation standards non-compliance may also be used as evidence of negligence.

Accreditation is not a form of window dressing. It is a status that sets apart human research programs from the competition. As such, it places a specific compliance responsibility on the institution, IRB, research administration, and research investigators.

It is reasonable to ask how do the major accreditation programs differ? Is there an advantage to going with one accreditation program over another? The new PHRP program focuses on organizational responsibilities, the individual structure and operations of an IRB, risks and benefits, and informed consent. The PHRP blends together self-assessment, off-site review of self-assessment results, and on-site surveys. It is not too dissimilar from the AAHRP program in terms of the process.

PHRP is the creation of two long-standing accreditation programs. AAHRP sprung from a number of prestigious groups interested in clinical research. Both are being impacted by Institute of Medicine Reports and consumer demand for subject safety in clinical research. PHRP sees its accreditation program as driving accountability at each level of a research organization. AAHRP, like PHRP, sees the accreditation approach as the basis for installing confidence in sponsors of clinical research that human research organizations are meeting important standards.

The accreditation programs require a disciplined approach that goes beyond meeting the basic standards set out in federal and state law. Over time, it remains to be seen what will happen with the evolution of the accreditation process.

. . . .

RISK MANAGEMENT

Risk management is a systemic process for identifying and handling actual and potential financial loss exposures that stem from clinical trial-related injury to the person, property, or reputation of a research subject, a healthcare professional, or institution. The same concept applies in other fields such as aviation, manufacturing, maritime shipping, and healthcare in general.

Risk management has long been associated with the insurance industry. In an attempt to stem the tide of losses, insurers have encouraged clients to pinpoint areas of actual and potential loss exposure. Once known, steps are taken to eliminate or prevent the risk from occurring. If this is not possible, measures are taken to reduce the likely frequency of occurrence, to minimize the severity of potential outcome, and, in many instances, to transfer the risk of loss. The latter step is associated with insurance coverages, contractual language that shifts the financial burden of loss, and other risk-financing alternatives.

Aside from risk-financing methodologies, risk management is premised on three major initiatives: education, communication, and documentation. As information is learned about potential risks and steps are taken to manage the loss exposure, the risk management system uses the data to refine education, communication, and processes to lessen the likelihood of adverse events. The process is illustrated in Figure 15.1.

It is a closed-loop process that when functioning enables effective management of risk exposures associated with clinical trials administration.

Risk Management in Clinical Trials

The risk management process has a direct application to clinical trials. Conducting research on human subjects involves risk-taking that might culminate in adverse outcomes. Lessening the likelihood of such results involves eliminating and preventing risks that need not be part of the study. Steps can also be built into clinical trials that can reduce the likelihood of adverse outcomes and, when research subjects experience reactions, mechanisms built into the study can lessen the scope of possible injury. Seen in this way, risk management has a direct application to clinical trials administration.

Risk management is also applicable to the loss exposures involved in non-compliance with regulatory and contractual requirements pertinent to clinical trials. Risk management is a system that can be structured to identify actual or potential deficiencies in consent procedures, monitoring practices, billing, coding, or that pinpoints undisclosed conflict-of-interest. Once identified, steps can be taken to mitigate potential harm that might otherwise result in the study being halted or subjected to in-depth regulatory scrutiny.

Risk Identifiers for a Clinical Trials Risk Management Program

Each entity should develop its own set of practical risk identifiers for clinical trials. The set used by a hospital will differ from identifiers used by a CRO or a sponsor of a research study. The differences reflect the types of risk exposures that each organization must use to pinpoint the opportunity for loss stemming from clinical research.

FIGURE 15.1.   The Risk Management Process

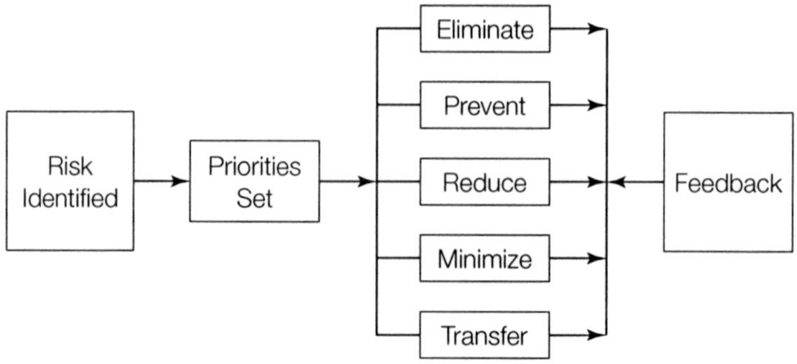

Common risk identifiers can be divided into those involving research subjects and clinical trials administration. Sample identifiers in terms of subject safety include the following:

- Adverse reaction to study device
- Adverse reaction to study medications
- Compliance with study protocol
- Consent deficiencies
- Dropping out of study
- Dietary non-compliance
- Enrollment of study subjects who do not meet entry criteria
- Medication non-compliance
- Missed appointments
- Unexpected death
- Unexpected disability
- Unexpected hospitalization

Identifiers that might be used for research administration include

- Adverse event
- Annual review of ongoing studies—non-compliance
- Billing errors—submitting accounts to sponsor and Medicare or private payer
- Claims
- Complaints
- Consent deficiencies
- Confidentiality deficiencies
- Conflict-of-interest issues
- Contractual non-compliance
- Documentation deficiencies
- Failure to obtain demonstrated competencies in education for IRB members, research investigators, and research staff
- Failure to report research subject injury
- Failure to manage research subject injury
- Occupational safety non-compliance
- Recruitment practices
- Regulatory non-compliance
- Research subject selection practices
- Scientific misconduct
- Study design deficiencies
- Workers compensation claims

Practical Examples of Risk Management in Clinical Trials

Risk management involves eliminating, preventing, reducing, and minimizing loss exposures. It also involves risk transfer arrangements such as purchasing selected insurance products to address potential risk exposures. The latter will be addressed later in the chapter. Illustrative cases help to demonstrate the value of risk management in clinical trials administration.

Research Subject Risk Elimination Example   Enrollment criteria for a medication study excludes individuals with a history of asthma. The pool of potential subjects completes a confidential healthcare inventory. One individual who answered, "yes" to the question, "Do you have a history of asthma" was nonetheless enrolled in the study. The study investigator reviewed the healthcare inventory documentation for those selected for inclusion in the study. When he found the positive answer to the asthma question, he rejected the person from the research trial. He also asked his associates to conduct a meticulous review of the completed healthcare inventory information to make certain that no one was enrolled in the study with a history of asthma.

Risk Management Intervention: By carefully examining the documentation, the principal investigator eliminated the risk of a potential subject experiencing an adverse reaction to the test medication.

Regulatory Compliance Risk Prevention Example   The research administrator conducted an orientation program for new clinical investigators. One of the topics was use of waiver provisions for access to confidential information. The orientation led to a discussion with a new clinical investigator who did not understand the process to follow for securing a waiver under application law. The study she was in the process of designing did not make it clear that a waiver was contemplated for the study.

Through the educational program, the problem was identified and non-compliance was prevented. The instructor referred the clinical investigator to the Chief Research Officer for assistance in revising the study for purposes of regulatory compliance.

Risk Management Intervention: Education helped to prevent regulatory non-compliance on the part of a research investigator unfamiliar with the requirements for securing a waiver from an IRB or Privacy Board.

Risk Reduction Example   A study involved a test medication with a high frequency of moderate to severe dizziness among research subjects. The symptoms were known to last for no more than three hours. Attempts to walk without assistance had culminated in twenty-five falls resulting in a least one fractured wrist. To reduce the frequency of falls, the study was modified to restrict ambulation until subjects were free of dizziness. The intervention led to a major reduction in injury-producing falls.

Risk Management Intervention: Modifying the ambulation component of the study dramatically lessened the likelihood of falls. Although the intervention did not eliminate the risk of falls, it did reduce the frequency of the loss exposure.

Risk Minimization Example   A research study resulted in a subject experiencing a severe drop in blood pressure during the course of the experimental protocol. It was the sixth such episode reported in a multicenter study involving 2500 subjects. The principal investigator worked with his colleagues at two of the centers to develop an early warning and intervention protocol to be used with any subject who appeared to have a similar reaction. Although the protocol did not reduce the frequency of the adverse event, it did minimize the likelihood of death and the need for hospitalization.

Risk Management Intervention: Communication of early indicators to pinpoint the onset of an adverse reaction coupled with intervention strategies minimized the likelihood of an outcome involving hospitalization or death.

The Role of the Risk Manager in Clinical Trials

Risk management professionals can be found throughout all manner of healthcare organizations, CROs, and pharmaceutical and medical device manufacturing firms. The role of the risk management professional is to help the entity handle actual and potential loss exposures. This is done through a combination of measures including education, designing effective communication and documentation practices, monitoring and surveillance for potential loss exposures, and mitigation efforts for risk that do occur. The risk management professional is often the responsible person for negotiating insurance coverages, arranging for alternate risk financing mechanisms, and managing claims.

In many hospitals and other healthcare organizations, the risk management professional is responsible for other departments or functions. Thus the person with the title risk manager may also be the Director of Information Services, the Infection Control Officer, the Process Improvement Director, Human Resources Director, or Corporate Compliance Officer. In larger organizations, however, a full-time risk management professional usually has as a sole or primary focus on loss prevention, loss control, and insurance programs. With the healthcare field focusing on patient safety strategies, including those focused on research subject effort, a gradual trend has begun in which the risk manager has moved up the corporate ranks to become the Chief Risk Officer.

In the clinical trial setting, the risk manager interfaces with research office administrative personnel, the IRB, principal investigators, and research study staff. The interactions may involve education, reviewing policies and procedures from a risk management perspective, handling complaints, or managing claims stemming from an adverse event that occurred in a study. The risk management professional might also be involved in handling workers compensation issues for research study staff or arranging insurance coverages for clinical trials.

In many facilities, the risk manager is *not* involved in research trials until there is an actual or potential claim. The risk manager is not a participant in education. Many are shut out from participating as institutional members of the IRB. It is a reflection of an attitude that risk managers are in place just to handle claims or so narrow in their viewpoints that given a role on IRBs, they would reject most protocols as containing an unacceptable level of risk.

Old attitudes about risk managers reflect a stereotype that is unjustly deserved. Indeed, it reflects a misunderstanding of the role and training of risk management professionals. Many risk management professionals come to their jobs with a broad range of clinical healthcare experience. Schooled in statistics, utilization of data, a broad knowledge of laws and regulations, education and training methodologies, their task is to *manage* the risks that come from business decisions made by corporate leadership. It is not the responsibility of the professional risk manager to stop studies from going forward or from precluding healthcare organizations from embarking on new treatment systems. Rather, it is the role of the risk management professional to operationalize the level of risk accepted by senior leadership. Thus an IRB may approve a study with a high level of risk for research subjects. The role of the risk management professional is to assist in creating an environment that helps to eliminate, prevent, reduce, and minimize potential risks involved in such an approved study. Concomitantly, the risk management professional works with the entity leadership to put in place appropriate insurance coverages to address claims stemming from adverse events.

Rather than being seen as an impediment to research, the healthcare risk management professional can help leadership control the opportunity for loss involved in clinical research. This can and should be part of a larger coordinated effort with corporate compliance and chief research officers of the healthcare organization. Seen as a facilitator, not an obstruction to research, the risk management professional can make a positive contribution for the benefit of the facility, the clinical research team, and the well being of research subjects.

Practical Risk Management Strategies to Follow in Terms of Developing Policies and Procedures for Clinical Trials Administration

Risk management strategies can either be incorporated into a stand-alone policy and procedure for clinical trials administration or blended into the fabric of existing policy and procedure governing research studies. There are some practitioners who favor the former approach, suggesting that the stand-alone philosophy reinforces the risk-prone nature of clinical trials and the need to pay particular attention to management of such potential loss exposures. Others take quite the opposite approach. They believe that it is best to include risk management strategies in daily operational policy and procedure. In doing so they claim that loss prevention, loss control, and mitigation become part of the routine for those involved in clinical trials.

The selection of one approach or another must be consistent with the culture and organizational framework of the CRO, hospital, or healthcare organization. The key is to include risk management strategies in the administration of clinical trials. To this end, there are a number of key risk management components to incorporate in policy and procedure. These include the following *general* considerations:

- Claims management
- Coordinated functions
- Credentialing
- Delineated approach for risk management functions and activities
- Delineated process for communication of risk management information, functions, and activities
- Delineated process for documenting risk management activities
- Education
- Performance measures for risk management program
- Procedures for risk elimination
- Procedures for risk minimization
- Procedures for risk prevention
- Procedures for risk reduction
- Process for risk identification
- Process for risk prioritization

- Regulatory compliance
- Reporting relationships
- Risk transfer arrangements

In terms of specific clinical trials risk management policy and procedure, a number of topics are ripe for consideration:

- Adverse event reporting
- Adverse event investigation
- Adverse event resolution
- Conflict-of-interest disclosure requirements
- Consent process
- Consent documentation
- Confidentiality process
- Confidentiality waiver
- Contract administration
- Contract review
- Coordinated management of claims for adverse events stemming from multisite clinical research trials
- Credentialing clinical trials investigators
- Data analysis
- Data collection and uses
- Data Safety Monitoring Boards (DSMBs)
- Device- or equipment-related events management
- Investigations
  - Management
  - Activities in coordination with corporate compliance officer
  - Activities in coordination with legal counsel
  - Cooperation with state and federal regulators
- Insurance coverages (see risk transfer)
- Integrity agreements—ongoing oversight and compliance
- IRB membership selection
- IRB activities
- Risk transfer arrangements for business interruption, directors and officers liability, errors and omission liability, key person, cyber risk, etc.
- Subject recruitment
- Subject safety
- Subject selection and retention

More can be added to the list of topics ripe for inclusion in a risk management–oriented policy and procedure for clinical trials administration. Much depends upon the setting, the nature of the trials under way, and planned activities for the future. When the healthcare organization is a satellite facility for research trials, the role of the local risk manager may be limited in terms of loss control and prevention activities. The primary facility leading a multicenter trial may have the greatest resources for purposes of risk management. However, local risk management participation is important, especially in terms of managing adverse events, compliance queries for government agencies, and handling claims.

Additional strategies are important in developing risk management–oriented policies and procedures. This includes using language that is clear, easy to understand, and leaves no doubt about intent or meaning. Policies and procedures should be concise and focused, obviating the need for lengthy reviews and interpretations. If standards, guidelines, or criteria are incorporated in policy and procedure, it is prudent not to set an expected level of performance that is difficult or impossible to achieve in clinical trials administration. The goal should be to set the standard that can be met by those expected to adhere to the policy and procedure. When changes are introduced to policy and procedure, education programs should be provided to those responsible for implementing the new requirements. Copies of outdated policies and procedures should be removed from the clinical trials office and new requirements should be provided to principal investigators and their personnel. The same is true for members of the IRB. Each version of the policy and procedure should be clearly identified (Version 1.5) along with the effective date of the new requirements. Taking these steps can go a long way toward managing the risk associated with clinical trials research policy and procedure.

Policy and procedure alone are not sufficient to create a successful risk management approach for clinical trials. Policies and procedures must be *implemented* and *followed.* Part of risk management surveillance is to make certain that policies and procedures are being used correctly. If deficiencies are identified, corrective action is important to address would-be risk exposure from non-compliance with such established practices. The reason for this approach goes well beyond a focus on rigid compliance with policy and procedures. The reason is that in some instances, policies and procedures can be portrayed as a standard of care. The failure to follow acknowledged standards, resulting in foreseeable harm or death, can lead to a finding of negligence.

Credentialing Principal Investigators and IRB Members: A Risk Management Perspective

Credentialing may be of great value as a risk management tool in clinical trials administration. Credentialing and privileging are systems tools used in hospitals, managed care organizations, many long-term care facilities, and integrated delivery systems. In essence, health professionals—especially physicians, dentists, podiatrists, and clinical psychologists—apply to become part of the medical staff. The concept was designed initially for independent contractors, but in many instances it is used to qualify salaried professionals to be part of the medical or health professional staff.

At the outset, a detailed review is made of an individual's qualifications. The screening mechanism includes a review of educational background, occupational history, a review of graduate training programs completed, professional liability history, current and past licensure history, and other detailed information. The applicant supplies a list of references with whom contact is made to confirm data supplied by the healthcare professional. Original, certified, or attested certificates are supplied to substantiate information provided in the application regarding education and training, licensure, and professional insurance coverage. Applicants are often asked about criminal history and the need for any consideration of accommodation under the Americans With

Disabilities Act (ADA) for disabilities and Section 504 of the 1973 Rehabilitation Act that addresses the requirements of the handicap.

Once the information is collected and verified, the application goes before a medical staff committee convened for the purpose of reviewing and making recommendations to the governance board of the healthcare organization. A favorable recommendation from the committee may result in the governance board granting appointment to the medical staff. In many instances, the appointment may be of a probationary nature, enabling clinical leadership to evaluate the individual in terms of clinical application, technique, and prescribing practices. The appointment also comes with a delineation of privileges that defines the scope of practice opportunity for the individual.

An appointment is usually for two years, and the individual must apply for a reappointment. Doing so triggers a recredentialing process which evaluates many of the same criteria reviewed initially, and clinical and practice information gathered at the local healthcare organization. It is also a time for the individual to request a greater scope of delineated privileges. As with the initial appointment process, a medical staff committee makes a recommendation to the governing body. On the basis of this recommendation, the governing body either reappoints or rejects the renewal application. If the application is accepted, the governing body also may expand or retain the current scope of delineated privileges.

Within each two-year cycle, steps can be taken to curtail, suspend, revoke or not renew the privileges granted to an individual. This is done in those situations in which the individual's practice or behavior jeopardizes the well being of patients, and nothing in terms of corrective action can be done but to remove the person from practicing at the healthcare organization in terms of suspending or revoking privileges. Sometimes, a suspension may be useful for other purposes, such as pending the outcome of a corporate compliance investigation or as a means of disciplining a caregiver who fails to follow established rules for charting healthcare information. Privileges may also be curtailed as a way of letting the caregiver continue to perform certain functions while relieving the individual of treatment opportunities in areas of identified deficient practice.

How would this process relate to clinical trials administration? With an increasing degree of oversight responsibility, healthcare organizations could use the credentialing process to qualify those conducting clinical trials on their premises or enrolling patients from their facility. There is much merit to using credentialing procedures for this purpose.

When a health plan, hospital, or integrated delivery system holds itself out as participating in or promoting clinical trials, it is in essence suggesting that the trials are acceptable. It is also implicitly saying that the health professionals involved in these trials are qualified for this purpose. In some instances, advertising or promotion may be quite explicit, stating that the facility is a leading research center, staffed by some of the most capable and leading researchers in the field.

When a facility knows or ought to know that the consumer relies upon such assertions, it should have a process in place to qualify those involved in clinical trials. If the facility knew or ought to know that such statements were false, it could be exposed to a claim of false advertising or misrepresentation. The failure to properly screen researchers to conduct trials could also be considered negligence on the part of the institution. This is especially the case if the facility knew or ought to have known that the research team lacks requisite qualifications to carry out their responsibilities.

There is another strong risk management rationale for credentialing professionals to conduct research trials. The skills needed for clinical trials are not necessarily the same as those required for therapeutic treatment. There are a number of legal and regulatory requirements bound up in clinical trials that are not found in routine treatment situations. The credentialing process serves as a way of identifying those who lack the requisite knowledge for conducting clinical trials in a compliant organization. Once identified, steps can be taken to help them obtain the needed training to achieve demonstrated competencies. This might mean taking an on-line course, participating in facility-sponsored seminars, or completing the program made available on-line by the Office of Human Research Protections (OHRP) ("Human Research Assurance Tutorial"). The latter is especially important since any institution involved in federally supported clinical trials must state in writing that it will adhere to the protection of research subjects. This written undertaking, assurance of compliance, must be approved by OHRP. OHRP must be confident that the Institutional Official, the Chairperson of the IRB, and the Human Protections Administrator know the responsibilities involved in an institutional program of human subject protection.

From a risk management standpoint, it would be prudent to extend the training requirements to principal investigators and key clinical trial personnel. It provides a useful way to explain their responsibilities, and, if made a prerequisite for credentialing, serves as a practical qualification for clinical trials oversight.

As indicated earlier, when deficiencies occur, the credentialing process has a built-in mechanism termed corrective action to enable the healthcare organization to address substandard practice or non-compliance. The corrective action mechanism provides an even-handed approach, according due process of the law to those under scrutiny. Applied to clinical trials, such an approach would be a useful tool for managing scientific misconduct and regulatory non-compliance. Moreover, it provides a degree of control or influence that serves as an incentive to achieve compliance by those specifically credentialed for this purpose.

Criteria for a Research Credentialing Program

Aside from the criteria mentioned earlier, there are several specific questions to include in the research professional credentialing process. These queries are linked to qualifications for clinical trials work and regulatory compliance:

- Have you completed specific training or fellowship work in clinical trial administration or study design? If so, please indicate the name and location of the training program, coordinator's name, and completion date.

- Have you ever conducted or had administrative responsibilities for clinical research trials? If the answer is yes, please list the name(s) and locations(s) of facilities where this work took place, research project name, topic, sponsor, and dates when it occurred. Provide a list of three references for each location in which you conducted or had administrative responsibilities for clinical trials.

- Have you ever been disciplined or sanctioned in conjunction with clinical trial work? If so, please describe the circumstances in an attachment.

- Have you even been debarred from completing clinical trial work by a sponsor? CRO? Federal government department or agency? If so, please describe the circumstances in an attachment.

- Have you even been disciplined, sanctioned, or debarred from receiving federal funds as a healthcare provider or clinical researcher?

- Have you even been found responsible for or admitted to scientific misconduct by a Sponsor? CRO? Research program? Institution? Federal department? If so, please describe the circumstances in an attachment.

- Have you published research findings? Have you ever had a research publication retracted? If so, please describe the circumstances in an attachment.

- Have you ever had a research study rejected on the basis of scientific misconduct? If so, please describe the circumstances in an attachment.

- Are you or any components of your research program/organization now under a corporate integrity program? If so, please describe the circumstances in an attachment.

- Are you now under investigation for scientific misconduct, corporate non-compliance, or either civil or criminal infractions under the Federal False Claims Act? If so, please describe the circumstances in an attachment.

- Have you ever been named in a lawsuit involving allegations of research misconduct, research fraud, negligent research consent, or injury stemming from research subject participation in a clinical trial? If so, please describe the circumstances in an attachment.

Aside from this line of questioning, it is useful to have the applicant sign a document in which the individual grants permission to check references and to conduct a background check. Such a statement should also spell out the consequences of supplying false or inaccurate information. The ongoing responsibility to abide by research policies and procedures and the duty to report debarment, claims, or complaints should also be part of the statement.

The rationale for such a detailed statement is that it puts the applicant on notice. If the requirements are unacceptable, the individual need not proceed with the credentialing process. If the individual does proceed with the process, it would be difficult to later claim that he or she did not know the consequences of nonconformity.

Insurance Coverages and Solutions for Clinical Trials

The types of insurance coverages needed for clinical trials vary from sponsors to CROs to clinical investigators to facilities in which research is conducted. An insurance broker or agent or an insurance consultant can provide useful guidance on the subject. The insurance expert will look at the clinical trials operation. The process will involve an examination of existing insurance policies, short-term and long-term needs, risk exposures, the insurance specifications prescribed by sponsors, and contractual risk obligations assumed by the client. It means that the insurance expert must have a complete understanding of the business operations in order to make prudent recommendations. This process may be particularly important if recent recommendations are adopted for a compensation program for inferred research participants (IOM, Responsible Research: A Systems Approach for Protections Research Participants, October, 2002).

There are a number of ways to finance the risks involved in clinical research trials. Some may take a moderate to large self-retention of risk for allegations based on negligence. This may translate into $25,000 to $75,000 per claim. Anything over that amount would be addressed through another risk financing strategy such as an insurance premium.

Risk financing strategies are based on factual information, including data obtained from actuaries and experience with similar claims known to insurance underwriters. Retaining "first dollar" coverage for a claim may bring down premium costs. The insurance expert will encourage the client to implement aggressive loss control and loss prevention strategies found in risk management. The recommendation will likely include financial reserve strategies to pay for first dollar claims up to the point that insurance coverages attach to the claim. The amount of reserves will vary with the likelihood and projected frequency of claims.

Insurance plans or policies are available for clinical trials research. Some may be as simple as getting a so-called endorsement to an existing policy to coverage some aspect of clinical trials. For example, an existing cyber risk policy may need an endorsement to address transmission of electronic clinical trials data files from one site to another in a multicenter trial. Once again, the insurance expert can provide guidance on the subject.

In other instances it may be apparent that the research facility lacks the requisite insurance coverage needed for potential losses stemming from clinical trials. For example, nothing may be in place to cover the members of the IRB for errors and omissions (E&O) stemming from negligent oversight of ongoing clinical trials. By identifying what is in place and what is needed, the insurance expert can assist in designing a risk financing program to match the needs of those involved in the clinical trials program.

In some instances, there will be room for different interpretations of what is covered under existing insurance policies or programs. For example, a physician group may have broadly worded coverage for professional liability for errors and omissions that occur in the diagnosis, treatment, and care of patients. Does the word care include circumstances in which the person is both a study subject *and* a patient? Some might say yes and others may say no. Because there is room for reaching opposite conclusions, the insurance agent, broker, or consultant may advise the client to obtain specific insurance coverage. This may take the form of an endorsement to an existing policy or a new type of insurance coverage.

Some may question the value of an insurance expert in the area of clinical trials research. This is an era of growing regulatory scrutiny, contractual prerequisites for insurance coverage in clinical trials, and growing litigation. To avoid being left without adequate coverage means financial risk for underinsured CROs, sponsors, clinical investigators, IRB members, and research facilities. To avoid such risk potential an insurance assessment is in order.

There are a number of questions and areas of review that go into an insurance assessment. These include the following:

- Have there been any claims? If so, what type of claims?
- Are there any claims outstanding?
- Is there insurance in place to cover these potential losses?
- Is the current program based on claims-made coverage (that is, coverage for claims reported while the insurance plan is in force, and the event occurred following the start date of the policy and prior to the termination of the insurance plan) or occurrence-based coverage (coverage for claims that occur while the policy is in force and that does not consider when the claim is reported or whether or not the insured party maintains the insurance)?
- Has anyone reviewed contracts in which the other party has shifted liability to the CRO, health plan, or hospital, integrated delivery system? If such contracts exist, is there insurance in place to cover potential losses?

- What is the current cost of insurance coverage?
- What is the potential for claims in this area?
- Has any thought been given to alternate risk financing solutions? If so, what was suggested?
- Is there a strong risk management program in place that offers loss control and loss prevention services geared to clinical trials?
- Does the existing insurance program match up with expected coverage needs such as
  - Business interruption or continuity
  - Cyber risks (electronic transmissions, cyber vandalism, etc.)
  - Directors and officers liability
  - Errors and omissions—Professional liability
  - General liability
  - Intellectual property
  - Regulatory investigations
- Has any thought been given to an insurance captive for those who meet the criteria for such an insurance program?

Based on the information gleaned from discussions, documentation review, and insurance program analysis, a solid insurance plan can be put in place as part of a risk management initiative for clinical trials.

....

RECORD MANAGEMENT AND REPORTING

Record management is an integral part of clinical trials research and human subject protection programs. Such information is important for purposes of continuity of research trials, coding, and billing for work done under a grant. It is equally important in terms of regulatory compliance.

A related issue is reporting adverse events in clinical trials. It is imperative that key individuals know when to report adverse events and to whom such information should be disseminated. Researchers, clinical research administration officials, institutional officials, and others must be knowledgeable in this regard.

Knowing "how" to document adverse events is an important consideration for the claims administration process. Not only is it important from the standpoint of litigation, it is an area of prime interest in terms of regulatory compliance. These issues are addressed below.

Record Retention and Clinical Trials

The record retention period is a function of the uses of the information. If a facility is engaged in twenty-five-year longitudinal studies involving the use of research subjects, the retention period will be that period of time plus the length of time that the institution is exposed to potential liability for the study. The term liability here connotes more than culpability for negligent clinical trials. A claim may involve breach of contract, fraud, misrepresentation, or deceit. It may involve breach of confidentiality, lack of informed consent, or battery. Each claim or civil wrong may have a different limitation period in which the litigant may bring suit. Hence, it is imperative to understand the requirements of applicable law to determine the requisite retention period for such purposes.

The record retention period may be lengthened under what is termed a tolling provision. If, for example, the study subjects were neonates involved in pharmaceutical study, the limitation period might be tolled (suspended) until the subjects are of the age of majority or can actively instruct counsel in possible claims linked to the research. Tolling provisions are important considerations when a study involves a vulnerable population such as minors or mentally ill or behaviorally challenged persons.

Aside from litigation, there may be other uses that attenuate the retention period for clinical trials records. For example, a study might run for a two-year period. Since several different funding sources were used for the study, it may be necessary to retain the documentation for more than the three-year limitation period for negligence claims under state law. Because the administrative records include financial data premised on the clinical trial, it would be important to retain the documents for the length of time that may be needed for an Internal Revenue Service (IRS) audit. The IRS limitation is seven years. Thus in this example, the retention period would be seven years beyond the conclusion of the study.

From a practical standpoint, it may be difficult to retain hard copy records for long periods of time. The law recognizes this fact and accommodation is made for record transfer to other long-term media such as backup tapes, microfilm, or CD-ROM. The key is to select a reliable long-term storage media and to follow a recognized process for data transfer. The same is true for electronic records. Useful resources can be found in CRO, hospital, health plan, or integrated delivery systems. These include The Chief Information Officer, Health Information Manager, and the risk management professional. Specific legal advice is also important especially in multicenter, multijurisdictional studies in which decisions must be made about retention periods and recognized storage media.

Documenting and Managing Clinical Trial-Related Adverse Events

An adverse event does not necessarily mean that one should anticipate a lawsuit. Rather, it is a signal that an undesirable outcome has occurred that merits careful review. The results of the review process may trigger a number of subsequent steps, including developing an adverse event management protocol to guide the process for handling such occurrences. The protocol should consider all the "next steps," including the following:

Notification Requirements—Delineate those who should be notified about the adverse event, including the IRB, sponsor, clinical trial administrators, clinical trial staff, DSMB, risk manager, leadership of the healthcare entity or CRO, and trial coordinators at other locations for the study.

Format for Notification—Define the way in which notification will be provided such as e-mail, completion of study forms, letters, documented telephone calls.

Investigation of Adverse Event—Define the steps to follow in determining what occurred and why, such as system failure analysis or root cause analysis, evaluation of equipment used in administering test articles, device inspections, interviews, photographs of the location of the event, equipment testing, analysis of tubing, syringes, etc.

Discussion with Research Subject and Family—Describe the process to follow in discussing the adverse event with the research subject and family, including treatment options and compensation arrangements per the approved research protocol.

Occupational Exposure Management—Define the process to follow when the adverse event involves an employee of the facility or the research study staff, including the parameters in place under Occupational Safety and Health Administration (OSHA) guidelines, state department of labor accident investigations, and workers compensation rules.

Decide About Suspending or Continuing the Study—If a major design fault is identified, or greater risk is discovered than previously linked to the study, a decision should be made whether to suspend or discontinue the study. The decision may come from others such as a study sponsor or the IRB. If a decision is made to halt the study, a determination must be made what to do regarding subjects currently enrolled in the clinical trial. Consideration must be given to the potential harm that could be done if a study is halted abruptly. An explanation must be given to subjects explaining the adverse event, the reason for halting the clinical trial, how long it may be stopped, and the options open to the study subjects. For those subjects who are also receiving treatment, an effort must be made to coordinate study stoppage with ongoing care of such patients.

Lessons Learned—Use the information gleaned from the investigation to improve the clinical trial process. This includes the procedures followed after an adverse event.

The Risk Management Challenges in Reporting Adverse Events

Several concerns come to light in reporting adverse events. One is that it might be construed as an admission of liability. A second is that it exposes sensitive proprietary information to those who would use the data to their own benefit. A third is a fear that it could lead to identification of individual subjects and their personal health information. A fourth is that the data could be used as part of a compliance investigation, a step that would otherwise be beyond the scope of regulatory officials absent the use of some formal legal process. A fifth is that such detailed information could lead to litigation based on negligence.

There may be merit in each of these concerns. However, from a risk management standpoint much can be done to contain the scope of potential loss stemming from reporting adverse events. Risk management professionals start from a worst-case standpoint. That is, what would be the likely loss potential if an adverse event report was used to prove a negligence claim? Identify a research subject and his or health history? Facilitate a regulatory review? Rather than try to thwart reporting—something that would be unlikely under sponsor contracts and regulatory law—the focus turns to how to develop and prepare for adverse events in a way that assumes the worst-case scenario. The approach is to avoid conjecture, speculation, or turning the adverse event report into a newspaper style opinion page. Factual, concise, and verified information is reported. Anything that needs further elucidation is noted, along with an indication that when this process is completed an addendum will be made available for this purpose. This enables the end-user to use clear, accurate information to fulfill his or her responsibilities. It avoids misunderstanding and reliance on speculative information that could lead to inappropriate decision-making about next steps. An example helps to demonstrate this point.

A 25-year-old diabetic research subject was enrolled in a study to test a new insulin pump. After two months, the man's condition was stable. On day 75, the man contacted the study coordinator and reported that he felt awful. He was hospitalized and went into diabetic shock. Efforts to save him failed, and he died. The death was reported to the study sponsor as a "possible adverse event linked to the insulin pump." The report noted that an autopsy was being performed, including a comprehensive biochemistry screen.

The device was to be examined by a panel of three experts, one from the sponsor, one selected by the clinical investigator, and a third chosen from an outside testing service. When the results were known from the biochemistry screen and the device evaluation, the information would be provided to the sponsor. The sponsor decided to send out an advisory to the other clinical study centers. Since this was the first death linked to the pump, it was decided to continue with the study.

Thirty days later the results were received from the biochemical screen. The tests demonstrated a substantial amount of "street drugs" were present at the time of death. There were only trace amounts of the diabetic preparations made available to all test subjects in the man's system at the time of his death. This information correlated with the quantity of unused study preparations returned by the subject's family. The report from the three experts suggested that the device was functioning correctly. The conclusion drawn from the autopsy, biochemical, and equipment evaluations was that the subject had been non-compliant with the study protocol. He had not properly self-medicated himself, and the combination of his underlying diabetic condition and use of illicit drugs led to his death.

The case example demonstrates that it is easy to jump to conclusions about a study-related adverse event. Until all the facts are known, drawing inferences or conclusions in an adverse event report could prove harmful and misleading. This is especially the case in adverse outcomes in which there is a likelihood of regulatory scrutiny or litigation. The risk management approach is to state the known facts, make the appropriate reports, but in doing so to provide no basis for drawing potentially errant conclusions. When investigations are completed and the facts are known, provision can be made to state a final conclusion about the causes of an adverse event. Such information can then be used for process improvements, enhanced screening techniques for subject selection, implementation of safety provisions for subjects, and in handling any claims that arise from the occurrence.

The Claims Management Process for a Clinical Trial Adverse Event

Beyond the usual, detailed claims management process, additional steps should be considered for handling claims stemming from a clinical trials–related adverse event. This is particularly important when an adverse event involves a person who is also receiving therapeutic treatment. It may be difficult to determine whether a negative outcome was the result of substandard therapeutic care, a consequence of the clinical trial, or a natural progression of the underlying disease. Additionally, there are many reporting demands for clinical trials adverse events. Consistency is important. The reports provided to one group, such as clinical sponsors or CROs, should provide information consistent with information provided to government regulatory officials.

An effective claims management process has many components. A part of the risk management program, claims management involves the interface with trial counsel, insurers, investigators, regulatory officials, and, possibly responding to media inquiries. Many healthcare organizations and health plans have a dedicated person or full-time equivalent serve as the claims manager. In some instances, in larger organizations such as an integrated delivery system, claims management may be outsourced to an outside firm that specializes in adjusting such claims. Information learned from the claims management process is used for purposes of process improvement, research subject safety, and education. Policies and procedures may also be modified subsequent to the lessons learned in the claims management process.

The claims management process for clinical trials would include the following:

- Investigation
- Interviews
- Securing equipment and documentation, including experimental devices
- Opening a claims management file
- Notifications and reporting (to sponsors, government departments and agencies, insurance carrier or captive manager, IRBs)
- Assignment of legal counsel
- Discovery
- Settlements
- Trial
- Appeals

Part of the claims management process entails monitoring the use of legal counsel. Legal fees can accumulate quickly if there is nothing in place to set forth the terms of engagement. The insurer often provides an attorney to handle the case or a list of selected individuals from which the insured can select a lawyer. The appointment should set forth the expectations for managing the claim, regular status reports, and project costs and fees. Lessons learned from the claim can be channeled into revisions of clinical trials management procedures and educational programs for IRB members, principal investigators, and research study staff. (For an excellent book on the subject see N. Acerbo-Avalone and K. Kremer, 1997.)

Claims management is an integral part of the risk management program for handling adverse events in clinical trials. It needs to be honed to meet the specific needs of research studies and facilities for whom there must be precise coordination in claims management while responding to regulatory inquiries or investigations stemming from the same event. Along with risk financing and loss control and prevention activities, much can be done to control the potential for financial loss in clinical trials administration.

··········

CONCLUSION

Quality improvement, accreditation and risk management programming play a pivotal role in the successful implementation of a human research protection program. At the very least, there is merit in designing a consistent approach from quality to risk management and to the accreditation process. Valuable information can be learned from doing a self-assessment of current practices relative to such norms as those found in the OHRP QI Program or the standards in the two clinical trials accreditation programs.

Having in place the appropriate insurance program is equally important. When problems occur, having the right coverages can make the difference between suspending a trial and the continuity of ongoing studies. A strong claims management process serves to reinforce the process for those instances in which a claim is made involving a clinical trial.

Much can be learned from the healthcare field regarding quality improvement, accreditation, and risk management. However, even with these lessons in hand, refinement will be necessary to shape such programs to meet the needs of human research protection plans. Once in place much can be done to enhance efficiency and effectiveness of the clinical trials process.

References

Acerbo-Avalone, K., & Kremer, K. (1997). *Medical Malpractice Claims Investigation.* Gaithersburg, Maryland: Aspen Publishers.

Association for the Accreditation of Human Research Protection Programs. "Accreditation Step-by-Step."

Association for the Accreditation of Human Research Protection Programs. (2002). "Final Accreditation Standards."

Koski, G. (2002). "An Open Letter to the Human Subject Research Community."

National Committee for Quality Assurance. (2001). Press Release. "NCQA, VA Launch First Ever Accreditation Program for Human Research Protection."

NCQA, JCAHO Form Partnership for Human Research Protection, Inc.; New Organization Will Accredit Human Research Protection Programs in U.S., Abroad," www.ncqa.org, January 16, 2003.

Office of Human Research Protection. "Human Research Assurance Tutorial."

Office of Human Research Protection. (2002). Objectives and Overview of the OHRP Quality Improvement Program.

Responsible Research: A Systems Approach to Protecting Research Participants, IDM, October, 2002.

FORMS

Quality Assurance Self-Assessment Tool
Instructions

Version Date 05/06/2002

Introduction

The purpose of this QA Self-Assessment Tool is to assist your institution or independent Institutional Review Board (IRB) in assessing your human subjects protection program. The questions presented are primarily designed to assess compliance with the federal regulations for the protection of human subjects in research. Additional information is requested to gain an understanding of your institution's or independent IRB's program, including: i) elements of the program that may go beyond the requirements of the federal regulations, ii) volume of work conducted by your IRB, and iii) available resources for your human subjects protection program. Therefore, not all questions require a positive (i.e., "yes") response. Please do not assume that a "yes" response means that your program is in compliance with a given federal regulation.

Instructions

This self-assessment tool should be completed by one or more individuals who are knowledgeable about your institution's or independent IRB's human subjects protection program, such as the IRB Chair(s), IRB Administrator(s), or Signatory Official.

While the intent of this tool is to be as comprehensive as possible, it was also designed with consideration for the amount of effort required to complete it. Some questions may involve discussion with your colleagues. In an effort to decrease the amount of time required for completion of this instrument, we offer the following suggestions. If a question requires review of information or appears difficult to answer, we recommend flagging it and moving on to the next question. You may also write draft responses in pencil and then erase them and write the final answer in pen. Once the tool is completed, you should review it and respond to any flagged, unanswered questions. In this manner the first pass through of the questions may be completed in less than two hours.

Most questions can be answered with a simple response, such as "yes," "no," or "not applicable." If you are unable to respond to a question, you may respond with answers such as "not known" or "not sure." Some questions may apply only to biomedical research and others only to behavioral research. If such questions are not applicable to your program, you may simply respond with "not applicable."

Once this tool is completed, your institution or independent IRB and OHRP should be able to begin assessment of your institution's or independent IRB's human subjects protection program, including its strengths and weaknesses. The tool may identify areas where clarification of regulatory requirements is needed or where to focus necessary education. Information regarding IRB workload and time allocation may increase an IRB's awareness of its resources, delegation of responsibility, and time management. This awareness may facilitate changes that in turn can increase efficiency. OHRP can assist your institution in this process and provide consultation toward increasing the performance, efficiency, and quality of your human subjects protection program.

If additional space is needed to answer any question, please copy the relevant page and attach it as an appendix.

---

*If you have questions about human subject research, click **ohrp@osophs.dhhs.gov***
*If you have questions/suggestions about this web page, click **Webmaster***

U.S. Department of Health and Human Services (DHHS)
Office for Human Research Protections (OHRP)

Description of the Quality Improvement Program - Stage 1: Quality Assurance

Version Date 05/06/2002

The OHRP Quality Improvement Program (QIP) is provided by the Division of Assurances and Quality Improvement (DAQI) and will include three stages: 1) Quality Assurance (QA), 2) Quality Improvement (QI), and 3) Continuous Quality Improvement (CQI). Through the QIP, DAQI offers assessment, instruction, education, and sharing of best practices. DAQI is currently offering the QIP on a voluntary basis to all institutions and independent IRBs.

In the first stage, DAQI will conduct activities intended to promote a solid foundation for a human subjects protection program. Before a program can be improved, an assessment of the program's strengths and weaknesses is needed. During this stage, DAQI will guide institutions in conducting a self assessment. To facilitate this process, DAQI has developed a self-assessment tool that will be available for use by institutions and independent (commercial) IRBs after approval is obtained by the Office of Management and Budget (OMB). The QA Self-Assessment Tool is primarily intended to help gauge an institution's compliance with the federal regulations for human subjects protection.

The QA Self-Assessment Tool and its instructions are posted on this website and are available for public comment. DAQI will not use or collect the QA Self-Assessment Tool until OMB approves this form. In the meantime, QA activities may involve review of a human subjects protection program's operating procedures and minutes of recent IRB meetings. Following the QA assessment, DAQI will continue the QIP process via any of the following three modes of communication: 1) written correspondence and teleconference, 2) videoconference, and 3) on-site consultation visit. Selection of the type of interaction will be made by DAQI based on the need and willingness of the institution, the overall demand and volume of requests received, and resources available at DAQI.

After evaluation by DAQI, the institution will be provided with appropriate guidance and recommendations for improving its system for protecting human subjects. Education and consultation will be offered by OHRP staff to improve the human subjects protection program in any necessary area(s). The process will include mechanisms to protect the confidentiality of information voluntarily provided by the institution to the greatest extent possible allowable by law.

---

*If you have questions about human subject research, click **ohrp@osophs.dhhs.gov***
*If you have questions/suggestions about this web page, click **Webmaster***
Updated May 8, 2002

U.S. Department of Health and Human Services (DHHS) Office for Human Research Protections (OHRP)

Sample Schedule for the OHRP QI Consultation Visit

Version Date 07/23/2002

Day 1 - Start approximately 1:00pm:

Interview with Institutional Official(s) - 20 minutes

Interview with Institutional Official(s) and IRB Chair(s), Director(s) of IRB - 20 minutes

Tour of IRB office, operation, and files - 20-30 minutes

Record review - approximately 2 hours (OHRP staff only)

Review of Operating Procedures, IRB Minutes (and/or QA Self-Assessment Tool after OMB approval is obtained) with IRB Director and appropriate staff - 1hour

Day 2 - Start approximately 9:00am:

Interview with IRB Chair(s) - 40 minutes

Interview with Director of IRB office and IRB coordinator(s) - 1 hour

Break 10-15 minutes

Interview with IRB members (at least 2-3) - 40 minutes

Lunch - approximately 1 hour

Interview with Investigators (Group A) - 40 minutes

Interview with Investigators (Group B) - 40 minutes

Break 10 - 15 minutes

Free-for-all Question & Answer Period - 60 to 90 minutes

Break - 15 minutes (QI Team preparation for Exit Interview)

Exit Interview [Institutional Official, IRB chair(s), Director of IRB] - 30 minutes

We would like to conclude by 5:00pm each day. You may rearrange the schedule to have the first day as the full day and the second day as a half-day. You may also have the flexibility to rearrange the meetings on either day. Please call OHRP to discuss altering starting or ending time.

*If you have questions about human subject research, click **ohrp@osophs.dhhs.gov***
*If you have questions/suggestions about this web page, click **Webmaster***
Updated July 23, 2002

OHRP QA Self-Assessment Tool

Date Completed: _____

SECTION A. <u>INSTITUTION'S HUMAN SUBJECTS PROTECTION PROGRAM</u>
This section collects information to assess your institution's or independent IRB's overall human subjects protection program.

1. Name of Institution or Organization:

2. Address:

3. Institutional Review Board (IRB) Organization Number (IORG #):

This number, assigned by OHRP, can be found on the OHRP website at <u>http://ohrp.osophs.dhhs.gov/</u>

4. a) Name of Contact Person: b) Title:
   c) Phone: d) Fax: e) E-mail:

     General Administrative Information on the IRB Component of the Human Subjects Protection Program

5. How many IRBs are operated or supported by your institution?
Include special situation IRBs (e.g., prisoner research, emergency use, etc.).

6. Who oversees the day-to-day operations of the human subjects protection program?
Provide name and title.

7. To whom does the IRB(s) report?
Provide name and title.

8. Does the IRB(s) have its own budget?

9. Who authorizes budget support for the IRB(s)?
Provide name and title or reference previous response (e.g., "same as Question 7").

10. Does the IRB(s) have a written Charter or Charge?

11. Does your institution or organization have an organizational chart for your human subjects protection program?
    If yes, please provide a copy as an attachment to this tool.

12. Who appoints the IRB Chair(s)?
Provide name and title or reference previous response (e.g., "same as Question 7").

13. Describe the criteria used to select the Chair(s).

14. Who selects and appoints IRB members?
Provide name and title or reference previous response (e.g., "same as Question 7").

15. Describe the criteria used to select IRB members.

16. Are conflict of interest issues with IRB members managed and eliminated or minimized?

    If yes, how?

General Information on Other Components of the Human Subjects Protection Program

17. Have senior officials ever issued a memo, to any or all of your institution's staff, about the institution's policy on human subjects protections and/or promoting the ethical conduct of human subject research?

18. Does your institution/IRB organization have a separate committee for review of non-compliance incidents?

   a) If yes, how are the findings and actions communicated to the IRB?

   b) If no, how are non-compliance incidents reviewed?

19. Does your institution/IRB organization have established policies and procedures for disclosure and management of potential conflicts of interest?

20. Does your institution/IRB organization have a separate committee for review of issues related to conflicts of interest?

   If yes and when applicable, how are the findings and actions communicated to the IRB?

21. Does your institution/IRB organization have an internal audit, quality assurance, or quality improvement program for human research activities?

If yes, describe what was done in the last year and any changes that were made as a result of an audit, QA, or QI program.

22. Does your institution/IRB organization have an advocacy program or ombudsman accessible to potential or enrolled research participants?

23. Does your institution/IRB organization ever receive complaints, questions, or concerns regarding human subject protections?

   If yes, approximately how many during the past year?

24. Does your institution/IRB organization have a centralized hotline or 800 number for potential or enrolled research participants to file complaints or direct questions regarding human subjects protection issues?

Workload of the IRB(s) and Staffing Resources
The information in questions 25 to 28 is collected to understand the workload of an IRB. This information in summary form can be used to help make recommendations, which may increase not only the performance and quality of an IRB, but also its efficiency.

25. Provide the following general information for each IRB.
For consistency throughout this tool, each IRB should be referenced when appropriate in all further responses by the sequential numbers 1, 2, 3, etc. below. IRB Registration Identifiers, Federalwide Assurance (FWA), Multiple Project Assurance (MPA), and Cooperative Project Assurance (CPA) Numbers assigned by OHRP can be found on the OHRP website at http://ohrp.osophs.dhhs.gov/. The table may be expanded if your institution/organization has more than 6 IRBs.

IRB #	IRB Registration Identifier	Type (e.g., biomedical, behavioral, both)	Number Years in Existence	How Often Does the IRB Regularly Meet (e.g., once/mo, twice/mo)	List, by Number, any FWA, MPA, or CPA That Designate This IRB
a) 1					
b) 2					
c) 3					
d) 4					
e) 5					
f) 6					

26. Please complete the following table to provide information on staffing resources available to the IRB. *Maintain reference to the respective IRBs from table in Question 25.*

IRB #	IRB Chair			IRB Administrator			Name(s) of Staff Members Supporting IRB (Indicate Full-Time or Part-Time Staff)
	Name(s)	# Years	% Effort to IRB	Name(s)	# Years	% Effort to IRB	
a) 1							
b) 2							
c) 3							
d) 4							
e) 5							
f) 6							

27. Does your IRB Chair(s) perform administrative functions for the IRB (e.g., prepare or assist in the development of letters to investigators)?

28. Please complete the following summary table to provide information on the volume of work over the past 12 months for each IRB. *Maintain reference to the respective IRBs from tables in Questions 25 and 26.*

IRB Workload Summary Table *Enter data for each IRB for the past 12 months*	IRB 1	IRB 2	IRB 3	IRB 4	IRB 5	IRB 6
a) Total number of active studies reviewed						
b) Total number of studies reviewed and found to be exempt						
c) Approximate average duration of an IRB meeting: (i.e., hours, minutes)						
d) Number of new protocols reviewed by full committee						
e) Number of new protocols approved by expedited review						
f) Number of continuing review protocols reviewed by full committee						
g) Number of continuing review protocols reviewed by expedited review						
h) Number of amendments requiring full committee review						
i) Number of amendments approved by expedited review						
j) Number of adverse reactions/unanticipated events reviewed						

Educational Training

29. Provide the following information regarding educational training in human subjects protection for each staff member.

	Training received before assuming position? (Y/N)	Training received after assuming position? (Y/N)	How often is training repeated? (e.g., 1/yr, 2x/yr, 1/2yrs, etc.)
a) Signatory Official			
b) IRB Chair(s)			
c) IRB administrator(s)			
d) IRB members			
e) Investigators			

30. Briefly describe the human subjects protection training each staff member typically received in the last year.

a) Signatory Official	
b) IRB Chair(s)	
c) IRB administrator(s)	
d) IRB members	
e) Investigators	

31. Does your institution/IRB organization maintain a log or in some other way document human subjects protection training received by each individual?

32. Does your institution/IRB organization review the training received by each individual and determine its adequacy for that person's role?

— — — — — — — — — — —

33. Name of person(s) completing Section A:

SECTION B. <u>INSTITUTIONAL REVIEW BOARD</u>

Complete a copy of this section for <u>each</u> IRB that reviews human subjects research for your institution.

IRB Number(s):
Reference the number (e.g., IRB 2) from Section A, Questions 25, 26, and 28.

1. Who manages the day-to-day operations of the IRB?
Provide name and title.

2. To whom does this person report?
Provide name and title.

3. How often does your IRB usually convene for full committee review of research studies?

       ___ > once/week ___ once/week ___ twice/month

       ___ once/month ___ >once/month ___ other: _____

4. Does your IRB have written operating procedures?

5. When were the written IRB operating procedures last reviewed?

6. When were the written IRB operating procedures last updated?

      What kinds of changes were made to the procedure (e.g., typographical errors, substantive, policy, etc.)?

7. Do the written IRB operating procedures indicate how frequently they should be reviewed and, if necessary, updated?

8. Who reviews and revises the IRB written operating procedures?
Provide name and title.

9. How long are IRB records (e.g., protocol files, minutes) stored on site and readily accessible to the IRB members and staff?

      How are records stored (e.g., paper, electronic)?

10. Are IRB records retained after this period?

      a) If yes, how?

      b) For how long?

11. Does your IRB organization use a computerized database for tracking all protocols?

      a) Identify the types of letters that can be produced by the database (e.g., continuing review notice, approval letters).

      b) Identify the types of reports you can generate from your database.

      c) What reports do you use routinely?

      d) Does the database track adverse events?

Submission Process for IRB Review

12. Does your IRB require investigators to use an IRB submission form for initial review of protocols?
If yes, please submit a copy of this form(s).

13. Does your IRB submission form request the name of the sponsor?

14. Does your IRB submission form request the approval and signature of the department chair (or supervisor) prior to submission to the IRB?

15. Does your IRB require the approval and signature of other individuals prior to submission to the IRB (e.g., pharmacy, nursing)?

16. What items are requested and distributed to each designated IRB member(s) for review? *Check all that apply.*

Items Collected for IRB Review		Distributed for Full Committee Review			
Item	Requested by IRB	IRB Chair	Primary Reviewer	Other IRB Members	Alternate Members
a) IRB submission form					
b) Full protocol					
c) Full grant or contract application (if federally funded)					
d) Protocol summary					
e) Informed consent form					
f) Scientific review					
g) Recruitment material (e.g., advertisements, recruitment letters, scripts for telephone conversation or focus groups, etc.)					
h) Investigator's qualifications (e.g., CV, medical license(s), etc.)					
i) Conflict of interests disclosure					
j) List of all investigators					
k) Questionnaires					
l) Other (*Describe*)					
Additional elements that may apply for biomedical research. *Check all that apply.*					
m) Investigator Brochure					
n) Package insert providing drug information					
o) Device manual					
p) IND/IDE number					
q) Copy of FDA 1572 form or Investigator Agreement (for device studies)					
r) Copy of case report forms					

Preparation for Full Committee Review Process

17. Does your IRB have a deadline for investigators to submit protocols that require full committee review? If yes, how many days are between the deadline and the scheduled IRB meeting?

18. How many days do IRB members have to review materials prior to the date of the IRB meeting?

19. Does your IRB(s) use a primary reviewer system for full committee reviews of new protocols?

   a) If yes, how many reviewers are assigned for each protocol?

   b) Is there an attempt to match the primary reviewer's expertise to the protocol's subject matter?

20. How often does the IRB bring in a consultant to provide scientific or other relevant expertise for review of a particular protocol?

21. Does your IRB ensure that the informed consent document includes input by a non-scientist (e.g., lay person(s))?

Preparation for Continuing Review

22. Does your IRB request a written status report from the investigator for continuing review?

   If yes, how long before expiration of IRB approval? *Select one. If no, go to question 24.*

   __>60 days   __45-59 days   __30-44 days   __<30days   __other:

23. What items are requested in the written status report? *Check all that apply.*

   a) ___ Number of subjects enrolled

   b) ___ Number of subjects screened

   c) ___ Number of subjects withdrawn

   d) ___ Reasons for withdrawal

   e) ___ Number of subjects dropped out of protocol

   f) ___ Reasons for drop-out

   g) ___ Number of subjects lost to follow-up

   h) ___ Gender and ethnic/racial breakdown of enrolled subjects

   i) ___ Verification that informed consent was obtained from all subjects and that all signed consent forms are on file (unless requirements were waived)

   j) ___ Number of serious adverse events (SAEs)

   k) ___ Description of SAEs

   l) ___ Number of unanticipated problems

   m) ___ A description of the unanticipated problems

   n) ___ List of amendments or modifications since last IRB review

   o) ___ Change in study personnel

   p) ___ Change in sponsor

   q) ___ Subject complaints

OHRP QA/QI Self-Assessment Tool

   r) ___ Summary of progress/preliminary findings

   s) ___ Other: _____

24. How many days prior to the IRB meeting date do IRB members have to review continuing review material?

25. What information is requested for continuing review? *Check all that apply.*

Items Collected for Continuing Review		Distributed for Full Committee Review			
Item	Requested by IRB	Chair	Primary Reviewer	Other IRB Members	Alternate Members
a) IRB's written status report form					
b) Full protocol					
c) Copy of informed consent form(s) used during the past approval period					
d) Protocol summary					
e) Protocol/project modifications					
f) Summary of recent literature					
g) NIH Progress Report					
h) DSMB Progress Report					
i) Other:					

26. Does your IRB use a primary reviewer system for continuing reviews requiring full committee review?

If yes, how many reviewers are assigned to each protocol?

IRB Review Process

27. After a brief review of three recent IRB minutes, complete the following table.
Start with "Meeting 1" representing the most recent meeting. However, if you convened more than one meeting per month, respond by using information from the first IRB meeting in each of the past 3 months.

IRB Workload Table	1st Meeting	2nd Meeting	3rd Meeting
a) Number of new protocols determined as exempt			
b) Number of new protocols approved by expedited review that were reported to the IRB			
c) Number of new protocols reviewed by full committee			
d) Number of continuing review protocols approved by expedited review that were reported to the IRB			
e) Number of continuing review protocols reviewed by full committee			
f) Number of amendments approved by expedited review that were reported to the IRB			
g) Number of amendments reviewed by full committee			
h) Number of adverse reactions/unanticipated events reviewed by full committee			

28. Provide information for the following IRB functions:
Check the appropriate boxes for each individual.

	IRB Chair(s)	IRB Administrator	IRB Staff	IRB Member	Other Person; If Other, Specify Who:
a) Performs administrative review					
b) Determines category for review (exempt, expedited, full board)					
c) Performs expedited review					
d) Performs initial review of adverse events					
e) Prepares IRB meeting agenda					
f) Prepares IRB meeting minutes					
g) Maintains IRB database					
h) Maintains IRB files					

29. Does your IRB review the entire grant, contract, or cooperative agreement application for federally supported research when providing review for the prime awardee of an application?

30. Does your IRB consider whether performance sites are engaged in human subject research supported by the federal government?

31. For federally supported human subject research, does your IRB inform the investigator of the need to obtain Assurances for performance sites engaged in the research; sites which do not have an appropriate OHRP or federally approved Assurance?

32. When your IRB reviews research to be conducted at other institutions, does your IRB consider characteristics of the local setting (i.e., race, gender, cultural backgrounds, and sensitivity to issues such as community attitudes, institutional policies and commitments, as well as applicable law and standards of professional conduct and practice)?

33. Who usually determines whether a protocol submitted for IRB review is to be reviewed by full committee or expedited review?

34. Who is authorized by your IRB/IRB chair to approve protocols by expedited review?

35. Approximately how much time does it usually take to review a new protocol by expedited procedures?

36. For each study, does your IRB determine who will be authorized to obtain informed consent from subjects?

37. Does your IRB require the PI to obtain IRB approval before delegating the responsibility to someone else to obtain informed consent from subjects?

For high-risk studies, does the IRB approve delegation to specific individuals by name?

38. Does your IRB have a sample consent form that investigators may use as a resource?

If yes, please submit a copy to OHRP as an attachment.

39. Does your IRB review the process by which informed consent will be obtained (e.g., conditions under which a subject is approached for recruitment)?

40. How does your IRB ensure that the informed consent document is comprehensible to the subject population (e.g., appropriate reading level)?

41. Does your IRB consider whether a translation to a foreign language (e.g., Spanish language) is needed?

42. Does your IRB ever waive the requirement to obtain informed consent from each prospective subject or the subject's legally authorized representative?

   If yes, what criteria does the IRB use to waive the requirement?

43 Does your IRB ever waive the requirement to document informed consent using a written consent form that is signed by the subject or the subject's legal representative?

   If yes, what criteria does the IRB use to waive the requirement?

44. How is waiver of informed consent documented for protocols undergoing expedited review?

45. Does your IRB have a policy for review of research involving deception?

46. Does your IRB explicitly consider how to minimize risks to subjects?

47. Does your IRB consider whether risks to subjects are reasonable in relation to anticipated benefits?

48. Does your IRB ever consider the long-range effects of applying the knowledge gained in the research as among the risks that fall within the purview of its responsibility?

49. Does your IRB review recruitment processes to ensure that the selection of subjects will be equitable (e.g., gender, age, race/ethnicity)?

50. Does your IRB review advertisements to be used for recruitment of subjects?

51. Does your IRB include awareness of, through consultation or representation on the IRB as appropriate, the additional concerns or issues of research involving vulnerable populations (such as, children, prisoners, women who are pregnant, persons with mental disabilities, or persons who are economically or educationally disadvantaged)?

52. Does your IRB require, when appropriate, that the research plan includes adequate provisions for monitoring the data collected to ensure the safety of subjects?

53. Does your IRB require, when appropriate, that there are adequate provisions to protect the privacy of subjects and to maintain confidentiality?

54. Does your IRB recommend or require, when appropriate, submission of a Certificate of Confidentiality?

   If yes, in what situations?

55. When some or all of the subjects are likely to be vulnerable to coercion or undue influence (such as, children, prisoners, women who are pregnant, persons with mental disabilities, or persons who are economically or educationally disadvantaged), does your IRB consider and require that additional safeguards be included in the study to protect the rights and welfare of the subjects?

56. Does your IRB determine at the initial review of a study the appropriate interval for continuing review based on the degree of risk?

57. Does your IRB consider and comply with the reporting requirements in accordance with 45 CFR §46?

   a) With 21 CFR §50, §56, §312?

   b) With 21 CFR §612, §812?

IRB Minutes

58. After a brief review of three recent IRB minutes, complete the following table.
Start with "Meeting 1" representing the most recent meeting. However, if you convened more than one meeting per month, respond by using information from the first IRB meeting in each of the past 3 months. Maintain reference to the same minutes used in Question 27.

IRB Minutes—Allocation of Time	Meeting 1	Meeting 2	Meeting 3
a) Date of meeting			
b) Time meeting started			
c) Time meeting ended			
d) Length of meeting			
e) Estimated amount of time for full committee protocols/meeting			
f) Estimated amount of time for modifications requiring full committee review/meeting			
g) Estimated amount of time for review of adverse reactions/ unanticipated events reported/meeting			
h) Estimated amount of time for continuing review protocols requiring full committee review/meeting			

59. Do the IRB minutes usually record the names of IRB members present?

60. Do the IRB minutes usually record the names of IRB members absent?

61. Do the IRB minutes usually record the names of consultants and visitors present?

62. Does the IRB usually approve the minutes from the prior meeting?

63. Are IRB members notified of all new sponsor- or investigator-initiated modifications/amendments to protocols (i.e., not changes requested by the full committee from a prior review) that were approved by expedited review since the prior meeting?

   If not done at the IRB meeting, how are these approvals communicated to IRB members?

64. Are all substantive sponsor- or investigator-initiated modifications/amendments to protocols reviewed and approved by the convened IRB (with quorum)?

65. Are IRB members notified of all protocols that were approved by expedited review since the prior meeting?

   If not done at the IRB meeting, how are these approvals communicated to IRB members?

66. For protocols undergoing continuing review by full committee, does the convened IRB (with quorum) review, deliberate, and vote for each study?

67. Are IRB members notified of all protocols undergoing continuing review by the expedited review process?

   If not done at the IRB meeting, how are these continuing reviews communicated to IRB members?

68. Do the minutes document IRB review of adverse events and unanticipated problems?

69. Do the minutes include IRB review of protocol violations or deviations?

Documentation of IRB Reviews in the Minutes

70. For each protocol reviewed by your IRB, do the minutes include written documentation of any discussion of controverted issues and their resolution?

71. For protocols in which your IRB waived the requirement of informed consent, was the justification for waiver documented in the minutes in accordance with 45 CFR §46.116(d)?

72. For research involving pregnant women and/or fetuses, do the minutes document IRB findings required under Subpart B of 45 CFR §46?

73. For research involving prisoners, does the composition of the IRB include a prisoner or a prisoner representative with appropriate background and experience?

74. For research involving prisoners, do the minutes document IRB findings as required under 45 CFR §46.305(a)?

75. For research involving children, do the minutes document IRB findings in accordance with Subpart D of 45 CFR §46?

76. Do the minutes document consideration of additional safeguards for vulnerable subjects when appropriate?

77. Do the minutes document that a quorum was present for all IRB actions requiring a vote?

78. Do the minutes document that at least a majority of the IRB members present voted on all actions requiring a vote?

79. Do the minutes document that all IRB actions included at least one scientist in the review and vote?

80. Do the minutes document that all IRB actions included at least one nonscientist in the review and vote?

81. Do the minutes document that all IRB actions included at least one noninstitutional member in the review and vote?

   If no, how frequently has the absence of this member occurred in the past 3 months?

82. Do the minutes record the name of IRB members who abstained from a vote and provide the reason for abstention?

83. Do the minutes record the name of IRB members who were excused from the discussion and vote due to a conflict of interest?

   If yes, was the reason for the conflict documented in the minutes?

84. When approval of a study has been deferred by your IRB, do the IRB minutes state who (e.g., chair, reviewers, full committee) will review and confirm that the investigator has completed the modifications requested by the IRB?

   Do subsequent minutes document that this review was done?

Post IRB Review

85. Does your IRB notify **investigators** in writing of its decision to approve or disapprove the proposed research activity or to require modifications in order to secure IRB approval?

86. Does your IRB notify the **institution** in writing of its decision to approve or disapprove the proposed research activity or to require modifications in order to secure IRB approval?

87. On average, how much time lapses between an IRB meeting and sending the above written notifications to the investigators?

   Who approves these letters before they are sent?

88. If your IRB decides to disapprove a research activity, does it include in its written notification a statement of the reason(s) for its decision and provide the investigator with an opportunity to respond in person or in writing?

89. Does your IRB Chair (or designee) review substantive changes required by the full committee and subsequently made by the investigator?

   If yes, in what situations?

90. Does the IRB monitor or require monitoring of any studies?

   If yes, please describe when and how.

Approval Letter

91. Does the approval letter or approval document from your IRB include the title of the study, protocol number, and version (or amendment) date?

   If no, what items are included?

92. For federally supported research, does the approval letter from your IRB include the grant, contract, or cooperative agreement number?

93. For protocols reviewed by full committee, does the approval letter from your IRB reference the date of the IRB meeting at which the protocol was approved?

94. If the IRB approved a study for one year, does the approval letter provide an expiration date that is one year from the date of the convened IRB meeting in which the study was approved?

95. Does the approval letter reference the requirement to use the IRB-approved informed consent form?

96. Is a copy of the IRB-approved informed consent form attached with the approval letter?

97. Is the IRB-approved informed consent form stamped with an approval date?

98. Is the IRB-approved informed consent form stamped with an expiration date?

— — — — — — — — — — —

99. Name of person(s) completing Section B:

NOTE: If you have any questions regarding this Self-Assessment Tool, please call the Division of Assurances and Quality Improvement at (301) 496-7005.

16

Corporate Compliance and Human Research

Overview 444
Corporate Compliance 444
   The Structure of Corporate Compliance 445
   The Corporate Compliance Officer 446
Federal Agencies and Compliance 446
   Federal Agencies Responsible for Compliance Enforcement 447
   Laws Implicated in Enforcement Actions 447
The Relationship Between Corporate Compliance and Clinical Trials Research 447
   Federal Administrative Provisions That Address Clinical Trials Non-Compliance 448
   New Requirements Anticipated for Responsible Research 451
   How the Government Decides Which Course of Action
   to Take for Non-Compliance 452
   Federal Regulatory Bodies Seek to Enforce the Rules or Help Research
   Entities and Investigators Maintain Compliance 453
A Research Compliance Plan 454
   The Core Elements of a Clinical Research Compliance Plan 454
   The Corporate Compliance Officer and Research Compliance 457
   The Research Integrity Officer as the Research Compliance Officer 458
   High-Risk Areas That Merit Close Attention 458
   Documentation Practices to Substantiate Thorough
   Evaluations and Compliance 459
Non-Compliance 460
   The Whistleblower in the Compliance Context 461
   Managing "Non-Compliance" in Clinical Trials 462
   The Possible Consequences of Non-Compliance in Clinical Trials Research 463
Medicare Compliance and Clinical Trials Research 463
   Clinical Trials Activity Under Medicare 464
   Billing Medicare When a Patient Is Also a Research Subject Under a Grant 464
Conclusion 464
Resources 465
References 465
Appendix 469

············
OVERVIEW

Clinical trials research is subject to a number of federal and state laws and regulations. In addition, sponsors set down their own requirements through contracts and protocol designs that require investigators to comply with or adhere to certain expectations in conducting clinical trials. The failure to achieve compliance can have many consequences. These include federal exclusions or debarment of individual investigators, civil monetary penalties, and, in some instances, criminal sanctions. The failure to achieve compliance may also be evidence of a breach of a standard of care. Thus, if a subject is injured as a result of the failure to meet such a standard resulting in foreseeable harm, non-compliance may be used to prove negligence. Non-compliance may also signal a breach of contract between a clinical investigator or research organization and the sponsor. The failure to abide by compliance standards in such instances could lead to withdrawal of funding for the research and termination of the clinical trials agreement. The subsequent adverse publicity from regulatory action or litigation may have additional consequences, such as adverse publicity in the community and a reticence on the part of researchers or sponsors to conduct trials at the healthcare organization.

Corporate compliance programs are seen as one way to avoid such programs. A voluntary set of guidelines, compliance programs embraced by healthcare organizations and clinical research organizations (CROs) can lead to conformity, good research practices, reduce the risk of participant injury and help to maintain the reputation of the institution and researchers. Adopting such programs involves more than paying lip service to a set of ethical principles. It means adhering to well-defined parameters of conduct. Once adopted, the expectation by regulators and sponsors is that the compliance plan will be followed by healthcare entities and CROs. Treating the plan as window dressing is unacceptable. There can be severe consequences for those who profess to have a culture of corporate compliance when in fact it is nothing more than a pretext for securing funding. This chapter examines corporate compliance, the idea of a research compliance plan, the operational aspects of such a program, and what steps can be taken when there is evidence of regulatory or contractual non-compliance.

············
CORPORATE COMPLIANCE

A corporate compliance program is a methodical approach to achieving and maintaining adherence to laws and regulations. In the healthcare field, much of the impetus for corporate compliance grew out of a concern about fraud and abuse. With the development of the Federal Fraud and Abuse Control Program in the 1990s, and subsequent publicity, healthcare entities realized that they needed to take concerted action. Healthcare facilities quickly understood the potential impact of heavy fines, civil penalties, and criminal sanctions.

In an effort to help the healthcare industry understand corporate compliance the Office of Inspector General (OIG) of the Department of Health and Human Services (HHS) issued a number of voluntary model compliance guidelines. These models set a minimum expectation for clinical labs, Medicare+Choice, physician practices, hospice, hospitals, long-term care, and durable medical equipment companies. While this has helped curb bad practices, it has not stopped all fraud and abuse in the healthcare field. There is ample room for more in-depth compliance activities.

The Structure of Corporate Compliance

Most compliance programs are modeled on the guidance provided by the OIG. The OIG model contains seven basic elements:

1. Written policies and procedures for all employees and agents of the healthcare organization with a particular focus on high-risk exposures.
2. Appointment of a high-level individual (such as an officer) to be responsible for the Corporate Compliance Program.
3. Education and training regarding the organization's compliance plan, standards, and applicable laws provided at a level understandable to those receiving such information.
4. Establishment of an effective *communication* system through which employees can report suspected instances of violations without the fear of retaliation or recrimination.
5. The healthcare organization should have in place an appropriate written, implemented disciplinary system to punish those who violate the standards or applicable law, and, at the same time, not delegate large amounts of discretionary authority to those that it should know had a propensity to participate in illegal actions.
6. Implementation of ongoing monitoring audits and surveillance to identify non-compliant activities.
7. The system should include an effective mechanism to respond to identified non-compliance and to correct it so that it does not reoccur in future.

In addition to the seven-step plan, there are a number of important operational ingredients in structuring a compliance plan. These include the following considerations:

- Creation of a Corporate Compliance Committee, including key individuals to help set policy, development standards, and facilitate implementation of the plan.
- A contract review process to identify terms and conditions that are incongruent with applicable law, regulation, or the compliance plan of the healthcare organization.
- A delineated communications process for the board and compliance officer, including how information should flow on a need-to-know basis when an officer of the healthcare organization is under review or suspicion for non-compliance.
- Employee handbook and employee contract language to address termination if the employee is found culpable of fraud and abuse or other non-compliant behavior by an outside agency or regulatory body.
- Bylaws provisions to address either suspension or revocation of privileges granted to a health professional found culpable of fraud and abuse or other non-compliant behavior by an outside agency or regulatory body.
- Documentation requirements for recording when employees and others participated in mandatory compliance education, including regular update training.
- Implementation of alternate, user-friendly communication systems such as hotlines or suggestion boxes for reporting known or suspected non-compliance.
- Practical strategies for investigating suspected cases of non-compliance, including securing sensitive information and interviewing key individuals.
- Decision algorithms for determining when to self-report identified cases of fraud and abuse.

- Process improvement when current systems require enhancements to detect or deter non-compliance.
- Procedures for personnel to follow when presented with a subpoena, search warrant, or request for a friendly chat by a regulatory body or law enforcement official relative to suspected fraud and abuse on any other type of non-compliance.

There is no set formula for developing a successful compliance plan. Much depends on the size of the healthcare organization, the number of employees, campuses, and structure of the entity. Thus it is possible to find a staff of Corporate Compliance Managers or Directors reporting to a Corporate Compliance Officer. This might be the case in a large academic medical center with numerous off-campus facilities or a complex integrated delivery system with a multiplicity of hospitals, long-term care centers, and day surgery units.

The Corporate Compliance Officer

There is much debate about the propriety of the chief financial officer (CFO) or general counsel serving as the corporate compliance officer. The reason is that with so much of the program focused on financial matters, it may be impossible for the CFO to investigate himself or his department. Similarly, it may be very difficult for the general counsel to give advice that puts her or her department in jeopardy under the compliance plan. Indeed, there may be a real question about evidentiary privilege if the general counsel has access to information that is for the purview of only the compliance officer. Having seen what is not protected, might leave the information open to discovery and use that would otherwise not occur in such matters.

Many healthcare organizations balk at the notion of hiring a full-time corporate compliance officer. They feel it is not necessary or that they cannot afford the costs. Thus the designated individual might wear a number of hats, including risk management or human resources, or chief operating officer. Even for these individuals there can be potential conflicts of interest if their competing responsibilities cross the line in terms of regulatory compliance.

What is most important is to set the job qualifications for the compliance officer. The individual must be articulate, have a facility for understanding financial information, statistics, and a good skill set for identifying and managing non-compliance. The compliance officer must be a respected individual, one who can easily converse with the chairman of the board and members of the medical staff. The ability to take a stand on an issue cannot be underestimated. Threats of retaliation or intimidation should not deter the compliance officer.

FEDERAL AGENCIES AND COMPLIANCE

Corporate compliance is largely a voluntary program undertaken by healthcare entities and organizations. However, with contractors and payers requiring healthcare organizations to have a compliance plan, it is becoming less and less an issue of whether an entity should have a program. Now the question is, what type of compliance plan is necessary?

Once a plan is in place, the failure to abide by it can prove worse than if the entity did not have a compliance program at all. The rationale is that regulators look upon sham compliance plans as a rouse to deflect their attention from serious fraud and abuse programs. Because an organization has held itself out as a compliance entity, the sham in such instances serves as a lightening rod to garner attention and punishment for the offending party.

Federal Agencies Responsible for Compliance Enforcement

A number of federal and state agencies are able and willing to enforce laws that surround corporate compliance. These include the departments and agencies that make up the Fraud and Abuse Control Program (e.g., the FBI, OIG of HHS, the Department of Justice, and state Medicaid Fraud Control Units). Some investigate or evaluate circumstances with a view to civil litigation or administrative action. In other situations, the focus may be on criminal activity stemming from regulatory non-compliance.

Laws Implicated in Enforcement Actions

There are several laws that can be used as the basis for civil or criminal actions based on non-compliance. These include the civil aspect of the False Claims Act (31 USC §§3729-3731), the criminal provisions of the False Claims Act (18 USC §§287, 371, and 1001) the fraud and abuse laws (the Social Security Act, §1128B(b) and also 42 USC §1320a-7b(b) as modified by the Health Insurance Portability and Accountability Act of 1996, P.L. 104-191, tit. II, §204, 110 Stat. 1936, 1999 (1996)), the *qui tam* provisions of the False Claims Act (31 USC §3730), and the Stark Provisions dealing with self-referrals (Ominbus Reconciliation Act of 1989, Pub. L. No. 101-239, 103 Stat. 2106 (1989) and Omnibus Reconciliation Act of 1993 Pub. L. No. 103-66, 107 Stat. 312 (1993) as amended by the Social Security Act Amendments of 1994, Pub. L. No. 103-432, 108 Stat. 4398 (1994)).

....

THE RELATIONSHIP BETWEEN CORPORATE COMPLIANCE AND CLINICAL TRIALS RESEARCH

Many aspects of clinical trials come within the scope of the laws used to combat fraud and abuse in Medicare, Medicaid, and other federal reimbursement programs. These include the False Claims Act, the Stark Self-Referral provisions, and the anti-kickback laws. Some examples help to explain how these laws pertain to clinical trials research.

Making False Statements—When a researcher, a healthcare entity, or another body signs an assurance that it is compliant with all federal requirements, making such assurances knowing that such statements are false implicates the False Claims Act. A researcher who knows, for example, that his study does not comport with Part A of the HHS regulations governing clinical trials could be in legal jeopardy by executing a false statement that the ongoing study is in compliance with the regulations.

Making A False Claim—When a healthcare organization bills a federal health program for a procedure that is actually a cost item covered under a federal grant, making such a submission is a false claim.

Falsified Research—Submitting a final report on a study to complete remuneration of study costs knowing that the data is false constitutes an infraction under the false statement component of the False Claims Act.

Anti-Kickback Provisions—Giving substantial sums of money for steering patients into clinical studies as part of a recruitment scheme or giving a physician money to participate in questionable research may violate the Anti-Kickback law, which prohibits transactions that lead a caregiver to make referrals or to compensate them for doing so. It should be noted that there are so-called Safe Harbor provisions under this law that permit activities that would otherwise be unlawful. Whether the clinical trial comes within the scope of safe harbor requires a thorough analysis of the study and transactions.

Self-Referral Provisions—Under the Stark provisions a clinician is precluded from making a referral of a Medicare or Medicaid recipient to a facility that provides certain designated healthcare services if the caregiver has a financial relationship with that entity. There are some exceptions under the Stark provisions. However, it is possible that a physician-researcher can have the type of financial relationship that triggers the application of the Stark law with respect to a patient-subject. Much depends upon careful evaluation of the legal relationship between the clinician and the facility.

There are other ways in which non-compliance can generate application of federal law, such as failing to report adverse events when required to do so under regulations, or violations of laws protecting the disabled or handicapped in terms of subject recruitment, or consent and failure to meet confidentiality provisions. Infractions in these instances provide evidence of a breach of Assurance and contract statements promising to meet federal protections and standards. It can go further too, especially if a researcher or sponsor claims to subscribe to nationally accepted standards for avoiding conflict-of-interest. A breach of these undertakings may constitute a breach of federal contracts or Assurance or private sponsorship contracts and become evidence of non-compliance under institutional programs.

Other laws may be pertinent, too. For example, using the U.S. Postal Service or electronic transmission of data across state lines may trigger the application of a different class of laws. Sending false reports in the postal system may amount to mail fraud (18 USC §1341) just as an e-mail of false data in a multicenter study (18 USC §1343) may trigger wire fraud when the intent is to use the information to secure grant funds or unlawful remuneration of costs.

The federal government has a cadre of civil and criminal tools to use to make researchers, sponsors, and healthcare facilities become compliant, which should not be needed if a good plan is in place to avoid improper conduct.

Federal Administrative Provisions That Address Clinical Trials Non-Compliance

Aside from civil and criminal action, there is a host of administrative authority vested in federal agencies with oversight responsibilities for clinical trials. Some of this activity is undertaken by NIH, the FDA, the PHS, and other regulatory bodies who support or have responsibility for human research trials. It is useful to see how some of these bodies handle compliance oversight.

OMA—Within the National Institutes of Health (NIH), the Office of Management Administration (OMA) reviews allegations of fraud, waste, and abuse involving internal matters within the NIH as well as those involving extramural grantees and contractors. In essence, the major focus of the OMA is on financial mismanagement in clinical trials. When serious misconduct or fraud becomes apparent to the OMA, the information may be shared with the Office of the Inspector General of HHS. It is also possible that the matter could go beyond administrative intervention. Thus instances of fraud and abuse in NIH-funded research could become the subject of criminal prosecution by U.S. Attorney.

OPERA—The office of Policy for Extramural Research Administration (OPERA) within NIH provides education and outreach programs for extramural grantees and contractors. The office also conducts site visits of grantees. These visits are done as part of the oversight responsibility of the office and can lead to identification of noncompliant practices. In such instances, OPERA may provide regular ongoing reviews until a grantee achieves compliance.

OER—The Office of Extramural Research of NIH handles an issue of growing importance in clinical trials: conflict-of-interest. As this topic impacts consent to participate in clinical trials research, subject recruitment, study design, data management and reporting, and a number of other concerns, it is bound to capture more attention in future. Not only is there the potential for findings of misconduct for failure to disclose a conflict-of-interest, there is a very real issue of possible criminal liability under the False Claims Act. This is especially the case when an investigator signs documentation assuring the PHS that he or she does not have a conflict-of-interest. Securing federal funding for clinical trials on the basis of a false statement (that is, where the researcher does have a conflict-of-interest), could form the basis for criminal proceedings.

ORA—In the Food and Drug Administration the Office of Research Affairs (ORA) has a broad mandate covering research misconduct involving the testing and evaluation of human and animal drugs, food and feed additives, human biological products, and medical devices. The ORA processes this misconduct work through its Division of Compliance Policy. Additionally, under compliance authority vested in ORA, the FDA can take steps to ensure the quality of data submitted to the agency with respect to safety and efficacy of regulated products and to determine that human research subjects are adequately protected. This is an important mandate. If an Establishment Inspection Report (EIR) documents violations of a serious nature that necessitate administrative or regulation action, the consequences can be quite burdensome. The FDA may start proceedings to disqualify the investigator or recommend criminal prosecution. Another option is a consent decree with the clinical investigator (21 CFR §312.70 et seq.). The FDA may seize nonexempted test articles or seek injunctive relief (7348.811 Chapter 48, Bioresearch Monitoring, Clinical Investigators, September 30, 2000).

ORI—The Office of Research Integrity (ORI) is the successor authority to the Office of Scientific Integrity (OSI) in the Office of the Director of NIH and the Office of Scientific Integrity Review (OSIR) that was in the Office of the Assistant Secretary for Health. The Office of Research Integrity includes the Division of Research Investigations (DRI), and the Division of Policy and Education (DPE). Legal services are furnished by the Office of the General Counsel of the Research Integrity Branch of HHS.

ORI handles research misconduct for biomedical and behavioral studies supported by the Public Health Service (PHS). It is noteworthy that the PHS comprises NIH, the Centers for Disease Control and Prevention (CDC), the FDA, the Substance Abuse and Mental Health Services Administration (SAMHSA), the Health Resources and Services Administration (HRSA), the Agency for Health Research and Quality (AHRQ), the Agency for Toxic Substances and Disease Registry (ATSDRO), and the Indian Health Service (HIS). With the exception of the FDA, ORI's responsibility encompasses all the entities under the Public Health Service.

In dealing with research-related scientific misconduct, ORI relies upon the definition found in the Federal Regulations. For this purpose, scientific misconduct means "fabrication, falsification, plagiarism, or other practices that seriously deviate from those that are commonly accepted within the scientific community for proposing, conducting, or reporting research" (42 CFR §50.102).

It is the Division of Research Investigations that assesses allegations of scientific misconduct, reviews inquiries and investigations from institutions, and carries out inquiries and investigations at extramural entities and PHS intramural investigations. Following a preliminary assessment of the situation, an inquiry may be conducted by the institution that has received PHS funding. This process is designed to evaluate available information to determine whether there is sufficient evidence to proceed with an investigation. The latter is a formal mechanism that culminates in a report and a determination by the institution. The final report, in turn, is to be submitted to ORI. After reviewing a report of scientific misconduct, the ORI may perform its own investigation. The institution may impose its own sanctions on the research investigator involved in scientific misconduct. Similarly, the ORI may impose sanctions on the investigator as well as the institution (42 CFR §50.104).

The regulations prompt notification of the ORI at any stage of the inquiry or investigatory process when it becomes apparent that there is an immediate health hazard, there is an immediate need to protect federal funds or equipment, there is an immediate need to protect the person making the allegations or who is the subject of these assertions, or it is probable that the alleged misconduct will be the subject of a public report. If there is a reasonable indication of criminal violation, the institution must report it to the ORI within twenty-four hours of learning this information. The office, then must turn the matter over to the Office of Inspector General (42 CFR §50.104).

The ORI makes recommendations to the Assistant Secretary of Health regarding administrative actions to be taken on research misconduct. If the Assistant Secretary accepts the recommendations of the ORI, the respondent (culpable individual) is given the opportunity to have a hearing before a Department Appeals Board (DAB) on the finding of misconduct and administrative actions. If the appeal is not taken, then the misconduct findings become final, and, along with the administrative actions, the information is published in the *Federal Register,* the *NIH Guide for Grants and Contracts,* the *ORI Newsletter,* and the *ORI Annual Report.* Debarments can be found in the *List of Parties Excluded from Federal Procurement and Nonprocurement Programs* published by the General Service Administration (GSA).

The administrative actions taken are dependent on a number of factors. The seriousness of the misconduct and its impact are considered along with whether or not it is part of a pattern of behavior. Administrative sanctions range from one to ten years.

OHPR—The Office of Human Research Protection is the successor to the Office for Protection from Research Risks (OPRR). Whereas OPRR was housed within NIH, OHRP is now in the office of the Secretary of HHS. The OHRP is responsible for human subjects protection in any research conducted or supported by any component of HHS. Its task is to coordinate HHS regulations, policies, and procedures within the department and with other federal departments and agencies. The OHRP has other responsibilities as well, including to develop and implement educational programs and materials and to enhance and improve research subject safety. The Officer of the Director of OHRP directs compliance oversight. The Division of Policy and Assurance negotiates Assurances of Compliance with research facilities. The Division of Compliance Oversight inquires into and investigates alleged noncompliant activities. It can recommend corrective action and oversee a compliance program for a grantee. There is also a Division of Education and Development that produces and coordinates conferences and workshops that focus on human research subject protection (*Federal Register,* 65(114): 37136-37137, June 13, 2000).

OHRP has developed a set of procedures for compliance oversight activities. (Compliance Oversight Procedures, 2000). It is made quite clear that by submitting a written Assurance of Compliance, the facility agrees to full compliance with the law on the part of its personnel and the institution. The OHRP places considerable responsibility on the clinical investigator, institutional officials, and others to make certain that there is compliance with the regulations and to protect the rights and welfare of human subjects under Section 491 of the Public Health Service Act.

In a compliance oversight evaluation, institutional authorities are apprised in writing by OHRP of what they are likely to find during the course of a review. In most instances OHRP will not take action against a facility without first giving the facility the opportunity to rebuff suggestions of non-compliance. Corrective action may be a possibility, and OHRP may decide to restrict the Assurance of Compliance by suspending some or all research projects pending the institution achieving compliance. In some instances OHRP may review some or all of the research projects under the entity's Assurance of Compliance. Corrective action may include education for committee members and institutional officials. In some cases, the OHRP may withdraw its approval of an entity's Assurance of Compliance. The consequence is that HHS cannot fund any of the institution's research projects until there is compliance. At the far end of the scale, corrective action may necessitate the removal of the investigator temporarily or permanently from participation in the research. Debarment is also a recourse in which an institution or an investigator is declared ineligible to take part in HHS-supported research. A debarment is usually government-wide.

Other federal departments and entities have the capacity to handle research misconduct under their authority. This includes the National Science Foundation, the Department of the Navy, the Veterans Administration, and others.

New Requirements Anticipated for Responsible Research

The Public Health Service published a document entitled, "PHS Policy for Instruction in the Responsible Conduct of Research (*Fed. Register,* 65(236): 76647, December 7, 2000). However, the new policy was suspended indefinitely in February 2001 in accordance with the President's Regulatory Review Plan. This was done to enable the new administration to review the substantive portions of the policy and the procedure followed in adopting it. The suspension included no definite time limit (*Fed. Register* 66(35): 11032, February 21, 2001).

The new policy (PHS Policy for Instruction in the Responsible Conduct of Research) places considerable emphasis on education, including core educational areas. These are

- Data acquisition, management, sharing, and ownership
- Mentor/Trainee responsibilities
- Public practices and responsible authorship
- Peer review
- Collaborative science
- Human subjects
- Research involving animals
- Research misconduct
- Conflict of interest and commitment

Aside from the core content, the institution must submit a written Assurance that the entity has an education plan and a written description of the program. This Assurance must accompany requests for PHS funds for research.

It is unclear when and if the new policy will take effect as there was some concern expressed by members of the U.S. House of Representatives about the way in which the new policy was adopted. Coupled with the Regulatory Review Plan implementation, it may be some time before the new policy becomes operational. Even at that stage, the policy incorporates a phase-in approach to implementation.

Many research entities are not waiting for a final disposition on the policy. They have begun to establish practical educational programs premised on the core content required in the PHS plan.

Looking further ahead, many observers believe that further inroads can be expected by the Federal government. One idea is the creation of a National Office of Human Research Oversight (NOHRO) that came from a draft report of the National Bioethics Advisory Committee (December 2000). Still others may be considered.

The key point is that there are a number of regulatory bodies already using existing laws, policies, and guidance to exercise authority geared to clinical trials compliance. Much more can be done within this envelope of regulation. Self-policing, monitoring, surveillance, education, corrective action, and discipline may obviate the need for regulatory intervention. Achieving a balance between regulatory oversight and internal surveillance and persistence may help to reduce onerous corrective action plans and possible civil and criminal liability.

How the Government Decides Which Course of Action to Take for Non-Compliance

There are a number of government departments and agencies with oversight and enforcement responsibilities. What might be a matter of documentation deficiencies that do not impact billing, accounting, or research subject safety might merit an on-site review, assistance with education, and follow-up compliance visits. When, however, research subject safety is of prime concern, much more intrusive action is warranted. On-site evaluations, suspending trials, working with the entity to develop and implement a corrective action plan, and then follow-up monitoring might be the hallmarks of government intervention. The Department of Justice may take action involving false claims, false statements, or fraudulent Assurances made as the basis for federal research funds. Fraud and abuse in terms of managing research funds, double-dipping in terms of Medicare or Medicaid payments for a treatment paid for under study grants, or misappropriation of federal research funds is likely to engender a criminal investigation and possibly indictments. Certainly, credible whistleblower assertions will trigger careful review, whether it is for scientific misconduct, research subject safety issues, or allegations of fraud in the management of research funds.

Once a major issue does bubble up to the surface, it may be seen as a marker requiring further scrutiny of the investigator or entity. For example, significant noncompliance with an FDA test article might trigger inquiries by OHRP or OMA if the same study comes within their respective jurisdictions. Sometimes too, the marker event may have nothing to do with clinical trials. The healthcare entity may be the subject of an IRS probe looking into possible tax evasion. In the course of an audit, discrepancies are detected that can be traced back to federally funded research. This may signal a backdoor investigation into potential research irregularities. On other occasions, it may be the actions of a sponsor or an accrediting body that spark a federal regulatory agency into action. A sponsor may report serious concerns regarding research subject safety or a reviewable event may occur involving serious harm to a subject-patient, triggering the need for a root cause analysis under the Joint Commission on Accreditation of Healthcare Organizations (JCAHO). If the event is serious enough, JCAHO may take stern action with respect to the facility, including placement of the entity on Accreditation Watch. As a facility that depends upon its JCAHO accreditation to participate in Medicare or Medicaid, significant accreditation action may set the stage for regulatory reviews by the Centers for Medicare and Medicaid Services (CMS), formerly the Healthcare Financing Administration or HCFA. That the event involved research subject safety may then trigger an agency to look into research compliance.

There are a number of ways in which a federal department or agency might pursue allegations of non-compliance in clinical trials. Depending upon the outcome of investigations, recourse may be to stop the research, debar an investigator, seek prosecution under the False Claims Act, suspend a clinical trial, or impose a corrective action plan. The facts of the case will play a large role in deciding what action is appropriate in the circumstance.

Federal Regulatory Bodies Seek to Enforce the Rules or Help Research Entities and Investigators Maintain Compliance

Do the federal entities seek to enforce the rules or be helpers to facilitate compliance? The answer depends upon whether there are deficiencies or requests for assistance in helping to rectify less-than-acceptable practices, or whether the matter comes within the scope of enforcement measures. With the changes announced in 2000 and the shift of OPRR from the NIH to a transformed unit in the Secretary's Office termed the Office for Human Research Protections (OHRP), there is a definite effort to provide assistance and also to pursue a traditional regulatory framework. The assistance component involves education, furnishing help in rectifying deficiencies, and hosting workshops. Some have even termed this a partnership approach between government and the private sector. At the same time, there is the regulatory model in operation. Agencies and departments with enforcement responsibilities will use an array of tools to deter fraud and abuse, punish those who engage in such activities, and preclude those who are found culpable of scientific conduct from engaging in federally funded or sponsored clinical trials. Even for the latter group, the debarment may be time-limited. Thus, the federal approach is a blend of assistance and enforcement in clinical trials.

. . . .

A RESEARCH COMPLIANCE PLAN

Given the amount of regulatory oversight exerted over human subject clinical trials, it is imperative to develop and implement a research compliance plan. For those facilities conducting animal studies, it would be beneficial to extend such a plan to encompass such research.

This section examines the core elements of a clinical research compliance plan, taking into consideration the role of both a research compliance officer and integrity officer. High-risk practices are discussed along with documentation methodologies.

The Core Elements of a Clinical Research Compliance Plan

Aside from the traditional seven elements of a compliance plan, there are very specific aspects that should be included in a program targeting clinical trials. There are also structural issues that affect the type of compliance plan put in place for clinical trials research. The special elements of a research compliance plan are addressed first and then the structural considerations.

In a traditional compliance plan, the core elements of the program include

1. Written policies and procedures
2. Appointment of a high-level individual as the Compliance Officer
3. Education and training regarding the organization's compliance plan, standards, and applicable laws provided at a level understandable to those receiving such information
4. Establishment of an effective communication system for reporting suspected violations of the law or the compliance plan
5. Development of a clearly written disciplinary system to punish those who violate the applicable standards or law
6. Implementation of ongoing monitoring audits and surveillance methods of identifying non-compliant activities
7. Establishment of an effective mechanism to respond to identified non-compliance and to correct it so that it does not reoccur in future

For a research compliance plan there are a number of specific elements that should be considered.

- *Written policies and procedures*
  - Definition of research compliance
  - Definition of non-compliance in clinical research
  - Research compliance role and responsibility of IRB members, research investigators, and clinical research staff
  - Reporting known or suspected non-compliance
  - Reporting known or suspected scientific misconduct

- Nonretaliation for good faith reporting
- Reporting known or suspected unsafe conditions or research practices
- Acceptable investigatory methods
- Surveillance and monitoring practices
- Incorporate by reference the "Model Policy for Responding to Allegations of Scientific Misconduct" and the "Model Procedures for Responding to Allegations of Scientific Misconduct" of the Office of Research Integrity (ORI) as part of a due process–oriented method for investigating and managing non-compliant practices
- Management of research subject safety issues (adverse events, unanticipated outcomes, relationship to and involvement of the Data Safety Monitoring Board)
- Acceptable corrective action methods

- *Appointment of a high-level individual as the Compliance Officer*
  - Role of the research compliance or Integrity Officer
  - Authority
  - Chain of command
  - Reporting hierarchy
  - Responsibilities of the corporate compliance officer and committee with respect to clinical trials research compliance
  - Responsibilities of the corporate research compliance or integrity officer in relations to the general counsel, outside counsel, and senior management of the healthcare entity or organization

- *Education and Training*
  - General compliance requirements
  - Specific research compliance requirements
    - ❑ Research design (use of placebo, randomization, double-blind studies)
    - ❑ Research subject recruitment and selection
    - ❑ Informed consent practices
    - ❑ Documentation of the consent process
    - ❑ Confidentiality of individually identifiable research subject information
  - Responsible conduct of research requirements
    - ❑ Acceptable methods for education and training
    - ❑ Documentation of participation in mandatory education
    - ❑ Measurement of understanding of core requirements
    - ❑ Documented participation in continuing education programs on responsible conduct of research practices
    - ❑ *Core Content curriculum development*
      - → Data acquisition, management, sharing and ownership
      - → Mentor/trainee responsibilities
      - → Publication practices and responsible authorship

→ Peer review

→ Collaborative science

→ Human and animal research

→ Research misconduct

→ Conflict of interest

- *Establishment of an effective communication system for reporting suspected violations of the law or the compliance plan*

  ❑ Research compliance hotline system

  ❑ Research compliance suggestion box

  ❑ Process for handling complaints, expressions of concern, or allegations of non-compliance (anonymous reporting or anonymous reporting with a tag number for follow-up discussion)

  ❑ Time line for processing allegations of suspected non-compliance

- *Development of a clearly written disciplinary system to punish those who violate the applicable standards or law*

  ❑ Notice provision in employment application and application for clinical privileges regarding consequence of scientific misconduct or non-compliance

  ❑ Bylaw provisions that delineate recourse for health professional found culpable of scientific misconduct or sanctioned for regulatory non-compliance. Model by law provisions are at the end of this chapter

  ❑ Recourse under collective agreements for handling scientific misconduct or regulatory non-compliance by union members

  ❑ Notice provision in employee handbook and human resources regarding consequence of scientific misconduct or non-compliance

  ❑ Contractual terms and conditions for management of non-compliance or debarment of clinical research contractor

  ❑ Terms and conditions for exclusion of research fellows, residents, and interns found accountable for scientific misconduct by a federal agency or department, a state agency, or an academic program

- *Implementation of ongoing monitoring audits and surveillance methods to identify non-compliant activities*

  ❑ Consent process monitoring

  ❑ Audits of consent documentation

  ❑ Randomized record audits of research files

  ❑ Unannounced audits

  ❑ Bioresearch monitoring for human drugs and medical devices under FDA-sponsored or funded clinical trials

  ❑ Coordinated billing, coding, and accounting practices for use of research funds with ongoing clinical studies

  ❑ Coordinated billing, coding, and accounting practices for Medicare-Medicaid funds used to support clinical trials

❑ Coordinated billing, coding, and accounting practices for clinical trials in which research subjects are also recipients of routine medical services

❑ Audits of adverse events documentation and reporting practices

❑ Audits of research subject complaints

- *Establishment of an effective mechanism to respond to identified non-compliance and to correct it so that it does not reoccur in future*

  ❑ Acceptable investigatory practices (interviews, collection of data)

  ❑ Use of investigation committees and hearings

  ❑ Preparation of an investigatory report with recommendations

  ❑ Report to outside entities of investigatory findings

    → Scientific misconduct

    → Request to retract published findings

    → Professional licensure bodies

    → Accreditation bodies

    → Regulatory bodies

    → Funding agencies

    → Sponsors

    → Multicenter coordinators

    → Insurance carrier or captive manager if litigation is anticipated for termination of study, termination of research investigator, contract with outside vendor or for injury to patients

  ❑ Lessons learned

    → Inclusion in ongoing education

    → Inclusion in enhanced policies and procedures

    → Inclusion in ongoing surveillance and monitoring strategies

The Corporate Compliance Officer and Research Compliance

No one set formula exists for determining whether a facility compliance officer should also be responsible for research compliance. A number of considerations need to be weighed in making a decision: budget, reporting structures, the volume of research activities, the funding sources for clinical trials research (private versus public or a blend of both), and also the specifications found in sponsorship contracts. The inherent responsibilities of the corporate compliance officer should be carefully considered, especially if the demands are such that the research compliance component will receive little attention if added to an already challenging portfolio. While the position should not be dependent upon the office holder, there is also a practical reality that needs to be considered. If the job description of the corporate compliance officer is heavily dependent upon financial acumen, the office holder may have a difficult time dealing with the nuances of study design, research assurance information, and clinical trials information. Certainly, these challenges can be overcome with input from individuals with a blend of appropriate skill sets. However, in contemporary healthcare circles developing such a critical mass of personnel can be burdensome when they, in turn, are drawn in several different directions. Thus many healthcare organizations and CROs are apt to place considerable credence on the clinical healthcare background of the person responsible for research compliance.

At the very least, the research compliance officer must have a solid orientation to the various laws, regulations, and guidelines for clinical trials research. The individual needs a thorough understanding of scientific and professional misconduct in clinical trials research, conflict-of-interest principles as applied to clinical research, and the type of investigatory skills required for teasing out honest mistakes from fraud, abuse, and other improprieties stemming from clinical trials. This knowledge requirement is *in addition to* the challenging informational requirements for traditional corporate compliance.

Some may argue that the research compliance officer should be a specialist or hold a deputy position to the overall compliance officer of the healthcare organization or CRO. This idea may have merit in some instances as it ensures a strong organizational communications and operational linkage for purposes of compliance. The actual structure will depend upon the nature of the entity and its corporate culture regarding compliance.

The Research Integrity Officer as the Research Compliance Officer

In both the "Model Policy for Responding to Allegations of Scientific Misconduct" and the "Model Procedures for Responding to Allegations of Scientific Misconduct," the Office of Research Integrity (ORI) defines the "Research Integrity Officer" as "the institutional official responsible for assessing allegations of scientific misconduct and determining when such allegations warrant inquiries and for overseeing any inquiries and investigations."

Given the description of the duties of the research integrity officer, it is quite possible that the RIO may be the same as the corporate compliance or research compliance officer. This is dependent upon organizational structure, too. If, for example, a particular matter necessitates specialized skills, a qualified individual may be specifically designated as the RIO. In other instances, the research compliance officer may call upon additional resources to assist him or her in acting in the capacity of the RIO.

The ORI model policy and procedures stress the importance of affording due process to those under review for scientific misconduct. Thus, someone acting in the capacity as RIO should not be the individual termed the Deciding Officer who makes the final determination on allegations regarding scientific misconduct and the response of the organization to it.

High-Risk Areas That Merit Close Attention

In September 2000, the Division of Compliance Oversight of the Office of Human Research Protections (OHRP) published a very useful tool to assist IRBs, researchers, and research compliance officers in pinpointing high-risk areas. The report, "OHRP Compliance Activities: Common Findings and Guidance," highlights eight key areas:

1. Initial and continuing review

2. Expedited review procedures

3. Reporting of unanticipated problems and IRB review of protocol changes

4. Application of exemptions

5. Informed consent

6. IRB Membership, expertise, staff, support, and workload

7. Documentation of IRB activities, findings, and procedures

8. Miscellaneous OHRP guidance

Within each broad category, the OHRP identified very specific issues. In total, seventy-five areas were listed by the OHRP. Working back from this list and the suggested guidance provided, IRBs, research compliance officers, sponsors, healthcare organizations, and CROs can develop strong compliance plans. The information can be used as a self-assessment tool. For example, one of the risk areas is entitled, "Documentation of Required IRB Findings in IRB Minutes" ("OHRP Compliance Activities: Common Findings and Guidance," item number 65). By turning this demonstrative statement into a question on a self-assessment tool, an IRB can do its own compliance systems check. Similarly, the research compliance officer could use the question to evaluate the IRB's performance relative to existing policy and procedure as well as OHRP expectations. As OHRP publishes additional reports, the information can be used to conduct a systems analysis with a view to compliance improvement.

At the same time, it is important for each institution, IRB, and CRO to evaluate its own high-risk areas. This can be done by means of a compliance inventory that includes information gleaned from hotlines, frequently asked questions, compliance audits, monitoring, and surveillance as well as the results of scientific misconduct investigations. Using the OHRP report as an audit tool may reveal that a CRO is in fine shape; however, its own review may disclose much more pressing risk-prone areas that merit immediate attention. Thus, it is a combination of both national experience and local knowledge that helps to pinpoint high-risk compliance issues.

Documentation Practices to Substantiate Thorough Evaluations and Compliance

Lawyers, compliance officers, and risk managers often talk in terms of a paper trail to substantiate compliance with rules, regulations, policies, and procedures. Indeed, in the therapeutic context, there is an old expression to the effect, "If it is not charted, it was not done." The same rationale applies to clinical trials research administration and compliance.

There are a number of practical documentation procedures to use in demonstrating not only compliance but sound research practices. The key is not to overwhelm researchers, sponsors, CROs, and IRB members with paper, since the sheer volume of documentation could obscure serious risk issues. Indeed, setting the bar too high in terms of documentation may create its own problem. The failure to complete a report or a series of documents could be construed as substandard practice.

One could look at what other institutions or CROs use for documentation practices. This may be a useful exercise. However, what others use may not match the peculiar needs of the local facility, CRO, or IRB. Taking this fact into consideration, there are some practical strategies to use with regard to clinical trials documentation:

Create a list of mandatory documentation for clinical trials research—This can be done by gleaning information from mandatory reporting forms found in grants, contracts, regulations, and statutory law. (See illustration at the end of this chapter.) The scope should not be too limited; thus, requirements for documenting the "Final National Coverage Decision" for Medicare Coverage of aspects of a clinical trial should be part of the documentation package if it is pertinent to the local human research enterprise. Some of the more common documentary information should include

✓ Adverse event reports

✓ Annual reports on ongoing studies

✓ Audit reports (financial, research subject safety, and specially required reports for data safety, compliance, etc.)

✓ Conflict-of-interest documentation (including mandatory education attendance, declarations as part of research trial applications, etc.)

✓ Consent monitoring reports (especially of same surveillance practices or special risk subjects)

✓ Field reports

✓ IRB minutes

✓ IRB follow-up actions

✓ Modification of study requests and disposition

✓ Monitoring reports

✓ Wrap-up reports for concluding or terminating studies

These are some illustrations; others will be dependent upon local needs and requirements.

Documentation Audit Results To Be Recorded—The paper trail should demonstrate that the documentation has been reviewed. This means a designated person should sign-off or attest to the fact that the documentation has been evaluated for completeness. The documentation audit may reflect glaring gaps, inconsistencies with established procedures, or compliance requirements. If this is the case, this audit safety net should trigger appropriate follow-up action to ensure compliance. If documentation is acceptable, the sign-off or attestation should reflect this fact.

Decision Trees Can Be Useful Documentation Tools—When trying to decide whether an event requires reporting to a sponsor or regulatory body, or in trying to determine if an item comes within Medicare clinical trials coverage, decision trees can be a useful tool. The decision tree, a stylized flowchart, consists of a series of Yes and No questions to a series of objective questions. Depending upon the answer, a determination may be to report an event or to disallow a service from coverage under the Medicare program. This objective approach can foster consistency in making determinations. It eliminates possible subjective information that could lead to inappropriate decision-making. Moreover, it can reduce the time required to generate a report and lessen the opportunity for conjecture, speculation, and needless information to be recorded in documentation.

NON-COMPLIANCE

The failure to comply with applicable federal requirements can have serious consequences. Research staff trained in regulatory requirements may signal their concerns to the hierarchy of an organization. If their concerns go unheeded, they may report suspected non-compliance to regulatory officials. In other instances they may file a *qui tam* action. Such whistleblower activities can generate rigorous scrutiny for an organization.

For entities under compliance review, it is imperative to have a method in place to respond to such investigations. Even with this process in place, the possible consequences of non-compliance can lead to undesirable results in terms of ongoing clinical trials.

The Whistleblower in the Compliance Context

In the research compliance context, a whistleblower may mean a person who makes an allegation regarding scientific misconduct (ORI publications, "Model Policy for Responding to Allegations of Scientific Misconduct" and the "Model Procedures for Responding to Allegations of Scientific Misconduct"). It also has a similar connotation albeit dealing with the False Claims Act (31 USC §3730(a)-(b)). Under the False Claims Act *any person* may bring an action. When the person is a private individual or entity, it is known as a *qui tam* action, and the party initiating it is referred to as the *qui tam* relator. Once the lawsuit is filed, the government must be furnished with information about the action. The complaint is sealed for at least two months, providing time for the government to decide if it wants to join the claim. Even if at this stage the government decides not to participate, it can decide to do so at a later stage. *Qui tam* relator actions may involve clinical trials research fraud for falsifying information or submitting false claims. Whether pursued as a matter of scientific misconduct under the ORI model policies and procedures or the False Claims Act, whistleblowers may have some level of protection against retaliation for bringing the claim. Section 3730(h) of the False Claims Act protects "any employee who is discharged, demoted, suspended, threatened, harassed, or in any other manner discriminated against" for bringing a False Claims Act. This may mean reinstatement with the same seniority and some degree of compensation. By comparison, under the ORI model policies and procedures, the whistleblower protection goes beyond employees. It states that

> The Research Integrity Officer will monitor the treatment of individuals who bring allegations of misconduct or of inadequate institutional response thereto . . . and will ensure that these persons will not be retaliated against in the terms and conditions of their employment *or other status at the institution.* . . . ["Model Policy for Responding to Allegations of Scientific Misconduct" and the "Model Procedures for Responding to Allegations of Scientific Misconduct"] (emphasis added)

In addition, the ORI model policy and procedures address the issue of privacy protection for the whistleblower and the individual's integrity. It is stated very clearly that, "Institutions are required to undertake diligent efforts to protect the positions and reputations of those persons who, in good faith, make allegations" ("Model Policy for Responding to Allegations of Scientific Misconduct" and the "Model Procedures for Responding to Allegations of Scientific Misconduct").

The rationale for whistleblower protection is the same whether under the False Claims Act or the ORI model policy and procedures. Those with knowledge of serious non-compliance are encouraged to step forward and take appropriate action to curb such improprieties. Both the False Claims Act and the ORI model policy and procedures serve as ways in which the knowledgeable individual can take appropriate action. Providing anti-retaliation protections helps to make it easier for the individual to blow the whistle on scientific misconduct or false claims. Under the False Claims Act, the successful *qui tam* relator is entitled to a substantial portion of what is recovered or reached in settlement. The amount varies depending upon whether the government intervenes in such cases. However, the prospect of substantial financial gain may also serve as an incentive for someone to be a *qui tam* relator.

Managing "Non-Compliance" in Clinical Trials

An allegation of non-compliance requires a careful analysis of the assertion. Facts must be gathered and evaluated. Conjecture, speculation, or idle gossip are insufficient grounds for making a determination of non-compliance. Much more is needed. A good approach to handling allegations of non-compliance can be found in the ORI Model Policy for Responding to Allegations of Scientific Misconduct and the Model Procedures for Responding to Allegations of Scientific Misconduct. A logical step-by-step process is mapped out by the ORI, from an inquiry through an investigation to administrative action recommended and then taken by the person responsible for making the decision on behalf of the institution or organization. The nature of the alleged misconduct may merit inclusion of others in the process. For example, if a whistleblower makes an allegation of Medicare fraud involving clinical trials research, the services of an outside forensic auditor may be needed to ascertain the validity of the claim. An allegation of misconduct involving data falsification or manipulation may necessitate an evaluation by a neutral, objective expert in biostatistics or epidemiology. The compliance investigatory rules should enable the CRO or facility to make use of such outside experts done under pertinent laws for peer review or, when appropriate, attorney-client privilege.

The rights of the alleged perpetrator must be respected. Due process should be afforded the individual. If culpability is found, appropriate action must be taken to redress non-compliance. An example demonstrates what is involved in such cases.

> A researcher signs a conflict-of-interest statement indicating that she had no financial ties or stock holdings in the company sponsoring the test article under investigation. The IRB received all relevant documentation for the study, including the signed conflict-of-interest statement. Nothing in the documentation suggested that there was any impropriety in the funding for the study and the clinical investigator's relationship with the sponsor. Six months later, the research compliance officer received an anonymous voice mail on the compliance hotline suggested that the principal investigator had given a false Assurance regarding conflict-of-interest. Following an inquiry and investigation, it was determined that the principal investigator had received 500 shares of stock from the sponsor contingent upon the study being successfully completed within a 15 percent savings of the specified budget for the research trial. IRB minutes documenting the review of the original protocol noted that the study involved more than minimal risk, and the IRB had insisted that additional protections be put in place for study subjects. The investigator had promised to do so. None of these measures were put in place. It was later learned that the added protections would have exceeded the 15 percent budget savings that would preclude the investigator from receiving the stock. This was seen as a conflict-of-interest for which the investigator could not profess ignorance. The decision was made to suspend the trial, prohibit the investigator from conducting studies for three years on the premises, and to complete a mandatory course in bioethics. A letter of reprimand was sent to the study sponsor indicating that the institution would not accept any further studies unless the financial structure did not create conflicts-of-interest for investigators or otherwise jeopardize the well-being of study subjects. The final outcome regarding the matter was reported to the ORI. Thus the action taken against the investigator was reported to ORI. The state board of medicine also

received information about possible unprofessional conduct stemming from the clinical trial. The institution also sent to ORI a copy of the letter sent to the sponsor. Along with it, the institution outlined its plan for corrective action that included advance training on conflict-of-interest for research investigators, the development of a new screening tool for conflict-of-interest in contracts, and a notification letter to be sent to all existing and new sponsors regarding conflict-of-interest.

This case example shows what can be done in a serious non-compliance matter. Not only was there a thorough investigation, there was a clear plan of action for handling the misconduct identified and practical steps to prevent similar cases in future. Taking such an approach signals a strong commitment to compliance, an important consideration when federal regulators are notified of misconduct on the part of a clinical investigator. Preventing the institution from being seen as a non-compliant organization is important so that it does not lose the opportunity for future grants or experience a litany of investigations looking for other non-compliant practices.

The Possible Consequences of Non-Compliance in Clinical Trials Research

There are several ripple effects that can occur as a consequence of non-compliance. The actions taken may be limited or more pronounced in certain cases. Much depends upon the nature of the non-compliant practices. For example

- Exclusion from future research for a period of time
- Debarment of an individual for misconduct
- Civil monetary penalties under civil False Claims Act litigation
- Criminal actions for fraud or abuse
- Removal of officials responsible for the stewardship of the clinical trials program
- Imposition of a corrective action plan
- Public notice of regulatory action taken with regard to non-compliance
- Cancellation by sponsors of contracts for non-compliance
- Civil lawsuits for breach of contract involving CROs or sponsors
- Termination of a healthcare organization from participation in a multicenter trial as an entity seen as non-compliant and therefore unacceptable to continue in a study
- Loss of funds, and, in some instances, a requirement to repay funds provided for studies that are terminated or suspended
- Larger compliance probes involving one or more of the Federal Fraud and Abuse Control Program or a state agency

....

MEDICARE COMPLIANCE AND CLINICAL TRIALS RESEARCH

A particular area of compliance involves Medicare and clinical trials research. Separating what is acceptable from non-Medicare qualified research is important in terms of coverage—a key issue for compliance. Avoiding double-billing to a clinical trial granting agency and Medicare is equally important in terms of regulatory compliance. Both issues are addressed in this section.

Clinical Trials Activity Under Medicare

Under the Final National Coverage of Clinical Trials Program, Medicare will cover some routine costs of a clinical trial as well as reasonable and necessary items and services needed to diagnose or treat complications that arise from participation in clinical trials. CMS has developed some guidance regarding what is and what is not covered. This applies to Medicare carriers, fiscal intermediaries, QIOs, HMOs, and Medicare+Choice organizations (CMS, "Clinical Coverages Manual, 30-1, 09-00).

There are apt to be many situations in which careful evaluations will have to be made in order to determine the propriety of Medicare coverage. The risk that this coverage could be abused demands meticulous analysis to avoid non-compliance in such financial matters.

Billing Medicare When a Patient Is Also a Research Subject Under a Grant

A major financial compliance issue is separating out what is appropriate routine billing for a Medicare patient from what is an allowable cost under a grant. The fact that the grant is from a private sponsor or a government agency should not make any difference. Coding, accounting, and billing practices should be set up to track items for appropriate allocation. Accounting and billing officials should document the assumptions for the coding and billing practices. If there is any concern or question about the practice, prior to implementing it, a formal written inquiry should be made to the fiscal intermediary, CMS, private sponsors, or any other relevant party to validate that the proposed system is acceptable. If it is not acceptable, knowing this in advance enables the entity to develop a permissible methodology. However, *all* relevant parties (private and public) should agree to it to avoid problems at a later time.

Audits should be structured to evaluate and verify that good accounting practices have been used to properly handle the Medicare component as compared with the grant funds. The same would be true for Medicaid and other federal health plans.

············

CONCLUSION

Compliance is a major topic for clinical trials research. It goes beyond traditional compliance issues dealing with financial matters. Scientific misconduct, research subject safety, research ethics, and the integrity of the healthcare organization are all important aspects to a compliance program. A plan requires careful review and upgrading. As laws and regulations change, so too should the compliance plan to keep it current. When this is done, educational opportunities should be provided to everyone, much the same way that Responsible Conduct in Research (RCR) initiatives are designed to achieve with respect to thwarting scientific misconduct. Taking these steps can go a long way toward avoiding rigorous scrutiny by regulators, adverse publicity, and possible litigation. It is these concerns and the desire to do the right thing that make a compelling argument for designing and implementing a comprehensive research compliance program. Resources for this purpose can be found in the appendix, including sample bylaw language for clinical investigators who are on staff of healthcare organizations, sample language for the employee handbook, and model terms and conditions for contracts with sponsors.

Resources

ORI Model Policy Scientific Misconduct
ORI Model Procedure Scientific Misconduct

References

21 CFR §312.70 et seq.

31 USC §287, §371, §1001

31 USC §3729-3731

42 CFR §50.102

Social Security Act 1128B(b)

Bioresearch Monitoring. Clinical Investigators. 7348.811. September 30, 2000.

18 USC 1341

42 USC 1320a-7b(b)

Federal Register. 65(114). 37136-37137. June 13, 2000.

Federal Register. 65(236). 76647, December 7, 2000.

Federal Register. 66(35). 11032 February 21, 2001.

Health Care Financing Administration. "Clinical Coverages Manual." (30-1, 09-00).

Health Insurance Portability and Accountability Act of 1996, P.L. 104-191, tit. II, 204, 110 Stat. 1936, 1999.

31 USC 3730.

National Bioethics Advisory Committee. (2000). Ethical and Policy Issues in Research Involving Human Participants (Draft report).

Omnibus Reconciliation Act of 1989. Pub. L No. 101-239 103 Stat. 2106 (1989).

Omnibus Reconciliation Act of 1993. Pub. L No. 103-66, 107 Stat. 312 (1993).

Social Security Act Amendments of 1994, Pub. L No. 103-432, 108 Stat. 4398 (1994).

Human Research Due Diliegence Checklist

Instructions: *Use this quality improvement tool to enhance research activity. Answers are expressed as* "Yes," "No," *and* "NA" *for not-applicable. A* "No" *response indicates an opportunity for compliance improvement.*

Organizational Component

	Yes	No	NA
There is a human research policy and procedure in effect in the healthcare organization			
The policy and procedure has been evaluated for internal consistency with the organizational compliance plan			
Human research trials are reviewed for scientific and ethical design			
Informed consent requirements are reviewed for each research project for regulatory compliance			
On-going research trials are reviewed on an annual basis by the IRB			
Changes in study design, or research population enrollment are reported to the IRB			
Adverse occurrences involving research subjects are reported within 12 hours to the IRB			
Random, unannounced surveillance is conducted of research subject enrollment and consent practices			
Random review is completed of research study records for compliance with pertinent federal and state laws			
Enrollment and consent practices are monitored for subjects in specially protected categories			
Measures are in place to address research subject complaints, self-disenrollment, and study-related injury			
Communications systems are in place among multiple project centers in approved research protocols			
Random surveillance is completed on communications system with multiple project centers			
Contracts with multiple project centers require notification of JCAHO de-accreditation or certification by Medicare or another federal or state regulatory body			
Human research regulatory compliance surveillance is carried out on a regulatory basis, minimally annually			
Reports of non-compliance are investigated and resolved promptly			

Research Subject Rights

	Yes	No	NA
A process is used to monitor coding and billing of patients enrolled in federally funded research trials			
A process is used to monitor coding and billing of patients enrolled in privately funded research trials			
Coding and billing personnel are oriented to specific practices used in entering code data for patients/subjects			
Consent practices and documentation are consistent with regulatory and organizational requirements			
Research subjects are enrolled in studies in a non-discriminatory manner			
EMTALA screening examination and treatment requirements are followed with potential research subjects in all emergency setting research trials			
Patient Self-Determination Act and applicable state laws regarding advance directives, proxies, substitute decision-making, and others-not-to resuscitate are followed in all emergency setting research trials			
Reasonable and appropriate accommodation is made for human subjects with linguistic, auditory, or visual impairments who require assistance as part of research protocols			
Procedures are followed to safeguard confidentiality of identifier-linked research subject data			
Consent to re-disclosure is obtained from research subjects when identifier-linked data is to be used by the principal investigator or is sought by the research funding source			

Contracts

	Yes	No	NA
Contracts and assurances are reviewed for conformance with applicable law and the organizational compliance plan on a regularly basis and minimally, annually			
Contracts contain clauses that require notification if a participating research facility or research team investigator is the subject of regulatory sanction or debarment with a provision for termination of the agreement			
Contracts require all participating facilities, clinics, and private medical offices to comply with applicable federal and state law			

Credentialing

	Yes	No	NA
Principal investigators are credentialed as a prerequisite to conducting human research trials			
Credentialing practices provide a mechanism to deal with principal investigators sanctioned or debarred by Medicare, Medicaid, Office of Professional Misconduct, other federal agencies, or state licensing or disciplinary boards			
Multiple project centers credential professional staff participating in approved research trials in a manner consistent with assurance and contract requirements			
Credentialing staff update information on a monthly basis from regulatory compliance databases, The Federal Register, and other resources for debarment or sanctions by federal funding sources and sources overseeing human research and research integrity			
Sanction and debarment information is reported to appropriate individuals in the healthcare organization for prompt action			

Orientation and Education

	Yes	No	NA
IRB members receive orientation education on compliance with federal and state laws			
IRB members receive orientation education on the organizational compliance program			
Research administrators, healthcare professionals, and other staff involved in the operational aspects of human research trials are oriented to their roles and responsibilities under applicable law and organizational compliance plans			
Research administrators, healthcare professionals, and other staff involved in the operational aspects of human research trials are trained in the appropriate steps to follow when responding to non-compliance with applicable law and the organizational compliance plan			
Regular in-service education is completed on a mandatory basis by IRB members, research administrators, healthcare professionals, and other staff involved in the operational aspects of human research trials			
Demonstrated competencies are required of IRB members, research administrators, healthcare professionals, and other staff involved in the operational aspects of human research trials in terms of regulatory compliance			

Communication/Documentation

	Yes	No	NA
Communication processes are in place to convey relevant information about principal investigators to the healthcare organization compliance officer, health professional staff committee, and risk management			
Documentation is retained in conformance with applicable state and federal law			
Documentation access is granted only in accordance with applicable laws and regulations			

Clinical Trial Review/Oversight Criteria	Federal Requirements Specify ___ CFR ___	Contractual Requirements Sponsor	Foreign Law/Guideline	Comment Section*
• Definitions • IRB Composition • IRB Review Requirements • Expedited Review • IRB Approval Criteria • Institutional Review • Protocol Monitoring • IRB Suspension or Termination of Research Approval • Cooperative Research • IRB Records • Informed Consent • Informed Consent Documentation • Use of Federal Funds • Early Termination of Research • Privacy • Confidentiality • Conflict-of-Interest Statements • Safety/Security Specifications • Adverse Event Reporting • Continuity of Research–Enterprise Disruption • Insurance Coverages • Quality Management				

Multi-Review Matrix Instructions

Place an "x" for each category in which there is a multiple review. In the Commentary Section provide details regarding overlap or inconsistency and explain how it has been addressed. If this requires a lengthy explanation, attach a separate sheet for referencing the applicable category.

Sample Bylaw Language

Corrective Action Subsequent to Regulatory Action—Clinical Trials

A finding of scientific misconduct or debarment from receipt of federal funding to pursue clinical trials or other research activities shall form the basis for corrective action proceedings under these bylaws [See section of the Medical Staff Bylaws].

Sample Employee Handbook Language

A finding of scientific misconduct or debarment from receipt of federal funding to pursue clinical trials or other research activities shall form the basis for review of employment status. Employment may be terminated when misconduct or debarment involves an infringement of federal law, clinical trials research subject safety, or regulatory non-compliance.

Sample Contract Language

Notification Provisions

Sponsor Responsibilities—The sponsor shall notify the principal investigator within 3 days of an adverse event. Notification may be through telephone, email, fax, courier or mail.

Principal Investigator—The principal investigator shall notify the sponsor within 3 days of an adverse event, breach in confidentiality, breach of research protocol, scientific misconduct or notification of withdrawal of status to receive federal funding for clinical trials or research. The principal investigator shall notify the sponsor within 3 days of becoming aware of his or her status of one under investigator for regulatory non-compliance, fraud or abuse by a federal or state regulatory agency. Notification may be through telephone, email, fax, courier or mail.

Model Sponsor Agreement

Obligations of Sponsor—The sponsor agrees to abide by: (a) all applicable Federal and state laws governing clinic trials research and (b) the healthcare facility clinical research compliance plan.

Termination of Sponsorship—A material breach of the terms and conditions relating to regulatory law or the healthcare facility clinical research compliance plan, constitute grounds for termination of the sponsorship agreement.

Model Policy
for Responding to Allegations
of Scientific Misconduct

Table of Contents

I.   Introduction 472
     A.   General Policy 472
     B.   Scope 472

II. Definitions 472

III. Rights and Responsibilities 474
     A.   Research Integrity Officer 474
     B.   Whistleblower 474
     C.   Respondent 475
     D.   Deciding Official 475

IV. General Policies and Principles 475
     A.   Responsibility to Report Misconduct 475
     B.   Protecting the Whistleblower 475
     C.   Protecting the Respondent 476
     D.   Cooperation with Inquiries and Investigations 476
     E.   Preliminary Assessment of Allegations 476

V.   Conducting the Inquiry 476
     A.   Initiation and Purpose of the Inquiry 476
     B.   Sequestration of the Research Records 477
     C.   Appointment of the Inquiry Committee 477
     D.   Charge to the Committee and the First Meeting 477
     E.   Inquiry Process 478

VI. The Inquiry Report 478
     A.   Elements of the Inquiry Report 478
     B.   Comments on the Draft Report by the Respondent and the Whistleblower 478
     C.   Inquiry Decision and Notification 479
     D.   Time Limit for Completing the Inquiry Report 479

VII. Conducting the Investigation 479
     A.   Purpose of the Investigation 479
     B.   Sequestration of the Research Records 479
     C.   Appointment of the Investigation Committee 480
     D.   Charge to the Committee and the First Meeting 480
     E.   Investigation Process 481

VIII. The Investigation Report 481
     A.   Elements of the Investigation Report 481
     B.   Comments on the Draft Report 481

C.   Institutional Review and Decision 482
D.   Transmittal of the Final Investigation Report to ORI 482
E.   Time Limit for Completing the Investigation Report 483

IX.   Requirements for Reporting to ORI 483

X.   Institutional Administrative Actions 484

XI.   Other Considerations 484
A.   Termination of Institutional Employment or Resignation Prior
      to Completing Inquiry or Investigation 484
B.   Restoration of the Respondent's Reputation 484
C.   Protection of the Whistleblower and Others 485
D.   Allegations Not Made in Good Faith 485
E.   Interim Administrative Actions 485

XII.   Record Retention 485

I.   Introduction*

A.   General Policy

[NOTE: **Institution should insert general statements about its philosophy and that
of the scientific community related to ethics in research in this section.
These might include institutional values related to scientific integrity, a
statement of principles, and the institution's position on preventing
misconduct in research and supporting good faith whistleblowers.**]

B.   Scope

This policy and the associated procedures apply to all individuals at [Institution]
engaged in research that is supported by or for which support is requested from PHS.
The PHS regulation at 42 C.F.R. Part 50, Subpart A applies to any research, research-
training or research-related grant or cooperative agreement with PHS. This policy
applies to any person paid by, under the control of, or affiliated with the institution,
such as scientists, trainees, technicians and other staff members, students, fellows,
guest researchers, or collaborators at [Institution].

The policy and associated procedures will normally be followed when an allegation
of possible misconduct in science is received by an institutional official. Particular
circumstances in an individual case may dictate variation from the normal procedure
deemed in the best interests of [Institution] and PHS. Any change from normal procedures also must ensure fair treatment to the subject of the inquiry or investigation.
Any significant variation should be approved in advance by the [designated official]
of [*Institution*].

II.   Definitions

A.   *Allegation* means any written or oral statement or other indication of possible
scientific misconduct made to an institutional official.

B.   *Conflict of interest* means the real or apparent interference of one person's interests
with the interests of another person, where potential bias may occur due to prior or
existing personal or professional relationships.

C.   *Deciding Official* means the institutional official who makes final determinations
on allegations of scientific misconduct and any responsive institutional actions.
[**Optional addition: The Deciding Official will not be the same individual as
the Research Integrity Officer and should have no direct prior involvement
in the institution's inquiry, investigation, or allegation assessment.**]

D.   *Good faith allegation* means an allegation made with the honest belief that scientific
misconduct may have occurred. An allegation is not in good faith if it is made with
reckless disregard for or willful ignorance of facts that would disprove the allegation.

---

*Sections that are based on requirements of the PHS regulations codified at 42 C.F.R. Part 50, Subpart A have endnotes that indicate the
applicable section number, *e.g.*, 42 C.F.R. §50.103(d)(1).

E. *Inquiry* means gathering information and initial fact-finding to determine whether an allegation or apparent instance of scientific misconduct warrants an investigation.[1]

F. *Investigation* means the formal examination and evaluation of all relevant facts to determine if misconduct has occurred, and, if so, to determine the responsible person and the seriousness of the misconduct.[2]

G. *ORI* means the Office of Research Integrity, the office within the U.S. Department of Health and Human Services (DHHS) that is responsible for the scientific misconduct and research integrity activities of the U.S. Public Health Service.

H. *PHS* means the U.S. Public Health Service, an operating component of the DHHS.

I. *PHS regulation* means the Public Health Service regulation establishing standards for institutional inquiries and investigations into allegations of scientific misconduct, which is set forth at 42 C.F.R. Part 50, Subpart A, entitled "Responsibility of PHS Awardee and Applicant Institutions for Dealing With and Reporting Possible Misconduct in Science."

J. *PHS support* means PHS grants, contracts, or cooperative agreements or applications therefore.

K. *Research Integrity Officer* means the institutional official responsible for assessing allegations of scientific misconduct and determining when such allegations warrant inquiries and for overseeing inquiries and investigations. **[Option: A multi-campus institution or an institution with several large research components may wish to delegate these functions to more than one individual.]**

L. *Research record* means any data, document, computer file, computer diskette, or any other written or non-written account or object that reasonably may be expected to provide evidence or information regarding the proposed, conducted, or reported research that constitutes the subject of an allegation of scientific misconduct. A research record includes, but is not limited to, grant or contract applications, whether funded or unfunded; grant or contract progress and other reports; laboratory notebooks; notes; correspondence; videos; photographs; X-ray film; slides; biological materials; computer files and printouts; manuscripts and publications; equipment use logs; laboratory procurement records; animal facility records; human and animal subject protocols; consent forms; medical charts; and patient research files.

M. *Respondent* means the person against whom an allegation of scientific misconduct is directed or the person whose actions are the subject of the inquiry or investigation. There can be more than one respondent in any inquiry or investigation.

N. *Retaliation* means any action that adversely affects the employment or other institutional status of an individual that is taken by an institution or an employee because the individual has in good faith, made an allegation of scientific misconduct or of inadequate institutional response thereto or has cooperated in good faith with an investigation of such allegation. **[Option: The institution may wish to define** more specifically the standard to be applied in its determination of whether an adverse action was taken in response to a good faith allegation or cooperation.]

O. *Scientific misconduct or misconduct in science* means fabrication, falsification, plagiarism, or other practices that seriously deviate from those that are commonly accepted within the scientific community for proposing, conducting, or reporting research. It does not include honest error or honest differences in interpretations or judgments of data.[3]

P. *Whistleblower* means a person who makes an allegation of scientific misconduct.

III. Rights and Responsibilities

A. Research Integrity Officer

The [designated institutional official] will appoint [**Option: will serve as**] the Research Integrity Officer who will have primary responsibility for implementation of the procedures set forth in this document. The Research Integrity Officer will be an institutional official who is well qualified to handle the procedural requirements involved and is sensitive to the varied demands made on those who conduct research, those who are accused of misconduct, and those who report apparent misconduct in good faith.

The Research Integrity Officer will appoint the inquiry and investigation committees and ensure that necessary and appropriate expertise is secured to carry out a thorough and authoritative evaluation of the relevant evidence in an inquiry or investigation. The Research Integrity Officer will attempt to ensure that confidentiality is maintained.

The Research Integrity Officer will assist inquiry and investigation committees and all institutional personnel in complying with these procedures and with applicable standards imposed by government or external funding sources. The Research Integrity Officer is also responsible for maintaining files of all documents and evidence and for the confidentiality and the security of the files.

The Research Integrity Officer [**Option: Deciding Official**] will report to ORI as required by regulation and keep ORI apprised of any developments during the course of the inquiry or investigation that may affect current or potential DHHS funding for the individual(s) under investigation or that PHS needs to know to ensure appropriate use of Federal funds and otherwise protect the public interest.[4]

B. Whistleblower

The whistleblower will have an opportunity to testify before the inquiry and investigation committees, to review portions of the inquiry and investigation reports pertinent to his/her allegations or testimony, to be informed of the results of the inquiry and investigation, and to be protected from retaliation. Also, if the Research Integrity Officer has determined that the whistleblower may be able to provide pertinent information on any portions of the draft report, these portions will be given to the whistleblower for comment.

The whistleblower is responsible for making allegations in good faith, maintaining confidentiality, and cooperating with an inquiry or investigation.

C. Respondent

The respondent will be informed of the allegations when an inquiry is opened and notified in writing of the final determinations and resulting actions. The respondent will also have the opportunity to be interviewed by and present evidence to the inquiry and investigation committees, to review the draft inquiry and investigation reports, and to have the advice of counsel.

The respondent is responsible for maintaining confidentiality and cooperating with the conduct of an inquiry or investigation. If the respondent is not found guilty of scientific misconduct, he or she has the right to receive institutional assistance in restoring his or her reputation.[5]

D. Deciding Official

The Deciding Official will receive the inquiry and/or investigation report and any written comments made by the respondent or the whistleblower on the draft report. The Deciding Official will consult with the Research Integrity Officer or other appropriate officials and will determine whether to conduct an investigation, whether misconduct occurred, whether to impose sanctions, or whether to take other appropriate administrative actions [see section X].

IV. **General Policies and Principles**

A. Responsibility to Report Misconduct

All employees or individuals associated with [Institution] should report observed, suspected, or apparent misconduct in science to the Research Integrity Officer **[Option: also list other officials]**. If an individual is unsure whether a suspected incident falls within the definition of scientific misconduct, he or she may call the Research Integrity Officer at [telephone number] to discuss the suspected misconduct informally. If the circumstances described by the individual do not meet the definition of scientific misconduct, the Research Integrity Officer will refer the individual or allegation to other offices or officials with responsibility for resolving the problem.

At any time, an employee may have confidential discussions and consultations about concerns of possible misconduct with the Research Integrity Officer **[Option: also list other officials]** and will be counseled about appropriate procedures for reporting allegations.

B. Protecting the Whistleblower

The Research Integrity Officer will monitor the treatment of individuals who bring allegations of misconduct or of inadequate institutional response thereto, and those who cooperate in inquiries or investigations. The Research Integrity Officer will ensure that these persons will not be retaliated against in the terms and conditions of their employment or other status at the institution and will review instances of alleged retaliation for appropriate action.

Employees should immediately report any alleged or apparent retaliation to the Research Integrity Officer.

Also the institution will protect the privacy of those who report misconduct in good faith[6] to the maximum extent possible. For example, if the whistleblower requests anonymity, the institution will make an effort to honor the request during the allegation assessment or inquiry within applicable policies and regulations and state and local laws, if any. The whistleblower will be advised that if the matter is referred to an investigation committee and the whistleblower's testimony is required, anonymity may no longer be guaranteed. Institutions are required to undertake diligent efforts to protect the positions and reputations of those persons who, in good faith, make allegations.[7]

C. Protecting the Respondent

Inquiries and investigations will be conducted in a manner that will ensure fair treatment to the respondent(s) in the inquiry or investigation and confidentiality to the extent possible without compromising public health and safety or thoroughly carrying out the inquiry or investigation.[8]

Institutional employees accused of scientific misconduct may consult with legal counsel or a non-lawyer personal adviser (who is not a principal or witness in the case) to seek advice and may bring the counsel or personal adviser to interviews or meetings on the case. [**Option: Some institutions do not permit the presence of lawyers at interviews or meetings with institutional officials.**]

D. Cooperation with Inquiries and Investigations

Institutional employees will cooperate with the Research Integrity Officer and other institutional officials in the review of allegations and the conduct of inquiries and investigations. Employees have an obligation to provide relevant evidence to the Research Integrity Officer or other institutional officials on misconduct allegations.

E. Preliminary Assessment of Allegations

Upon receiving an allegation of scientific misconduct, the Research Integrity Officer will immediately assess the allegation to determine whether there is sufficient evidence to warrant an inquiry, whether PHS support or PHS applications for funding are involved, and whether the allegation falls under the PHS definition of scientific misconduct.

V. Conducting the Inquiry

A. Initiation and Purpose of the Inquiry

Following the preliminary assessment, if the Research Integrity Officer determines that the allegation provides sufficient information to allow specific follow-up, involves

476

PHS support, and falls under the PHS definition of scientific misconduct, he or she will immediately initiate the inquiry process. In initiating the inquiry, the Research Integrity Officer should identify clearly the original allegation and any related issues that should be evaluated. The purpose of the inquiry is to make a preliminary evaluation of the available evidence and testimony of the respondent, whistleblower, and key witnesses to determine whether there is sufficient evidence of possible scientific misconduct to warrant an investigation. The purpose of the inquiry is **not** to reach a final conclusion about whether misconduct definitely occurred or who was responsible. The findings of the inquiry must be set forth in an inquiry report.

B. Sequestration of the Research Records

After determining that an allegation falls within the definition of misconduct in science and involves PHS funding, the Research Integrity Officer must ensure that all original research records and materials relevant to the allegation are immediately secured. The Research Integrity Officer may consult with ORI for advice and assistance in this regard.

C. Appointment of the Inquiry Committee

The Research Integrity Officer, in consultation with other institutional officials as appropriate, will appoint an inquiry committee and committee chair within [suggested: 10 days] of the initiation of the inquiry. The inquiry committee should consist of individuals who do not have real or apparent conflicts of interest in the case, are unbiased, and have the necessary expertise to evaluate the evidence and issues related to the allegation, interview the principals and key witnesses, and conduct the inquiry. These individuals may be scientists, subject matter experts, administrators, lawyers, or other qualified persons, and they may be from inside or outside the institution. **[Option: As an alternative, the institution may appoint a standing committee authorized to add or reuse members or use experts when necessary to evaluate specific allegations.]**

The Research Integrity Officer will notify the respondent of the proposed committee membership in [suggested: 10 days]. If the respondent submits a written objection to any appointed member of the inquiry committee or expert based on bias or conflict of interest within [suggested: 5 days], the Research Integrity Officer will determine whether to replace the challenged member or expert with a qualified substitute.

D. Charge to the Committee and the First Meeting

The Research Integrity Officer will prepare a charge for the inquiry committee that describes the allegations and any related issues identified during the allegation assessment and states that the purpose of the inquiry is to make a preliminary evaluation of the evidence and testimony of the respondent, whistleblower, and key witnesses to determine whether there is sufficient evidence of possible scientific misconduct to warrant an investigation as required by the PHS regulation. The purpose is not to determine whether scientific misconduct definitely occurred or who was responsible.

At the committee's first meeting, the Research Integrity Officer will review the charge with the committee, discuss the allegations, any related issues, and the appropriate procedures for conducting the inquiry, assist the committee with organizing plans for the inquiry, and answer any questions raised by the committee. The Research Integrity Officer and institutional counsel will be present or available throughout the inquiry to advise the committee as needed.

E. Inquiry Process

The inquiry committee will normally interview the whistleblower, the respondent, and key witnesses as well as examining relevant research records and materials. Then the inquiry committee will evaluate the evidence and testimony obtained during the inquiry. After consultation with the Research Integrity Officer and institutional counsel, the committee members will decide whether there is sufficient evidence of possible scientific misconduct to recommend further investigation. The scope of the inquiry does not include deciding whether misconduct occurred or conducting exhaustive interviews and analyses.

VI. The Inquiry Report

A. Elements of the Inquiry Report

A written inquiry report must be prepared that states the name and title of the committee members and experts, if any; the allegations; the PHS support; a summary of the inquiry process used; a list of the research records reviewed; summaries of any interviews; a description of the evidence in sufficient detail to demonstrate whether and investigation is warranted or not; and the committee's determination as to whether an investigation is recommended and whether any other actions should be taken if an investigation is not recommended. Institutional counsel will review the report for legal sufficiency.

B. Comments on the Draft Report by the Respondent and the Whistleblower

The Research Integrity Officer will provide the respondent with a copy of the draft inquiry report for comment and rebuttal and will provide the whistleblower, if he or she is identifiable, with portions of the draft inquiry report that address the whistleblower's role and opinions in the investigation. **[Option: The institution may provide the whistleblower with a summary of the inquiry findings for comment instead of portions of the draft report.]**

1. Confidentiality

The Research Integrity Officer may establish reasonable conditions for review to protect the confidentiality of the draft report.

2. Receipt of Comments

Within [suggested: 14] calendar days of their receipt of the draft report, the whistleblower and respondent will provide their comments, if any, to the inquiry committee. Any comments that the whistleblower or respondent submits on the draft report will become part of the final inquiry report and record.[9] Based on the comments, the inquiry committee may revise the report as appropriate.

C. Inquiry Decision and Notification

1. Decision by Deciding Official

The Research Integrity Officer will transmit the final report and any comments to the Deciding Official, who will make the determination of whether findings from the inquiry provide sufficient evidence of possible scientific misconduct to justify conducting an investigation. The inquiry is completed when the Deciding Official makes this determination, which will be made within 60 days of the first meeting of the inquiry committee. Any extension of this period will be based on good cause and recorded in the inquiry file.

2. Notification

The Research Integrity Officer will notify both the respondent and the whistleblower in writing of the Deciding Official's decision of whether to proceed to an investigation and will remind them of their obligation to cooperate in the event an investigation is opened. The Research Integrity Officer will also notify all appropriate institutional officials of the Deciding Official's decision.

D. Time Limit for Completing the Inquiry Report

The inquiry committee will normally complete the inquiry and submit its report in writing to the Research Integrity Officer no more than 60 calendar days following its first meeting,[10] unless the Research Integrity Officer approves an extension for good cause. If the Research Integrity Officer approves an extension, the reason for the extension will be entered into the records of the case and the report.[11] The respondent also will be notified of the extension.

VII. **Conducting the Investigation**

A. Purpose of the Investigation

The purpose of the investigation is to explore in detail the allegations, to examine the evidence in depth, and to determine specifically whether misconduct has been committed, by whom, and to what extent. The investigation will also determine whether there are additional instances of possible misconduct that would justify broadening the scope beyond the initial allegations. This is particularly important where the alleged misconduct involves clinical trials or potential harm to human subjects or the general public or if it affects research that forms the basis for public policy, clinical practice, or public health practice. The findings of the investigation will be set forth in an investigation report.

B. Sequestration of the Research Records

The Research Integrity Officer will immediately sequester any additional pertinent research records that were not previously sequestered during the inquiry. This sequestration should occur before or at the time the respondent is notified that an investigation has begun. The need for additional sequestration of records may occur for any number of reasons, including the institution's decision to investigate additional allegations not considered during the inquiry stage or the identification of records during the inquiry process that had not been previously secured. The procedures to be followed for sequestration during the investigation are the same procedures that apply during the inquiry.

C. Appointment of the Investigation Committee

The Research Integrity Officer, in consultation with other institutional officials as appropriate, will appoint an investigation committee and the committee chair within [suggest: 10 days] of the notification to the respondent that an investigation is planned or as soon thereafter as practicable. The investigation committee should consist of at least three individuals who do not have real or apparent conflicts of interest in the case, are unbiased, and have the necessary expertise to evaluate the evidence and issues related to the allegations, interview the principals and key witnesses, and conduct the investigation.[12] These individuals may be scientists, administrators, subject matter experts, lawyers, or other qualified persons, and they may be from inside or outside the institution. Individuals appointed to the investigation committee may also have served on the inquiry committee. [**Option: As an alternative, the institution may appoint a standing committee authorized to add or reuse members or use consultants when necessary to evaluate specific allegations**].

The Research Integrity Officer will notify the respondent of the proposed committee membership within [suggest: 5 days]. If the respondent submits a written objection to any appointed member of the investigation committee or expert, the Research Integrity Officer will determine whether to replace the challenged member or expert with a qualified substitute.

D. Charge to the Committee and the First Meeting

1. Charge to the Committee

The Research Integrity Officer will define the subject matter of the investigation in a written charge to the committee that describes the allegations and related issues identified during the inquiry, defines scientific misconduct, and identifies the name of the respondent. The charge will state that the committee is to evaluate the evidence and testimony of the respondent, whistleblower, and key witnesses to determine whether, based on a preponderance of the evidence, scientific misconduct occurred and, if so, to what extent, who was responsible, and its seriousness.

During the investigation, if additional information becomes available that substantially changes the subject matter of the investigation or would suggest additional respondents, the committee will notify the Research Integrity Officer, who will determine whether it is necessary to notify the respondent of the new subject matter or to provide notice to additional respondents.

2. The First Meeting

The Research Integrity Officer, with the assistance of institutional counsel, will convene the first meeting of the investigation committee to review the charge, the inquiry report, and the prescribed procedures and standards for the conduct of the investigation, including the necessity for confidentiality and for developing a specific investigation plan. The investigation committee will be provided with a copy of these instructions and, where PHS funding is involved, the PHS regulation.

E. Investigation Process

The investigation committee will be appointed and the process initiated within 30 days of the completion of the inquiry, if findings from that inquiry provide a sufficient basis for conducting an investigation.[13]

The investigation will normally involve examination of all documentation including, but not necessarily limited to, relevant research records, computer files, proposals, manuscripts, publications, correspondence, memoranda, and notes of telephone calls.[14] Whenever possible, the committee should interview the whistleblower(s), the respondents(s), and other individuals who might have information regarding aspects of the allegations.[15] Interviews of the respondent should be tape recorded or transcribed. All other interviews should be transcribed, tape recorded, or summarized. Summaries or transcripts of the interviews should be prepared, provided to the interviewed party for comment or revision, and included as part of the investigatory file.[16]

VIII. The Investigation Report

A. Elements of the Investigation Report

The final report submitted to ORI must describe the policies and procedures under which the investigation was conducted, describe how and from whom information relevant to the investigation was obtained, state the findings, and explain the basis for the findings. The report will include the actual text or an accurate summary of the views of any individual(s) found to have engaged in misconduct as well as a description of any sanctions imposed and administrative actions taken by the institution.[17]

B. Comments on the Draft Report

1. Respondent

The Research Integrity Officer will provide the respondent with a copy of the draft investigation report for comment and rebuttal. The respondent will be allowed [ ] days to review and comment on the draft report. The respondent's comments will be attached to the final report. The findings of the final report should take into account the respondent's comments in addition to all the other evidence.

2. Whistleblower

The Research Integrity Officer will provide the whistleblower, if he or she is identifiable, with those portions of the draft investigation report that address the whistleblower's role and opinions in the investigation. The report should be modified, as appropriate, based on the whistleblower's comments.

3. Institutional Counsel

The draft investigation report will be transmitted to the institutional counsel for a review of its legal sufficiency. Comments should be incorporated into the report as appropriate.

4. Confidentiality

In distributing the draft report, or portions thereof, to the respondent and whistleblower, the Research Integrity Officer will inform the recipient of the confidentiality under which the draft report is made available and may establish reasonable conditions to ensure such confidentiality. For example, the Research Integrity Officer may request the recipient to sign a confidentiality statement or to come to his or her office to review the report.

C. Institutional Review and Decision

Based on a preponderance of the evidence, the Deciding Official will make the final determination whether to accept the investigation report, its findings, and the recommended institutional actions. If this determination varies from that of the investigation committee, the Deciding Official will explain in detail the basis for rendering a decision different from that of the investigation committee in the institution's letter transmitting the report to ORI. The Deciding Official's explanation should be consistent with the PHS definition of scientific misconduct, the institution's policies and procedures, and the evidence reviewed and analyzed by the investigation committee. The Deciding Official may also return the report to the investigation committee with a request for further fact-finding or analysis. The Deciding Official's determination, together with the investigation committee's report, constitutes the final investigation report for purposes of ORI review.

When a final decision on the case has been reached, the Research Integrity Officer will notify both the respondent and the whistleblower in writing. In addition, the Deciding Official will determine whether law enforcement agencies, professional societies, professional licensing boards, editors of journals in which falsified reports may have been published, collaborators of the respondent in the work, or other relevant parties should be notified of the outcome of the case. The Research Integrity Officer is responsible for ensuring compliance with all notification requirements of funding or sponsoring agencies.

D. Transmittal of the Final Investigation Report to ORI

After comments have been received and the necessary changes have been made to the draft report, the investigation committee should transmit the final report with attachments, including the respondent's and whistleblower's comments, to the Deciding Official, through the Research Integrity Officer.

E. Time Limit for Completing the Investigation Report

An investigation should ordinarily be completed within 120 days of its initiation,[18] with the initiation being defined as the first meeting of the investigation committee. This includes conducting the investigation, preparing the report of findings, making the draft report available to the subject of the investigation for comment, submitting the report to the Deciding Official for approval, and submitting the report to the ORI.[19]

IX. **Requirements for Reporting to ORI**

A. An institution's decision to initiate an investigation must be reported in writing to the Director, ORI, on or before the date the investigation begins.[20] At a minimum, the notification should include the name of the person(s) against whom the allegations have been made, the general nature of the allegation as it relates to the PHS definition of scientific misconduct, and the PHS applications or grant number(s) involved.[21] ORI must also be notified of the final outcome of the investigation and must be provided with a copy of the investigation report.[22] Any significant variations from the provisions of the institutional policies and procedures should be explained in any reports submitted to ORI.

B. If an institution plans to terminate an inquiry or investigation for any reason without completing all relevant requirements of the PHS regulation, the Research Integrity Officer will submit a report of the planned termination to ORI, including a description of the reasons for the proposed termination.[23]

C. If the institution determines that it will not be able to complete the investigation in 120 days, the Research Integrity Officer will submit to ORI a written request for an extension that explains the delay, reports on the progress to date, estimates the date of completion of the report, and describes other necessary steps to be taken. If the request is granted, the Research Integrity Officer will file periodic progress reports as requested by the ORI.[24]

D. When PHS funding or applications for funding are involved and an admission of scientific misconduct is made, the Research Integrity Officer will contact ORI for consultation and advice. Normally, the individual making the admission will be asked to sign a statement attesting to the occurrence and extent of misconduct. When the case involves PHS funds, the institution cannot accept an admission of scientific misconduct as a basis for closing a case or not undertaking an investigation without prior approval from ORI.[25]

E. The Research Integrity Officer will notify ORI at any stage of the inquiry or investigation if:

1. there is an immediate health hazard involved;[26]

2. there is an immediate need to protect Federal funds or equipment;[27]

3. there is an immediate need to protect the interests of the person(s) making the allegations or of the individual(s) who is the subject of the allegations as well as his/her co-investigators and associates, if any;[28]

4. it is probable that the alleged incident is going to be reported publicly;[29] or

5. the allegation involves a public health sensitive issue, *e.g.*, a clinical trial; or

6. there is a reasonable indication of possible criminal violation. In this instance, the institution must inform ORI within 24 hours of obtaining that information.[30]

X.   Institutional Administrative Actions

[Institution] will take appropriate administrative actions against individuals when an allegation of misconduct has been substantiated.[31]

If the Deciding Official determines that the alleged misconduct is substantiated by the findings, he or she will decide on the appropriate actions to be taken, after consultation with the Research Integrity Officer. The actions may include:

- withdrawal or correction of all pending or published abstracts and papers emanating from the research where scientific misconduct was found.

- removal of the responsible person from the particular project, letter of reprimand, special monitoring of future work, probation, suspension, salary reduction, or initiation of steps leading to possible rank reduction or termination of employment;

- restitution of funds as appropriate.

XI.   Other Considerations

A.   Termination of Institutional Employment or Resignation Prior to Completing Inquiry or Investigation

The termination of the respondent's institutional employment, by resignation or other-wise, before or after an allegation of possible scientific misconduct has been reported, will not preclude or terminate the misconduct procedures.

If the respondent, without admitting to the misconduct, elects to resign his or her position prior to the initiation of an inquiry, but after an allegation has been reported, or during an inquiry or investigation, the inquiry or investigation will proceed. If the respondent refuses to participate in the process after resignation, the committee will use its best efforts to reach a conclusion concerning the allegations, noting in its report the respondent's failure to cooperate and its effect on the committee's review of all the evidence.

B.   Restoration of the Respondent's Reputation

If the institution finds no misconduct and ORI concurs, after consulting with the respondent, the Research Integrity Officer will undertake reasonable efforts to restore the respondent's reputation. Depending on the particular circumstances, the Research Integrity Officer should consider notifying those individuals aware of or involved in the investigation of the final outcome, publicizing the final outcome in forums in which the allegation of scientific misconduct was previously publicized, or expunging all reference to the scientific misconduct allegation from the respondent's personnel file. Any institutional actions to restore the respondent's reputation must first be approved by the Deciding Official.

C. Protection of the Whistleblower and Others[32]

Regardless of whether the institution or ORI determines that scientific misconduct occurred, the Research Integrity Officer will undertake reasonable efforts to protect whistleblowers who made allegations of scientific misconduct in good faith and others who cooperate in good faith with inquiries and investigations of such allegations. Upon completion of an investigation, the Deciding Official will determine, after consulting with the whistleblower, what steps, if any, are needed to restore the position or reputation of the whistleblower. The Research Integrity Officer is responsible for implementing any steps the Deciding Official approves. The Research Integrity Officer will also take appropriate steps during the inquiry and investigation to prevent any retaliation against the whistleblower.

D. Allegations Not Made in Good Faith

If relevant, the Deciding Official will determine whether the whistleblower's allegations of scientific misconduct were made in good faith. If an allegation was not made in good faith, the Deciding Official will determine whether any administrative action should be taken against the whistleblower.

E. Interim Administrative Actions

Institutional officials will take interim administrative actions, as appropriate, to protect Federal funds and ensure that the purposes of the Federal financial assistance are carried out.[33]

XII. Record Retention

After completion of a case and all ensuing related actions, the Research Integrity Officer will prepare a complete file, including the records of any inquiry or investigation and copies of all documents and other materials furnished to the Research Integrity Officer or committees. The Research Integrity Officer will keep the file for three years after completion of the case to permit later assessment of the case. ORI or other authorized DHHS personnel will be given access to the records upon request.[34]

Issued April 1995
Revised February 1997

NOTES:

---

1. 42 C.F.R. §50.102.
2. 42 C.F.R. §50.102.
3. 42 C.F.R. §50.102.
4. 42 C.F.R. §50.103(d)(12).
5. 42 C.F.R. §50.103(d)(13).
6. 42 C.F.R. §50.103(d)(2).
7. 42 C.F.R. §50.103(d)(13).
8. 42 C.F.R. §50.103(d)(3).
9. 42 C.F.R. §50.103(d)(1).
10. 42 C.F.R. §50.103(d)(1).
11. 42 C.F.R. §50.103(d)(1).
12. 42 C.F.R. §50.103(d)(8).
13. 42 C.F.R. §50.103(d)(7).
14. 42 C.F.R. §50.103(d)(7).
15. 42 C.F.R. §50.103(d)(7).
16. 42 C.F.R. §50.103(d)(7).
17. 42 C.F.R. §50.104(a)(4); 42 C.F.R. §50.103(d)(15).
18. 42 C.F.R. §50.104(a)(2).
19. 42 C.F.R. §50.104(a)(2).
20. 42 C.F.R. §50.104(a)(1).
21. 42 C.F.R. §50.104(a)(1).
22. 42 C.F.R. §50.103(d)(15).
23. 42 C.F.R. §50.104(a)(3).
24. 42 C.F.R. §50.104(a)(5).
25. 42 C.F.R. §50.104(a)(3).
26. 42 C.F.R. §50.104(b)(1).
27. 42 C.F.R. §50.104(b)(2).
28. 42 C.F.R. §50.104(b)(3).
29. 42 C.F.R. §50.104(b)(4).
30. 42 C.F.R. §50.104(b)(5).
31. 42 C.F.R. §50.103(d)(14).
32. 42 C.F.R. §50.103(d)(14).
33. 42 C.F.R. §50.103(d)(11).
34. 42 C.F.R. §50.103(d)(10).

Model Procedures for Responding
To Allegations of Scientific Misconduct

Table of Contents

I.   Introduction. 489

II.   Definitions 489

III. General Procedures and Principles 491
    A.   Responsibility to Report Misconduct 491
    B.   Protecting the Whistleblower 491
    C.   Protecting the Respondent 491
    D.   Confidentiality 491
    E.   Responding to Allegations 491
    F.   Employee Cooperation 492
    G.   Evidentiary Standards 492
    H.   Completion of Process 493
    I.   Early Termination 493
    J.   Referral of Non-Scientific Misconduct Issues 493
    K.   Requirements for Reporting to ORI 494

IV. Preliminary Assessment of Allegations 495
    A.   Allegation Assessment 495
    B.   Referral of Other Issues 496

V.   Conducting the Inquiry 496
    A.   Initiation and Purpose of the Inquiry 496
    B.   First Steps If an Inquiry Is Necessary 496
    C.   Sequestration of the Research Records 497
    D.   Notification of the Respondent 498
    E.   Designation of an Official or a Committee to Conduct the Inquiry 498
    F.   Appointment of the Inquiry Committee 499
    G.   Charge to the Committee and the First Meeting 501
    H.   General Approaches to Conducting the Inquiry 501
    I.   General Approaches to Conducting an Interview 501

VI. The Inquiry Report 504
    A.   Elements of the Inquiry Report 504
    B.   Comments on the Draft Report by the Respondent and the Whistleblower 504
    C.   Inquiry Decision and Notification 504
    D.   Time Limit for Completing the Inquiry Report 505

VII. ORI Oversight 505
    A.   Decision to Investigate 505
    B.   Decision Not to Investigate 505
    C.   Access to Evidence 505

VIII. Referral to Other Agencies 505

IX. Conducting the Investigation 505
    A. Purpose of the Investigation 505
    B. Sequestration of the Research Records 506
    C. Notification of the Respondent 506
    D. Designation of an Official or a Committee to Conduct the Investigation 506
    E. Appointment of the Investigation Committee 507
    F. Charge to the Committee and the First Meeting 508
    G. Developing an Investigation Plan 508
    H. General Approaches to Conducting the Investigation 509
    I. Reviewing the Evidence 509
    J. Conducting Interviews 509
    K. Committee Deliberations 510

X. The Investigation Report 511
    A. Outline for an Investigation Report 511
    B. Standard Format of the Investigation Report 514
    C. Documenting the Investigative File 515
    D. Comments on the Draft Report 516
    E. Institutional Review and Decision 516
    F. Transmittal of the Final Investigation Report to ORI 517
    G. Time Limit for Completing the Investigation Report 517

XI. Institutional Administrative Actions 517

XII. Other Considerations 518
    A. Termination of Institutional Employment or Resignation
       Prior to Completing Inquiry or Investigation 518
    B. Restoration of the Respondent's Reputation 518
    C. Protection of the Whistleblower and Others 518
    D. Allegations Not Made in Good Faith 518
    E. Interim Administrative Actions 518

XIII. ORI Review of the Investigation Report and Follow-up 518
    A. Purpose of ORI Review 518
    B. Cooperation with ORI Review 519
    C. Request for Additional Documents and Information 519
    D. Notification of ORI Determination 519
    E. Cooperation in Appealed Cases 520

XIV. Record Retention 520

I.   **Introduction**

The purpose of these procedures is to provide advice to institutional officials on the methods and principles for assessing allegations and conducting inquiries and investigations related to possible scientific misconduct in research proposed to or supported by the U.S. Public Health Service. These procedures also address requirements for reporting scientific misconduct investigations to PHS, adopting institutional actions in response to findings of scientific misconduct, and cooperating with the Office of Research Integrity in its review of institutional actions and reports.

These procedures are intended to guide institutional officials responsible for assessing allegations, conducting inquiries and investigations, and reporting the results to ORI. The procedures do not create any right or benefit, substantive or procedural, enforceable at law by a party against the institution, its agencies, officers, or employees.

These procedures should be read in conjunction with the General Institutional Policies for Dealing with Scientific Misconduct (General Policies) [**if applicable**].

II.   **Definitions**[1]

A.   *Allegation* means any written or oral statement or other indication of possible scientific misconduct made to an institutional official.

B.   *Deciding Official* means the institutional official who makes final determinations on allegations of scientific misconduct and any responsive institutional actions. [**Optional addition: The Deciding Official will not be the same individual as the Research Integrity Officer and should have no direct prior involvement in the institution's inquiry, investigation, or allegation assessment.**]

C.   *Employee* means, for the purpose of these instructions only, any person paid by, under the control of, or affiliated with the institution, including but not limited to scientists, physicians, trainees, students, fellows, technicians, nurses, support staff, and guest researchers.

D.   *Good faith allegation* means an allegation made with the honest belief that scientific misconduct may have occurred. An allegation is not in good faith if it is made with reckless disregard for or willful ignorance of facts that would disprove the allegation.

E.   *Inquiry* means information-gathering and initial fact-finding to determine whether an allegation or apparent instance of scientific misconduct warrants an investigation.

F.   *Institutional counsel* means legal counsel who represents the institution during the scientific misconduct inquiry and investigation and who is responsible for advising the Research Integrity Officer, the inquiry and investigation committees, and the Deciding Official on relevant legal issues. The institutional counsel does not represent the respondent, the whistleblower, or any other person participating during the inquiry, investigation, or any follow-up action, except the institutional officials responsible for managing or conducting the institutional scientific misconduct process as part of their official duties.

G. *Investigation* means the formal examination and evaluation of all relevant facts
    to determine if scientific misconduct has occurred and, if so, to determine the
    responsible person and the seriousness of the misconduct.

H. *ORI* means the Office of Research Integrity, the office within the U.S. Department of
    Health and Human Services (DHHS) that is responsible for the scientific misconduct
    and research integrity activities of the U.S. Public Health Service.

I. *PHS* means the U.S. Public Health Service, an operating component of the U.S.
    Department of Health and Human Services.

J. *PHS regulation* means the Public Health Service regulation establishing standards for
    institutional inquiries and investigations into allegations of scientific misconduct,
    which is set forth at 42 C.F.R. Part 50, Subpart A, entitled "Responsibility of PHS
    Awardee and Applicant Institutions for Dealing With and Reporting Possible
    Misconduct in Science."

K. *PHS support* means Public Health Service grants, contracts, or cooperative
    agreements, or applications therefor.

L. *Research Integrity Officer* means the institutional official responsible for assessing
    allegations of scientific misconduct and determining when such allegations warrant
    inquiries and for overseeing any inquiries and investigations. **[Option: A multi-
    campus institution or an institution with several large research components
    may wish to delegate this function to more than one individual.]**

M. *Research record* means any data, document, computer file, computer diskette, or
    any other written or non-written account or object that reasonably may be expected
    to provide evidence or information regarding the proposed, conducted, or reported
    research that constitutes the subject of an allegation of scientific misconduct.
    A research record includes, but is not limited to, grant or contract applications,
    whether funded or unfunded; grant or contract progress and other reports; laboratory
    notebooks; notes; correspondence; videos; photographs; X-ray film; slides; biological
    materials; computer files and printouts; manuscripts and publications; equipment use
    logs; laboratory procurement records; animal facility records; human and animal
    subject protocols; consent forms; medical charts; and patient research files.

N. *Respondent* means the person against whom an allegation of scientific misconduct is
    directed or the person who is the subject of the inquiry or investigation. There can be
    more than one respondent in any inquiry or investigation.

O. *Retaliation*[2] means any action that adversely affects the employment or other status
    of an individual that is taken by an institution or an employee because the individual
    has, in good faith, made an allegation of scientific misconduct or of inadequate
    institutional response thereto, or has cooperated in good faith with an investigation of
    such allegation. **[Option: The institution may wish to define more specifically
    the standard to be applied in its determination of whether an adverse
    action was taken in response to a good faith allegation or cooperation.]**

P. *Scientific misconduct or misconduct in science* means fabrication, falsification,
    plagiarism, or other practices that seriously deviate from those that are commonly

accepted within the scientific community for proposing, conducting, or reporting research. It does not include honest error or honest differences in interpretations or judgments of data.

Q. *Whistleblower* means a person who makes an allegation of scientific misconduct

III. General Procedures and Principles

A. Responsibility to Report Misconduct

Institutional employees who receive or learn of an allegation of scientific misconduct will immediately report the allegation to the Research Integrity Officer for appropriate action. The Research Integrity Officer will promptly engage in an assessment of the allegation to determine whether it falls within the definition of scientific misconduct, involves PHS support, and provides sufficient information to proceed with an inquiry. **[Option: If the institution does not wish to mandate reporting of allegations, it may wish to "strongly encourage" such reporting. Nevertheless, ORI believes that supervisors and management officials should be required to forward all allegations to the Research Integrity Officer.]**

B. Protecting the Whistleblower[3]

Institutional employees who receive or learn of an allegation of scientific misconduct will treat the whistleblower with fairness and respect and, when the allegation has been made in good faith, will take reasonable steps to protect the position and reputation of the whistleblower and other individuals who cooperate with the institution against retaliation. Employees will immediately report any alleged or apparent retaliation to the Research Integrity Officer.

C. Protecting the Respondent[4]

Institutional employees who receive or learn of an allegation of scientific misconduct will treat the respondent with fairness and respect and will take reasonable steps to ensure that the procedural safeguards in the PHS regulation, 42 C.F.R. Part 50, Subpart A, and these procedures are followed. Employees will report significant deviations from these instructions to the Research Integrity Officer. The Research Integrity Officer will report any allegation not made in good faith to the Deciding Official for appropriate action.

D. Confidentiality[5]

Institutional employees who make, receive, or learn of an allegation of scientific misconduct will protect, to the maximum extent possible, the confidentiality of information regarding the whistleblower, the respondent, and other affected individuals. The Research Integrity Officer may establish reasonable conditions to ensure the confidentiality of such information.

E. Responding to Allegations

In responding to allegations of scientific misconduct, the Research Integrity Officer and any other institutional official with an assigned responsibility for handling such allegations will make diligent efforts to ensure that the following functions are performed.

1. Any allegation assessment, inquiry, or investigation is conducted in a timely, objective, thorough, and competent manner.[6]

2. Reasonable precautions are taken to avoid bias and real or apparent conflicts of interest on the part of those involved in conducting the inquiry or investigation.[7]

3. Immediate notification is provided to ORI if[8]:

   a. there is an immediate health hazard involved;

   b. there is an immediate need to protect Federal funds or equipment;

   c. there is an immediate need to protect the interests of the person(s) making the allegations or of the individual(s) who is the subject of the allegations as well as his/her coinvestigators and associates, if any;

   d. it is probable that the alleged incident is going to be reported publicly;

   e. the allegation involves a public health sensitive issue, *e.g.*, a clinical trial;

   f. there is a reasonable indication of a possible Federal criminal violation. In this instance, the institution must inform ORI within 24 hours of obtaining that information.

4. Interim administrative actions are taken, as appropriate, to protect Federal funds and the public health, and to ensure that the purposes of the Federal financial assistance are carried out.[9]

F. Employee Cooperation[10]

Institutional employees will cooperate with the Research Integrity Officer and other institutional officials in the review of allegations and the conduct of inquiries and investigations. Employees have an obligation to provide relevant evidence to the Research Integrity Officer or other institutional officials on misconduct allegations. Further, employees will cooperate with ORI in its conduct of inquiries and investigations, its oversight of institutional inquiries and investigations, and any follow up actions.

G. Evidentiary Standards[11]

The following evidentiary standards apply to findings of scientific misconduct made under the PHS regulation.

1. Burden of Proof

   The burden of proof for making a finding of scientific misconduct is on the institution. [**Note: If ORI adopts the institutional finding of scientific misconduct or makes an ORI finding, the burden of proof is on ORI for purposes of its finding and administrative actions.**]

2. Standard of Proof

Any institutional or ORI finding of scientific misconduct will be established by a preponderance of the evidence. This means that the evidence shows that it is more likely than not that the respondent committed scientific misconduct. **[Option: institutional findings not related to PHS funding may adopt a different burden and standard of proof.]**

H. Completion of Process

The Research Integrity Officer is responsible for ensuring that the inquiry/investigation process and all other steps required by this instruction and the PHS regulation are completed even in those cases where the respondent leaves the institution after allegations are made.

I. Early Termination[12]

If the institution plans to terminate an inquiry or investigation prior to completion of all the steps required by the PHS regulation, the Research Integrity Officer will notify ORI of the planned termination and the reasons therefore. ORI will review the information provided and advise the institution whether further investigation should be undertaken.

J. Referral of Non-Scientific Misconduct Issues

When the institution's review of the allegation identifies non-scientific misconduct issues, the Research Integrity Officer should refer these matters to the proper institutional or Federal office for action. Issues requiring referral are described below.

1. HHS Criminal Violations[13]

Potential violation of criminal law under HHS grants and contracts should be referred to the Office of Inspector General, HHS-OIG Hot line, P.O. Box 17303, Baltimore, MD 21203-7303, telephone (800) 368-5779. If the possible criminal violation is identical to the alleged scientific misconduct (*e.g.,* alleged false statements in a PHS grant application), the criminal charge should be reported to ORI. ORI will then refer it to OIG.

2. Violation of Human and Animal Subject Regulations

Potential violations of human subject regulations should be referred to the Office of Human Research Protections, Department of Health and Human Services, 6100 Executive Boulevard, Suite 3B01, Rockville, MD 20892-7507. Phone: 301-496-7005. Email: ohrp@osophs.dhhs.gov.

Potential violations of animal subject regulations should be referred to the Office of Laboratory Animal Welfare, National Institutes of Health, 6705 Rockledge Drive, RKL1, Suite 1050, MSC 7982, Bethesda, MD 20892-7982, Phone: 301-402-5913.

3.   Violation of FDA Regulations

Potential violations of Food and Drug Administration regulated research require-
ments should be referred to the FDA Office of Regulatory Affairs, Division of
Compliance Policy, Bioresearch Program Coordination, 5600 Fishers Lane,
HFC-230 TWBK 715, Rockville, MD 20857, telephone (301) 827-0420.

4.   Fiscal Irregularities

Potential violations of cost principles or other fiscal irregularities should be
referred as follows:

a.   For all NIH Agencies—Office of Management Assessment, NIH, Building 31,
Room 1B05, Bethesda, MD 20892, telephone (301) 496-1361.

b.   For all other PHS Agencies—PHS Office of Grants and Contracts, 5600
Fishers Lane, Room 17A39, Rockville, MD 20857, telephone (301) 443-
6630.

If there are any questions regarding the proper referral of non-scientific misconduct
issues, the Research Integrity Officer may call the ORI Division of Research
Investigations at (301) 443-5330 to obtain advice.

K.   Requirements for Reporting to ORI

1.   An institution's decision to initiate an investigation must be reported in writing
to the Director, ORI, on or before the date the investigation begins.[14] At a
minimum, the notification should include the name of the person(s) against
whom the allegations have been made, the general nature of the allegation as it
relates to the PHS definition of scientific misconduct, and the PHS applications or
grant number(s) involved.[15] ORI must also be notified of the final outcome of the
investigation and must be provided with a copy of the investigation report.[16]
Any significant variations from the provisions of the institutional policies and
procedures should be explained in any reports submitted to ORI.

2.   If an institution plans to terminate an inquiry or investigation for any reason
without completing all relevant requirements of the PHS regulation, the Research
Integrity Officer will submit a report of the planned termination to ORI, including
a description of the reasons for the proposed termination.[17]

3.   If the institution determines that it will not be able to complete the investigation
in 120 days, the Research Integrity Officer will submit to ORI a written request
for an extension that explains the delay, reports on the progress to date, estimates
the date of completion of the report, and describes other necessary steps to be
taken. If the request is granted, the Research Integrity Officer will file periodic
progress reports as requested by the ORI.[18]

4.   When PHS funding or applications for funding are involved and an admission of
scientific misconduct is made, the Research Integrity Officer will contact ORI for

consultation and advice. Normally, the individual making the admission will be asked to sign a statement attesting to the occurrence and extent of misconduct. When the case involves PHS funds, the institution cannot accept an admission of scientific misconduct as a basis for closing a case or not undertaking an investigation without prior approval from ORI.[19]

5.   The Research Integrity Officer will notify ORI at any stage of the inquiry or investigation if:

    a.   there is an immediate health hazard involved;[20]

    b.   there is an immediate need to protect Federal funds or equipment;[21]

    c.   there is an immediate need to protect the interests of the person(s) making the allegations or of the individual(s) who is the subject of the allegations as well as his/her co-investigators and associates, if any;[22]

    d.   it is probable that the alleged incident is going to be reported publicly;[23] or

    e.   the allegation involves a public health sensitive issue, *e.g.,* a clinical trial; or

    f.   there is a reasonable indication of possible criminal violation. In this instance, the institution must inform ORI within 24 hours of obtaining that information.[24]

IV.   Preliminary Assessment of Allegations

A.   Allegation Assessment

Upon receiving an allegation of scientific misconduct, the Research Integrity Officer will immediately assess the allegation to determine whether there is sufficient evidence to warrant an inquiry, whether PHS support or PHS applications for funding are involved, and whether the allegation falls under the PHS definition of scientific misconduct.

1.   PHS Support

Allegations involving research supported by PHS-funded grants, contracts, or cooperative agreements, or applications for PHS funding connote PHS support. If the allegation does not involve PHS support, it should be handled under the institution's own definition of scientific misconduct and procedures [**if applicable**] without regard to the PHS regulation at 42 C.F.R. Part 50, Subpart A.

2.   PHS Definition

The allegation should be carefully reviewed to determine whether it potentially constitutes fabrication, falsification, plagiarism, or other serious deviation from commonly accepted practices for proposing, conducting, or reporting research. In case of doubt, the Research Integrity Officer should consult with the institutional counsel or ORI on whether the allegation falls within the PHS definition of scientific misconduct.

3. Sufficient evidence to proceed

There is not always sufficient evidence or information to permit further inquiry into the allegation. For example, an allegation that a scientist's work should be subjected to general examination for possible misconduct is not sufficiently substantial or specific to initiate an inquiry. In case of such a vague allegation, an effort should be made to obtain more information before initiating an inquiry. This information may be sought from any reasonable source, including the whistleblower, if known.

B. Referral of Other Issues

Regardless of whether it is determined that a scientific misconduct inquiry is warranted, if the allegation involves PHS support and concerns possible failure to protect human or animal subjects, financial irregularities, or criminal activity, the allegation should be referred to the appropriate PHS or DHHS office. See section III-J.

V. Conducting the Inquiry[25]

A. Initiation and Purpose of the Inquiry[26]

Following the preliminary assessment, if the Research Integrity Officer determines that the allegation provides sufficient information to allow specific follow-up, involves PHS support, and falls under the PHS definition of scientific misconduct, he or she will immediately initiate the inquiry process. In initiating the inquiry, the Research Integrity Officer should identify clearly the original allegation and any related issues that should be evaluated. The purpose of the inquiry is to make a preliminary evaluation of the available evidence and testimony of the respondent, whistleblower, and key witnesses to determine whether there is sufficient evidence of possible scientific misconduct to warrant an investigation. The purpose of the inquiry is **not** to reach a final conclusion about whether misconduct definitely occurred or who was responsible. The findings of the inquiry must be set forth in an inquiry report.

B. First Steps If an Inquiry Is Necessary

As soon as practicable after the Research Integrity Officer determines that an inquiry is required, he or she will:

1. secure the relevant research records;

2. notify the [**appropriate institutional officials**], institutional counsel, the respondent, and ORI (if the request to open the inquiry originated from ORI);

3. appoint and charge the inquiry committee; and

4. notify ORI if any of the conditions listed in section III.E.3 of these procedures are present.

The Research Integrity Officer or institutional counsel may consult with ORI at any time regarding appropriate procedures to be followed.

C. Sequestration of the Research Records

1. Immediate Sequestration

If the relevant research records have not been obtained at the assessment stage, the Research Integrity Officer will immediately locate, collect, inventory, and secure them to prevent the loss, alteration, or fraudulent creation of records.

2. Institutional Access

Research records produced under PHS grants and cooperative agreements are the property of the institution, and employees cannot interfere with the institution's right of access to them. Under contracts, certain research records may belong to PHS, but the institution will be provided access to contract records in the custody of the institution for purposes of reviewing misconduct allegations.

3. Original Records

The documents and materials to be sequestered will include all the original items (or copies if originals cannot be located) that may be relevant to the allegations. These include, but are not limited to, research records as defined in section II.N of this document.

4. Sequestration of the Records from the Respondent

The Research Integrity Officer should notify the respondent that an inquiry is being initiated simultaneously with the sequestration so that the respondent can assist with location and identification of the research records. The Research Integrity Officer should obtain the assistance of the respondent's supervisor and institutional counsel in this process, as necessary. If the respondent is not available, sequestration may begin in the respondent's absence. The respondent should not be notified in advance of the sequestration of research records to prevent questions being raised later regarding missing documents or materials and to prevent accusations against the respondent of tampering with or fabricating data or materials after the notification. In addition to securing records under the control of the respondent, the Research Integrity Officer may need to sequester records from other individuals, such as coauthors, collaborators, or whistleblowers. As soon as practicable, a copy of each sequestered record will be provided to the individual from whom the record is taken if requested.

5. Inventory of the Records

A dated receipt should be signed by the sequestering official and the person from whom an item is collected, and a copy of the receipt should be given to the person from whom the record is taken. If it is not possible to prepare a complete inventory list at the time of collection, one should be prepared as soon as possible, and then a copy should be given to the person from whom the items were collected.

6. Security and Chain of Custody

The Research Integrity Officer will lock records and materials in a secure place. The persons from whom items are collected may be provided with a copy of any item. Where feasible, that person will have access to his or her own original items under the direct and continuous supervision of an institutional official. This will ensure that a proper chain of custody is maintained and that the originals are kept intact and unmodified. Questions about maintaining the chain of custody of records should be referred to the institutional counsel.

D. Notification of the Respondent

1. Contents of Notification

The Research Integrity Officer will notify the respondent in writing of the opening of the inquiry. The notification should identify the research project in question and the specific allegations, define scientific misconduct, identify the PHS funding involved, list the names of the members of the inquiry committee (if appointed) and experts (if any), explain the respondent's opportunity to challenge the appointment of a member of the committee or expert for bias or conflict of interest, to be assisted by counsel, to be interviewed, to present evidence to the committee, and to comment on the inquiry report; address the respondent's obligation as an employee of the institution to cooperate; describe the institution's policy on protecting the whistleblower against retaliation and the need to maintain the whistleblower's confidentiality during the inquiry and any subsequent proceedings.

2. Potential Respondents

If no specific respondent has been identified at this stage of the process, the Research Integrity Officer will notify each potential respondent that an inquiry will be undertaken, *e.g.*, each coauthor on a questioned article or each investigator on a questioned grant application. **[Option: Advise the Research Integrity Officer to consult with the institutional counsel on the proper notification under the circumstances.]**

E. Designation of an Official or a Committee to Conduct the Inquiry

The Research Integrity Officer is responsible for conducting or designating others to conduct the inquiry.

1. Use of an Inquiry Committee

In complex cases, the Research Integrity Officer will normally appoint a committee of three or more persons to conduct the inquiry, following the procedures set forth in section V.E.

2. Use of an Inquiry Official

   In cases in which the allegations and apparent evidence are straightforward, such as an allegation of plagiarism or simple falsification or an admission of misconduct by the respondent, the Research Integrity Officer may choose to conduct the inquiry directly or designate another qualified individual to do so. In such cases, the inquiry official will nevertheless obtain the necessary expert and technical advice to consider properly all scientific issues.

3. Inquiry Process

   The inquiry, whether conducted by a committee or an individual, will follow each procedural step set forth below.

F. Appointment of the Inquiry Committee

   If an inquiry committee is to be appointed, the Research Integrity Officer will use the following procedures:

1. Committee Membership

   The Research Integrity Officer, in consultation with other institutional officials as appropriate, will appoint the committee and committee chair within [suggested: 10 days] of the initiation of the inquiry. The inquiry committee should consist of at least three individuals who do not have real or apparent conflicts of interest in the case, are unbiased, and have the necessary expertise to evaluate the evidence and issues related to the allegation, interview the principals and key witnesses, and conduct the inquiry. These individuals may be scientists, subject matter experts, administrators, lawyers, or other qualified persons, and they may be from inside or outside of the institution. [**Option: As an alternative, the institution may appoint a standing committee authorized to add or reuse members or use experts when necessary to evaluate specific allegations.**]

2. Experts

   The Research Integrity Officer, in consultation with the committee, will determine whether additional experts other than those appointed to the committee need to be consulted during the inquiry to provide special expertise to the committee regarding the analysis of specific evidence. In this case, the experts provide a strictly advisory function to the committee; they do not vote and generally do not interview witnesses. The experts chosen may be from inside or outside of the institution.

3. Bias or Conflict of Interest

   The Research Integrity Officer will take reasonable steps to ensure that the members of the committee and experts have no bias or personal or professional conflict of interest with the respondent, whistleblower, or the case in question. In

making this determination, the Research Integrity Officer will consider whether
the individual (or any members of his or her immediate family):

a. has any financial involvement with the respondent or whistleblower;

b. has been a coauthor on a publication with the respondent or whistleblower;

c. has been a collaborator or coinvestigator with the respondent or
    whistleblower;

d. has been a party to a scientific controversy with the respondent or
    whistleblower;

e. has a supervisory or mentor relationship with the respondent or
    whistleblower;

f. has a special relationship, such as a close personal friendship, kinship, or a
    physician/patient relationship with the respondent or whistleblower; or

g. falls within any other circumstance that might appear to compromise the
    individual's objectivity in reviewing the allegations.

4. Objection by Respondent

    The Research Integrity Officer will notify the respondent of the proposed commit-
    tee membership within [suggested: 10 days]. If the respondent submits a written
    objection to any appointed member of the inquiry committee or expert based on
    bias or conflict of interest within [suggested: 5 days], the Research Integrity
    Officer will immediately determine whether to replace the challenged member or
    expert with a qualified substitute.

5. Confidentiality

    Members of the committee and experts will agree in writing to observe the
    confidentiality of the proceeding and any information or documents reviewed as
    part of the inquiry. Outside of the official proceedings of the committee, they may
    not discuss the proceedings with the respondent, whistleblower, witnesses, or
    anyone not authorized by the Research Integrity Officer to have knowledge of the
    inquiry.

6. Provision of Assistance

    The Research Integrity Officer, in consultation with the institutional counsel, will
    provide staff assistance and guidance to the committee and the experts on the
    procedures for conducting and completing the inquiry, including procedures for
    maintaining confidentiality, conducting interviews, analyzing data, and preparing
    the inquiry report.

G. Charge to the Committee and the First Meeting

The Research Integrity Officer will prepare a charge for the inquiry committee that describes the allegations and any related issues identified during the allegation assessment and states that the purpose of the inquiry is to make a preliminary evaluation of the evidence and testimony of the respondent, whistleblower, and key witnesses to determine whether there is sufficient evidence of possible scientific misconduct to warrant an investigation, as required by the PHS regulation. The purpose is not to determine whether scientific misconduct definitely occurred or who was responsible.

At the committee's first meeting, the Research Integrity Officer will review the charge with the committee, discuss the allegations, any related issues, and the appropriate procedures for conducting the inquiry, assist the committee with organizing plans for the inquiry, and answer any questions raised by the committee. The Research Integrity Officer and institutional counsel will be present or available throughout the inquiry to advise the committee as needed.

H. General Approaches to Conducting the Inquiry

During the inquiry, the committee will take the following steps:

1. Avoid Bias or Conflict of Interest

All necessary steps must be taken to avoid bias or conflict of interest between the committee and experts and the respondent, whistleblower, and witnesses.

2. Refer Other Issues

The Research Integrity Officer must be advised of any necessary interim actions to protect the research funds, human or animal subjects, or other steps required by regulation or policy. See section III.E.3 and III.J.

I. General Approaches to Conducting an Interview

1. Purpose of the Interview

The purpose of an interview at the inquiry stage is to allow each respondent, whistleblower, or witness to tell his or her side of the story. The committee should not attempt to speculate about what happened or might have happened or put words in the witnesses' mouths. Also, the committee should not disclose information obtained from others interviewed unless this is necessary and can be done without identifying the source of the information.

2. Issues to Cover

Before an interview, the committee should provide each witness with a summary of the matters or issues intended to be covered at the interview. If the committee raises additional matters, the witness should be given an opportunity to supplement the record in writing or in another interview. The witness should be informed that his or her cooperation and truthful answers are expected.

3. Confrontation

Witnesses should not be told at this stage whether other testimony conflicts with theirs, although questions may be asked for purposes of clarifying the testimony. Avoid leading questions such as, "You must have made a mistake and thought it was actually this way, right?"

4. Using Experts

The committee may request that experts attend or participate in interviews to assist in its evaluation of the allegations and related issues. If the committee determines that such participation is not appropriate, it may ask an expert to prepare questions for the committee to use at the interview. Any expert retained to assist the committee may read the transcripts or summaries of the interviews.

5. Transcribing Interviews

Interviews with the respondent will be transcribed or recorded. Interviews with anyone else will be summarized, tape-recorded, or transcribed. A transcript or summary of the interview will be provided to each witness for review and correction of errors. Witnesses may add comments or information. Changes to the transcript or summary will be made only to correct factual errors.

6. Confidentiality of Interviews

Witnesses should be advised that the proceedings are confidential and that they should not discuss the inquiry or their interview with anyone else other than their counsel or adviser.

7. Access to Counsel

Witnesses may be accompanied and advised by legal counsel or by a non-legal adviser who is not a principal or witness in the case. However, the counsel or adviser may only advise the witness and may not participate directly in the interview. Witnesses will respond directly to the interview questions. **[Option: Some institutional policies do not permit the presence of counsel during interviews.]**

8. Order of Interviews

The inquiry committee should interview, if possible, the whistleblower, key witnesses, and the respondent, in that order. Witnesses should be asked to provide, in advance if possible, any relevant evidence including their own notes, manuscripts, research records, or other documents that were not sequestered previously but are relevant to the allegation.

9.   Interviewing the Whistleblower

In interviewing the whistleblower, the inquiry committee should attempt to obtain as much additional evidence regarding the substance of the allegation as possible and to determine the whistleblower's view of the significance and impact of the alleged misconduct. However, it is not the whistleblower's responsibility to prove his or her allegations.

10.   Interviewing the Respondent

The respondent should be asked to provide his or her own response to the allegations, including any analysis of the primary data. If the respondent claims that an honest error or difference of scientific judgement occurred, he or she should provide any evidence to support that claim. If he or she requests, the respondent may make a closing statement at the end of the interview.

11.   Recording Admissions

If the respondent admits to the misconduct, the respondent should be asked immediately to sign a statement attesting to the occurrence and extent of the misconduct. Normally, an admission is a sufficient basis to proceed directly to an investigation. However, the admission may not be a sufficient basis for closing a case. Further investigation may be needed to determine the extent of the misconduct or to explore additional issues. If an admission is made, the Research Integrity Officer or institutional counsel may seek advice from ORI in determining whether there is a sufficient basis to close a case, after the admission is fully documented and all appropriate procedural steps are taken. If the case is closed, the report should be forwarded to the Deciding Official with recommendations for appropriate institutional sanctions and then submitted to ORI for review. **[Option: If the respondent admits to the misconduct, the institution may wish to advise the committee to consult with the institutional counsel immediately, with the option of seeking advice from ORI as needed.]**

12.   Committee Deliberations

The inquiry committee will evaluate the evidence and testimony obtained during the inquiry. After consultation with the Research Integrity Officer and institutional counsel, the committee members will decide whether there is sufficient evidence of possible scientific misconduct to recommend further investigation. The scope of the inquiry does not include deciding whether misconduct occurred or conducting exhaustive interviews and analyses.

Committee deliberations should never be held in the presence of the interviewee. During the interview, the committee members should not debate among themselves or with witnesses over possible scientific interpretations. These questions should be reserved for private discussions among the inquiry committee members and expert consultants.

VI.   The Inquiry Report[27]

A.   Elements of the Inquiry Report

A written inquiry report must be prepared that states the name and title of the committee members and experts, if any; the allegations; the PHS support; a summary of the inquiry process used; a list of the research records reviewed; summaries of any interviews; a description of the evidence in sufficient detail to demonstrate whether an investigation is warranted; and the committee's determination as to whether an investigation is recommended and whether any other actions should be taken if an investigation is not recommended. Institutional counsel will review the report for legal sufficiency. All relevant dates should be included in the report.

B.   Comments on the Draft Report by the Respondent and the Whistleblower[28]

The Research Integrity Officer will provide the respondent with a copy of the draft inquiry report for comment and rebuttal and will provide the whistleblower, if he or she is identifiable, with those portions of the draft report that address the whistleblower's role and opinions in the investigation. **[Option: The institution may provide the whistleblower with a summary of the inquiry findings for comment instead of portions of the draft report.]**

1.   Confidentiality

The Research Integrity Officer may establish reasonable conditions for review to protect the confidentiality of the draft report.

2.   Receipt of Comments

Within [ ] calendar days of their receipt of the draft report, the whistleblower and respondent will provide their comments, if any, to the inquiry committee. Any comments that the whistleblower or respondent submits on the draft report will become part of the final report and record.[29] Based on the comments, the inquiry committee may revise the report as appropriate.

C.   Inquiry Decision and Notification[30]

1.   Decision by Deciding Official

The Research Integrity Officer will transmit the final report and any comments to the Deciding Official, who will make the determination of whether findings from the inquiry provide sufficient evidence of possible scientific misconduct to justify conducting an investigation. The inquiry is completed when the Deciding Official makes this determination, which will be made within 60 days of the first meeting of the inquiry committee. Any extension of this period will be based on good cause and recorded in the inquiry file.

2.   Notification

The Research Integrity Officer will notify both the respondent and the whistle-blower in writing of the Deciding Official's decision of whether to proceed to an investigation and will remind them of their obligation to cooperate in the event an investigation is opened. The Research Integrity Officer will also notify all appropriate institutional officials of the Deciding Official's decision.

D. Time Limit for Completing the Inquiry Report

The inquiry committee will complete the inquiry and submit its report in writing to the Research Integrity Officer no more than 60 calendar days following its first meeting,[31] unless the Research Integrity Officer approves an extension for good cause. If the Research Integrity Officer approves an extension, the reason for the extension will be entered into the records of the case and the report. The respondent will also be notified of the extension.

VII. ORI Oversight[32]

A. Decision to Investigate

If the Deciding Official decides that an investigation will be conducted, the Research Integrity Officer [or other designated official, if applicable] will notify ORI and will forward a copy of the final inquiry report and the institution's policies and procedures for conducting investigations to ORI.

B. Decision Not to Investigate

If the Deciding Official decides not to proceed to an investigation and the inquiry was begun at the request of ORI or if ORI requests a copy, the Research Integrity Officer [or other designated official] will send a copy of the final inquiry report and the institutional decision to ORI. Otherwise, the case may be closed without notice to ORI.

C. Access to Evidence

If ORI is performing an oversight review of the institution's determination not to proceed to an investigation, the Research Integrity Officer, if so requested, will provide ORI with the report and the inquiry file including, but not limited to, sequestered evidence, analyses, and transcripts of interviews. The Research Integrity Officer will keep all records secure until ORI makes its final decision on its oversight of the institutional inquiry or investigation.

VIII. Referral to Other Agencies

Information obtained during the inquiry regarding allegations other than scientific misconduct involving PHS funds should be referred to the responsible institutional officials or government agencies. See section III.J.

IX. Conducting the Investigation[33]

A. Purpose of the Investigation

The purpose of the investigation is to explore in detail the allegations, to examine the evidence in depth, and to determine specifically whether misconduct has been committed, by whom, and to what extent. The investigation will also determine whether there are additional instances of possible misconduct that would justify broadening the scope beyond the initial allegations. This is particularly important where the alleged misconduct involves clinical trials or potential harm to human subjects or the general public or if it affects research that forms the basis for public policy, clinical practice, or public health practice. The findings of the investigation will be set forth in an investigation report.

B. Sequestration of the Research Records

The Research Integrity Officer will immediately sequester any additional pertinent research records that were not previously sequestered during the inquiry. This sequestration should occur before or at the time the respondent is notified that an investigation has begun. The need for additional sequestration of records may occur for any number of reasons, including the institution's decision to investigate additional allegations not considered during the inquiry stage or the identification of records during the inquiry process that had not been previously secured. The procedures to be followed for sequestration during the investigation are the same procedures that apply during the inquiry. See section V.B.

C. Notification of the Respondent

The Research Integrity Officer will notify the respondent as soon as reasonably possible after the determination is made to open an investigation. The notification should include: a copy of the inquiry report; the specific allegations; the sources of PHS funding; the definition of scientific misconduct; the procedures to be followed in the investigation, including the appointment of the investigation committee and experts; the opportunity of the respondent to be interviewed, to provide information, to be assisted by counsel, to challenge the membership of the committee and experts based on bias or conflict of interest, and to comment on the draft report; the fact that ORI will perform an oversight review of the report regarding PHS issues; and an explanation of the respondent's right to request a hearing before the DHHS Departmental Appeals Board if there is an ORI finding of misconduct under the PHS definition.

D. Designation of an Official or a Committee to Conduct the Investigation

The Research Integrity Officer is responsible for conducting or designating others to conduct the investigation.

1. Use of an Investigation Committee

In complex cases, the Research Integrity Officer will normally appoint a committee of three or more persons to conduct the investigation, following the procedures set forth in section IX.E.

2. Use of an Investigation Official

In cases in which the allegations and apparent evidence are straightforward, such as an allegation of plagiarism or simple falsification or an admission of misconduct by the respondent, the Research Integrity Officer may choose to conduct the investigation directly or designate another qualified individual to do so. In such cases, the investigation official will nevertheless obtain the necessary expert and technical advice to consider properly all scientific issues.

3. Investigation Process

The investigation, whether conducted by a committee or an individual, will follow each procedural step set forth below.

E. Appointment of the Investigation Committee

If an investigation committee is to be appointed, the Research Integrity Officer will use the following procedures:

1. Committee Membership

The Research Integrity Officer, in consultation with other institutional officials as appropriate, will appoint the investigation committee and the committee chair within **[suggest: 10 days]** of the notification to the respondent or as soon thereafter as practicable. The investigation committee should consist of at least three individuals who do not have real or apparent conflicts of interest in the case, are unbiased, and have the necessary expertise to evaluate the evidence and issues related to the allegations, interview the principals and key witnesses, and conduct the investigation.[34] These individuals may be scientists, administrators, subject matter experts, lawyers, or other qualified persons, and they may be from inside or outside the institution. Individuals appointed to the investigation committee may also have served on the inquiry committee. **[Option: As an alternative, the institution may appoint a standing committee authorized to add or reuse members or use consultants when necessary to investigate specific allegations.]**

2. Experts

Experts may be appointed as noted in section V.E.2-4 (or carried over from the inquiry) to advise the committee on scientific or other issues.

3. Bias or Conflict of Interest

The Research Integrity Officer will take reasonable steps to ensure that the members of the committee and the experts have no bias or personal or professional conflict of interest with the respondent, whistleblower, or the case in question. See section V.E.3.

4. Objection to Committee or Experts by Respondent

The Research Integrity Officer will notify the respondent of the proposed committee membership within **[suggest: 5 days]**. If the respondent submits a written objection to any appointed member of the investigation committee or expert based on bias or conflict of interest, the Research Integrity Officer will immediately determine whether to replace the challenged member or expert with a qualified substitute.

5. Confidentiality

Members of the committee and experts will agree in writing to observe the confidentiality of the proceedings and any information or documents reviewed as part of the investigation. Outside of the official proceedings of the committee, they may not discuss the proceedings with the respondent, whistleblower, witnesses, or anyone not authorized by the Research Integrity Officer to have knowledge of the investigation.

F.   Charge to the Committee and the First Meeting

1. Charge to the Committee

The Research Integrity Officer will define the subject matter of the investigation in a written charge to the committee that describes the allegations and related issues identified during the inquiry, defines scientific misconduct, and identifies the name of the respondent. The charge will state that the committee is to evaluate the evidence and testimony of the respondent, whistleblower, and key witnesses to determine whether, based on a preponderance of the evidence, scientific misconduct occurred and, if so, to what extent, who was responsible, and its seriousness.

During the investigation, if additional information becomes available that substantially changes the subject matter of the investigation or would suggest additional respondents, the committee will notify the Research Integrity Officer, who will determine whether it is necessary to notify the respondent of the new subject matter or to provide notice to additional respondents.

2. The First Meeting

The Research Integrity Officer, with the assistance of institutional counsel, will convene the first meeting of the investigation committee to review the charge, the inquiry report, and the prescribed procedures and standards for the conduct of the investigation, including the necessity for confidentiality and for developing a specific investigation plan. The investigation committee will be provided with a copy of these instructions and, where PHS funding is involved, the PHS regulation.

G.   Developing an Investigation Plan

At the initial meeting, the committee should begin development of its investigative plan and complete it as soon as reasonably possible. The investigation plan will include an inventory of all previously secured evidence and testimony; a determination of whether additional evidence needs to be secured; what witnesses need to be interviewed, including the whistleblower, respondent, and other witnesses with knowledge of the research or events in question; a proposed schedule of meetings, briefing of experts, and interviews; anticipated analyses of evidence (scientific, forensic, or other); and a plan for the investigative report.

H. General Approaches to Conducting the Investigation

During the investigation, the committee will take the following steps:

1. Avoid Bias or Conflict of Interest

    All necessary steps must be taken to avoid bias or conflict of interest between the
    committee and experts and the respondent, whistleblower, and witnesses.

2. Refer Other Issues

    The Research Integrity Officer must be advised of any necessary interim actions to
    protect the research funds, human or animal subjects, or other steps required by
    regulation or policy. See section III.E.3 and III.J.

3. Consult with the Research Integrity Officer and institutional counsel

    The Research Integrity Officer and institutional counsel should be consulted
    throughout the investigation on compliance with these procedures and PHS regu-
    lations, appropriate investigatory and interviewing methods and strategies, legal
    issues, and the standard of proof. The Research Integrity Officer and institutional
    counsel will be present or available throughout the investigation to advise the
    committee.

I. Reviewing the Evidence

The investigation committee will obtain and review all relevant documentation and
perform or cause to be performed necessary analyses of the evidence, including
scientific, forensic, statistical, or other analyses as needed.

J. Conducting Interviews

The investigation committee will conform to the following guidelines:

1. Conducting the Interviews

    The investigation committee will conduct the interviews as described in section
    V.G., except that at the investigative stage interviews should be in-depth and all
    significant witnesses should be interviewed. Each witness should have the
    opportunity to respond to inconsistencies between his or her testimony and
    the evidence or other testimony, subject to the need to take reasonable steps to
    maintain the confidentiality of the testimony of the respondent and other
    witnesses.

2. Preparing for Interviews

    The investigation committee will prepare carefully for each interview. All relevant
    documents and research data should be reviewed in advance and specific
    questions or issues that the committee wants to cover during the interview should
    be identified. The committee should appoint one individual to take the lead on

each interview. If significant questions or issues arise during an interview that require committee deliberation, the committee should take a short recess to discuss the issues. Committee deliberations should never be held in the presence of the interviewee.

3. Objectivity

The investigation committee will conduct all interviews in a professional and objective manner, without implying guilt or innocence on the part of any individual.

4. Transcribing Interviews

Any interview with the respondent will be transcribed or recorded. Interviews with anyone else will be summarized, tape-recorded, or transcribed. A transcript or summary of the interview will be provided to each witness for review and correction of errors. Witnesses may add comments or additional information, but changes to the transcript or summary will only be made to correct factual errors.

5. Recording Admissions

If the respondent admits to the misconduct, he or she should be asked immediately to sign a statement attesting to the occurrence and extent of the misconduct, acknowledging that the statement was voluntary and stating that the respondent was advised of his or her right to seek the advice of counsel. The committee should consult with the institutional counsel on the specific form and procedure for obtaining this statement. The admission may not be used as a basis for closing the investigation unless the committee has adequately determined the extent and significance of the misconduct and all procedural steps for completion of the investigation have been met. The committee may ask the Research Integrity Officer or institutional counsel to consult with ORI when deciding whether an admission has adequately addressed all the relevant issues such that the investigation can be considered completed. The investigation should not be closed unless the respondent has been appropriately notified and given an opportunity to comment on the investigative report. If the case is considered complete, it should be forwarded to the Deciding Official with recommendations for appropriate institutional actions and then to ORI for review. **[Option: If the respondent admits to the misconduct, the institution may wish to advise the committee to consult with the institutional counsel immediately, with the option of seeking advice from ORI as needed.]**

K. Committee Deliberations

1. Burden and Standard of Proof

In reaching a conclusion on whether there was scientific misconduct and who committed it, the burden of proof is on the institution to support its conclusions and findings by a preponderance of the evidence. See section III.G. **[Option: The institution may apply a different burden and standard of proof for non-PHS findings.]**

2. Definition of Scientific Misconduct

The committee will consider whether falsification, fabrication, or plagiarism occurred in proposing, conducting, or reporting research or whether and why there was a serious deviation from accepted practices in the scientific community at the time the actions were committed.

3. Sufficient Evidence

The committee will consider whether there is sufficient evidence of intent such that the institution can meet its burden of proving misconduct by a preponderance of the evidence. The committee will also consider whether the respondent has presented substantial evidence of honest error or honest differences in interpretations or judgments of data, such that scientific misconduct cannot be proven by a preponderance of the evidence.

X. The Investigation Report

A. Outline for an Investigation Report

The following annotated outline may prove useful in preparing the Investigation Report required by the Office of Research Integrity (42 C.F.R. Part 50, Subpart A), except when special factors suggest a different approach.

1. Background

Include sufficient background information to ensure a full understanding of the issues that concern the PHS under its definition of scientific misconduct. This section should detail the facts leading to the institutional inquiry, including a description of the research at issue, the persons involved in the alleged misconduct, the role of the whistleblower, and any associated public health issues. All relevant dates should be included.

2. Allegations

List all the allegations of scientific misconduct raised by the whistleblower and any additional scientific misconduct allegations that arose during the inquiry and investigation. The source and basis for each allegation or issue should be cited except to the extent that the confidentiality of a whistleblower requesting anonymity is compromised or where the identity of the source is irrelevant or unnecessary. The allegations identified in this section will form the structure or context in which the subsequent analysis and findings are presented.

3. PHS Support

For each allegation of scientific misconduct under the PHS definition, identify the PHS support for the research or report (*e.g.*, publication) at issue or the application containing the falsification/fabrication or plagiarism.

4. Institutional Inquiry: Process and Recommendations

    Summarize the inquiry process, including the composition of the committee
    (names, degrees, departmental affiliation, and expertise), and the charge to the
    committee. List the persons interviewed, the evidence secured and reviewed and
    the measures taken to ensure its security, the policies and procedures used
    (or citation to the pertinent section of the institution's policies and procedures),
    and any other factors that may have influenced the proceedings.

5. Institutional Investigation: Process

    Summarize the investigation process, including the composition of the committee
    (names, degrees, departmental affiliation, and expertise), and the charge to the
    committee. List the persons interviewed, the evidence secured and reviewed and
    the measures taken to ensure its security, the policies and procedures used
    (or citation to the pertinent section of the institution's policies and procedures),
    and any other factors that may have influenced the proceedings.

6. Institutional Investigation: Analysis

    For each allegation:

    Background

       Describe the particular matter (*e.g.*, experiment or component of a clinical
       protocol) in which the alleged misconduct occurred and why and how the
       issue came to be under investigation.

    Analysis

       The analysis should take into account all the relevant statements, claims
       (*e.g.*, a claim of a significant positive result in an experiment), rebuttals,
       documents, and other evidence, including circumstantial evidence, related to
       the issue. The source of each statement, claim, or other evidence should be
       cited (*e.g.*, laboratory notebook with page and date, medical chart
       documents and dates, relevant manuscripts, transcripts of interview, etc.).

       Any use of additional expert analysis should be noted (forensic, statistical, or
       special analysis of the physical evidence, such as similarity of features or
       background in contested figures).

       Summarize or quote relevant statements, including rebuttals, made by the
       whistleblower, respondent, and other pertinent witnesses and reference/cite
       the appropriate sources.

       Summarize each argument that the respondent raised in his or her defense
       against the scientific misconduct allegation and cite the source of each argu-
       ment. Any inconsistencies among the respondent's various arguments should
       be noted.

The analysis should be consistent with the terms of PHS definition of scientific misconduct. It should describe the relative weight given to the various witnesses and pieces of evidence, noting inconsistencies, credibility, and persuasiveness.

Describe any evidence that shows that the respondent acted with intent, that is, any evidence that the respondent knowingly engaged in the alleged falsification, fabrication, plagiarism, or other conduct that constitutes a serious deviation from commonly accepted practices.

Similarly, describe the evidence supporting the possibility that honest error or differences of scientific opinion occurred with respect to the issue.

Conclusions

a. Findings of Misconduct or No Misconduct

Concisely state the investigation committee's finding for each identified issue. The investigation report should make separate findings as to whether or not each issue constitutes scientific misconduct, using the PHS definition.

A finding of scientific misconduct should be supported by a preponderance of the evidence. Institutions may have their own standard of proof under their scientific misconduct policies and procedures, one that may be higher than preponderance of the evidence. In such cases, ORI has requested institutions to reexamine the evidence and report to ORI what their conclusions would have been under a preponderance of the evidence standard.

If the investigation committee finds scientific misconduct on one or more issues, the report should identify the type of misconduct for each issue (fabrication, falsification, plagiarism, or other practices that seriously deviate from those that are commonly accepted within the scientific community). The report should indicate the extent and seriousness of the fabrication, falsification, or plagiarism, including its effect on research findings, publications, research subjects, and the laboratory or project in which the misconduct occurred.

If the investigation committee determines that the respondent committed scientific misconduct by seriously deviating from "other commonly accepted practices," the report should thoroughly document the commonly accepted practice of the relevant scientific community at the time the misconduct occurred and indicate the extent of the respondent's deviation from that standard. Publications, standards of the institution or relevant professional societies, State and Federal regulations, expert opinion, and other sources should be described and cited as the basis for the commonly accepted practice. The serious deviation therefrom should be described in detail, indicating why the alleged act was a serious deviation.

b. Misconduct under the Institution's Policies

The investigation committee may determine that an action that does not constitute scientific misconduct under the PHS definition is, nevertheless, scientific misconduct under the institution's own definition (*e.g.*, clinical protocol deviations or other violations of human subjects protection; documented animal welfare concerns; substandard data management practices; deficient mentoring of trainees). Any issue that the investigation committee determines to be scientific misconduct solely under the institution's own definition should be identified as such. These findings are not subject to ORI's jurisdiction if ORI agrees that they do not meet the PHS definition or jurisdictional basis.

7. Recommended Institutional Actions

Based on its findings, the investigation committee should recommend administrative actions that it believes the institution should take consistent with its policies and procedures, including appropriate actions against the respondent, such as a letter of reprimand, special supervision, probation, termination, etc. The institution should also identify any published research reports or other sources of scientific information (such as data bases) that should be retracted or corrected and take steps to ensure that appropriate officials who can effect these corrections or retractions are notified.

Attachments

Copies of all significant documentary evidence that is referenced in the report should be appended to the report, if possible (relevant notebook pages or other research records, relevant committee or expert analyses of data, transcripts or summary of each interview, respondent and whistleblower responses to the draft report(s), manuscripts, publications or other documents, including grant progress reports and applications, etc.). It is also helpful to include a "List of Attachments."

It is useful to identify allegedly false statements, misrepresentations in figures or parts of figures, areas of plagiarism, etc., on a copy of the page or section of the questioned document (*e.g.*, a page from a research notebook). A side-by-side comparison with the actual data or material that is alleged to have been plagiarized is helpful.

B. Standard Format of the Investigation Report

The following outline should be used in preparing the Investigation Report, except when special factors suggest a different approach. The report should incorporate all of the elements described in section X.A.

1. Background

   – Chronology of events
   – Include public health issues

2. Allegations

3. PHS Support or Application(s) (by allegation)

4. Institutional Inquiry: Process and Recommendations

   – Composition of committee
   – Individuals interviewed
   – Evidence sequestered and reviewed

5. Institutional Investigation: Process

   – Composition of committee
   – Individuals interviewed
   – Evidence sequestered and reviewed

6. Institutional Investigation: Analysis

   For each allegation:

   – Background
   – Analysis of all the relevant evidence and specific identification of evidence
     supporting the finding
   – Conclusion: scientific misconduct or no scientific misconduct
   – Effect of misconduct (*e.g.*, potential harm to research subjects, reliability of
     data, publications that need to be corrected or retracted, etc.)

7. Recommended Institutional Actions

8. Attachments

C. Documenting the Investigative File

   1. Index of Evidence

      The investigation committee should maintain an index of all the relevant evidence
      it secured or examined in conducting the investigation, including any evidence that
      may support or contradict the report's conclusions. Evidence includes, but is not
      limited to, research records, transcripts or recordings of interviews, committee
      correspondence, administrative records, grant applications and awards,
      manuscripts, publications, and expert analyses.

   2. Purpose of Documentation

      The purpose of the documentation is to substantiate the investigation's findings.

   3. Record Retention

      After completion of a case and all ensuing related actions, the Research Integrity
      Officer will prepare a complete file, including the records of any inquiry or
      investigation and copies of all documents and other materials furnished to the
      Research Integrity Officer or committees. The Research Integrity Officer will

keep the file for three years after completion of the case to permit later assessment of the case. ORI or other authorized DHHS personnel will be given access to the records upon request.[35]

D.   Comments on the Draft Report

1.   Respondent

The Research Integrity Officer will provide the respondent with a copy of the draft investigation report for comment and rebuttal. The respondent will be allowed [ ] days to review and comment on the draft report. The respondent's comments will be attached to the final report. The findings of the final report should take into account the respondent's comments in addition to all the other evidence.

2.   Whistleblower

The Research Integrity Officer will provide the whistleblower, if he or she is identifiable, with those portions of the draft investigation report that address the whistleblower's role and opinions in the investigation. The report should be modified, as appropriate, based on the whistleblower's comments.

3.   Institutional Counsel

The draft investigation report will be transmitted to the institutional counsel for a review of its legal sufficiency. Comments should be incorporated into the report as appropriate.

4.   Confidentiality

In distributing the draft report, or portions thereof, to the respondent and whistleblower, the Research Integrity Officer will inform the recipient of the confidentiality under which the draft report is made available and may establish reasonable conditions to ensure such confidentiality. For example, the Research Integrity Officer may request the recipient to sign a confidentiality statement or to come to his or her office to review the report.

E.   Institutional Review and Decision

Based on a preponderance of the evidence, the Deciding Official will make the final determination whether to accept the investigation report, its findings, and the recommended institutional actions. If this determination varies from that of the investigation committee, the Deciding Official will explain in detail the basis for rendering a decision different from that of the investigation committee in the institution's letter transmitting the report to ORI. The Deciding Official's explanation should be consistent with the PHS definition of scientific misconduct, the institution's policies and procedures, and the evidence reviewed and analyzed by the investigation committee. The Deciding Official may also return the report to the investigation committee with a request for further fact-finding or analysis. The Deciding Official's determination, together with the investigation committee's report, constitutes the final investigation report for purposes of ORI review.

When a final decision on the case has been reached, the Research Integrity Officer will notify both the respondent and the whistleblower in writing. In addition, the Deciding Official will determine whether law enforcement agencies, professional societies, professional licensing boards, editors of journals in which falsified reports may have been published, collaborators of the respondent in the work, or other relevant parties should be notified of the outcome of the case. The Research Integrity Officer is responsible for ensuring compliance with all notification requirements of funding or sponsoring agencies.

F.   Transmittal of the Final Investigation Report to ORI

After comments have been received and the necessary changes have been made to the draft report, the investigation committee should transmit the final report with attachments, including the respondent's and whistleblower's comments, to the Deciding Official, through the Research Integrity Officer.

G.   Time Limit for Completing the Investigation Report

The final investigation report will be submitted to ORI within 120 days of the first meeting of the investigation committee, unless the institution requests a written request for extension and ORI grants the extension. All attachments to the final report should be submitted with the report. The Research Integrity Officer should maintain all other evidence and materials for possible ORI review.

XI.   Institutional Administrative Actions

[Institution] will take appropriate administrative actions against individuals when an allegation of misconduct has been substantiated.[36]

If the Deciding Official determines that the alleged misconduct is substantiated by the findings, he or she will decide on the appropriate actions to be taken, after consultation with the Research Integrity Officer. The actions may include:

- withdrawal or correction of all pending or published abstracts and papers emanating from the research where scientific misconduct was found.

- removal of the responsible person from the particular project, letter of reprimand, special monitoring of future work, probation, suspension, salary reduction, or initiation of steps leading to possible rank reduction or termination of employment;

- restitution of funds as appropriate.

XII.   Other Considerations

A.   Termination of Institutional Employment or Resignation Prior to Completing Inquiry or Investigation

The termination of the respondent's institutional employment, by resignation or other-wise, before or after an allegation of possible scientific misconduct has been reported, will not preclude or terminate the misconduct procedures.

517

If the respondent, without admitting to the misconduct, elects to resign his or her position prior to the initiation of an inquiry, but after an allegation has been reported, or during an inquiry or investigation, the inquiry or investigation will proceed. If the respondent refuses to participate in the process after resignation, the committee will use its best efforts to reach a conclusion concerning the allegations, noting in its report the respondent's failure to cooperate and its effect on the committee's review of all the evidence.

B.   Restoration of the Respondent's Reputation[37]

If the institution finds no misconduct and ORI concurs, after consulting with the respondent, the Research Integrity Officer will undertake reasonable efforts to restore the respondent's reputation. Depending on the particular circumstances, the Research Integrity Officer should consider notifying those individuals aware of or involved in the investigation of the final outcome, publicizing the final outcome in forums in which the allegation of scientific misconduct was previously publicized, or expunging all reference to the scientific misconduct allegation from the respondent's personnel file. Any institutional actions to restore the respondent's reputation must first be approved by the Deciding Official.

C.   Protection of the Whistleblower and Others[38]

Regardless of whether the institution or ORI determines that scientific misconduct occurred, the Research Integrity Officer will undertake reasonable efforts to protect whistleblowers who made allegations of scientific misconduct in good faith and others who cooperate in good faith with inquiries and investigations of such allegations. Upon completion of an investigation, the Deciding Official will determine, after consulting with the whistleblower, what steps, if any, are needed to restore the position or reputation of the whistleblower. The Research Integrity Officer is responsible for implementing any steps the Deciding Official approves. The Research Integrity Officer will also take appropriate steps during the inquiry and investigation to prevent any retaliation against the whistleblower.

D.   Allegations Not Made in Good Faith

If relevant, the Deciding Official will determine whether the whistleblower's allegations of scientific misconduct were made in good faith. If an allegation was not made in good faith, the Deciding Official will determine whether any administrative action should be taken against the whistleblower.

E.   Interim Administrative Actions

Institutional officials will take interim administrative actions, as appropriate, to protect Federal funds and ensure that the purposes of the Federal financial assistance are carried out.[39]

XIII.   ORI Review of the Investigation Report and Follow-up[40]

A.   Purpose of ORI Review

ORI reviews the final investigation report, the supporting materials, and the Deciding Official's determinations to decide whether the investigation has been performed in a timely manner and with sufficient objectivity, thoroughness, and competence. Based on its review, ORI may:

1. request additional information from the institution;

2. accept all the findings and conclusions of the report;

3. accept all or part of the factual findings of the report and make its own conclusions;

4. request additional investigation by the institution;

5. reject the report and conduct its own investigation;

6. impose administrative actions on the respondent beyond those recommended by the institution;

7. refer the case to the Division of Policy and Education, ORI, for a review of the institution's regulatory compliance;[41] or

8. take any other action deemed to be in the public interest and within ORI's authority.

ORI will attempt to complete its review of the institution's report within 180 days of its receipt, except where additional follow up activities are required, such as an ORI request for additional information or analysis or where further investigation is necessary.

B. Cooperation with ORI Review[42]

ORI is authorized by statute and PHS regulations to review institutional reports on allegations of scientific misconduct. In reviewing an institution's report, ORI may request additional information or other assistance from the Research Integrity Officer or other institutional officials. If the institutional official receiving the ORI request is unsure how to respond, he or she should consult with the Research Integrity Officer or institutional counsel. Institutional counsel may consult with ORI counsel prior to advising the institutional official on how to respond.

C. Request for Additional Documents and Information

The Research Integrity Officer will cooperate with any ORI request for additional documents and information by responding to all requests in a timely and responsive fashion. The Research Integrity Officer may consult with institutional counsel for advice as needed.

D. Notification of ORI Determination

1. ORI Concurrence

If ORI concurs with the institution's findings, ORI will notify the respondent and appropriate institutional officials in writing and will send the respondent and appropriate institutional official a summary or copy of the concurrence and notice of any additional PHS actions. If there is an ORI finding of scientific misconduct, the respondent will be notified of his or her opportunity to appeal to the DHHS Departmental Appeals Board (DAB). See 59 *Fed. Reg.* 29809 (1994).

2. ORI Nonconcurrence

    If ORI does not concur with the institution's findings, ORI will notify the appropriate institutional official of the basis for that decision. If ORI does not concur with a finding of no misconduct, the institution may be requested to conduct a further investigation, either with the same or a different investigation committee, or ORI may conduct its own investigation. In the latter instance, ORI will notify the appropriate individuals of its investigation.

E. Cooperation in Appealed Cases[43]

For cases in which ORI concurs with the institution's findings of scientific misconduct under the PHS definition or makes its own finding of scientific misconduct, ORI will request institutional employees to cooperate in presenting ORI findings of misconduct before the DAB if the respondent appeals the findings. Cooperation includes providing evidence, testimony, or any other information needed to assist in the preparation and presentation of ORI's case before the DAB. Institutional employees may consult with the Research Integrity Officer or institutional counsel in responding to ORI's request for cooperation.

XIV. Record Retention[44]

After completion of a case and all ensuing related actions, the Research Integrity Officer will prepare a complete file, including the records of any inquiry or investigation and copies of all documents and other materials furnished to the Research Integrity Officer of Committees. The Research Integrity Officer will keep the file for at least three years after completion of the case to permit later assessment of the case. ORI or other authorized DHHS personnel will be given access to the records upon request.

Issued April 1995
Revised February 1997

NOTES:

---

1. Some of the definitions in this section are based on the Public Health Service regulations. 42 C.F.R. §50.102.

2. 42 C.F.R. §50.103(d)(13); See also, 42 U.S.C. §289b(e).

3. Id.

4. 42 C.F.R. §§50.103(d)(3) and (13) and §50.104(a)(2).

5. 42 C.F.R. §§50.103(d)(2) and (3).

6. 42 C.F.R. §50.104(a)(6).

7. 42 C.F.R. §50.103(d)(9).

8. 42 C.F.R. §50.103(d)(5) and §50.104(b)(1)-(5).

9. 42 C.F.R. §50.103(d)(11).

10. 42 C.F.R. §50.103(c)(3) and (4) and §50.104(a)(6).

11. Section XI of the Hearing Procedures for Scientific Misconduct, 59 Fed. Reg. 29809, 29811, June 9, 1994; 45 C.F.R. §§76.313(c)(1) and (2).

12. 42 C.F.R. §50.104(a)(3).

13. 42 C.F.R. §50.104(b)(5).

14. 42 C.F.R. §50.104(a)(1).

15. 42 C.F.R. §50.104(a)(1).

16. 42 C.F.R. §50.103(d)(15).

17. 42 C.F.R. §50.104(a)(3).

18. 42 C.F.R. §50.104(a)(5).

19. 42 C.F.R. §50.104(a)(3).

20. 42 C.F.R. §50.104(b)(1).

21. 42 C.F.R. §50.104(b)(2).

22. 42 C.F.R. §50.104(b)(3).

23. 42 C.F.R. §50.104(b)(4).

24. 42 C.F.R. §50.104(b)(5).

25. 42 C.F.R. §50.103(d).

26. 42 C.F.R. §50.103(d)(1).

27. 42 C.F.R. §50.103(d)(1).

28. 42 C.F.R. §§50.103(d)(1) and (3).

29. 42 C.F.R. §50.103(d)(1).

30. 42 C.F.R. §§50.103(d)(4) and (7).

31. 42 C.F.R. §50.103(d)(1).

32. 42 C.F.R. §50.103(d)(6) and 42 C.F.R. §50.103(d)(10).

33. 42 C.F.R. §50.103(d) and §50.104.

34. 42 C.F.R. §50.103(d)(8)

35. 42 C.F.R. §50.103(d)(10).

36. 42 C.F.R. §50.103(d)(14).

37. 42 C.F.R. §50.103(d)(13).

38. 42 C.F.R. §50.103(d)(13).

39. 42 C.F.R. §50.103(d)(11).

40. 42 C.F.R. §50.103(d)(11).

41. 42 C.F.R. §50.105.

42. 42 C.F.R. §50.104(a)(6); 42 C.F.R. §50.103(c)(4).

43. 42 C.F.R. §50.103(d)(4).

44. 42 C.F.R. §50.103(d)(4).

17

Ethics in Human Research

Bernard H. Adelson, M.D., Ph.D., F.A.C.P.
with Rodney K. Adams, Esquire

Introduction 524
Frequently Used Theories of Ethics 524
    Normative Ethics 524
        Nonmaleficence 524
        Beneficence 524
        Respect for Autonomy 525
        Justice 525
        Prioritizing Moral Factors 525
    Consequentialism (Utilitarianism) 525
    Deontology 525
    Casuistry 526
    Virtue Ethics 526
Translational Ethics in Human Research 526
Guidelines to the Ethics of Human Research 526
    The Nuremberg Code 527
    The Declaration of Helsinki 527
    The Belmont Report 527
    The International Ethical Guidelines 527
A Framework for Ethics in Clinical Research 528
    Scientific Value and Validity as Ethical Issues 528
    Fair Selection of Subjects as an Ethical Issue 528
    Favorable Risk/Benefit Ratio as an Ethical Issue 529
    Independent Review as an Ethical Issue 529
    Respect for Potential and Enrolled Subjects as an Ethical Issue 529
    The Reporting of Study Findings as an Ethical Issue 530
Conflict of Interest Issues 530
    Potential Fiscal Conflicts of Interest for the Investigator 530
    Potential Conflict of Interest Between the Role of the Scientist Versus
    the Role of the Physician 530
    Potential for Conflicts of Interest for an IRB 531
The Ethics of Placebo in Human Research 531
References 532

INTRODUCTION

Resolving ethical issues is one of the core purposes of the Institutional Review Board (IRB). Ethics can be defined as the disciplined study of the rightness and wrongness of human actions with emphasis on the consequences of these actions to the individual and to society. This definition, of necessity, includes the scholarly effort to analyze the rules, customs, and beliefs of society. Medical ethics, sometimes referred to as bioethics, is an ancient subspecialty of ethics, dating back at least twenty-five centuries to the Hippocratic Corpus. The central concept of the term medical ethics is that the physician shall serve as the moral fiduciary of the patient. This basic fact tends to be vitiated today by powerful forces, such as super-specialists, rapidly evolving technology, and of equal importance, the increasing financial and regulatory role defined by the government, third-party payers, managed care organizations, and the like. We must never lose sight of the primacy of the physician-patient dyad. Moses Maimonides most eloquently states this in the Physician's Prayer, "Let me see in the sufferer, the man alone."

A framework of moral principles to guide human experimentation (Heifetz, 1996) should be:

1. Prescriptive in the sense of giving direction as to how the researcher should act
2. Proscriptive in the sense of suggesting what would be unacceptable behavior
3. Potentially applicable to all areas of the human condition
4. Acceptable to diverse cultures and thereby have universal application
5. Suggestive that adherence to them generally functions to the long-term benefit of the individual and society
6. In harmony with human nature

Unfortunately, there is no easy answer to the essence of ethics, which is the balancing of individual autonomy against societal needs and desires.

FREQUENTLY USED THEORIES OF ETHICS

Medical ethics draws heavily from classical theories of ethics. A brief discussion of frequently utilized ethics theories follows.

Normative Ethics

Normative ethics (also called principle-based ethics) include certain principles upon which most American ethicists agree in their analysis of medical ethics issues. These consist of nonmaleficence, beneficence, respect for autonomy, and justice (Beauchamp, 1994). *The Belmont Report,* discussed here, appears to be based primarily on this school of ethics. The primary criticism of principle-based ethics is that it has no hierarchical order of principles. Thus, the ethicist is left to an arbitrary ranking of principles in any given situation.

Nonmaleficence   Nonmaleficence is the principle of doing no harm to a patient. In clinical research, the risks associated with a research protocol should be minimized.

Beneficence   Beneficence is the quality or character of being good or doing good. In medical ethics, the principle entails an obligation to protect persons from harm. It can be expressed in two general rules: (1) do not harm; and (2) protect from harm by maximizing possible benefits and minimizing possible risks of harm.

Respect for Autonomy Respect for autonomy (also called respect for persons) is the fundamental belief that each individual should have the right to determine what will and will not be done to him. It underlies the duty to obtain informed consent from participants. In fact, one commentator observed that informed consent should more aptly be called informed choice, as the participant or patient should be given all the available options from which to choose (Weijer et al., 1997).

Justice In the context of medical ethics, the term justice most commonly refers to distributive justice in which equals are treated equally and unequals are treated unequally proportionate to the moral differences between the individuals. As Justinian put it, justice is "the constant and perpetual wish to render every one his due." The challenge, of course, is trying to determine what is done to who and why. Fair distribution can include "(1) to each person an equal share; (2) to each person according to individual need; (3) to each person according to individual effort; (4) to each person according to societal contributions; and (5) to each person according to merit" (*The Belmont Report,* 1979).

When used in the context of selecting research participants, justice requires that the benefits and burdens of research be fairly distributed, often expressed in terms of treating persons of similar circumstances or characteristics similarly. Vulnerable people must not be exploited. Eligible candidates who may benefit from participation should not be excluded without good cause. One might also include the obligation of designing studies in a way to ensure that studies are of sufficient importance to warrant the risk to participants and that valid findings will be obtained.

Prioritizing Moral Factors It is not possible to precisely prioritize nonmaleficence, autonomy, justice, and beneficence. These factors usually are ranked in the order they are listed in the preceding sentence. However, they all must be considered in healthcare decision-making. One should not be given undue importance over another. Unfortunately, there are no clear-cut rules on how to apply or weight these factors to a particular situation.

Consequentialism (Utilitarianism)

Utilitarianism, expressed by Jeremy Benthem and James Mill, requires that all actions shall be directed toward achieving the greatest happiness for the greatest number of people. The rightness or wrongness of a given action is judged exclusively by its consequences. A utilitarian ignores motive and responsibility and focuses solely on outcome. Individual action and public policy should maximize utility (happiness or preference satisfaction) for the greatest number of people.

Deontology

Deontology, as expressed by Emanuel Kant, is a duty-based theory based upon his categorical imperative. The worth of an action is determined by its conformity to some binding rule rather than by its consequences. An act is judged by motive and not consequence. This approach is often expressed in the form of rules, such as "Do not kill." For example, a deontologist would conclude that the life of an innocent person should not be taken, no matter what the benefit to others. A utilitarian may conclude that killing an innocent person is acceptable to save the lives of others. Traditional duty-based ethics involved a list of prescribed duties. The self-evident duties of seventeenth and eighteenth centuries, such as the duty to not commit suicide, are less self-evident today. An additional problem is that deontology does not have a clear procedure for resolving conflicts between duties.

Casuistry

Casuistry is a case-based ethics that requires that a case be evaluated on its individual merits with reference to a paradigm or ideal case that takes into account the various conflicting ethical theories that are inherent in the case. In other words, it is the application of general principles of ethics to specific problems of right and wrong in conduct, in order to solve or clarify them.

Virtue Ethics

In recent years, virtue ethics has been revived and cited as an important part of medical ethics. Extolled by Aristotle, it is the oldest of the normative philosophies. Virtue theory contends that the basis of morality is the development of good character traits such as compassion, humility, confidentiality, prudence, temperance, courage, and truthfulness. Some commentators cite more than a hundred virtues to be considered. Attempting to apply so many elements is a bit challenging in the clinical setting. Virtue ethics does not try to examine the rightness or wrongness of a specific act but tries to inquire of attributes of the person. Unfortunately, critics would say, this does not give much guidance to particular situations.

TRANSLATIONAL ETHICS IN HUMAN RESEARCH

Translational research is the translating of laboratory studies to applications in human healthcare. This ranges from the development of new screening tests for particular conditions, as in a genetic testing for a predisposition to breast cancer, to new therapeutic techniques, as in the use of stem cells to regenerate damaged cells in an adult, to using animal tissue in humans (transgenics or xenotransplantation). The examples chosen were intended to highlight the potential controversy of each. The role of ethics, religion, economics, and law will all come into consideration when pondering such issues. The crucible for considering the ethics of scientific innovation is often the clinical research setting. Almost daily the news media carries stories on cloning, stem cell research, and other cutting-edge research that is under social scrutiny. In modern society, very few limits have been placed on the advancement of knowledge through translational research.

GUIDELINES TO THE ETHICS OF HUMAN RESEARCH

The history of the ethical implications of human research is of great importance, and we can only allude to them here in a brief fashion. The basic codes established for the conduct of human subject research stem from *The Nuremberg Code* (1947), which resulted from the war crimes tribunal in Nuremberg at the end of World War II, in which German physicians were held liable for egregious disrespect for human rights in the conduct of scientific experiments. This was followed by *The Declaration of*

Helsinki in 1964, *The Belmont Report* in 1979, and *The International Ethical Guidelines for Biomedical Research Involving Human Subjects* in 1982.

The Nuremberg Code

The Nuremburg Code was developed as part of the judicial decision during the trials of Nazi war criminals following World War II. It was the first international framework describing ethical limitations for clinical research. The code was widely adopted as a standard during the 1950s and 1960s for protecting human subjects. It focused on the need for informed consent and favorable risk/benefit analysis in clinical research.

The Declaration of Helsinki

The Declaration of Helsinki was approved by the World Medical Association in 1964 and widely adopted by medical associations in various countries to establish standards for clinical research. It focuses on favorable risk/benefit analysis and independent review in clinical research. The distinction between therapeutic and nontherapeutic research is also highlighted. The Declaration has been revised several times, most recently during a World Medical Association General Assembly meeting in Edinburgh (2000).

The Edinburgh revision of the Declaration was substantial and controversial. The distinction between therapeutic and nontherapeutic research was dropped. The applicability of the Declaration was changed from solely physicians to include anyone who may be conducting research. The term "best current methods" was adopted in the discussion of the standard of care in lieu of "best proven methods" or "highest standard of care." No resolution was reached as to the appropriate standard of care for control arms of studies. The independence of ethics committees was reinforced, and additional emphasis has been placed on protecting study participants.

The Belmont Report

The Belmont Report is a statement of basic ethical principles governing research involving human subjects that was issued by the National Commission for the Protection of Human Subjects in 1979. Informed consent, favorable risk/benefit analysis, and protection of vulnerable populations are the focus of the Report (National Commission for the Protection of Human Subjects of Biomedical and Behavioral Research, 1979). This has become the guiding ethical document for American clinical research.

The International Ethical Guidelines

The International Ethical Guidelines for Biomedical Research Involving Human Subjects was developed by the Council for International Organizations of Medical Sciences as a form of guidance for large-scale trials of vaccines and drugs in developing countries. It has been revised several times since its genesis in 1982. Unlike other ethics statements, it considers compensation for research injuries and wrestles more openly with the quandary of conducting clinical research in settings where the highest quality of medical care may not be routinely available (Council for International Organizations of Medical Sciences, 1993).

············

A FRAMEWORK FOR ETHICS IN CLINICAL RESEARCH

After considering *The Nuremberg Code, The Declaration of Helsinki, The Belmont Report,* and *The International Guidelines,* Emanual, Wendler, and Grady (2000) have created a simple framework for use by researchers and IRB members to consider whether clinical research meets appropriate ethical standards:

1. Value: Enhancements of health or knowledge must be derived from the research
2. Scientific validity: The research must be methodologically rigorous
3. Fair subject selection: Scientific objectives, not vulnerability or privilege, and the potential for and distribution of risks and benefits should determine communities selected as study sites and the inclusion criteria for individual subjects
4. Favorable risk/benefit ratio: Within the context of standard clinical practice and the research protocol, risks must be minimized, potential benefits enhanced, and the potential benefits to individuals and knowledge gained for society must outweigh the risks
5. Independent review: Unaffiliated individuals must review the research and approve, amend, or terminate it
6. Informed consent: Individuals should be informed about the research and provide their voluntary consent
7. Respect for enrolled subjects: Subjects should have their privacy protected, the opportunity to withdraw, and their well being monitored

A researcher and an IRB would be well advised to consider all of these points when developing a research protocol. Informed consent, while currently receiving a lot of attention, is not the sole criteria for determining whether a protocol meets ethical requirements. A well-drafted research protocol will address these ethical issues.

Scientific Value and Validity as Ethical Issues

Scientific validity requires that accepted scientific principles and methods be included, and that every effort be made to avoid "junk science." "Shoddy science is never ethical" (Weijer et al., 1997). There should be some indication that the study will lead to scientific and social value. Otherwise, the risk of harm to the study participants cannot be justified. Further, studies using small numbers of participants may be unethical. Such underpowered studies may expose participants to risk while not leading to valid scientific conclusions. Halpern, Karlawish, and Berlin (2002) conclude that underpowered clinical trials are ethical only in two situations: in studies of rare disease in which the investigators explicitly intend to add their data with similar trials in a prospective meta-analysis, and in early-phase drug or device studies with sufficient participants to test the defined hypothesis other than randomized treatment comparisions.

Fair Selection of Subjects as an Ethical Issue

Fair subject selection is given in satisfaction to the demands of justice. The selection of participants should be carefully described as to who will be included or excluded in the recruitment of subjects. This is particularly important with regard to vulnerable and disadvantaged groups, such as children, prisoners, socially disadvantaged individuals, and cognitively impaired individuals. Participant selection requires that individuals who bear the risks and burdens of the study should be in the position to enjoy its benefits and that those who may benefit should share in some of the risks and burdens.

Favorable Risk/Benefit Ratio as an Ethical Issue

The participant must be assured that the study has been formulated in such a way that its hypothesis and protocol minimize the risk of harm and damage to the participant. The principles of beneficence and nonmaleficence require that there be a favorable risk/benefit ratio with minimal risks to the extent that it is possible in enhancement of potential benefits to the participant and to society.

Independent Review as an Ethical Issue

A researcher usually acts with only the highest ideals, but everyone suffers from personal bias. Review by individuals independent of the proposed research will bring objectivity not only as to the technical aspects of the protocol but also as to ethical issues, legal implications, and community concerns. A diverse review committee will ensure the best opportunity for contrasting perspectives to be heard and considered. Ongoing review is important to ensure that the risk/benefit ratio remains favorable. Consideration of ethical principles should continue to be compared against the study data as it develops.

Respect for Potential and Enrolled Subjects as an Ethical Issue

Respect for persons is defined as an ethical principle discussed in *The Belmont Report,* requiring that individual autonomy be respected and that persons with diminished autonomy be protected. This includes protecting the study participant through informed consent, minimization of risk, and confidentiality. Even before enrolling participants, autonomy should be considered in defining the potential participant population.

The ethical precepts of informed consent include those principles common to medical ethics: respect for autonomy; beneficence; nonmaleficence; and justice.

The ethical obligation of a researcher goes beyond obtaining informed consent. The researcher must be continually vigilant to minimize risk of injury to the participants. This ranges from carefully designing the study to careful monitoring of each participant's health to terminating a study when the data demonstrates that either (1) the benefits of one research arm are superior to another or (2) the risks to the participants outweighs the potential benefits.

Confidentiality pertains to the treatment of information that an individual has disclosed in a relationship of trust and with the expectation that it will not be divulged to others without permission in ways that are inconsistent with the understanding of the original disclosure. In contrast, privacy is defined as one's control over the extent, timing, and circumstances of sharing oneself (physically, behaviorally, or intellectually) with others. A researcher has an obligation to protect both privacy and confidentiality of study participants. Breaching either should only occur with the express consent of the participant.

Respect for persons requires that individuals be thoroughly assured of confidentiality, that they be informed of newly discovered risks or benefits from the study, that they are permitted to withdraw from the study without prejudice, and that every effort be made to maintain their welfare.

The Reporting of Study Findings as an Ethical Issue

An additional, but often overlooked, ethical consideration is that study findings will be reported accurately, completely, promptly, and in such a way that clinicians can utilize the information in practice (Weijer et al., 1997). By doing so, patients or future study participants are not exposed to injury needlessly. NIH has proposed that its grantee researchers be required to set forth their plan for sharing resultant data. (NIH, 2002).

············

CONFLICT OF INTEREST ISSUES

A conflict of interest can occur in many ways. The importance of justice has been alluded to in the function of the IRB. This is particularly interpreted as distributive justice, namely the distribution of risks and benefits shared alike by the participants in a study and carefully explained to them in the consent for that study.

Potential Fiscal Conflicts of Interest for the Investigator

A conflict of interest occurs in the arena of financial affairs. Investigators frequently have a financial stake in the sponsor of their study and thereby are prejudiced in the conduct and the outcome of the study. This is a difficult matter, the resolution of which is subject to many different interpretations and recommendations. In essence, a financial conflict of interest can be best handled by complete candor and revelation of financial ties with the sponsor of the study. This is an attitude that has been documented in the current thinking in medical ethics, and in its absence are found many egregious examples of conflicts of interest.

Potential Conflict of Interest Between the Role of the Scientist Versus the Role of the Physician

In healthcare, a physician's ethical obligation to his patient is fairly explicit. This is often characterized as a fiduciary duty to the patient to obtain informed consent, provide good care, and maintain confidentiality. In clinical research, a physician also has the obligation to ensure that the study findings are valid and reproducible. To this end, the physician has an ethical obligation to enroll a sufficient number of participants to obtain statistical power. Successful completion of studies has important implications for the clinician and his institution, which may have broad social benefits such as increased funding for further research to benefit society, improved resources for patients at the institution, or other laudable results. However, under the current ethics rubric, the clinician's primary concern must be the safety of the participant. All other considerations are secondary.

One of the more frequent conflicts of interest occurs when the investigator is also playing the role of a physician. As investigator, he has an interest in enrolling subjects, conducting a reasoned study, analyzing the data, and ultimately using this data to draw conclusions that may be publishable, which may be a source of income or a source of academic promotion. These interests sometimes will conflict with his role as a physician, in which it is his fiduciary duty to care for the patient in the best possible way. When this way is cloudy, the decision between the two routes that the investigator/physician must take becomes very difficult.

It is particularly important to remember that the physician/investigator has a dual role with possible inherent conflicts of interest, in that on the one hand he becomes the physician for the patient and thereby assumes the moral fiduciary responsibility, while on the other hand he will become an advocate for the study itself and thereby be tempted to include or manipulate participants in order to obtain a more favorable study population.

The IRB must carefully consider the distinctions between experimentation and treatment. Research involves trying new interventions of unknown benefit and risk, whereas standard practice involves tested procedures with known benefits and risks. This gives rise to problematic situations, particularly in the instance when seriously ill patients are being treated, as in emergency rooms and intensive care units, wherein the pressures of time and medical urgency diminish the ability of an investigator to fully explain the purposes of his research. One must always be aware of this and of the fact that much of what is called standard treatment has not yet met the test of randomized clinical trials. Whether an intervention is research or standard practice can be determined by answering a series of questions, such as whether or not there is an intent to advance knowledge, whether patients will be randomized, whether there is an intent to disseminate the results, or whether the intervention deviates from standard practice. Research is more tightly regulated than practice because experimental interventions raise more serious ethical issues than standard practice. In general, being a research subject is more risky than being a patient. Research differs from standard practice, in that the physician has serious conflicts of interest.

Potential for Conflicts of Interest for an IRB

An IRB, as an entity or through individual members, may also suffer from conflicts of interest. For example, various members may have financial relationships with a sponsor, such as significant stock ownership, funding for other research protocols, or employment positions. An IRB member might be in competition with a fellow researcher, either financially or academically. As an entity, an IRB may be biased by the current or potential level of support provided by the sponsor to the institution. A researcher, through the size of his funding sources or his position in the organization, may have undue influence over the IRB. When these influences cannot be effectively removed from the deliberation of an IRB, then consideration should be given to having an outside IRB consider the research proposal.

Further discussion of this topic is in Chapter Nine.

. . . .

THE ETHICS OF PLACEBO IN HUMAN RESEARCH

Placebo is defined as a chemically inert substance given in the guise of medicine for its psychologically suggestive effect. A placebo may be used in controlled clinical trials to determine whether improvement and side effects reflect imagination or anticipation rather than actual power of a drug. The ethical ambiguities of the comparison of a study drug with a placebo, or no treatment, in lieu of a comparison with a known therapeutic agent should be discussed with a research participant. Many ethicists argue that a placebo is never an appropriate part of a clinical trial because it violates the duty of honesty by the researcher. Many participants do not appreciate that they may be in the placebo group. (See Reicken et al., "Informed consent to biomedical research in

Veteran's Administration hospitals," and Appelbaum, "False hopes and best data: Consent to research and the therapeutic misconception." A participant's health should never be placed at risk by giving a placebo. To this end, most ethics codes mandate that when a proven therapy is available, a placebo should not be used. Historical controls should be used. As will be discussed in Chapter Eighteen, much controversy has arisen over whether this standard should be observed in countries where the proven therapy is not readily available.

Weijer (1997) has developed the following criteria for when a non-validated treatment may be compared to a placebo control:

1. No standard therapy exists

2. Standard therapy exists but it has been shown to be no better than placebo

3. Standard therapy is placebo

4. Standard therapy is toxic and of marginal benefit

5. Validated treatment exists but is not available because of cost or limited supplies

The last point remains controversial.

References

Applebaum. (1995). "False hopes and best data: Consent to research and the therapeutic misconception." Hastings Center Report.

Beauchamp. (1994). *The 'Four Principles' Approach"* in Gillon, *Principles of Healthcare Ethics.*

Beecher, H. K. "Ethics and Clinical Research." New England Journal of Medicine. 74 (1966) 1354–1360.

Council for International Organizations of Medical Sciences. (1993). *International Ethical Guidelines for Biomedical Research Involving Human Subjects.* Geneva, Switzerland.

Emanuel, E. J., Wendler, D., Grady, C. (2000). "What Makes Clinical Research Ethical?" *JAMA* 283: 2701–2711.

Fost, N. "Ethical Dilemmas in Medical Innovation and Research: Distinguishing Experimentation from Practice Seminars in Perinatology." 22 (1998) 223–232.

Halpern, Karlawish, and Berlin. (2002). "The Continuing Unethical Conduct of Underpowered Clinical Trials," *JAMA* 288: 358–362.

Hayny, M. "Ethics Committee, Principles and Consequences." Journal of Medical Ethics. 24 (1998) 81–85.

Heifetz, Ethics in Medicine. (1996).

Kagarish, M. J., Sheldon, G. F. "Translational Ethics: A Perspective for the New Millinium." Archive of Surgery. 135: 39–45. January 2000.

National Commission for the Protection of Human Subjects of Research (1979). *The Belmont Report: Ethical Principles and Guidelines for the Protection of Human Subjects of Research.* Washington, D.C.: U.S. Government Printing Office.

National Institutes of Health, Draft Statement on Sharing Research Data (March 2002), http://grants1.nih.gov/grants/policy/data_sharing/index.htm

NIH database on ethics in clinical research: http://www.nlm.nih.gov/pubs/cbm/hum_exp.html#10

The Nuremberg Code. 1947.

Reicken et al. "Informed Consent to Biomedical Research in Veterans Administration Hospitals." *JAMA* 248: 344–350. (1982).

Rothman, D. J. *Strangers at the Bedside*. Basic Book. 1991.

Veotch, R. M. "Medical Ethics." Jones and Bartlett, 2nd Edition. 1997.

Weijer. (1997). "The Placebo Effect [Response]," *CMAJ;* 157: 1019.

Weijer et al. (1997). "Bioethics for Clinicians: 10, Research Ethics." *CMAJ,* 156: 1153–1157.

World Medical Association (1964). Code of Ethics, *Declaration of Helsinki*: Recommendations Guiding Medical Doctors in Biomedical Research Involving Human Subjects. Revised, 2000.

Zion, D., Gillem, L., and Loff, B. "The Declaration of Helsinki, CIOMS and the Ethics of Research on Vulnerable Populations." Nature Medicine. 6(6): 615–617. June 2000.

18

International Research

American Investigator Compliance with U.S. Regulations When
Conducting Research Outside the United States 535
The Guidelines for Good Clinical Practice (GCP) 536
The International Ethical Guidelines for Biomedical
Research Involving Human Subjects 536
Controversial Issues for American Researchers Conducting
Clinical Trials Outside the United States 538
The Role of an American IRB in International Research 539
Concerns That an American IRB Should Consider
When Reviewing an Overseas Study 539
Concerns That a Sponsor or Investigator Should Consider
in Conducting a Study Outside the United States 539
FDA Consideration of Data Collected Outside
the United States in Support of an IND or IDE 539
Proposals as to Research Conducted Outside
the United States by American Scientists 540
References 540

American scientists often find themselves participating in international research activities. This may take the form of research taking place simultaneously at several different locations around the world or research being conducted solely at non–U.S. sites. What regulations apply to such projects? What regulations apply to clinical investigations of a drug by an American company at a foreign site? The answer may vary depending on the surrounding circumstances.

American Investigator Compliance with U.S. Regulations When Conducting Research Outside the United States

If the American investigator's study is being conducted or funded by a U.S. government agency, then the investigator must comply with the federal agency's guidelines regardless of the physical location of all or part of the study. If the agency has not adopted the U.S. Federal Policy for the Protection of Human Subjects ("The Common Rule") (e.g. 45 CFR Part 46), then the study protocol should comply with internationally recognized standards for the protection of human subjects. Variance from the Common Rule may be approved by a federal agency if the procedures in the foreign country afford protections that are at least equivalent to those in the Common Rule (45 CFR §46.101(h)). HHS requires that written policies and procedures implementing international standards, such as *The Declaration of Helsinki* or *The Nuremberg Code,* must be submitted for review to determine if "protections that are at least equivalent" actually exist (OPRR, *Institutional Review Board Guidebook*).

Research that is not funded or conducted by a federal agency may still be subject to U.S. regulations under an institution's Assurance (see Chapter Nine). This may bind the investigator to complying with U.S. regulations even when actually conducting research in another country. The institution may face disciplinary action for a faculty member's research conducted abroad. Pharmaceutical research almost always will need to comply with U.S. regulations or their equivalent in order to obtain FDA marketing approval.

An emerging question is the reach of accreditation programs by organizations such as Association for Accreditation of Human Research Protection Programs (AAHRPP) and Partnership for Human Research Protection (PHRP). Application of U.S. accreditation programs in other countries may raise many further questions and major administrative burdens.

The Guidelines for Good Clinical Practice (GCP)

The International Conference for Harmonisation (ICH) is sponsored by the European Commission, the European Federation of Pharmaceutical Industries Associations, the Japanese Ministry of Health and Welfare, the Japanese Pharmaceutical Manufacturers Association, the Centers for Drug Evaluation and Research and Biologics Evaluation and Research of the U.S. Food and Drug Administration, and the Pharmaceutical Research and Manufacturers of America to standardize pharmaceutical product development in the European Union, the United States, and Japan. The goal is to bring international uniformity in the pharmaceutical industry, including the conduct of investigational drug trials. Toward this end, ICH has generated the Guidelines for Good Clinical Practice (GCP). Compliance with GCP is generally considered to be a minimum for meeting the ethical and regulatory requirements of American research, as they reflect the current position of the FDA (1997). Most nations have adopted or recognized GCP as the baseline for study design, conduct, and reporting. However, a researcher should be careful to seek out any local variations.

The International Ethical Guidelines for Biomedical Research Involving Human Subjects

The Council for International Organizations of Medical Sciences (CIOMS) published *The International Ethical Guidelines for Biomedical Research Involving Human Subjects* in 1993. Draft revisions were being considered in 2001 and are included in this discussion. The guidelines use *The Declaration of Helsinki* as its primary basis but address concerns not discussed in most regulatory schemes.

Guideline 6 is notable for stating that "the sponsor and the researcher must make every effort to ensure that the research is responsive to the health needs and the priorities of the population or community in which it is to be carried out; and any product developed will be made reasonably available to that population or community." The commentary to the guideline states that it is unethical to conduct research on a new product in a population that is unlikely to have the marketed product reasonably available.

The guidelines also address the use of placebo-controlled studies. Guideline 7 repeats the common observation that placebo or no-treatment control groups should not be used where effective treatment is known. However, the commentary notes two sound scientific and ethical reasons for departing from this mandate: "1) withholding the best current treatment will result in only temporary discomfort and no serious adverse consequences; and 2) a comparative study of two treatments will yield no reliable scientific results." The commentary then tackles the hotly debated issue of whether "best current therapeutic method" is that of a technologically developed country or of the host country:

> In some such cases it may be appropriate to compare the new inexpensive alternative with a locally available product rather than with the locally unavailable "best proven therapeutic method." Although there is no general agreement on this point, there are commentators who have concluded that in such circumstances use of a control other than the best current method is justified if: 1) the scientific and ethical review committees in both the country of the sponsoring institution and the host country determine that use of the best current method as a control would be likely to invalidate the results of the research or make the results inapplicable in the host country; 2) plans to make the therapeutic product reasonably available in the host country or community are securely established; and 3) a process of planning and negotiation, including justification of a study in regard to local healthcare needs, has taken place with the health authorities in the host country before the research begins.

The commentary to Guideline 8, which generally addresses informed consent, discusses the issue of genetic sampling:

> Studies of genetic variation should be conducted only after consultation with the communities or subpopulations that may be liable to stigmatization or otherwise harmed as a result of the information obtained; the communities or subpopulations concerned must have identifiable leadership. In all cases, however, the consent of the individual subjects must be obtained.
>
> Studies of particular genetic diseases also require the consent of the individual. Community consultation may be appropriate, but in no case may community consultation or permission substitute for, or override, individual informed consent.

Guideline 11 describes that a participant may be paid for the inconvenience and time spent. However, the guideline forbids payments or other inducements that are so great as to induce consent by an individual against his better judgment. The commentary acknowledges that what is unacceptable recompense is very subjective. For example, an unemployed person or a student may find $100 to be significant while a researcher may not. "Monetary and in-kind recompense must, therefore, be evaluated in the light of the traditions of the particular culture and population in which they are offered, to determine whether they constitute undue influence." To avoid exploitation of incompetent persons, the commentary states that a guardian should not be offered any remuneration beyond out-of-pocket expenses. The selective recruitment of impoverished people to participate in studies simply because they can be more easily induced to enroll for small payments is unjust, observes the commentary to Guideline 12. Subject to some controversy, Guideline 20 states that research participants are entitled to free medical care and such other assistance as would compensate them equitably for any impairment suffered as a result of a study. In the case of death, this would include compensation to dependants. Only explicit waiver by the ethics review committee would limit the participant's right to compensation. The commentary to Guideline 20 places the obligation to pay on the sponsor, whether it is a pharmaceutical company, a government, or an institution.

In considering special populations, Guideline 16 mandates that women of reproductive age should not be generally excluded from participating in biomedical research. However, potential effects on a fetus if a participant were to become pregnant during the study should be considered in the research protocol. The commentary goes on to further water down the guideline by stating: "The exclusion of such women can be justified only on such grounds as evidence *or suspicion* that a particular drug or vaccine is liable to cause deformities, other birth defects, or mutations" (emphasis added). With the overwhelming fear in the United States of potential teratogenic effects of almost any substance, a researcher could likely maneuver to exclude women in virtually any study.

The sponsor and researcher, under Guideline 21, have an obligation to help the local venue develop capacity for ethical and scientific review of biomedical research. This mandate is intended to curb the perception that sponsors and researchers seek out less-developed countries to avoid regulatory systems and thus avoid the expense of compliance. Guideline 23 also places an obligation on external sponsors to provide facilities and personnel to make healthcare services available to the population from which the research participants are recruited. It also invites consideration of whether the sponsor should be required to continue the services after the study is completed.

Controversial Issues for American Researchers Conducting Clinical Trials Outside the United States

American researchers have drawn strong criticism for several studies in developing nations that have received publicity. One is the use of observational studies in third-world nations for diseases that are treated in developed nations. For example, researchers observed couples in Uganda where one partner was known to be HIV positive. The infected partner was not treated. Researchers contended that the local population could not afford the available therapies, which were proved to be effective only after the end of the study.

Second is use of no treatment as the control arm of studies in undeveloped countries when accepted treatment would be the standard control in developed nations. For example, researchers conducted an HIV treatment trial in Thailand where the control was placebo.

Third is the use of investigational drugs in third-world nations before adequate safety and efficacy studies have been completed. For example, Doctors without Borders chastised Pfizer for sending a medical team to treat a meningitis epidemic in Nigeria with a promising but untested antibiotic. Pfizer countered that 176 of the 187 treated patients survived. This was in stark contrast to the more than 15,000 Africans that died in the epidemic, even when receiving traditional care as offered by the Doctors without Borders. Recently a university was criticized for running a clinical study using an anticancer drug (an antioxidant) that had been removed from the list of Generally Recognized as Safe substances.

A continuing debate is what standard of medical care should be used as the control for a study: the local healthcare available or the best healthcare available? In developing nations, expensive medications, such as "combination therapy" for treating AIDS, is not readily available or affordable. Some commentators contend that the local standard of care is determined by the prices set by Western pharmaceutical companies. After a new therapy is developed through use of the citizens of a developing nation, does the manufacturer have an obligation to provide that product to the developing country at an affordable price? Should care continue to be provided to participants even after the study terminates?

The Role of an American IRB in International Research

An IRB is responsible for all studies conducted by the institution. The institution's Assurance usually affirms this, and the mandate includes studies conducted at off-site locations. Many universities have been chagrined to find out that research conducted overseas by faculty members must have the same approval process as domestic studies. In some circumstances, the institution's IRB must approve a study as well as a local ethics committee.

The World Health Organization has developed "Operational Guidelines for Ethics Committees That Review Biomedical Research" (2000). The stated objective of the Operational Guidelines is to contribute to the development of quality and consistency in the ethical review of biomedical research. Unfortunately, it does not have the specificity of the U.S. regulations.

Concerns That an American IRB Should Consider When Reviewing an Overseas Study

At first blush, a study being conducted at a non–U.S. site would be the same as a domestic study. However, a non–U.S. study brings additional ethical issues to be considered. For example, how does the proposed population from which participants will be recruited compare with those who will be the end-users? How will informed consent be ensured using the local language and customs? What is reasonable compensation for participation: the local wage or the American wage? Will the control group be treated with the medical standard locally or that found in developed countries? What medical care will be made available to participants during the study? Is the motive for conducting the study outside the United States ethically sound? Does any physiological difference exist between the study population and the end-users? What recourse will a participant have if he is injured by the study?

Concerns That a Sponsor or Investigator Should Consider in Conducting a Study Outside the United States

A sponsor or investigator should consider all local law, insurance coverage, and product liability issues before initiating a study anywhere. This requires even more deliberation when a study is being organized outside the home venue of the sponsor or investigator. As well, the sponsor and investigator should consider the issues listed above for IRBs.

FDA Consideration of Data Collected Outside the United States in Support of an IND or IDE

The FDA (21 CFR §312.120(a); §312.120(c)) will accept data on safety and efficacy from foreign clinical studies for Investigational New Drug (IND) or Investigational Device Exemption (IDE) of market approval applications if the studies are

- Well designed
- Done by qualified investigators

- Carefully performed
- Conducted in accordance with the world community's ethical principles (*The Revised Declaration of Helsinki*) or the laws and regulations of the country in which the studies were carried out, whichever offers individuals the most protection

However, "[b]ecause IND and IDE studies are intended, from the outset, to be reported to FDA to support marketing in the United States, the Agency requires that all such studies meet the regulations which have been established under standards of this country. FDA does not accept a lesser level of human subject protection for studies solely because they are to be conducted at foreign sites" (FDA, Information Sheets, 1998 Update). Thus, FDA standards for conducting research must be met regardless of where the study is conducted. Compliance with GCP is a good starting point. The OIG has criticized pharmaceutical companies and contract research organizations for rapidly expanding clinical trials to countries that have limited experience and expertise in protecting human participants (OIG, "The Globalization of Clinical Trials: A Growing Challenge in Protecting Human Subjects").

Proposals as to Research Conducted Outside the United States by American Scientists

The National Bioethics Advisory Commission (2000) has proposed that:

1. American researchers conducting drug trials in foreign countries should offer treatment of participants even after the research has ended.
2. Participants in the control group should be offered "an established, effective treatment," even if such treatment is not readily available in the host country.
3. Any research in a foreign country should deal with its health needs and directly benefit local residents.
4. Researchers should confront the question of how to make any drug developed from a study available to "some or all of the host country."
5. A study should not be done outside the United States solely for the sake of research or because it is easier to perform outside the United States.

References

Council for International Organizations of Medical Sciences (CIOMS). (2001). International Ethical Guidelines for Biomedical Research Involving Human Subjects (Draft revisions, 2001) [http://www.cioms.ch/draftguidelines_may_2001.htm]; (1993 Guidelines) [http://www.cioms.ch/frame_1993_texts_of_guidelines.htm].

FDA, *Federal Register:* May 9, 1997. (Volume 62, Number 90).

International Conference in Harmonization (ICH), Guidelines for Good Clinical Practice (GCP) [http://www.ifpma.org/pdfifpma/e6.pdf].

McLemee, "Federal Agency Criticizes Harvard U. Studies Involving Human Subjects in China." The Chronicle of Higher Education, April 1, 2002.

National Bioethics Advisory Commission. (2000). "Ethical & Policy Issues in International Research."

OHRP, Letters to Harvard University's School of Public Health, Brigham & Women's Hospital and The Massachusetts Mental Health Center, March 28, 2002, cited in *Washington Fax,* April 3, 2002.

OIG. (2001). The Globilization of Clinical Trials: A Growing Challenge in Protecting Human Subjects (OEI-01-00-00190).

OPRR, Institutional Review Board Guidebook, Section K.

Stephens, Flaherty, and Nelson. "The Body Hunters: Testing Drugs on the World," *Washington Post*. December 17–December 22, 2000.

The World Health Organization. (2000). Operational Guidelines for Ethics Committees That Review Biomedical Research. [http://www.who.int/tdr/publications/publications/pdf/ethics.pdf].

Glossary

This is a compilation of terms used in clinical research regulation. The primary source of these definitions is glossaries created by the involved government agencies, particularly the predecessor of the Office of Human Research Protection.

ABUSE-LIABLE Pharmacological substances that have the potential for creating abusive dependency. Abuse-liable substances can include both illicit drugs (heroine) and licit drugs (methamphetamines).

ADAMHA Alcohol, Drug Abuse, and Mental Health Administration; reorganized in October 1992 as the Substance Abuse and Mental Health Services Administration (SAMHSA). ADAMHA included the National Institute of Mental Health (NIMH), the National Institute on Alcohol Abuse and Alcoholism (NIAAA), the National Institute on Drug Abuse (NIDA), the Office for Substance Abuse Prevention (OSAP), and the Office for Treatment Intervention (OTI). NIMH, NIAAA, and NIDA are now part of the National Institutes of Health (NIH). (*See also SAMHSA.*)

ADJUVANT THERAPY Therapy provided to enhance the effect of a primary therapy; auxiliary therapy.

ADVERSE EFFECT An undesirable and unintended, although not necessarily unexpected, result of therapy or other intervention (headache following spinal tap or intestinal bleeding associated with aspirin therapy).

ASSENT Agreement by an individual not competent to give legally valid informed consent (a child or cognitively impaired person) to participate in research.

ASSURANCE A formal written, binding commitment that is submitted to a federal agency in which an institution promises to comply with applicable regulations governing research with human subjects and stipulates the procedures through which compliance will be achieved (45 CFR §46.103).

AUTHORIZED INSTITUTIONAL OFFICIAL An officer of an institution with the authority to speak for and legally commit the institution to adherence to the requirements of the federal regulations regarding the involvement of human subjects in biomedical and behavioral research.

AUTONOMY Personal capacity to consider alternatives, make choices, and act without undue influence or interference of others.

AUTOPSY Examination by dissection of the body of an individual to determine cause of death and other medically relevant facts.

BELMONT REPORT, THE A statement of basic ethical principles governing research involving human subjects issued by the National Commission for the Protection of Human Subjects in 1978.

BENEFICENCE An ethical principle discussed in *The Belmont Report* that entails an obligation to protect persons from harm. The principle of beneficence can be expressed in two general rules: (1) do not harm; and (2) protect from harm by maximizing possible benefits and minimizing possible risks of harm.

BENEFIT A valued or desired outcome; an advantage.

BIOLOGIC Any therapeutic serum, toxin, antitoxin, or analogous microbial product applicable to the prevention, treatment, or cure of diseases or injuries.

BLIND STUDY DESIGNS *See Masked Study Designs; Double-Masked Design;* and *Single-Masked Design.*

CADAVER The body of a deceased person.

CASE-CONTROL STUDY A study comparing persons with a given condition or disease (the cases) and persons without the condition or disease (the controls) with respect to antecedent factors. (*See also Retrospective Studies.*)

CAT SCAN Computerized Axial Tomography, an X-ray technique for producing images of internal bodily structures through the assistance of a computer.

CDC Centers for Disease Control and Prevention; an agency within the Public Health Service, Department of Health and Human Services.

CHILDREN Persons who have not attained the legal age for consent to treatment or procedures involved in the research, as determined under the applicable law of the jurisdiction in which the research will be conducted (45 CFR §46.401(a)).

CLASS I, II, III, DEVICES Classification by the Food and Drug Administration of medical devices according to potential risks or hazards.

CLINICAL TRIAL A controlled study involving human subjects, designed to evaluate prospectively the safety and effectiveness of new drugs or devices or of behavioral interventions.

CENTER FOR MEDICARE & MEDICAID SERVICES (CMS): The agency within HHS that administers Medicare & Medicaid. Formerly known as HCFA.

COGNITIVELY IMPAIRED Having either a psychiatric disorder (psychosis, neurosis, personality or behavior disorders, or dementia) or a developmental disorder (mental retardation) that affects cognitive or emotional functions to the extent that capacity for judgment and reasoning is significantly diminished. Others, including persons under the influence of or dependent on drugs or alcohol, those suffering from degenerative diseases affecting the brain, terminally ill patients, and persons with severely disabling physical handicaps, may also be compromised in their ability to make decisions in their best interests.

COHORT A group of subjects initially identified as having one or more characteristics in common who are followed over time. In social science research, this term may refer to any group of persons who are born at about the same time and share common historical or cultural experiences.

COMMON RULE The federal policy that provides regulations for the involvement of human subjects in research. The Policy applies to all research involving human subjects conducted, supported, or otherwise subject to regulation by any federal department or agency that takes appropriate administrative action to make the Policy applicable to such research. Currently, sixteen federal agencies have adopted the Federal Policy. The DHHS version of this is found at 45 CFR Part 46.

COMPENSATION Payment or medical care provided to subjects injured in research; does not refer to payment (remuneration) for participation in research. (*Compare Remuneration.*)

COMPETENCE Technically, a legal term, used to denote capacity to act on one's own behalf; the ability to understand information presented, to appreciate the consequences of acting (or not acting) on that information, and to make a choice. (*See also Incompetence; Incapacity.*)

CONFIDENTIALITY Pertains to the treatment of information that an individual has disclosed in a relationship of trust and with the expectation that it will not be divulged to others without permission in ways that are inconsistent with the understanding of the original disclosure.

CONSENT *See Informed Consent.*

CONTRACT An agreement; as used here, an agreement that a specific research activity will be performed at the request, and under the direction, of the agency providing the funds. Research performed under contract is more closely controlled by the agency than research performed under a grant. (*Compare: Grant.*)

CONTRACT RESEARCH ORGANIZATION (CRO): An entity that conducts clinical trials usually for a pharmaceutical company.

CONTROL (SUBJECTS) or **CONTROLS** Subjects used for comparison who are not given a treatment under study or who do not have a given condition, background, or risk factor that is the object of study. Control conditions may be concurrent (occurring more or less simultaneously with the condition under study) or historical (preceding the condition under study). When the present condition of subjects is compared with their own condition on a prior regimen or treatment, the study is considered historically controlled.

CONTRAINDICATED Disadvantageous, perhaps dangerous; a treatment that should not be used in certain individuals or conditions due to risks (a drug may be contraindicated for pregnant women and persons with high blood pressure).

CORRELATION COEFFICIENT A statistical index of the degree of relationship between two variables. Values of correlation coefficients range from −1.00 through zero to +1.00. A correlation coefficient of 0.00 indicates no relationship between the variables. Correlations approaching −1.00 or +1.00 indicate strong relationships between the variables. However, causal inferences about the relationship between two variables can never be made on the basis of correlation coefficients, no matter how strong a relationship is indicated.

CROSS-OVER DESIGN A type of clinical trial in which each subject experiences, at different times, both the experimental and control therapy. For example, half of the subjects might be randomly assigned first to the control group and then to the experimental intervention, while the other half would have the sequence reversed.

DATA AND SAFETY MONITORING BOARD (DSMB) A committee of scientists, physicians, statisticians, and others that collects and analyzes data during the course of a clinical trial to monitor for adverse effects and other trends (such as an indication that one treatment is significantly better than another, particularly when one arm of the trial involves a placebo control) that would warrant modification or termination of the trial or notification of subjects about new information that might affect their willingness to continue in the trial.

DEAD FETUS An expelled or delivered fetus that exhibits no heartbeat, spontaneous respiratory activity, spontaneous movement of voluntary muscles, or pulsation of the umbilical cord (if still attached) (45 CFR §46.203(f)). Generally, some organs, tissues, and cells (referred to collectively as fetal tissue) remain alive for varying periods of time after the total organism is dead.

DEBRIEFING Giving subjects previously undisclosed information about the research project following completion of their participation in research. (Note that this usage, which occurs within the behavioral sciences, departs from standard English, in which debriefing is obtaining rather than imparting information.)

DECLARATION OF HELSINKI A code of ethics for clinical research approved by the World Medical Association in 1964 and widely adopted by medical associations in various countries. It was revised several times, most recently in Edinburgh, 2001.

DEPARTMENT OF APPEALS BOARD (DAB) An administrative hearing panel that reviews any ORI determination of scientific misconduct involving research (57 *Fed. Reg.* 53125 (1992)). It conducts a trial-like hearing at which HHS has the burden of proving scientific misconduct by a preponderance of the evidence (59 *Fed. Reg.* 29809, 29811 (1994)).

DEPENDENT VARIABLES The outcomes that are measured in an experiment. Dependent variables are expected to change as a result of an experimental manipulation of the independent variable(s).

DESCRIPTIVE STUDY Any study that is not truly experimental (*e.g.*, quasi-experimental studies, correlational studies, record reviews, case histories, and observational studies).

DEVICE (MEDICAL) *See Medical Device.*

DIAGNOSTIC (PROCEDURE) Tests used to identify a disorder or disease in a living person.

DOUBLE-MASKED DESIGN A study design in which neither the investigators nor the subjects know the treatment group assignments of individual subjects. Sometimes referred to as "double-blind."

DRUG Any chemical compound that may be used on or administered to humans as an aid in the diagnosis, treatment, cure, mitigation, or prevention of disease or other abnormal conditions.

EMANCIPATED MINOR A legal status conferred upon persons who have not yet attained the age of legal competency as defined by state law (for such purposes as consenting to medical care), but who are entitled to treatment as if they had by virtue of assuming adult responsibilities such as being self-supporting and not living at home, marriage, or procreation. (*See also Mature Minor.*)

EMBRYO Early stages of a developing organism, broadly used to refer to stages immediately following fertilization of an egg through implantation and very early pregnancy (from conception to the eighth week of pregnancy). (*See also Fetus.*)

EPIDEMIOLOGY A scientific discipline that studies the factors determining the causes, frequency, and distribution of diseases in a community or given population.

EQUITABLE Fair or just; used in the context of selection of subjects to indicate that the benefits and burdens of research are fairly distributed (45 CFR §46.111(a)(3)).

ETHICS ADVISORY BOARD An interdisciplinary group that advises the Secretary, HHS, on general policy matters and on research proposals (or classes of proposals) that pose ethical problems.

ETHNOGRAPHIC RESEARCH Ethnography is the study of people and their culture. Ethnographic research, also called fieldwork, involves observation of and interaction with the persons or group being studied in the group's own environment, often for long periods of time. (*See also Fieldwork.*)

EXPANDED AVAILABILITY Policy and procedure that permits individuals who have serious or life-threatening diseases for which there are no alternative therapies to have access to investigational drugs and devices that may be beneficial to them. Examples of expanded availability mechanisms include Treatment INDs, Parallel Track, and open study protocols.

EXPEDITED REVIEW Review of proposed research by the IRB chair or a designated voting member or group of voting members rather than by the entire IRB. Federal rules permit expedited review for certain kinds of research involving no more than minimal risk and for minor changes in approved research (45 CFR §46.110).

EXPERIMENTAL Term often used to denote a therapy (drug, device, procedure) that is unproven or not yet scientifically validated with respect to safety and efficacy. A procedure may be considered "experimental" without necessarily being part of a formal study (research) to evaluate its usefulness. (*See also Research.*)

EXPERIMENTAL STUDY A true experimental study is one in which subjects are randomly assigned to groups that experience carefully controlled interventions manipulated by the experimenter according to a strict logic allowing causal inference about the effects of the interventions under investigation. (*See also Quasi-Experimental Study.*)

FALSE NEGATIVE When a test wrongly shows an effect or condition to be absent (that a woman is not pregnant when, in fact, she is).

FALSE POSITIVE When a test wrongly shows an effect or condition to be present (that a woman is pregnant when, in fact, she is not).

FDA Food and Drug Administration; an agency of the federal government established by Congress in 1912 to improve safety and purity under the Food, Drug & Cosmetic Act and presently part of the Department of Health and Human Services.

FETAL MATERIAL The placenta, amniotic fluid, fetal membranes, and umbilical cord.

FETUS The product of conception from the time of implantation until delivery. If the delivered or expelled fetus is viable, it is designated an infant (45 CFR §46.203(c)). The term "fetus" generally refers to later phases of development; the term "embryo" is usually used for earlier phases of development. (*See also Embryo.*)

FIELDWORK Behavioral, social, or anthropological research involving the study of persons or groups in their own environment and without manipulation for research purposes (distinguished from laboratory or controlled settings). (*See also Ethnographic Research.*)

510(K) DEVICE A medical device that is considered substantially equivalent to a device that was or is being legally marketed. A sponsor planning to market such a device must submit notification to the FDA ninety days in advance of placing the device on the market. If the FDA concurs with the sponsor, the device may then be marketed. 510(k) is the section of the Food, Drug & Cosmetic Act that describes premarket notification; hence the designation "510(k) device."

FRAUD & ABUSE: A term usually applied to violations of federal healthcare regulations.

FULL BOARD REVIEW Review of proposed research at a convened meeting at which a majority of the membership of the IRB are present, including at least one member whose primary concerns are in nonscientific areas. For the research to be approved, it must receive the approval of a majority of those members present at the meeting (45 CFR §46.108).

GENE THERAPY The treatment of genetic disease accomplished by altering the genetic structure of either somatic (nonreproductive) or germline (reproductive) cells.

GENERAL ASSURANCE Obsolete term, previously used to denote an institutional Assurance covering multiple research projects. (*See also Assurance.*)

GENERAL CONTROLS Certain FDA statutory provisions designed to control the safety of marketed drugs and devices. The general controls include provisions on adulteration, misbranding, banned devices, good manufacturing practices, notification and record keeping, and other sections of the Medical Device Amendments to the Food, Drug & Cosmetic Act (21 U.S. Code §360(c) (Food, Drug & Cosmetic Act §513)).

GENETIC SCREENING Tests to identify persons who have an inherited predisposition to a certain phenotype or who are at risk of producing offspring with inherited diseases or disorders.

GENOTYPE The genetic constitution of an individual.

GRANT Financial support provided for research study designed and proposed by the principal investigator(s). The granting agency exercises no direct control over the conduct of approved research supported by a grant. (*Compare Contract.*)

GUARDIAN An individual who is authorized under applicable state or local law to give permission on behalf of a child to general medical care (45 CFR §46.402(3)).

HELSINKI DECLARATION *See Declaration of Helsinki.*

HHS A federal agency: U.S. Department of Health and Human Services; formerly the Department of Health, Education and Welfare (DHEW).

HIPAA Health Insurance Portability & Accountability Act of 1996.

HISTORICAL CONTROLS Control subjects (followed at some time in the past or for whom data are available through records) who are used for comparison with subjects being treated concurrently. The study is considered historically controlled when the present condition of subjects is compared with their own condition on a prior regimen or treatment.

HUMAN IN VITRO FERTILIZATION Any fertilization involving human sperm and ova that occurs outside the human body.

HUMAN SUBJECTS Individuals whose physiologic or behavioral characteristics and responses are the object of study in a research project. Under the federal regulations, human subjects are defined as living individual(s) about whom an investigator conducting research obtains (1) data through intervention or interaction with the individual; or (2) identifiable private information (45 CFR §46.102(f)).

IDE *See Investigational Device Exemptions.*

INCAPACITY Refers to a person's mental status and means inability to understand information presented, to appreciate the consequences of acting (or not acting) on that information, and to make a choice. Often used as a synonym for incompetence. (*See also Incompetence.*)

INCOMPETENCE Technically, a legal term meaning inability to manage one's own affairs. Often used as a synonym for incapacity. (*See also Incapacity.*)

IND *See Investigational New Drug or Device.*

INDEPENDENT VARIABLES The conditions of an experiment that are systematically manipulated by the investigator.

INFORMED CONSENT A person's voluntary agreement, based upon adequate knowledge and understanding of relevant information, to participate in research or to undergo a diagnostic, therapeutic, or preventive procedure. In giving informed consent, subjects may not waive or appear to waive any of their legal rights, or release or appear to release the investigator, the sponsor, the institution, or agents thereof from liability for negligence (Federal Policy §116; 21 CFR §50.20 and §50.25).

INSTITUTION (1) Any public or private entity or agency (including federal, state, and local agencies) (45 CFR §46.102(b)).

INSTITUTION (2) A residential facility that provides food, shelter, and professional services (including treatment, skilled nursing, intermediate or long-term care, and custodial or residential care). Examples include general, mental, or chronic disease hospitals; inpatient community mental health centers; halfway houses and nursing homes; alcohol and drug addiction treatment centers; homes for the aged or dependent; residential schools for the mentally or physically handicapped; and homes for dependent and neglected children.

INSTITUTIONAL REVIEW BOARD A specially constituted review body established or designated by an entity to protect the welfare of human subjects recruited to participate in biomedical or behavioral research (45 CFR §46.102(g), §46.108, §46.109).

INSTITUTIONALIZED Confined, either voluntarily or involuntarily (a hospital, prison, or nursing home).

INSTITUTIONALIZED COGNITIVELY IMPAIRED Persons who are confined, either voluntarily or involuntarily, in a facility for the care of the mentally or otherwise disabled (a psychiatric hospital, home, or school for the retarded).

INVESTIGATIONAL DEVICE EXEMPTIONS (IDE) Exemptions from certain regulations found in the Medical Device Amendments that allow shipment of unapproved devices for use in clinical investigations (21 CFR §812.20).

INVESTIGATIONAL NEW DRUG OR DEVICE A drug or device permitted by the FDA to be tested in humans but not yet determined to be safe and effective for a particular use in the general population and not yet licensed for marketing.

INVESTIGATOR In clinical trials, an individual who actually conducts an investigation (21 CFR §312.3). Any interventions (such as drugs) involved in the study are administered to subjects under the immediate direction of the investigator. (*See also Principal Investigator.*)

IN VITRO Literally, "in glass" or "test tube"; used to refer to processes that are carried out outside the living body, usually in the laboratory, as distinguished from in vivo.

IN VIVO Literally, "in the living body"; processes, such as the absorption of a drug by the human body, carried out in the living body rather than in a laboratory (in vitro).

IRB *See Institutional Review Board.*

JUSTICE An ethical principle discussed in *The Belmont Report* requiring fairness in distribution of burdens and benefits; often expressed in terms of treating persons of similar circumstances or characteristics similarly.

LACTATION The period of time during which a woman is providing her breast milk to an infant or child.

LEGALLY AUTHORIZED REPRESENTATIVE A person authorized either by statute or by court appointment to make decisions on behalf of another person. In human subjects research, an individual or judicial or other body authorized under applicable law to consent on behalf of a prospective subject to the subject's participation in the procedure(s) involved in the research (45 CFR §46.102(c)).

LOD SCORE An expression of the probability that a gene and a marker are linked.

LONGITUDINAL STUDY A study designed to follow subjects forward through time.

MASKED STUDY DESIGNS Study designs comparing two or more interventions in which either the investigators, the subjects, or some combination thereof do not know the treatment group assignments of individual subjects. Sometimes called "blind" study designs. (*See also Double-Masked Design; Single-Masked Design.*)

MATURE MINOR Someone who has not reached adulthood (as defined by state law) but who may be treated as an adult for certain purposes (consenting to medical care). Note that a mature minor is not necessarily an emancipated minor. (*See also Emancipated Minor.*)

MEDICAL DEVICE A diagnostic or therapeutic article that does not achieve any of its principal intended purposes through chemical action within or on the body. Such devices include diagnostic test kits, crutches, electrodes, pacemakers, arterial grafts, intraocular lenses, and orthopedic pins or other orthopedic equipment.

MEDICAL DEVICE AMENDMENTS (MDA) Amendments to the Federal Food, Drug & Cosmetic Act passed in 1976 to regulate the distribution of medical devices and diagnostic products.

MENTALLY DISABLED *See Cognitively Impaired.*

METABOLISM (OF A DRUG) The manner in which a drug is acted upon (taken up, converted to other substances, and excreted) by various organs of the body.

MINIMAL RISK A risk is minimal where the probability and magnitude of harm or discomfort anticipated in the proposed research are not greater, in and of themselves, than those ordinarily encountered in daily life or during the performance of routine physical or psychological examinations or tests (45 CFR §46.102(i)). For example, the risk of drawing a small amount of blood from a healthy individual for research purposes is no greater than the risk of doing so as part of routine physical examination.

The definition of minimal risk for research involving prisoners differs somewhat from that given for noninstitutionalized adults. (See 45 CFR §46.303(d) and OPRR, Guidebook Chapter 6, Section E, "Prisoners.")

MONITORING The collection and analysis of data as the project progresses to ensure the appropriateness of the research, its design, and subject protections.

NATIONAL COMMISSION National Commission for the Protection of Human Subjects of Biomedical and Behavioral Research. An interdisciplinary advisory body, established by Congressional legislation in 1974, which was in existence until 1978, and which issued a series of reports and recommendations on ethical issues in research and medicine, many of which are now embodied in federal regulations.

NDA *See New Drug Application.*

NEW DRUG APPLICATION Request for FDA approval to market a new drug.

NIAAA National Institute on Alcohol Abuse and Alcoholism; an institute in NIH.

NIDA National Institute on Drug Abuse; an institute in NIH.

NIH National Institutes of Health: a federal agency within the Public Health Service of DHHS, comprising twenty-one institutes and centers. It is responsible for carrying out and supporting biomedical and behavioral research.

NIMH National Institute of Mental Health; an institute in NIH.

NONAFFILIATED MEMBER Member of an Institutional Review Board who has no ties to the parent institution, its staff, or faculty. This individual is usually from the local community (minister, business person, attorney, teacher, homemaker).

NONSIGNIFICANT RISK DEVICE An investigational medical device that does not present significant risk to the patient. (*See also Significant Risk Device.*)

NONTHERAPEUTIC RESEARCH Research that has no likelihood or intent of producing a diagnostic, preventive, or therapeutic benefit to the current subjects, although it may benefit subjects with a similar condition in the future.

NONVIABLE FETUS An expelled or delivered fetus which, although it is living, cannot possibly survive to the point of sustaining life independently, even with the support of available medical therapy (45 CFR §46.203(d) and (e)). Although it may be presumed that an expelled or delivered fetus is nonviable at a gestational age less than twenty weeks and weight less than 500 grams (*Federal Register* 40 (August 8, 1975): 33552), a specific determination as to viability must be made by a physician in each instance. (*See also Viable Infant.*)

NORMAL VOLUNTEERS Volunteer subjects used to study normal physiology and behavior or who do not have the condition under study in a particular protocol, used as comparisons with subjects who do have the condition. "Normal" may not mean normal in all respects. For example, patients with broken legs (if not on medication that will affect the results) may serve as normal volunteers in studies of metabolism, cognitive development, and the like. Similarly, patients with heart disease but without diabetes may be the "normals" in a study of diabetes complicated by heart disease.

NULL HYPOTHESIS The proposition, to be tested statistically, that the experimental intervention has "no effect," meaning that the treatment and control groups will not differ as a result of the intervention. Investigators usually hope that the data will demonstrate some effect from the intervention, thereby allowing the investigator to reject the null hypothesis.

NUREMBERG CODE A code of research ethics developed during the trials of Nazi war criminals following World War II and widely adopted as a standard during the 1950s and 1960s for protecting human subjects.

OFFICE FOR HUMAN RESEARCH PROTECTION (OHRP) The office under the Secretary of HHS responsible for implementing HHS regulations (45 CFR Part 46) involving human subjects. OHRP replaced the Office for Protection from Research Risks (OPRR).

OFFICE OF INSPECTOR GENERAL (OIG) The office under the Secretary of HHS provides auditing and consultative services as to the application and enforcement of HHS regulations.

OFFICE FOR PROTECTION OF RESEARCH RISKS (OPRR) The former office within the National Institutes of Health, an agency of the Public Health Service, Department of Health and Human Services, responsible for implementing HHS regulations (45 CFR Part 46) governing research involving human subjects. This office has now been replaced by the Office for Human Research Protection (OHRP) under the Secretary of HHS.

OFFICE OF RESEARCH INTEGRITY (ORI) The office formerly responsible for investigating allegations of scientific misconduct and to take administrative steps to protect the integrity of Public Health Service research (45 CFR §50.102). It replaced the Office of Scientific Integrity in 1992 (52 *Fed. Reg.* §24262 (1992)).

OFFICE OF SCIENTIFIC INTEGRITY (OSI) The office formerly responsible for investigation allegations of scientific misconduct and to take administrative steps to protect the integrity of Public Health Service research. It was succeeded by the Office of Research Integrity in 1992.

OHRP *See Office for Human Research Protection.*

OIG *See Office of Inspector General.*

OPEN DESIGN An experimental design in which both the investigator(s) and the subjects know the treatment group(s) to which subjects are assigned.

OPRR *See Office for Protection of Research Risks.*

PARTNERSHIP FOR HUMAN RESEARCH PROTECTION (PHRP): A joint effort of JACHO and NACQ for accreditation of research programs.

PATERNALISM Making decisions for others against or apart from their wishes with the intent of doing them good.

PERMISSION The agreement of parent(s) or guardian to the participation of their child or ward in research (45 CFR §46.402(c)).

PHARMACOLOGY The scientific discipline that studies the action of drugs on living systems (animals or human beings).

PHASE 1, 2, 3, 4 DRUG TRIALS Different stages of testing drugs in humans, from first application in humans (Phase 1) through limited and broad clinical tests (Phase 3), to postmarketing studies (Phase 4).

PHASE 1 DRUG TRIAL Phase 1 trials include the initial introduction of an investigational new drug into humans. These studies are typically conducted with healthy volunteers; sometimes, where the drug is intended for use in patients with a particular disease, however, such patients may participate as subjects. Phase 1 trials are designed to determine the metabolic and pharmacological actions of the drug in humans, the side effects associated with increasing doses (to establish a safe dose range), and, if possible, to gain early evidence of effectiveness; they are typically closely monitored. The ultimate goal of Phase 1 trials is to obtain sufficient information about the drug's pharmacokinetics and pharmacological effects to permit the design of well-controlled, sufficiently valid Phase 2 studies. Other examples of Phase 1 studies include studies of drug metabolism, structure-activity relationships, and mechanisms of actions in humans, as well as studies in which investigational drugs are used as research tools to explore biological phenomena or disease processes. The total number of subjects involved in Phase 1 investigations is generally in the range of 20–80.

PHASE 2 DRUG TRIAL Phase 2 trials include controlled clinical studies conducted to evaluate the drug's effectiveness for a particular indication in patients with the disease or condition under study, and to determine the common short-term side effects and risks associated with the drug. These studies are typically well-controlled, closely monitored, and conducted with a relatively small number of patients, usually involving no more than several hundred subjects.

PHASE 3 DRUG TRIAL Phase 3 trials involve the administration of a new drug to a larger number of patients in different clinical settings to determine its safety, efficacy, and appropriate dosage. They are performed after preliminary evidence of effectiveness has been obtained, and are intended to gather necessary additional information about effectiveness and safety for evaluating the overall benefit-risk relationship of the drug, and to provide an adequate basis for physician labeling. In Phase 3 studies, the drug is used the way it would be administered when marketed. When these studies are completed and the sponsor believes that the drug is safe and effective under specific conditions, the sponsor applies to the FDA for approval to market the drug. Phase 3 trials usually involve several hundred to several thousand patient-subjects.

PHASE 4 DRUG TRIAL Concurrent with marketing approval, FDA may seek agreement from the sponsor to conduct certain postmarketing (Phase 4) studies to delineate additional information about the drug's risks, benefits, and optimal use. These studies could include, but would not be limited to, studying different doses or schedules of administration than were used in Phase 2 studies, use of the drug in other patient populations or other stages of the disease, or use of the drug over a longer period of time (21 CFR §312.85).

PHENOTYPE The physical manifestation of a gene function.

PHS Public Health Service. Part of the U.S. Department of Health and Human Services, it includes FDA, NIH, CDC, SAMHSA, and HRSA.

PLACEBO A chemically inert substance given in the guise of medicine for its psychologically suggestive effect; used in controlled clinical trials to determine whether improvement and side effects may reflect imagination or anticipation rather than the actual power of a drug.

POSTAMENDMENTS DEVICES Medical devices marketed after enactment of the 1976 Medical Device Amendments.

PREAMENDMENTS DEVICES Medical devices marketed before enactment of the 1976 Medical Device Amendments.

PRECLINICAL INVESTIGATIONS Laboratory and animal studies designed to test the mechanisms, safety, and efficacy of an intervention prior to its applications to humans.

PREDICATE DEVICES Currently legally marketed devices to which new devices may be found substantially equivalent under the 510(k) process.

PREGNANCY The period of time from confirmation of implantation of a fertilized egg within the uterus until the fetus has entirely left the uterus (has been delivered). Implantation is confirmed through a presumptive sign of pregnancy such as missed menses or a positive pregnancy test (45 CFR §46.203(b)). This "confirmation" may be in error, but, for research purposes, investigators would presume that a living fetus was present until evidence to the contrary was clear. Although fertilization occurs a week or more before implantation, the current inability to detect the fertilization event or the presence of a newly fertilized egg makes a definition of pregnancy based on implantation necessary.

PREMARKET APPROVAL (PMA) Process of scientific and regulatory review by the FDA to ensure the safety and effectiveness of Class III devices.

PRESIDENT'S COMMISSION President's Commission for the Study of Ethical Problems in Medicine and Biomedical and Behavioral Research. An interdisciplinary advisory group, established by congressional legislation in 1978, which was in existence until 1983, and which issued reports on ethical problems in healthcare and in research involving human subjects.

PRINCIPAL INVESTIGATOR The scientist or scholar with primary responsibility for the design and conduct of a research project. (*See also Investigator.*)

PRISONER An individual involuntarily confined in a penal institution, including persons (1) sentenced under a criminal or civil statue; (2) detained pending arraignment, trial, or sentencing; and (3) detained in other facilities (for drug detoxification or treatment of alcoholism) under statutes or commitment procedures providing such alternatives to criminal prosecution or incarceration in a penal institution (45 CFR §46.303(c)).

PRIVACY Control over the extent, timing, and circumstances of sharing oneself (physically, behaviorally, or intellectually) with others.

PROBAND The person whose case serves as the stimulus for the study of other members of the family to identify the possible genetic factors involved in a given disease, condition, or characteristic.

PROPHYLACTIC Preventive or protective; a drug, vaccine, regimen, or device designed to prevent, or provide protection against, a given disease or disorder.

PROSPECTIVE STUDIES Studies designed to observe outcomes or events that occur subsequent to the identification of the group of subjects to be studied. Prospective studies need not involve manipulation or intervention but may be purely observational or involve only the collection of data.

PROTOCOL The formal design or plan of an experiment or research activity; specifically, the plan submitted to an IRB for review and to an agency for research support. The protocol includes a description of the research design or methodology to be employed, the eligibility requirements for prospective subjects and controls, the treatment regimen(s), and the proposed methods of analysis that will be performed on the collected data.

PURITY The relative absence of extraneous matter in a drug or vaccine that may or may not be harmful to the recipient or deleterious to the product.

QUASI-EXPERIMENTAL STUDY A study that is similar to a true experimental study except that it lacks random assignments of subjects to treatment groups. (*See also Experimental Study.*)

RADIOACTIVE DRUG Any substance defined as a drug in §201(b)(1) of the Federal Food, Drug & Cosmetic Act that exhibits spontaneous disintegration of unstable nuclei with the emission of nuclear particles or photons (21 CFR §310.3(n)). Included are any nonradioactive reagent kit or nuclide generator that is intended to be used in the preparation of a radioactive drug and "radioactive biological products," as defined in 21 CFR §600.3(ee). Drugs such as carbon-containing compounds or potassium-containing salts containing trace quantities of naturally occurring radionuclides are not considered radioactive drugs.

RADIOACTIVE DRUG RESEARCH COMMITTEE (RDRC) An institutional committee responsible for the use of radioactive drugs in human subjects for research purposes. Research involving human subjects that proposes to use radioactive drugs must meet various FDA requirements, including limitations on the pharmacological dose and the radiation dose. Furthermore, the exposure to radiation must be justified by the quality of the study and the importance of the information it seeks to obtain. The committee is also responsible for continuing review of the drug use to ensure that the research continues to comply with FDA requirements, including reporting obligations. The committee must include experts in nuclear medicine and the use of radioactive drugs, as well as other medical and scientific members (21 CFR §36.1).

RADIOPAQUE CONTRAST AGENTS Materials that stop or attenuate radiation that is passed through the body, creating an outline on film of the organ(s) being examined. Contrast agents, sometimes called "dyes," do not contain radioisotopes. When such agents are used, exposure to radiation results only from the X-ray equipment used in the examination. The chemical structure of radiopaque contrast agents can produce a variety of adverse reactions, some of which may be severe—and possibly life-threatening—in certain individuals.

RADIOPHARMACEUTICALS Drugs (compounds or materials) that may be labeled or tagged with a radioisotope. These materials are largely physiological or subpharmacological in action, and, in many cases, function much like materials found in the body. The principal risk associated with these materials is the consequent radiation exposure to the body or to specific organ systems when they are injected into the body.

RANDOM, RANDOM ASSIGNMENT, RANDOMIZATION, RANDOMIZED Assignment of subjects to different treatments, interventions, or conditions according to chance rather than systematically (as dictated by the standard or usual response to their condition, history, or prognosis, or according to demographic characteristics). Random assignment of subjects to conditions is an essential element of experimental research because it makes more likely the probability that differences observed between subject groups are the result of the experimental intervention.

RECOMBINANT DNA TECHNOLOGY "The ability to chop up DNA, the stuff of which genes are made, and move the pieces, [which] permits the direct examination of the human genome," and the identification of the genetic components of a wide variety of disorders (Holtzman (1989), p. 1). Recombinant DNA technology is also used to develop diagnostic screens and tests, as well as drugs and biologics for treating diseases with genetic components. See Guidebook Chapter 5, Section H, "Human Genetic Research."

REM Acronym for Roentgen Equivalent in Man; the unit of measurement for a dose of an ionizing radiation that produces the same biological effect as a unit of absorbed does (1 rad) of ordinary X rays. One millirem is equal to 1/1000 of a rem.

REMISSION A period in which the signs and symptoms of a disease are diminished or in abeyance. The term "remission" is used when one cannot say with confidence that the disease has been cured.

REMUNERATION Payment for participation in research. (NOTE: It is wise to confine use of the term "compensation" to payment or provision of care for research-related injuries.) (*Compare Compensation.*)

RESEARCH A systematic investigation (the gathering and analysis of information) designed to develop or contribute to generalizable knowledge (45 CFR §46.102(d)).

RESPECT FOR PERSONS An ethical principle discussed in *The Belmont Report* requiring that individual autonomy be respected and that persons with diminished autonomy be protected.

RETROSPECTIVE STUDIES Research conducted by reviewing records from the past (birth and death certificates, medical records, school records, or employment records) or by obtaining information about past events elicited through interviews or surveys. Case control studies are an example of this type of research.

REVIEW (OF RESEARCH) The concurrent oversight of research on a periodic basis by an IRB. In addition to the at least annual reviews mandated by the federal regulations, reviews may, if deemed appropriate, also be conducted on a continuous or periodic basis (45 CFR §46.108(e)).

RISK The probability of harm or injury (physical, psychological, social, or economic) occurring as a result of participation in a research study. Both the probability and magnitude of possible harm may vary from minimal to significant. Federal regulations define only "minimal risk." (*See also Minimal Risk.*)

SAMHSA Substance Abuse and Mental Health Services Administration; includes the Center for Substance Abuse Prevention, the Center for Substance Abuse Treatment, and the Center on Mental Health Services. Previously the Alcohol, Drug Abuse, and Mental Health Administration (ADAMHA). (*See also ADAMHA.*)

SCIENTIFIC REVIEW GROUP A group of highly regarded experts in a given field, convened by NIH to advise NIH on the scientific merit of applications for research grants and contracts. Scientific review groups are also required to review the ethical aspects of proposed involvement of human subjects. Various kinds of scientific review groups exist and are known by different names in different institutes of the NIH (Study Sections, Initial Review Groups, Contract Review Committees, or Technical Evaluation Committees).

SECRETARY A U.S. Cabinet Officer. In the context of HHS-conducted or -supported research, usually refers to the Secretary of Health and Human Services.

SIGNIFICANT RISK DEVICE An investigational medical device that presents a potential for serious risk to the health, safety, or welfare of the subject.

SINGLE-MASKED DESIGN Typically, a study design in which the investigator, but not the subject, knows the identity of the treatment assignment. Occasionally the subject, but not the investigator, knows the assignment. Sometimes called "single-blind design."

SITE VISIT A visit by agency officials, representatives, or consultants to the location of a research activity to assess the adequacy of IRB protection of human subjects or the capability of personnel to conduct the research.

SOCIAL EXPERIMENTATION Systematic manipulation of, or experimentation in, social or economic systems; used in planning public policy.

SPONSOR (OF A DRUG TRIAL) A person or entity that initiates a clinical investigation of a drug—usually the drug manufacturer or research institution that developed the drug. The sponsor does not actually conduct the investigation, but rather distributes the new drug to investigators and physicians for clinical trials. The drug is administered to subjects under the immediate direction of an investigator who is not also a sponsor. A clinical investigator may, however, serve as a sponsor-investigator. The sponsor assumes responsibility for investigating the new drug, including responsibility for compliance with applicable laws and regulations. The sponsor, for example, is responsible for obtaining FDA approval to conduct a trial and for reporting the results of the trial to the FDA.

SPONSOR-INVESTIGATOR An individual who both initiates and actually conducts, alone or with others, a clinical investigation. Corporations, agencies, or other institutions do not qualify as sponsor-investigators.

STATISTICAL SIGNIFICANCE A determination of the probability of obtaining the particular distribution of the data on the assumption that the null hypothesis is true. Or, more simply put, the probability of coming to a false positive conclusion. If the probability is less than or equal to a predetermined value (0.05 or 0.01), then the null hypothesis is rejected at that significance level (0.05 or 0.01).

STERILITY (1) The absence of viable contaminating microorganisms; aseptic state; (2) The inability to procreate; the inability to conceive or induce conception.

STUDY SECTION *See Scientific Review Group.*

SUBJECTS (HUMAN) *See Human Subjects.*

SURVEYS Studies designed to obtain information from a large number of respondents through written questionnaires, telephone interviews, door-to-door canvassing, or similar procedures.

THERAPEUTIC INTENT The research physician's intent to provide some benefit to improving a subject's condition (prolongation of life, shrinkage of tumor, or improved quality of life, even though cure or dramatic improvement cannot necessarily be effected). This term is sometimes associated with Phase 1 drug studies in which potentially toxic drugs are given to an individual with the hope of inducing some improvement in the patient's condition as well as assessing the safety and pharmacology of a drug.

THERAPY Treatment intended and expected to alleviate a disease or disorder.

UNIFORM ANATOMICAL GIFT ACT Legislation adopted by all fifty States and the District of Columbia that indicates procedures for donation of all or part of a decedent's body for such activities as medical education, scientific research, and organ transplantation.

VACCINE A biologic product generally made from an infectious agent or its components—a virus, bacterium, or other microorganism—that is killed (inactive) or live-attenuated (active, although weakened). Vaccines may also be biochemically synthesized or made through recombinant DNA techniques.

VARIABLE An element or factor that the research is designed to study, either as an experimental intervention or a possible outcome (or factor affecting the outcome) of that intervention.

VIABLE INFANT When referring to a delivered or expelled fetus, the term "viable infant" means likely to survive to the point of sustaining life independently, given the benefit of available medical therapy (45 CFR §46.203(d)). This judgment is made by a physician. In accordance with HHS regulations, the Secretary, HHS, may publish guidelines to assist in the determination of viability. Such guidelines were published in 1975 and specify an estimated gestational age of twenty weeks or more and a body weight of 500 grams or more as indices of fetal viability (*Federal Register* 40 (August 8, 1975): 33552). These indices depend on the state of present technology and may be revised periodically. (*See also Nonviable Fetus*.)

VOLUNTARY Free of coercion, duress, or undue inducement. Used in the research context to refer to a subject's decision to participate (or to continue to participate) in a research activity.

Appendix

The "Common Rule": 45 CFR 46 562
FDA regulations 590
   21 CFR Part 50 590
   21 CFR Part 56 601
International Guidelines 612
   The Nuremberg Code 612
   The Declaration of Helsinki (Edinburgh Revision, 2000) 614
   The Belmont Report 617
   Additional Resources 628

THE "COMMON RULE": 45 CFR 46

CODE OF FEDERAL REGULATIONS

TITLE 45
PUBLIC WELFARE

DEPARTMENT OF HEALTH AND HUMAN SERVICES
NATIONAL INSTITUTES OF HEALTH
OFFICE FOR PROTECTION FROM RESEARCH RISKS

PART 46
PROTECTION OF HUMAN SUBJECTS

* * *

Revised June 18, 1991
Effective August 19, 1991

* * *

<table>
<tr><td><u>Subpart A —</u></td><td>Federal Policy for the Protection of Human Subjects (Basic DHHS Policy for Protection of Human Research Subjects)</td></tr>
</table>

Sec.

<u>46.101</u>	To what does this policy apply?
<u>46.102</u>	Definitions.
<u>46.103</u>	Assuring compliance with this policy—research conducted or supported by any Federal Department or Agency.
<u>46.104-</u> <u>46.106</u>	[Reserved]
<u>46.107</u>	IRB membership.
<u>46.108</u>	IRB functions and operations.
<u>46.109</u>	IRB review of research.
<u>46.110</u>	Expedited review procedures for certain kinds of research involving no more than minimal risk, and for minor changes in approved research.
<u>46.111</u>	Criteria for IRB approval of research.
<u>46.112</u>	Review by institution.
<u>46.113</u>	Suspension or termination of IRB approval of research.
<u>46.114</u>	Cooperative research.
<u>46.115</u>	IRB records.

46.116	General requirements for informed consent.
46.117	Documentation of informed consent.
46.118	Applications and proposals lacking definite plans for involvement of human subjects.
46.119	Research undertaken without the intention of involving human subjects.
46.120	Evaluation and disposition of applications and proposals for research to be conducted or supported by a Federal Department or Agency.
46.121	[Reserved]
46.122	Use of Federal funds.
46.123	Early termination of research support: Evaluation of applications and proposals.
46.124	Conditions.

Subpart B —   **Additional DHHS Protections Pertaining to Research, Development, and Related Activities Involving Fetuses, Pregnant Women, and Human In Vitro Fertilization**

Sec.

46.201	Applicability.
46.202	Purpose.
46.203	Definitions.
46.204	Ethical Advisory Boards.
46.205	Additional duties of the Institutional Review Boards in connection with activities involving fetuses, pregnant women, or human in vitro fertilization.
46.206	General limitations.
46.207	Activities directed toward pregnant women as subjects.
46.208	Activities directed toward fetuses *in utero* as subjects.
46.209	Activities directed toward fetuses *ex utero*, including nonviable fetuses, as subjects.
46.210	Activities involving the dead fetus, fetal material, or the placenta.
46.211	Modification or waiver of specific requirements.

Subpart C —   **Additional DHHS Protections Pertaining to Biomedical and Behavioral Research Involving Prisoners as Subjects**

Sec.

46.301	Applicability.
46.302	Purpose.
46.303	Definitions.

46.304   Composition of Institutional Review Boards where prisoners are involved.

46.305   Additional duties of the Institutional Review Boards where prisoners are involved.

46.306   Permitted research involving prisoners.

Subpart D —   **Additional DHHS Protections for Children Involved as Subjects in Research**

Sec.

46.401   To what do these regulations apply?

46.402   Definitions.

46.403   IRB duties.

46.404   Research not involving greater than minimal risk.

46.405   Research involving greater than minimal risk but presenting the prospect of direct benefit to the individual subjects.

46.406   Research involving greater than minimal risk and no prospect of direct benefit to individual subjects, but likely to yield generalizable knowledge about the subject's disorder or condition.

46.407   Research not otherwise approvable which presents an opportunity to understand, prevent, or alleviate a serious problem affecting the health or welfare of children.

46.408   Requirements for permission by parents or guardians and for assent by children.

46.409   Wards.

Authority: 5 U.S.C. 301; Sec. 474(a), 88 Stat. 352 (42 U.S.C. 2891-3(a)).

Note: As revised, Subpart A of the DHHS regulations incorporates the Common Rule (Federal Policy) for the Protection of Human Subjects (56 FR 28003). Subpart D of the HHS regulations has been amended at Section 46.401(b) to reference the revised Subpart A.

The Common Rule (Federal Policy) is also codified at

7 CFR Part 1c	**Department of Agriculture**
10 CFR Part 745	**Department of Energy**
14 CFR Part 1230	**National Aeronautics and Space Administration**
15 CFR Part 27	**Department of Commerce**
16 CFR Part 1028	**Consumer Product Safety Commission**
22 CFR Part 225	**International Development Cooperation Agency, Agency for International Development**
24 CFR Part 60	**Department of Housing and Urban Development**
28 CFR Part 46	**Department of Justice**

32 CFR Part 219	Department of Defense
34 CFR Part 97	Department of Education
38 CFR Part 16	Department of Veterans Affairs
40 CFR Part 26	Environmental Protection Agency
45 CFR Part 690	National Science Foundation
49 CFR Part 11	Department of Transportation

TITLE 45
CODE OF FEDERAL REGULATIONS

* * *

PART 46
PROTECTION OF HUMAN SUBJECTS

* * *

Revised June 18, 1991
Effective August 19, 1991

* * *

Subpart A	Federal Policy for the Protection of Human Subjects (Basic DHHS Policy for Protection of Human Research Subjects)
	Source: 56 FR 28003, June 18, 1991.

§46.101 To what does this policy apply?

(a) Except as provided in paragraph (b) of this section, this policy applies to all research involving human subjects conducted, supported or otherwise subject to regulation by any Federal Department or Agency which takes appropriate administrative action to make the policy applicable to such research. This includes research conducted by Federal civilian employees or military personnel, except that each Department or Agency head may adopt such procedural modifications as may be appropriate from an administrative standpoint. It also includes research conducted, supported, or otherwise subject to regulation by the Federal Government outside the United States.

(1) Research that is conducted or supported by a Federal Department or Agency, whether or not it is regulated as defined in §46.102(e), must comply with all sections of this policy.

(2) Research that is neither conducted nor supported by a Federal Department or Agency but is subject to regulation as defined in §46.102(e) must be reviewed and approved, in compliance with §46.101, §46.102, and §46.107 through §46.117 of this policy, by an Institutional Review Board (IRB) that operates in accordance with the pertinent requirements of this policy.

(b) Unless otherwise required by Department or Agency heads, research activities in which the only involvement of human subjects will be in one or more of the following categories are exempt from this policy:[1]

> (1) Research conducted in established or commonly accepted educational settings, involving normal educational practices, such as (i) research on regular and special education instructional strategies, or (ii) research on the effectiveness of or the comparison among instructional techniques, curricula, or classroom management methods.

> (2) Research involving the use of educational tests (cognitive, diagnostic, aptitude, achievement), survey procedures, interview procedures or observation of public behavior, unless: (i) information obtained is recorded in such a manner that human subjects can be identified, directly or through identifiers linked to the subjects; and (ii) any disclosure of the human subjects' responses outside the research could reasonably place the subjects at risk of criminal or civil liability or be damaging to the subjects' financial standing, employability, or reputation.

> (3) Research involving the use of educational tests (cognitive, diagnostic, aptitude, achievement), survey procedures, interview procedures, or observation of public behavior that is not exempt under paragraph (b)(2) of this section, if: (i) the human subjects are elected or appointed public officials or candidates for public office; or (ii) Federal statute(s) require(s) without exception that the confidentiality of the personally identifiable information will be maintained throughout the research and thereafter.

> (4) Research involving the collection or study of existing data, documents, records, pathological specimens, or diagnostic specimens, if these sources are publicly available or if the information is recorded by the investigator in such a manner that subjects cannot be identified, directly or through identifiers linked to the subjects.

> (5) Research and demonstration projects which are conducted by or subject to the approval of Department or Agency heads, and which are designed to study, evaluate, or otherwise examine: (i) Public benefit or service programs; (ii) procedures for obtaining benefits or services under those programs; (iii) possible changes in or alternatives to those programs or procedures; or (iv) possible changes in methods or levels of payment for benefits or services under those programs.

> (6) Taste and food quality evaluation and consumer acceptance studies, (i) if wholesome foods without additives are consumed or (ii) if a food is consumed that contains a food ingredient at or below the level and for a use found to be safe, or agricultural chemical or environmental contaminant at or below the level found to be safe, by the Food and Drug Administration or approved by the Environmental Protection Agency or the Food Safety and Inspection Service of the U.S. Department of Agriculture.

(c) Department or Agency heads retain final judgment as to whether a particular activity is covered by this policy.

(d) Department or Agency heads may require that specific research activities or classes of research activities conducted, supported, or otherwise subject to regulation by the Department or Agency but not otherwise covered by this policy, comply with some or all of the requirements of this policy.

(e) Compliance with this policy requires compliance with pertinent Federal laws or regulations which provide additional protections for human subjects.

(f) This policy does not affect any State or local laws or regulations which may otherwise be applicable and which provide additional protections for human subjects.

(g) This policy does not affect any foreign laws or regulations which may otherwise be applicable and which provide additional protections to human subjects of research.

(h) When research covered by this policy takes place in foreign countries, procedures normally followed in the foreign countries to protect human subjects may differ from those set forth in this policy. [An example is a foreign institution which complies with guidelines consistent with the World Medical Assembly Declaration (Declaration of Helsinki amended 1989) issued either by sovereign states or by an organization whose function for the protection of human research subjects is internationally recognized.] In these circumstances, if a Department or Agency head determines that the procedures prescribed by the institution afford protections that are at least equivalent to those provided in this policy, the Department or Agency head may approve the substitution of the foreign procedures in lieu of the procedural requirements provided in this policy. Except when otherwise required by statute, Executive Order, or the Department or Agency head, notices of these actions as they occur will be published in the **Federal Register** or will be otherwise published as provided in Department or Agency procedures.

(i) Unless otherwise required by law, Department or Agency heads may waive the applicability of some or all of the provisions of this policy to specific research activities or classes or research activities otherwise covered by this policy. Except when otherwise required by statute or Executive Order, the Department or Agency head shall forward advance notices of these actions to the Office for Protection from Research Risks, National Institutes of Health, Department of Health and Human Services (DHHS), and shall also publish them in the **Federal Register** or in such other manner as provided in Department or Agency procedures.[1]

> [1] Institutions with DHHS-approved assurances on file will abide by provisions of Title 45 CFR Part 46 Subparts A-D. Some of the other departments and agencies have incorporated all provisions of Title 45 CFR Part 46 into their policies and procedures as well. However, the exemptions at 45 CFR §46.101(b) do not apply to research involving prisoners, fetuses, pregnant women, or human in vitro fertilization, Subparts B and C. The exemption at 45 CFR §46.101(b)(2), for research involving survey or interview procedures or observation of public behavior, does not apply to research with children, <u>Subpart D</u>, except for research involving observations of public behavior when the investigator(s) do not participate in the activities being observed.

§46.102 Definitions.

(a) *Department or Agency* head means the head of any Federal Department or Agency and any other officer or employee of any Department or Agency to whom authority has been delegated.

(b) *Institution* means any public or private entity or Agency (including Federal, State, and other agencies).

(c) *Legally authorized representative* means an individual or judicial or other body authorized under applicable law to consent on behalf of a prospective subject to the subject's participation in the procedure(s) involved in the research.

(d) *Research* means a systematic investigation, including research development, testing and evaluation, designed to develop or contribute to generalizable knowledge. Activities which meet this definition constitute research for purposes of this policy, whether or not they are conducted or supported under a program which is considered research for other purposes. For example, some demonstration and service programs may include research activities.

(e) *Research subject to regulation*, and similar terms are intended to encompass those research activities for which a Federal Department or Agency has specific responsibility for regulating as a research activity, (for example, Investigational New Drug requirements administered by the Food and Drug Administration). It does not include research activities which are incidentally regulated by a Federal Department or Agency solely as part of the Department's or Agency's broader responsibility to regulate certain types of activities whether research or non-research in nature (for example, Wage and Hour requirements administered by the Department of Labor).

(f) *Human subject* means a living individual about whom an investigator (whether professional or student) conducting research obtains

> (1) data through intervention or interaction with the individual, or
>
> (2) identifiable private information.

Intervention includes both physical procedures by which data are gathered (for example, venipuncture) and manipulations of the subject or the subject's environment that are performed for research purposes. *Interaction* includes communication or interpersonal contact between investigator and subject. *Private information* includes information about behavior that occurs in a context in which an individual can reasonably expect that no observation or recording is taking place, and information which has been provided for specific purposes by an individual and which the individual can reasonably expect will not be made public (for example, a medical record). Private information must be individually identifiable (i.e., the identity of the subject is or may readily be ascertained by the investigator or associated with the information) in order for obtaining the information to constitute research involving human subjects.

(g) *IRB* means an Institutional Review Board established in accord with and for the purposes expressed in this policy.

(h) *IRB approval* means the determination of the IRB that the research has been reviewed and may be conducted at an institution within the constraints set forth by the IRB and by other institutional and Federal requirements.

(i) *Minimal risk* means that the probability and magnitude of harm or discomfort anticipated in the research are not greater in and of themselves than those ordinarily encountered in daily life or during the performance of routine physical or psychological examinations or tests.

(j) *Certification* means the official notification by the institution to the supporting Department or Agency, in accordance with the requirements of this policy, that a research project or activity involving human subjects has been reviewed and approved by an IRB in accordance with an approved assurance.

§46.103 Assuring compliance with this policy—research conducted or supported by any Federal Department or Agency.

(a) Each institution engaged in research which is covered by this policy and which is conducted or supported by a Federal Department or Agency shall provide written assurance satisfactory to the

Department or Agency head that it will comply with the requirements set forth in this policy. In lieu of requiring submission of an assurance, individual Department or Agency heads shall accept the existence of a current assurance, appropriate for the research in question, on file with the Office for Protection from Research Risks, National Institutes Health, DHHS, and approved for Federalwide use by that office. When the existence of an DHHS-approved assurance is accepted in lieu of requiring submission of an assurance, reports (except certification) required by this policy to be made to Department and Agency heads shall also be made to the Office for Protection from Research Risks, National Institutes of Health, DHHS.

(b) Departments and agencies will conduct or support research covered by this policy only if the institution has an assurance approved as provided in this section, and only if the institution has certified to the Department or Agency head that the research has been reviewed and approved by an IRB provided for in the assurance, and will be subject to continuing review by the IRB. Assurances applicable to federally supported or conducted research shall at a minimum include:

(1) A statement of principles governing the institution in the discharge of its responsibilities for protecting the rights and welfare of human subjects of research conducted at or sponsored by the institution, regardless of whether the research is subject to Federal regulation. This may include an appropriate existing code, declaration, or statement of ethical principles, or a statement formulated by the institution itself. This requirement does not preempt provisions of this policy applicable to Department- or Agency-supported or regulated research and need not be applicable to any research exempted or waived under §46.101 (b) or (i).

(2) Designation of one or more IRBs established in accordance with the requirements of this policy, and for which provisions are made for meeting space and sufficient staff to support the IRB's review and recordkeeping duties.

(3) A list of IRB members identified by name; earned degrees; representative capacity; indications of experience such as board certifications, licenses, etc., sufficient to describe each member's chief anticipated contributions to IRB deliberations; and any employment or other relationship between each member and the institution; for example: full-time employee, part-time employee, member of governing panel or board, stockholder, paid or unpaid consultant. Changes in IRB membership shall be reported to the Department or Agency head, unless in accord with §46.103(a) of this policy, the existence of a DHHS-approved assurance is accepted. In this case, change in IRB membership shall be reported to the Office for Protection from Research Risks, National Institutes of Health, DHHS.

(4) Written procedures which the IRB will follow (i) for conducting its initial and continuing review of research and for reporting its findings and actions to the investigator and the institution; (ii) for determining which projects require review more often than annually and which projects need verification from sources other than the investigators that no material changes have occurred since previous IRB review; and (iii) for ensuring prompt reporting to the IRB of proposed changes in a research activity, and for ensuring that such changes in approved research, during the period for which IRB approval has already been given, may not be initiated without IRB review and approval except when necessary to eliminate apparent immediate hazards to the subject.

(5) Written procedures for ensuring prompt reporting to the IRB, appropriate institutional officials, and the Department or Agency head of (i) any unanticipated problems involving risks to subjects or others or any serious or continuing non-compliance with this policy or the requirements or determinations of the IRB; and (ii) any suspension or termination of IRB approval.

(c) The assurance shall be executed by an individual authorized to act for the institution and to assume on behalf of the institution the obligations imposed by this policy and shall be filed in such form and manner as the Department or Agency head prescribes.

(d) The Department or Agency head will evaluate all assurances submitted in accordance with this policy through such officers and employees of the Department or Agency and such experts or consultants engaged for this purpose as the Department or Agency head determines to be appropriate. The Department or Agency head's evaluation will take into consideration the adequacy of the proposed IRB in light of the anticipated scope of the institution's research activities and the types of subject populations likely to be involved, the appropriateness of the proposed initial and continuing review procedures in light of the probable risks, and the size and complexity of the institution.

(e) On the basis of this evaluation, the Department or Agency head may approve or disapprove the assurance, or enter into negotiations to develop an approvable one. The Department or Agency head may limit the period during which any particular approved assurance or class of approved assurances shall remain effective or otherwise condition or restrict approval.

(f) Certification is required when the research is supported by a Federal Department or Agency and not otherwise exempted or waived under §46.101 (b) or (i). An institution with an approved assurance shall certify that each application or proposal for research covered by the assurance and by §46.103 of this policy has been reviewed and approved by the IRB. Such certification must be submitted with the application or proposal or by such later date as may be prescribed by the Department or Agency to which the application or proposal is submitted. Under no condition shall research covered by §46.103 of the policy be supported prior to receipt of the certification that the research has been reviewed and approved by the IRB. Institutions without an approved assurance covering the research shall certify within 30 days after receipt of a request for such a certification from the Department or Agency, that the application or proposal has been approved by the IRB. If the certification is not submitted within these time limits, the application or proposal may be returned to the institution.
(Approved by the Office of Management and Budget under Control Number 9999-0020.)

§§46.104—46.106 [Reserved]

§46.107 IRB membership.

(a) Each IRB shall have at least five members, with varying backgrounds to promote complete and adequate review of research activities commonly conducted by the institution. The IRB shall be sufficiently qualified through the experience and expertise of its members, and the diversity of the members, including consideration of race, gender, and cultural backgrounds and sensitivity to such issues as community attitudes, to promote respect for its advice and counsel in safeguarding the rights and welfare of human subjects. In addition to possessing the professional competence necessary to review specific research activities, the IRB shall be able to ascertain the acceptability of proposed research in terms of institutional commitments and regulations, applicable law, and standards of professional conduct and practice. The IRB shall therefore include persons knowledgeable in these areas. If an IRB regularly reviews research that involves a vulnerable category of subjects, such as children, prisoners, pregnant women, or handicapped or mentally disabled persons, consideration shall be given to the inclusion of one or more individuals who are knowledgeable about and experienced in working with these subjects.

(b) Every nondiscriminatory effort will be made to ensure that no IRB consists entirely of men or entirely of women, including the institution's consideration of qualified persons of both sexes, so long as no selection is made to the IRB on the basis of gender. No IRB may consist entirely of members of one profession.

(c) Each IRB shall include at least one member whose primary concerns are in scientific areas and at least one member whose primary concerns are in nonscientific areas.

(d) Each IRB shall include at least one member who is not otherwise affiliated with the institution and who is not part of the immediate family of a person who is affiliated with the institution.

(e) No IRB may have a member participate in the IRB's initial or continuing review of any project in which the member has a conflicting interest, except to provide information requested by the IRB.

(f) An IRB may, in its discretion, invite individuals with competence in special areas to assist in the review of issues which require expertise beyond or in addition to that available on the IRB. These individuals may not vote with the IRB.

§46.108 IRB functions and operations.

In order to fulfill the requirements of this policy each IRB shall:

(a) Follow written procedures in the same detail as described in §46.103(b)(4) and to the extent required by §46.103(b)(5).

(b) Except when an expedited review procedure is used (see §46.110), review proposed research at convened meetings at which a majority of the members of the IRB are present, including at least one member whose primary concerns are in nonscientific areas. In order for the research to be approved, it shall receive the approval of a majority of those members present at the meeting.

§46.109 IRB review of research.

(a) An IRB shall review and have authority to approve, require modifications in (to secure approval), or disapprove all research activities covered by this policy.

(b) An IRB shall require that information given to subjects as part of informed consent is in accordance with §46.116. The IRB may require that information, in addition to that specifically mentioned in §46.116, be given to the subjects when in the IRB's judgment the information would meaningfully add to the protection of the rights and welfare of subjects.

(c) An IRB shall require documentation of informed consent or may waive documentation in accordance with §46.117.

(d) An IRB shall notify investigators and the institution in writing of its decision to approve or disapprove the proposed research activity, or of modifications required to secure IRB approval of the research activity. If the IRB decides to disapprove a research activity, it shall include in its written notification a statement of the reasons for its decision and give the investigator an opportunity to respond in person or in writing.

(e) An IRB shall conduct continuing review of research covered by this policy at intervals appropriate to the degree of risk, but not less than once per year, and shall have authority to observe or have a third party observe the consent process and the research.
(Approved by the Office of Management and Budget under Control Number 9999-0020.)

§46.110 Expedited review procedures for certain kinds of research involving no more than minimal risk, and for minor changes in approved research.

(a) The Secretary, HHS, has established, and published as a Notice in the **Federal Register,** a list of categories of research that may be reviewed by the IRB through an expedited review procedure. The list will be amended, as appropriate, after consultation with other departments and agencies, through periodic republication by the Secretary, HHS, in the Federal Register. A copy of the list is available from the Office for Protection from Research Risks, National Institutes of Health, DHHS, Bethesda, Maryland 20892.

(b) An IRB may use the expedited review procedure to review either or both of the following:

(1) some or all of the research appearing on the list and found by the reviewer(s) to involve no more than minimal risk,

(2) minor changes in previously approved research during the period (of one year or less) for which approval is authorized.

Under an expedited review procedure, the review may be carried out by the IRB chairperson or by one or more experienced reviewers designated by the chairperson from among members of the IRB. In reviewing the research, the reviewers may exercise all of the authorities of the IRB except that the reviewers may not disapprove the research. A research activity may be disapproved only after review in accordance with the non-expedited procedure set forth in §46.108(b).

(c) Each IRB which uses an expedited review procedure shall adopt a method for keeping all members advised of research proposals which have been approved under the procedure.

(d) The Department or Agency head may restrict, suspend, terminate, or choose not to authorize an institution's or IRB's use of the expedited review procedure.

§46.111 Criteria for IRB approval of research.

(a) In order to approve research covered by this policy the IRB shall determine that all of the following requirements are satisfied:

(1) Risks to subjects are minimized: (i) by using procedures which are consistent with sound research design and which do not unnecessarily expose subjects to risk, and (ii) whenever appropriate, by using procedures already being performed on the subjects for diagnostic or treatment purposes.

(2) Risks to subjects are reasonable in relation to anticipated benefits, if any, to subjects, and the importance of the knowledge that may reasonably be expected to result. In evaluating risks and benefits, the IRB should consider only those risks and benefits that may result from the research (as distinguished from risks and benefits of therapies subjects would receive even if not participating in the research). The IRB should not consider possible long-range effects of applying knowledge gained in the research (for example, the possible effects of the research on public policy) as among those research risks that fall within the purview of its responsibility.

(3) Selection of subjects is equitable. In making this assessment the IRB should take into account the purposes of the research and the setting in which the research will be conducted and should be particularly cognizant of the special problems of research involving vulnerable populations, such as children, prisoners, pregnant women, mentally disable persons, or economically or educationally disadvantaged persons.

(4) Informed consent will be sought from each prospective subject or the subject's legally authorized representative, in accordance with, and to the extent required by §46.116.

(5) Informed consent will be appropriately documented, in accordance with, and to the extent required by §46.117.

(6) When appropriate, the research plan makes adequate provision for monitoring the data collected to ensure the safety of subjects.

(7) When appropriate, there are adequate provisions to protect the privacy of subjects and to maintain the confidentiality of data.

(b) When some or all of the subjects are likely to be vulnerable to coercion or undue influence, such as children, prisoners, pregnant women, mentally disabled persons, or economically or educationally disadvantaged persons, additional safeguards have been included in the study to protect the rights and welfare of these subjects.

§46.112 Review by institution.

Research covered by this policy that has been approved by an IRB may be subject to further appropriate review and approval or disapproval by officials of the institution. However, those officials may not approve the research if it has not been approved by an IRB.

§46.113 Suspension or termination of IRB approval of research.

An IRB shall have authority to suspend or terminate approval of research that is not being conducted in accordance with the IRB's requirements or that has been associated with unexpected serious harm to subjects. Any suspension or termination or approval shall include a statement of the reasons for the IRB's action and shall be reported promptly to the investigator, appropriate institutional officials, and the Department or Agency head.
(Approved by the Office of Management and Budget under Control Number 9999-0020.)

§46.114 Cooperative research.

Cooperative research projects are those projects covered by this policy which involve more than one institution. In the conduct of cooperative research projects, each institution is responsible for safeguarding the rights and welfare of human subjects and for complying with this policy. With the approval of the Department or Agency head, an institution participating in a cooperative project may enter into a joint review arrangement, rely upon the review of another qualified IRB, or make similar arrangements for avoiding duplication of effort.

§46.115 IRB records.

(a) An institution, or when appropriate an IRB, shall prepare and maintain adequate documentation of IRB activities, including the following:

> (1) Copies of all research proposals reviewed, scientific evaluations, if any, that accompany the proposals, approved sample consent documents, progress reports submitted by investigators, and reports of injuries to subjects.

> (2) Minutes of IRB meetings which shall be in sufficient detail to show attendance at the meetings; actions taken by the IRB; the vote on these actions including the number of members voting for, against, and abstaining; the basis for requiring changes in or disapproving research; and a written summary of the discussion of controverted issues and their resolution.

> (3) Records of continuing review activities.

> (4) Copies of all correspondence between the IRB and the investigators.

> (5) A list of IRB members in the same detail as described in §46.103(b)(3).

> (6) Written procedures for the IRB in the same detail as described in §46.103(b)(4) and §46.103(b)(5).

> (7) Statements of significant new findings provided to subjects, as required by §46.116(b)(5).

(b) The records required by this policy shall be retained for at least 3 years, and records relating to research which is conducted shall be retained for at least 3 years after completion of the research. All records shall be accessible for inspection and copying by authorized representatives of the Department or Agency at reasonable times and in a reasonable manner.
(Approved by the Office of Management and Budget under Control Number 9999-0020.)

§46.116 General requirements for informed consent.

Except as provided elsewhere in this policy, no investigator may involve a human being as a subject in research covered by this policy unless the investigator has obtained the legally effective informed consent of the subject or the subject's legally authorized representative. An investigator shall seek such consent only under circumstances that provide the prospective subject or the representative sufficient opportunity to consider whether or not to participate and that minimize the possibility of coercion or undue influence. The information that is given to the subject or the representative shall be in language understandable to the subject or the representative. No informed consent, whether oral or written, may include any exculpatory language through which the subject or the representative is made to waive or appear to waive any of the subject's legal rights, or releases or appears to release the investigator, the sponsor, the institution or its agents from liability for negligence.

(a) Basic elements of informed consent. Except as provided in paragraph (c) or (d) of this section, in seeking informed consent the following information shall be provided to each subject:

(1) a statement that the study involves research, an explanation of the purposes of the research and the expected duration of the subject's participation, a description of the procedures to be followed, and identification of any procedures which are experimental;

(2) a description of any reasonably foreseeable risks or discomforts to the subject;

(3) a description of any benefits to the subject or to others which may reasonably be expected from the research;

(4) a disclosure of appropriate alternative procedures or courses of treatment, if any, that might be advantageous to the subject;

(5) a statement describing the extent, if any, to which confidentiality of records identifying the subject will be maintained;

(6) for research involving more than minimal risk, an explanation as to whether any compensation and an explanation as to whether any medical treatments are available if injury occurs and, if so, what they consist of, or where further information may be obtained;

(7) an explanation of whom to contact for answers to pertinent questions about the research and research subjects' rights, and whom to contact in the event of a research-related injury to the subject; and

(8) a statement that participation is voluntary, refusal to participate will involve no penalty or loss of benefits to which the subject is otherwise entitled, and the subject may discontinue participation at any time without penalty or loss of benefits to which the subject is otherwise entitled.

(b) additional elements of informed consent. When appropriate, one or more of the following elements of information shall also be provided to each subject:

(1) a statement that the particular treatment or procedure may involve risks to the subject (or to the embryo or fetus, if the subject is or may become pregnant) which are currently unforeseeable;

(2) anticipated circumstances under which the subject's participation may be terminated by the investigator without regard to the subject's consent;

(3) any additional costs to the subject that may result from participation in the research;

(4) the consequences of a subject's decision to withdraw from the research and procedures for orderly termination of participation by the subject;

(5) A statement that significant new findings developed during the course of the research which may relate to the subject's willingness to continue participation will be provided to the subject; and

(6) the approximate number of subjects involved in the study.

(c) An IRB may approve a consent procedure which does not include, or which alters, some or all of the elements of informed consent set forth above, or waive the requirement to obtain informed consent provided the IRB finds and documents that:

> (1) the research or demonstration project is to be conducted by or subject to the approval of state or local government officials and is designed to study, evaluate, or otherwise examine: (i) public benefit or service programs; (ii) procedures for obtaining benefits or services under those programs; (iii) possible changes in or alternatives to those programs or procedures; or (iv) possible changes in methods or levels of payment for benefits or services under those programs; and

> (2) the research could not practicably be carried out without the waiver or alteration.

(d) An IRB may approve a consent procedure which does not include, or which alters, some or all of the elements of informed consent set forth in this section, or waive the requirements to obtain informed consent provided the IRB finds and documents that:

> (1) the research involves no more than minimal risk to the subjects;

> (2) the waiver or alteration will not adversely affect the rights and welfare of the subjects;

> (3) the research could not practicably be carried out without the waiver or alteration; and

> (4) whenever appropriate, the subjects will be provided with additional pertinent information after participation.

(e) The informed consent requirements in this policy are not intended to preempt any applicable Federal, State, or local laws which require additional information to be disclosed in order for informed consent to be legally effective.

(f) Nothing in this policy is intended to limit the authority of a physician to provide emergency medical care, to the extent the physician is permitted to do so under applicable Federal, State, or local law.
(Approved by the Office of Management and Budget under Control Number 9999-0020.)

§46.117 Documentation of informed consent.

(a) Except as provided in paragraph (c) of this section, informed consent shall be documented by the use of a written consent form approved by the IRB and signed by the subject or the subject's legally authorized representative. A copy shall be given to the person signing the form.

(b) Except as provided in paragraph (c) of this section, the consent form may be either of the following:

> (1) A written consent document that embodies the elements of informed consent required by §46.116. This form may be read to the subject or the subject's legally authorized representative, but in any event, the investigator shall give either the subject or the representative adequate opportunity to read it before it is signed; or

(2) A short form written consent document stating that the elements of informed consent required by §46.116 have been presented orally to the subject or the subject's legally authorized representative. When this method is used, there shall be a witness to the oral presentation. Also, the IRB shall approve a written summary of what is to be said to the subject or the representative. Only the short form itself is to be signed by the subject or the representative. However, the witness shall sign both the short form and a copy of the summary, and the person actually obtaining consent shall sign a copy of the summary. A copy of the summary shall be given to the subject or the representative, in addition to a copy of the short form.

(c) An IRB may waive the requirement for the investigator to obtain a signed consent form for some or all subjects if it finds either:

(1) That the only record linking the subject and the research would be the consent document and the principal risk would be potential harm resulting from a breach of confidentiality. Each subject will be asked whether the subject wants documentation linking the subject with the research, and the subject's wishes will govern; or

(2) That the research presents no more than minimal risk of harm to subjects and involves no procedures for which written consent is normally required outside of the research context.

In cases in which the documentation requirement is waived, the IRB may require the investigator to provide subjects with a written statement regarding the research.
(Approved by the Office of Management and Budget under Control Number 9999-0020.)

§46.118 Applications and proposals lacking definite plans for involvement of human subjects.

Certain types of applications for grants, cooperative agreements, or contracts are submitted to departments or agencies with the knowledge that subjects may be involved within the period of support, but definite plans would not normally be set forth in the application or proposal. These include activities such as institutional type grants when selection of specific projects is the institution's responsibility; research training grants in which the activities involving subjects remain to be selected; and projects in which human subjects' involvement will depend upon completion of instruments, prior animal studies, or purification of compounds. These applications need not be reviewed by an IRB before an award may be made. However, except for research exempted or waived under §46.101 (b) or (i), no human subjects may be involved in any project supported by these awards until the project has been reviewed and approved by the IRB, as provided in this policy, and certification submitted, by the institution, to the Department or Agency.

§46.119 Research undertaken without the intention of involving human subjects.

In the event research is undertaken without the intention of involving human subjects, but it is later proposed to involve human subjects in the research, the research shall first be reviewed and approved by an IRB, as provided in this policy, a certification submitted, by the institution, to the Department or Agency, and final approval given to the proposed change by the Department or Agency.

§46.120 Evaluation and disposition of applications and proposals for research to be conducted or supported by a Federal Department or Agency.

(a) The Department or Agency head will evaluate all applications and proposals involving human subjects submitted to the Department or Agency through such officers and employees of the Department or Agency and such experts and consultants as the Department or Agency head determines to be appropriate. This evaluation will take into consideration the risks to the subjects, the adequacy of protection against these risks, the potential benefits of the research to the subjects and others, and the importance of the knowledge gained or to be gained.

(b) On the basis of this evaluation, the Department or Agency head may approve or disapprove the application or proposal, or enter into negotiations to develop an approvable one.

§46.121 [Reserved]

§46.122 Use of Federal funds.

Federal funds administered by a Department or Agency may not be expended for research involving human subjects unless the requirements of this policy have been satisfied.

§46.123 Early termination of research support: Evaluation of applications and proposals.

(a) The Department or Agency head may require that Department or Agency support for any project be terminated or suspended in the manner prescribed in applicable program requirements, when the Department or Agency head finds an institution has materially failed to comply with the terms of this policy.

(b) In making decisions about supporting or approving applications or proposals covered by this policy the Department or Agency head may take into account, in addition to all other eligibility requirements and program criteria, factors such as whether the applicant has been subject to a termination or suspension under paragraph (a) of this section and whether the applicant or the person or persons who would direct or has/have directed the scientific and technical aspects of an activity has/have, in the judgment of the Department or Agency head, materially failed to discharge responsibility for the protection of the rights and welfare of human subjects (whether or not the research was subject to Federal regulation).

§46.124 Conditions.

With respect to any research project or any class of research projects the Department or Agency head may impose additional conditions prior to or at the time of approval when in the judgment of the Department or Agency head additional conditions are necessary for the protection of human subjects.

Subpart B	Additional DHHS Protections Pertaining to Research, Development, and Related Activities Involving Fetuses, Pregnant Women, and Human In Vitro Fertilization
	Source: 40 FR 33528, Aug. 8, 1975; 43 FR 1758, January 11, 1978; 43 FR 51559, November 3, 1978.

§46.201 Applicability.

(a) The regulations in this subpart are applicable to all Department of Health and Human Services grants and contracts supporting research, development, and related activities involving: (1) the fetus, (2) pregnant women, and (3) human *in vitro* fertilization.

(b) Nothing in this subpart shall be construed as indicating that compliance with the procedures set forth herein will in any way render inapplicable pertinent State or local laws bearing upon activities covered by this subpart.

(c) The requirements of this subpart are in addition to those imposed under the other subparts of this part.

§46.202 Purpose.

It is the purpose of this subpart to provide additional safeguards in reviewing activities to which this subpart is applicable to assure that they conform to appropriate ethical standards and relate to important societal needs.

§46.203 Definitions.

As used in this subpart:

(a) "Secretary" means the Secretary of Health and Human Services and any other officer or employee of the Department of Health and Human Services (DHHS) to whom authority has been delegated.

(b) "Pregnancy" encompasses the period of time from confirmation of implantation (through any of the presumptive signs of pregnancy, such as missed menses, or by a medically acceptable pregnancy test), until expulsion or extraction of the fetus.

(c) "Fetus" means the product of conception from the time of implantation (as evidenced by any of the presumptive signs of pregnancy, such as missed menses, or a medically acceptable pregnancy test), until a determination is made, following expulsion or extraction of the fetus, that it is viable.

(d) "Viable" as it pertains to the fetus means being able, after either spontaneous or induced delivery, to survive (given the benefit of available medical therapy) to the point of independently maintaining heart beat and respiration. The Secretary may from time to time, taking into account medical advances, publish in the **Federal Register** guidelines to assist in determining whether a fetus is viable for purposes of this subpart. If a fetus is viable after delivery, it is a premature infant.

(e) "Nonviable fetus" means a fetus *ex utero* which, although living, is not viable.

(f) "Dead fetus" means a fetus *ex utero* which exhibits neither heartbeat, spontaneous respiratory activity, spontaneous movement of voluntary muscles, nor pulsation of the umbilical cord (if still attached).

(g) "*In vitro* fertilization" means any fertilization of human ova which occurs outside the body of a female, either through admixture of donor human sperm and ova or by any other means.

§46.204 Ethical Advisory Boards.

(a) One or more Ethical Advisory Boards shall be established by the Secretary. Members of these Board(s) shall be so selected that the Board(s) will be competent to deal with medical, legal, social, ethical, and related issues and may include, for example, research scientists, physicians, psychologists, sociologists, educators, lawyers, and ethicists, as well as representatives of the general public. No Board member may be a regular, full-time employee of the Department of Health and Human Services.

(b) At the request of the Secretary, the Ethical Advisory Board shall render advice consistent with the policies and requirements of this part as to ethical issues, involving activities covered by this subpart, raised by individual applications or proposals. In addition, upon request by the Secretary, the Board shall render advice as to classes of applications or proposals and general policies, guidelines, and procedures.

(c) A Board may establish, with the approval of the Secretary, classes of applications or proposals which: (1) must be submitted to the Board, or (2) need not be submitted to the Board. Where the Board so establishes a class of applications or proposals which must be submitted, no application or proposal within the class may be funded by the Department or any component thereof until the application or proposal has been reviewed by the Board and the Board has rendered advice as to its acceptability from an ethical standpoint.

(d) *[Nullified under Public Law 103-43, June 10, 1993]*

§46.205 Additional duties of the Institutional Review Boards in connection with activities involving fetuses, pregnant women, or human in vitro fertilization.

(a) In addition to the responsibilities prescribed for Institutional Review Boards under Subpart A of this part, the applicant's or offeror's Board shall, with respect to activities covered by this subpart, carry out the following additional duties:

(1) determine that all aspects of the activity meet the requirements of this subpart;

(2) determine that adequate consideration has been given to the manner in which potential subjects will be selected, and adequate provision has been made by the applicant or offeror for monitoring the actual informed consent process (e.g., through such mechanisms, when appropriate, as participation by the Institutional Review Board or subject advocates in: (i) overseeing the actual process by which individual consents required by this subpart are secured either by approving induction of each individual into the activity or verifying, perhaps through sampling, that approved procedures for induction of individuals into the activity are being followed, and (ii) monitoring the progress of the activity and intervening as necessary through such steps as visits to the activity site and continuing evaluation to determine if any unanticipated risks have arisen);

(3) carry out such other responsibilities as may be assigned by the Secretary.

(b) No award may be issued until the applicant or offeror has certified to the Secretary that the Institutional Review Board has made the determinations required under paragraph (a) of this section and the Secretary has approved these determinations, as provided in §46.120 of Subpart A of this part.

(c) Applicants or offerors seeking support for activities covered by this subpart must provide for the designation of an Institutional Review Board, subject to approval by the Secretary, where no such Board has been established under Subpart A of this part.

§46.206 General limitations.

(a) No activity to which this subpart is applicable may be undertaken unless:

(1) appropriate studies on animals and nonpregnant individuals have been completed;

(2) except where the purpose of the activity is to meet the health needs of the mother or the particular fetus, the risk to the fetus is minimal and, in all cases, is the least possible risk for achieving the objectives of the activity;

(3) individuals engaged in the activity will have no part in: (i) any decisions as to the timing, method, and procedures used to terminate the pregnancy, and (ii) determining the viability of the fetus at the termination of the pregnancy; and

(4) no procedural changes which may cause greater than minimal risk to the fetus or the pregnant woman will be introduced into the procedure for terminating the pregnancy solely in the interest of the activity.

(b) No inducements, monetary or otherwise, may be offered to terminate pregnancy for purposes of the activity.
Source: 40 FR 33528, Aug. 8, 1975, as amended at 40 FR 51638, Nov. 6, 1975.

§46.207 Activities directed toward pregnant women as subjects.

(a) No pregnant woman may be involved as a subject in an activity covered by this subpart unless: (1) the purpose of the activity is to meet the health needs of the mother and the fetus will be placed at risk only to the minimum extent necessary to meet such needs, or (2) the risk to the fetus is minimal.

(b) An activity permitted under paragraph (a) of this section may be conducted only if the mother and father are legally competent and have given their informed consent after having been fully informed regarding possible impact on the fetus, except that the father's informed consent need not be secured if: (1) the purpose of the activity is to meet the health needs of the mother; (2) his identity or whereabouts cannot reasonably be ascertained; (3) he is not reasonably available; or (4) the pregnancy resulted from rape.

§46.208 Activities directed toward fetuses *in utero* as subjects.

(a) No fetus *in utero* may be involved as a subject in any activity covered by this subpart unless: (1) the purpose of the activity is to meet the health needs of the particular fetus and the fetus will be placed at risk only to the minimum extent necessary to meet such needs, or (2) the risk to the fetus imposed by the research is minimal and the purpose of the activity is the development of important biomedical knowledge which cannot be obtained by other means.

(b) An activity permitted under paragraph (a) of this section may be conducted only if the mother and father are legally competent and have given their informed consent, except that the father's consent need not be secured if: (1) his identity or whereabouts cannot reasonably be ascertained, (2) he is not reasonably available, or (3) the pregnancy resulted from rape.

§46.209 Activities directed toward fetuses *ex utero*, including nonviable fetuses, as subjects.

(a) Until it has been ascertained whether or not a fetus *ex utero* is viable, a fetus *ex utero* may not be involved as a subject in an activity covered by this subpart unless:

> (1) there will be no added risk to the fetus resulting from the activity, and the purpose of the activity is the development of important biomedical knowledge which cannot be obtained by other means, or

> (2) the purpose of the activity is to enhance the possibility of survival of the particular fetus to the point of viability.

(b) No nonviable fetus may be involved as a subject in an activity covered by this subpart unless:

> (1) vital functions of the fetus will not be artificially maintained,

> (2) experimental activities which of themselves would terminate the heartbeat or respiration of the fetus will not be employed, and

> (3) the purpose of the activity is the development of important biomedical knowledge which cannot be obtained by other means.

(c) In the event the fetus *ex utero* is found to be viable, it may be included as a subject in the activity only to the extent permitted by and in accordance with the requirements of other subparts of this part.

(d) An activity permitted under paragraph (a) or (b) of this section may be conducted only if the mother and father are legally competent and have given their informed consent, except that the father's informed consent need not be secured if: (1) his identity or whereabouts cannot reasonably be ascertained, (2) he is not reasonably available, or (3) the pregnancy resulted from rape.

§46.210 Activities involving the dead fetus, fetal material, or the placenta.

Activities involving the dead fetus, macerated fetal material, or cells, tissue, or organs excised from a dead fetus shall be conducted only in accordance with any applicable State or local laws regarding such activities.

§46.211 Modification or waiver of specific requirements.

Upon the request of an applicant or offeror (with the approval of its Institutional Review Board), the Secretary may modify or waive specific requirements of this subpart, with the approval of the Ethical Advisory Board after such opportunity for public comment as the Ethical Advisory Board considers appropriate in the particular instance. In making such decisions, the Secretary will consider whether the risks to the subject are so outweighed by the sum of the benefit to the subject and the importance of the knowledge to be gained as to warrant such modification or waiver and that such benefits cannot be gained except through a modification or waiver. Any such modifications or waivers will be published as notices in the **Federal Register.**

Subpart C	Additional DHHS Protections Pertaining to Biomedical and Behavioral Research Involving Prisoners as Subjects
	Source: 43 FR 53655, Nov. 16, 1978.

§46.301 Applicability.

(a) The regulations in this subpart are applicable to all biomedical and behavioral research conducted or supported by the Department of Health and Human Services involving prisoners as subjects.

(b) Nothing in this subpart shall be construed as indicating that compliance with the procedures set forth herein will authorize research involving prisoners as subjects, to the extent such research is limited or barred by applicable State or local law.

(c) The requirements of this subpart are in addition to those imposed under the other subparts of this part.

§46.302 Purpose.

Inasmuch as prisoners may be under constraints because of their incarceration which could affect their ability to make a truly voluntary and uncoerced decision whether or not to participate as subjects in research, it is the purpose of this subpart to provide additional safeguards for the protection of prisoners involved in activities to which this subpart is applicable.

§46.303 Definitions.

As used in this subpart:

(a) "Secretary" means the Secretary of Health and Human Services and any other officer or employee of the Department of Health and Human Services to whom authority has been delegated.

(b) "DHHS" means the Department of Health and Human Services.

(c) "Prisoner" means any individual involuntarily confined or detained in a penal institution. The term is intended to encompass individuals sentenced to such an institution under a criminal or civil statute, individuals detained in other facilities by virtue of statutes or commitment procedures which provide alternatives to criminal prosecution or incarceration in a penal institution, and individuals detained pending arraignment, trial, or sentencing.

(d) "Minimal risk" is the probability and magnitude of physical or psychological harm that is normally encountered in the daily lives, or in the routine medical, dental, or psychological examination of healthy persons.

§46.304 Composition of Institutional Review Boards where prisoners are involved.

In addition to satisfying the requirements in §46.107 of this part, an Institutional Review Board, carrying out responsibilities under this part with respect to research covered by this subpart, shall also meet the following specific requirements:

(a) A majority of the Board (exclusive of prisoner members) shall have no association with the prison(s) involved, apart from their membership on the Board.

(b) At least one member of the Board shall be a prisoner, or a prisoner representative with appropriate background and experience to serve in that capacity, except that where a particular research project is reviewed by more than one Board only one Board need satisfy this requirement.

§46.305 Additional duties of the Institutional Review Boards where prisoners are involved.

(a) In addition to all other responsibilities prescribed for Institutional Review Boards under this part, the Board shall review research covered by this subpart and approve such research only if it finds that:

(1) the research under review represents one of the categories of research permissible under §46.306(a)(2);

(2) any possible advantages accruing to the prisoner through his or her participation in the research, when compared to the general living conditions, medical care, quality of food, amenities and opportunity for earnings in the prison, are not of such a magnitude that his or her ability to weigh the risks of the research against the value of such advantages in the limited choice environment of the prison is impaired;

(3) the risks involved in the research are commensurate with risks that would be accepted by nonprisoner volunteers;

(4) procedures for the selection of subjects within the prison are fair to all prisoners and immune from arbitrary intervention by prison authorities or prisoners. Unless the principal investigator provides to the Board justification in writing for following some other procedures, control subjects must be selected randomly from the group of available prisoners who meet the characteristics needed for that particular research project;

(5) the information is presented in language which is understandable to the subject population;

(6) adequate assurance exists that parole boards will not take into account a prisoner's participation in the research in making decisions regarding parole, and each prisoner is clearly informed in advance that participation in the research will have no effect on his or her parole; and

(7) where the Board finds there may be a need for follow-up examination or care of participants after the end of their participation, adequate provision has been made for such examination or care, taking into account the varying lengths of individual prisoners' sentences, and for informing participants of this fact.

(b) The Board shall carry out such other duties as may be assigned by the Secretary.

(c) The institution shall certify to the Secretary, in such form and manner as the Secretary may require, that the duties of the Board under this section have been fulfilled.

§46.306 Permitted research involving prisoners.

(a) Biomedical or behavioral research conducted or supported by DHHS may involve prisoners as subjects only if:

   (1) the institution responsible for the conduct of the research has certified to the Secretary that the Institutional Review Board has approved the research under §46.305 of this subpart; and

   (2) in the judgment of the Secretary the proposed research involves solely the following:

      (A) study of the possible causes, effects, and processes of incarceration, and of criminal behavior, provided that the study presents no more than minimal risk and no more than inconvenience to the subjects;

      (B) study of prisons as institutional structures or of prisoners as incarcerated persons, provided that the study presents no more than minimal risk and no more than inconvenience to the subjects;

      (C) research on conditions particularly affecting prisoners as a class (for example, vaccine trials and other research on hepatitis which is much more prevalent in prisons than elsewhere; and research on social and psychological problems such as alcoholism, drug addiction, and sexual assaults) provided that the study may proceed only after the Secretary has consulted with appropriate experts including experts in penology, medicine, and ethics, and published notice, in the **Federal Register,** of his intent to approve such research; or

      (D) research on practices, both innovative and accepted, which have the intent and reasonable probability of improving the health or well-being of the subject. In cases in which those studies require the assignment of prisoners in a manner consistent with protocols approved by the IRB to control groups which may not benefit from the research, the study may proceed only after the Secretary has consulted with appropriate experts, including experts in penology, medicine, and ethics, and published notice, in the **Federal Register,** of the intent to approve such research.

(b) Except as provided in paragraph (a) of this section, biomedical or behavioral research conducted or supported by DHHS shall not involve prisoners as subjects.

Subpart D	Additional DHHS Protections for Children Involved as Subjects in Research
	Source: 48 FR 9818, March 8, 1983; 56 FR 28032, June 18, 1991.

§46.401 To what do these regulations apply?

(a) This subpart applies to all research involving children as subjects, conducted or supported by the Department of Health and Human Services.

> (1) This includes research conducted by Department employees, except that each head of an Operating Division of the Department may adopt such nonsubstantive, procedural modifications as may be appropriate from an administrative standpoint.

> (2) It also includes research conducted or supported by the Department of Health and Human Services outside the United States, but in appropriate circumstances, the Secretary may, under paragraph (i) of §46.101 of Subpart A, waive the applicability of some or all of the requirements of these regulations for research of this type.

(b) Exemptions at §46.101(b)(1) and (b)(3) through (b)(6) are applicable to this subpart. The exemption at §46.101(b)(2) regarding educational tests is also applicable to this subpart. However, the exemption at §46.101(b)(2) for research involving survey or interview procedures or observations of public behavior does not apply to research covered by this subpart, except for research involving observation of public behavior when the investigator(s) do not participate in the activities being observed.

(c) The exceptions, additions, and provisions for waiver as they appear in paragraphs (c) through (i) of §46.101 of Subpart A are applicable to this subpart.

§46.402 Definitions.

The definitions in §46.102 of Subpart A shall be applicable to this subpart as well. In addition, as used in this subpart:

(a) "Children" are persons who have not attained the legal age for consent to treatments or procedures involved in the research, under the applicable law of the jurisdiction in which the research will be conducted.

(b) "Assent" means a child's affirmative agreement to participate in research. Mere failure to object should not, absent affirmative agreement, be construed as assent.

(c) "Permission" means the agreement of parent(s) or guardian to the participation of their child or ward in research.

(d) "Parent" means a child's biological or adoptive parent.

(e) "Guardian" means an individual who is authorized under applicable State or local law to consent on behalf of a child to general medical care.

§46.403 IRB duties.

In addition to other responsibilities assigned to IRBs under this part, each IRB shall review research covered by this subpart and approve only research which satisfies the conditions of all applicable sections of this subpart.

§46.404 Research not involving greater than minimal risk.

DHHS will conduct or fund research in which the IRB finds that no greater than minimal risk to children is presented, only if the IRB finds that adequate provisions are made for soliciting the assent of the children and the permission of their parents or guardians, as set forth in §46.408.

§46.405 Research involving greater than minimal risk but presenting the prospect of direct benefit to the individual subjects.

DHHS will conduct or fund research in which the IRB finds that more than minimal risk to children is presented by an intervention or procedure that holds out the prospect of direct benefit for the individual subject, or by a monitoring procedure that is likely to contribute to the subject's well-being, only if the IRB finds that:

(a) the risk is justified by the anticipated benefit to the subjects;

(b) the relation of the anticipated benefit to the risk is at least as favorable to the subjects as that presented by available alternative approaches; and

(c) adequate provisions are made for soliciting the assent of the children and permission of their parents or guardians, as set forth in §46.408.

§46.406 Research involving greater than minimal risk and no prospect of direct benefit to individual subjects, but likely to yield generalizable knowledge about the subject's disorder or condition.

DHHS will conduct or fund research in which the IRB finds that more than minimal risk to children is presented by an intervention or procedure that does not hold out the prospect of direct benefit for the individual subject, or by a monitoring procedure which is not likely to contribute to the well-being of the subject, only if the IRB finds that:

(a) the risk represents a minor increase over minimal risk;

(b) the intervention or procedure presents experiences to subjects that are reasonably commensurate with those inherent in their actual or expected medical, dental, psychological, social, or educational situations;

(c) the intervention or procedure is likely to yield generalizable knowledge about the subjects' disorder or condition which is of vital importance for the understanding or amelioration of the subjects' disorder or condition; and

(d) adequate provisions are made for soliciting assent of the children and permission of their parents or guardians, as set forth in §46.408.

§46.407 Research not otherwise approvable which presents an opportunity to understand, prevent, or alleviate a serious problem affecting the health or welfare of children.

DHHS will conduct or fund research that the IRB does not believe meets the requirements of §46.404, §46.405, or §46.406 only if:

(a) the IRB finds that the research presents a reasonable opportunity to further the understanding, prevention, or alleviation of a serious problem affecting the health or welfare of children; and

(b) the Secretary, after consultation with a panel of experts in pertinent disciplines (for example: science, medicine, education, ethics, law) and following opportunity for public review and comment, has determined either:

(1) that the research in fact satisfies the conditions of §46.404, §46.405, or §46.406, as applicable, or (2) the following:

(i) the research presents a reasonable opportunity to further the understanding, prevention, or alleviation of a serious problem affecting the health or welfare of children;

(ii) the research will be conducted in accordance with sound ethical principles;

(iii) adequate provisions are made for soliciting the assent of children and the permission of their parents or guardians, as set forth in §46.408.

§46.408 Requirements for permission by parents or guardians and for assent by children.

(a) In addition to the determinations required under other applicable sections of this subpart, the IRB shall determine that adequate provisions are made for soliciting the assent of the children, when in the judgment of the IRB the children are capable of providing assent. In determining whether children are capable of assenting, the IRB shall take into account the ages, maturity, and psychological state of the children involved. This judgment may be made for all children to be involved in research under a particular protocol, or for each child, as the IRB deems appropriate. If the IRB determines that the capability of some or all of the children is so limited that they cannot reasonably be consulted or that the intervention or procedure involved in the research holds out a prospect of direct benefit that is important to the health or well-being of the children and is available only in the context of the research, the assent of the children is not a necessary condition for proceeding with the research. Even where the IRB determines that the subjects are capable of assenting, the IRB may still waive the assent requirement under circumstances in which consent may be waived in accord with §46.116 of Subpart A.

(b) In addition to the determinations required under other applicable sections of this subpart, the IRB shall determine, in accordance with and to the extent that consent is required by §46.116 of Subpart A, that adequate provisions are made for soliciting the permission of each child's parents or guardian. Where parental permission is to be obtained, the IRB may find that the permission of one parent is sufficient for research to be conducted under §46.404 or §46.405. Where research is covered by §46.406 and §46.407 and permission is to be obtained from parents, both parents must give their permission unless one parent is deceased, unknown, incompetent, or not reasonably available, or when only one parent has legal responsibility for the care and custody of the child.

(c) In addition to the provisions for waiver contained in §46.116 of Subpart A, if the IRB determines that a research protocol is designed for conditions or for a subject population for which parental or guardian permission is not a reasonable requirement to protect the subjects (for example, neglected or abused children), it may waive the consent requirements in Subpart A of this part and paragraph (b) of this section, provided an appropriate mechanism for protecting the children who will participate as subjects in the research is substituted, and provided further that the waiver is not inconsistent with Federal, State, or local law. The choice of an appropriate mechanism would depend upon the nature and purpose of the activities described in the protocol, the risk and anticipated benefit to the research subjects, and their age, maturity, status, and condition.

(d) Permission by parents or guardians shall be documented in accordance with and to the extent required by §46.117 of Subpart A.

(e) When the IRB determines that assent is required, it shall also determine whether and how assent must be documented.

§46.409 Wards.

(a) Children who are wards of the State or any other agency, institution, or entity can be included in research approved under §46.406 or §46.407 only if such research is:

(1) related to their status as wards; or

(2) conducted in schools, camps, hospitals, institutions, or similar settings in which the majority of children involved as subjects are not wards.

(b) If the research is approved under paragraph (a) of this section, the IRB shall require appointment of an advocate for each child who is a ward, in addition to any other individual acting on behalf of the child as guardian or in loco parents. One individual may serve as advocate for more than one child. The advocate shall be an individual who has the background and experience to act in, and agrees to act in, the best interests of the child for the duration of the child's participation in the research and who is not associated in any way (except in the role as advocate or member of the IRB) with the research, the investigator(s), or the guardian organization.

FDA REGULATIONS

21 CFR Part 50

21 CFR PART 50—PROTECTION OF HUMAN SUBJECTS

Subpart A General Provisions

50.1 Scope.
50.3 Definitions.

Subpart B Informed Consent of Human Subjects

50.20 General requirements for informed consent.
50.21 Effective date.
50.23 Exception from general requirements.
50.24 Exception from informed consent requirements for emergency research
50.25 Elements of informed consent.
50.27 Documentation of informed consent.

[Source: 45 FR 36390, May 30, 1980, unless otherwise noted.]

Subpart A—General Provisions

ß 50.1 Scope.

(a) This part applies to all clinical investigations regulated by the Food and Drug Administration under sections 505(i) 507(d), and 520(g) of the Federal Food, Drug, and Cosmetic Act, as well as clinical investigations that support applications for research or marketing permits for products regulated by the Food and Drug Administration, including food and color additives, drugs for human use, medical devices for human use, biological products for human use, and electronic products. Additional specific obligations and commitments of, and standards of conduct for, persons who sponsor or monitor clinical investigations involving particular test articles may also be found in other parts (e.g., 21 CFR parts 312 and 812). Compliance with these parts is intended to protect the rights and safety of subjects involved in investigations filed with the Food and Drug Administration pursuant to sections 406, 409, 502, 503, 505, 506, 507, 510, 513-516, 518, 520, 706, and 801 of the Federal Food, Drug and Cosmetic Act and sections 351 and 354, 360F of the Public Health Service Act.

(b) References in this part to regulatory sections of the Code of Federal Regulations are to chapter I of title 21, unless otherwise noted.

[45 FR 36390, May 30, 1980; 46 FR 8979, Jan. 27, 1981]

ß 50.3 Definitions.

As used in this part:

(a) **Act** means the Federal Food, Drug, and Cosmetic Act, as amended (secs. 201-902, 52 Stat. 1040 et seq. as amended (21 U.S.C. 321-392)).

(b) Application for research or marketing permit includes:

(1) A color additive petition, described in part 71.

(2) A food additive petition, described in parts 171 and 571.

(3) Data and information about a substance submitted as part of the procedures for establishing that the substance is generally recognized as safe for use that results or may reasonably be expected to result, directly or indirectly, in its becoming a component or otherwise affecting the characteristics of any food, described in ßß 170.30 and 570.30.

(4) Data and information about a food additive submitted as part of the procedures for food additives permitted to be used on an interim basis pending additional study, described in ß 180.1.

(5) Data and information about a substance submitted as part of the procedures for establishing a tolerance for unavoidable contaminants in food and food-packaging materials described in section 406 of the act.

(6) An investigational new drug application, described in part 312 of this chapter.

(7) A new drug application, described in part 314.

(8) Data and information about the bioavailability or bioequivalence of drugs for human use submitted as part of the procedures for issuing, amending, or repealing a bioequivalence requirement, described in part 320.

(9) Data and information about an over-the-counter drug for human use submitted as part of the procedures for classifying these drugs as generally recognized as safe and effective and not misbranded, described in part 330.

(10) Data and information about a prescription drug for human use submitted as part of the procedures for classifying these drugs as generally recognized as safe and effective and not misbranded, described in this chapter.

(11) Data and information about an antibiotic drug submitted as part of the procedures for issuing, amending or repealing regulations for these drugs, described in ß 314.300 of this chapter.

(12) An application for a biological product license, described in part 601.

(13) Data and information about a biological product submitted as part of the procedures for determining that licensed biological products are safe and effective and not misbranded, described in part 601.

(14) Data and information about an *in vitro* diagnostic product submitted as part of the procedures for establishing, amending, or repealing a standard for these products, described in part 809.

(15) An *Application for an Investigational Device Exemption,* described in part 812.

(16) Data and information about a medical device submitted as part of the procedures for classifying these devices, described in section 513.

(17) Data and information about a medical device submitted as part of the procedures for establishing, amending, or repealing a standard for these devices, described in section 514.

(18) An application for premarket approval of a medical device, described in section 515.

(19) A product development protocol for a medical device, described in section 515.

(20) Data and information about an electronic product submitted as part of the procedures for establishing, amending or repealing a standard for these products, described in section 358 of the Public Health Service Act.

(21) Data and information about an electronic product submitted as part of the procedures for obtaining a variance from any electronic product performance standard, as described in ß 1010.4.

(22) Data and information about an electronic product submitted as part of the procedures for granting amending, or extending an exemption from a radiation safety performance standard, as described in ß 1010.5.

(c) **Clinical investigation** means any experiment that involves a test article and one or more human subjects and that either is subject to requirements for prior submission to the Food and Drug Administration under section 505(i), 507(d), or 520(g) of the act, or is not subject to requirements for prior submission to the Food and Drug Administration under these sections of the act, but the results of which are intended to be submitted later to, or held for inspection by, the Food and Drug Administration as part of an application for a research or marketing permit. The term does not include experiments that are subject to the provisions of part 58 of this chapter, regarding nonclinical laboratory studies.

(d) **Investigator** means an individual who actually conducts a clinical investigation, i.e., under whose immediate direction the test article is administered or dispensed to or used involving, a subject, or, in the event of an investigation conducted by a team of individuals, is the responsible leader of that team.

(e) **Sponsor** means a person who initiates a clinical investigation, but who does not actually conduct the investigation, i.e., the test article is administered or dispensed to or used involving, a subject under the immediate direction of another individual. A person other than an individual (e.g., corporation or agency) that uses one or more of its own employees to conduct a clinical investigation it has initiated is considered to be a sponsor (not a sponsor-investigator) and the employees are considered to be investigators.

(f) **Sponsor-investigator** means an individual who both initiates and actually conducts, alone or with others a clinical investigation, i.e., under whose immediate direction the test article is administered or dispensed to, or used involving, a subject. The term does not include any person other than an individual, e.g., corporation or agency.

(g) **Human subject** means an individual who is or becomes a participant in research, either as a recipient of the test article as a control. A subject may be either a healthy human or a patient.

(h) **Institution** means any public or private entity or Agency (including Federal, State, and other agencies). The word facility as used in section 520(g) of the act is deemed to be synonymous with the term institution for purposes of this part.

(i) **Institutional review board (IRB)** means any board, committee, or other group formally designated by an institution to review biomedical research involving humans as subjects, to approve the initiation of and conduct periodic review of such research. The term has the same meaning as the phrase institutional review committee as used in section 520(g) of the act.

(j) Test article means any drug (including a biological product for human use), medical device for human use, human food additive, color additive, electronic product, or any other article subject to regulation under the act or under sections 351 and 354-360F of the Public Health Service Act (42 U.S.C. 262 and 263b-263n).

(k) Minimal risk means that the probability and magnitude of harm or discomfort anticipated in the research are not greater in and of themselves than those ordinarily encountered in daily life or during the performance of routine physical or psychological examinations or tests.

(l) Legally authorized representative means an individual or judicial or other body authorized under applicable law to consent on behalf of a prospective subject to the subject's participation in the procedure(s) involved in the research.

(m) Family member means any one of the following legally competent persons: Spouse; parents; children (including adopted children); brothers and sisters; and any individual related by blood or affinity whose close association with the subject is the equivalent of a family relationship.

[45 FR 36390, May 30, 1980, as amended at 46 FR 8950 Jan. 27, 1981; 54 FR 9038, Mar. 3, 1989; 56 FR 28028, June 18, 1991; 61 FR 51497, Oct. 2, 1996; 62 FR 39440, July 23, 1997]

Subpart B—Informed Consent of Human Subjects

Source: 46 FR 8951, Jan. 27, 1981, unless otherwise noted.

Sec. 50.20 General requirements for informed consent.

Except as provided in Secs. 50.23 and 50.24, no investigator may involve a human being as a subject in research covered by these regulations unless the investigator has obtained the legally effective informed consent of the subject or the subject's legally authorized representative. An investigator shall seek such consent only under circumstances that provide the prospective subject or the representative sufficient opportunity to consider whether or not to participate and that minimize the possibility of coercion or undue influence. The information that is given to the subject or the representative shall be in language understandable to the subject or the representative. No informed consent, whether oral or written, may include any exculpatory language through which the subject or the representative is made to waive or appear to waive any of the subject's legal rights, or releases or appears to release the investigator, the sponsor, the institution, or its agents from liability for negligence.

[46 FR 8951, Jan. 27, 1981, as amended at 64 FR 10942, Mar. 8, 1999]

Sec. 50.23 Exception from general requirements.

(a) The obtaining of informed consent shall be deemed feasible unless, before use of the test article (except as provided in paragraph **(b)** of this section), both the investigator and a physician who is not otherwise participating in the clinical investigation certify in writing all of the following:

(1) The human subject is confronted by a life-threatening situation necessitating the use of the test article.

(2) Informed consent cannot be obtained from the subject because of an inability to communicate with, or obtain legally effective consent from, the subject.

(3) Time is not sufficient to obtain consent from the subject's legal representative.

(4) There is available no alternative method of approved or generally recognized therapy that provides an equal or greater likelihood of saving the life of the subject.

(b) If immediate use of the test article is, in the investigator's opinion, required to preserve the life of the subject, and time is not sufficient to obtain the independent determination required in paragraph (a) of this section in advance of using the test article, the determinations of the clinical investigator shall be made and, within 5 working days after the use of the article, be reviewed and evaluated in writing by a physician who is not participating in the clinical investigation.

(c) The documentation required in paragraph (a) or (**b**) of this section shall be submitted to the IRB within 5 working days after the use of the test article.

(d)(1) Under 10 U.S.C. 1107(f) the President may waive the prior consent requirement for the administration of an investigational new drug to a member of the armed forces in connection with the member's participation in a particular military operation. The statute specifies that only the President may waive informed consent in this connection and the President may grant such a waiver only if the President determines in writing that obtaining consent: Is not feasible; is contrary to the best interests of the military member; or is not in the interests of national security. The statute further provides that in making a determination to waive prior informed consent on the ground that it is not feasible or the ground that it is contrary to the best interests of the military members involved, the President shall apply the standards and criteria that are set forth in the relevant FDA regulations for a waiver of the prior informed consent requirements of section 505(i)(4) of the Federal Food, Drug, and Cosmetic Act (21 U.S.C. 355(i)(4)). Before such a determination may be made that obtaining informed consent from military personnel prior to the use of an investigational drug (including an antibiotic or biological product) in a specific protocol under an investigational new drug application (IND) sponsored by the Department of Defense (DOD) and limited to specific military personnel involved in a particular military operation is not feasible or is contrary to the best interests of the military members involved the Secretary of Defense must first request such a determination from the President, and certify and document to the President that the following standards and criteria contained in paragraphs (d)(1) through (d)(4) of this section have been met.

(i) The extent and strength of evidence of the safety and effectiveness of the investigational new drug in relation to the medical risk that could be encountered during the military operation supports the drug's administration under an IND.

(ii) The military operation presents a substantial risk that military personnel may be subject to a chemical, biological, nuclear, or other exposure likely to produce death or serious or life-threatening injury or illness.

(iii) There is no available satisfactory alternative therapeutic or preventive treatment in relation to the intended use of the investigational new drug.

(iv) Conditioning use of the investigational new drug on the voluntary participation of each member could significantly risk the safety and health of any individual member who would decline its use, the safety of other military personnel, and the accomplishment of the military mission.

(v) A duly constituted institutional review board (IRB) established and operated in accordance with the requirements of paragraphs (d)(2) and (d)(3) of this section, responsible for review of the study, has reviewed and approved the investigational new drug protocol and the administration of the investigational new drug without informed consent. DOD's request is to include the documentation required by Sec. 56.115(a)(2) of this chapter.

(vi) DOD has explained:

> (A) The context in which the investigational drug will be administered, e.g., the setting or whether it will be self-administered or it will be administered by a health professional;

> (B) The nature of the disease or condition for which the preventive or therapeutic treatment is intended; and

> (C) To the extent there are existing data or information available, information on conditions that could alter the effects of the investigational drug.

(vii) DOD's recordkeeping system is capable of tracking and will be used to track the proposed treatment from supplier to the individual recipient.

(viii) Each member involved in the military operation will be given, prior to the administration of the investigational new drug, a specific written information sheet (including information required by 10 U.S.C. 1107(d)) concerning the investigational new drug, the risks and benefits of its use, potential side effects, and other pertinent information about the appropriate use of the product.

(ix) Medical records of members involved in the military operation will accurately document the receipt by members of the notification required by paragraph (d)(1)(viii) of this section.

(x) Medical records of members involved in the military operation will accurately document the receipt by members of any investigational new drugs in accordance with FDA regulations including part 312 of this chapter.

(xi) DOD will provide adequate followup to assess whether there are beneficial or adverse health consequences that result from the use of the investigational product.

(xii) DOD is pursuing drug development, including a time line, and marketing approval with due diligence.

(xiii) FDA has concluded that the investigational new drug protocol may proceed subject to a decision by the President on the informed consent waiver request.

(xiv) DOD will provide training to the appropriate medical personnel and potential recipients on the specific investigational new drug to be administered prior to its use.

(xv) DOD has stated and justified the time period for which the waiver is needed, not to exceed one year, unless separately renewed under these standards and criteria.

(xvi) DOD shall have a continuing obligation to report to the FDA and to the President any changed circumstances relating to these standards and criteria (including the time period referred to in paragraph (d)(1)(xv) of this section) or that otherwise might affect the determination to use an investigational new drug without informed consent.

(xvii) DOD is to provide public notice as soon as practicable and consistent with classification requirements through notice in the Federal Register describing each waiver of informed consent determination, a summary of the most updated scientific information on the products used, and other pertinent information.

(xviii) Use of the investigational drug without informed consent otherwise conforms with applicable law.

(2) The duly constituted institutional review board, described in paragraph (d)(1)(v) of this section, must include at least 3 nonaffiliated members who shall not be employees or officers of the Federal Government (other than for purposes of membership on the IRB) and shall be required to obtain any necessary security clearances. This IRB shall review the proposed IND protocol at a convened meeting at which a majority of the members are present including at least one member whose primary concerns are in nonscientific areas and, if feasible, including a majority of the nonaffiliated members. The information required by Sec. 56.115(a)(2) of this chapter is to be provided to the Secretary of Defense for further review.

(3) The duly constituted institutional review board, described in paragraph (d)(1)(v) of this section, must review and approve:

(i) The required information sheet;

(ii) The adequacy of the plan to disseminate information, including distribution of the information sheet to potential recipients, on the investigational product (e.g., in forms other than written);

(iii) The adequacy of the information and plans for its dissemination to healthcare providers, including potential side effects, contraindications, potential interactions, and other pertinent considerations; and

(iv) An informed consent form as required by part 50 of this chapter, in those circumstances in which DOD determines that informed consent may be obtained from some or all personnel involved.

(4) DOD is to submit to FDA summaries of institutional review board meetings at which the proposed protocol has been reviewed.

(5) Nothing in these criteria or standards is intended to preempt or limit FDA's and DOD's authority or obligations under applicable statutes and regulations.

[46 FR 8951, Jan. 27, 1981, as amended at 55 FR 52817, Dec. 21, 1990; 64 FR 399, Jan. 5, 1999; 64 FR 54188, Oct. 5, 1999]

Sec. 50.24 Exception from informed consent requirements for emergency research.

(a) The IRB responsible for the review, approval, and continuing review of the clinical investigation described in this section may approve that investigation without requiring that informed consent of all research subjects be obtained if the IRB (with the concurrence of a licensed physician who is a member of or consultant to the IRB and who is not otherwise participating in the clinical investigation) finds and documents each of the following:

(1) The human subjects are in a life-threatening situation, available treatments are unproven or unsatisfactory, and the collection of valid scientific evidence, which may include evidence

obtained through randomized placebo-controlled investigations, is necessary to determine the safety and effectiveness of particular interventions.

(2) Obtaining informed consent is not feasible because:

(i) The subjects will not be able to give their informed consent as a result of their medical condition;

(ii) The intervention under investigation must be administered before consent from the subjects' legally authorized representatives is feasible; and

(iii) There is no reasonable way to identify prospectively the individuals likely to become eligible for participation in the clinical investigation.

(3) Participation in the research holds out the prospect of direct benefit to the subjects because:

(i) Subjects are facing a life-threatening situation that necessitates intervention;

(ii) Appropriate animal and other preclinical studies have been conducted, and the information derived from those studies and related evidence support the potential for the intervention to provide a direct benefit to the individual subjects; and

(iii) Risks associated with the investigation are reasonable in relation to what is known about the medical condition of the potential class of subjects, the risks and benefits of standard therapy, if any, and what is known about the risks and benefits of the proposed intervention or activity.

(4) The clinical investigation could not practicably be carried out without the waiver.

(5) The proposed investigational plan defines the length of the potential therapeutic window based on scientific evidence, and the investigator has committed to attempting to contact a legally authorized representative for each subject within that window of time and, if feasible, to asking the legally authorized representative contacted for consent within that window rather than proceeding without consent. The investigator will summarize efforts made to contact legally authorized representatives and make this information available to the IRB at the time of continuing review.

(6) The IRB has reviewed and approved informed consent procedures and an informed consent document consistent with Sec. 50.25. These procedures and the informed consent document are to be used with subjects or their legally authorized representatives in situations where use of such procedures and documents is feasible. The IRB has reviewed and approved procedures and information to be used when providing an opportunity for a family member to object to a subject's participation in the clinical investigation consistent with paragraph (a)(7)(v) of this section.

(7) Additional protections of the rights and welfare of the subjects will be provided, including, at least:

(i) Consultation (including, where appropriate, consultation carried out by the IRB) with representatives of the communities in which the clinical investigation will be conducted and from which the subjects will be drawn;

(ii) Public disclosure to the communities in which the clinical investigation will be conducted and from which the subjects will be drawn, prior to initiation of the clinical investigation, of plans for the investigation and its risks and expected benefits;

(iii) Public disclosure of sufficient information following completion of the clinical investigation to apprise the community and researchers of the study, including the demographic characteristics of the research population, and its results;

(iv) Establishment of an independent data monitoring committee to exercise oversight of the clinical investigation; and

(v) If obtaining informed consent is not feasible and a legally authorized representative is not reasonably available, the investigator has committed, if feasible, to attempting to contact within the therapeutic window the subject's family member who is not a legally authorized representative, and asking whether he or she objects to the subject's participation in the clinical investigation. The investigator will summarize efforts made to contact family members and make this information available to the IRB at the time of continuing review.

(b) The IRB is responsible for ensuring that procedures are in place to inform, at the earliest feasible opportunity, each subject, or if the subject remains incapacitated, a legally authorized representative of the subject, or if such a representative is not reasonably available, a family member, of the subject's inclusion in the clinical investigation, the details of the investigation and other information contained in the informed consent document. The IRB shall also ensure that there is a procedure to inform the subject, or if the subject remains incapacitated, a legally authorized representative of the subject, or if such a representative is not reasonably available, a family member, that he or she may discontinue the subject's participation at any time without penalty or loss of benefits to which the subject is otherwise entitled. If a legally authorized representative or family member is told about the clinical investigation and the subject's condition improves, the subject is also to be informed as soon as feasible. If a subject is entered into a clinical investigation with waived consent and the subject dies before a legally authorized representative or family member can be contacted, information about the clinical investigation is to be provided to the subject's legally authorized representative or family member, if feasible.

(c) The IRB determinations required by paragraph (a) of this section and the documentation required by paragraph (e) of this section are to be retained by the IRB for at least 3 years after completion of the clinical investigation, and the records shall be accessible for inspection and copying by FDA in accordance with Sec. 56.115(**b**) of this chapter.

(d) Protocols involving an exception to the informed consent requirement under this section must be performed under a separate investigational new drug application (IND) or investigational device exemption (IDE) that clearly identifies such protocols as protocols that may include subjects who are unable to consent. The submission of those protocols in a separate IND/IDE is required even if an IND for the same drug product or an IDE for the same device already exists. Applications for investigations under this section may not be submitted as amendments under Secs. 312.30 or 812.35 of this chapter.

(e) If an IRB determines that it cannot approve a clinical investigation because the investigation does not meet the criteria in the exception provided under paragraph (a) of this section or because of other relevant ethical concerns, the IRB must document its findings and provide these findings promptly in writing to the clinical investigator and to the sponsor of the clinical investigation. The sponsor of the clinical investigation must promptly disclose this information to FDA and to the sponsor's clinical investigators who are participating or are asked to participate in this or a substantially equivalent clinical investigation of the sponsor, and to other IRB's that have been, or are, asked to review this or a substantially equivalent investigation by that sponsor.

[61 FR 51528, Oct. 2, 1996]

Sec. 50.25 Elements of informed consent.

(a) Basic elements of informed consent. In seeking informed consent, the following information shall be provided to each subject:

(1) A statement that the study involves research, an explanation of the purposes of the research and the expected duration of the subject's participation, a description of the procedures to be followed, and identification of any procedures which are experimental.

(2) A description of any reasonably foreseeable risks or discomforts to the subject.

(3) A description of any benefits to the subject or to others which may reasonably be expected from the research.

(4) A disclosure of appropriate alternative procedures or courses of treatment, if any, that might be advantageous to the subject.

(5) A statement describing the extent, if any, to which confidentiality of records identifying the subject will be maintained and that notes the possibility that the Food and Drug Administration may inspect the records.

(6) For research involving more than minimal risk, an explanation as to whether any compensation and an explanation as to whether any medical treatments are available if injury occurs and, if so, what they consist of, or where further information may be obtained.

(7) An explanation of whom to contact for answers to pertinent questions about the research and research subjects' rights, and whom to contact in the event of a research-related injury to the subject.

(8) A statement that participation is voluntary, that refusal to participate will involve no penalty or loss of benefits to which the subject is otherwise entitled, and that the subject may discontinue participation at any time without penalty or loss of benefits to which the subject is otherwise entitled.

(b) Additional elements of informed consent. When appropriate, one or more of the following elements of information shall also be provided to each subject:

(1) A statement that the particular treatment or procedure may involve risks to the subject (or to the embryo or fetus, if the subject is or may become pregnant) which are currently unforeseeable.

(2) Anticipated circumstances under which the subject's participation may be terminated by the investigator without regard to the subject's consent.

(3) Any additional costs to the subject that may result from participation in the research.

(4) The consequences of a subject's decision to withdraw from the research and procedures for orderly termination of participation by the subject.

(5) A statement that significant new findings developed during the course of the research which may relate to the subject's willingness to continue participation will be provided to the subject.

(6) The approximate number of subjects involved in the study.

(c) The informed consent requirements in these regulations are not intended to preempt any applicable Federal, State, or local laws which require additional information to be disclosed for informed consent to be legally effective.

(d) Nothing in these regulations is intended to limit the authority of a physician to provide emergency medical care to the extent the physician is permitted to do so under applicable Federal, State, or local law.

Sec. 50.27 Documentation of informed consent.

(a) Except as provided in Sec. 56.109(c), informed consent shall be documented by the use of a written consent form approved by the IRB and signed and dated by the subject or the subject's legally authorized representative at the time of consent. A copy shall be given to the person signing the form.

(b) Except as provided in Sec. 56.109(c), the consent form may be either of the following:

(1) A written consent document that embodies the elements of informed consent required by Sec. 50.25. This form may be read to the subject or the subject's legally authorized representative, but, in any event, the investigator shall give either the subject or the representative adequate opportunity to read it before it is signed.

(2) A short form written consent document stating that the elements of informed consent required by Sec. 50.25 have been presented orally to the subject or the subject's legally authorized representative. When this method is used, there shall be a witness to the oral presentation. Also, the IRB shall approve a written summary of what is to be said to the subject or the representative. Only the short form itself is to be signed by the subject or the representative. However, the witness shall sign both the short form and a copy of the summary, and the person actually obtaining the consent shall sign a copy of the summary. A copy of the summary shall be given to the subject or the representative in addition to a copy of the short form.

[46 FR 8951, Jan. 27, 1981, as amended at 61 FR 57280, Nov. 5, 1996]

[61FR 51497, October 2, 1996]

21 CFR Part 56

21 CFR PART 56—INSTITUTIONAL REVIEW BOARDS

Subpart A General Provisions

56.101 Scope.
56.102 Definitions.
56.103 Circumstances in which IRB review is required.
56.104 Exemptions from IRB requirement.
56.105 Waiver of IRB requirement.

Subpart B Organization and Personnel

56.107 IRB membership.

Subpart C IRB Functions and Operations

56.108 IRB functions and operations.
56.109 IRB review of research.
56.110 Expedited review procedures for certain kinds of . . . research.
56.111 Criteria for IRB approval of research.
56.112 Review by institution.
56.113 Suspension or termination of IRB approval of research.
56.114 Cooperative research.

Subpart D Records and Reports

56.115 IRB records.

Subpart E Administrative Action for Non-compliance
56.120 Lesser administrative actions.
56.121 Disqualification of an IRB or an institution.
56.122 Public disclosure of information regarding revocation.
56.123 Reinstatement of an IRB or an institution.
56.124 Actions alternative or additional to disqualification.
[Source: 46 FR 8975, Jan. 27, 1981, unless otherwise noted.]

Subpart A—General Provisions

ß 56.101 Scope.

(a) This part contains the general standards for the composition operation, and responsibility of an Institutional Review Board (IRB) that reviews clinical investigations regulated by the Food and Drug Administration under sections 505(i) 507(d), and 520(g) of the act, as well as clinical investigations that support applications for research or marketing permits for products regulated by the Food and Drug Administration including food and color additives, drugs for human use medical devices for human use, biological products for human use, and electronic products. Compliance with this part is intended to protect the rights and welfare of human subjects involved in such investigations.

(b) References in this part to regulatory sections of the Code of Federal Regulations are to Chapter I of Title 21, unless otherwise noted.

ß 56.102 Definitions.

As used in this part:

(a) Act means the Federal Food, Drug, and Cosmetic Act, as amended (secs. 201-902, 52 Stat. 1040 et seq., as amended (21 U.S.C. 321-392)).

(b) Application for research or marketing permit includes:

(1) A color additive petition, described in part 71.

(2) Data and information regarding a substance submitted as part of the procedures for establishing that a substance is generally recognized as safe for a use which results or may reasonably be expected to result, directly or indirectly, in its becoming a component or otherwise affecting the characteristics of any food, described in ß 170.35.

(3) A food additive petition, described in part 171.

(4) Data and information regarding a food additive submitted as part of the procedures regarding food additives permitted to be used on an interim basis pending additional study, described in ß 180.1.

(5) Data and information regarding a substance submitted as part of the procedures for establishing a tolerance for unavoidable contaminants in food and food-packaging materials described in section 406 of the act.

(6) An investigational new drug application, described in part 312 of this chapter.

(7) A new drug application, described in part 314.

(8) Data and information regarding the bioavailability or bioequivalence of drugs for human use submitted as part of the procedures for issuing, amending, or repealing a bioequivalence requirement, described in part 320.

(9) Data and information regarding an over-the-counter drug for human use submitted as part of the procedures for classifying such drugs as generally recognized as safe and effective and not misbranded, described in part 330.

(10) Data and information regarding an antibiotic drug submitted as part of the procedures for issuing amending, or repealing regulations for such drugs, described in ß 314.300 of this chapter.

(11) An application for a biological product license, described in part 601.

(12) Data and information regarding a biological product submitted as part of the procedures for determining that licensed biological products are safe and effective and not misbranded, as described in part 601.

(13) An Application for an Investigational Device Exemption, described in parts 812 and 813.

(14) Data and information regarding a medical device for human use submitted as part of the procedures for classifying such devices, described in part 860.

(15) Data and information regarding a medical device for human use submitted as part of the procedures for establishing, amending, or repealing a standard for such device, described in part 861.

(16) An application for premarket approval of a medical device for human use, described in section 515 of the act.

(17) A product development protocol for a medical device for human use, described in section 515 of the act.

(18) Data and information regarding an electronic product submitted as part of the procedures for establishing, amending, or repealing a standard for such products, described in section 358 of the Public Health Service Act.

(19) Data and information regarding an electronic product submitted as part of the procedures for obtaining a variance from any electronic product performance standard, as described in ß 1010.4.

(20) Data and information regarding an electronic product submitted as part of the procedures for granting, amending, or extending an exemption from a radiation safety performance standard as described in ß 1010.5.

(21) Data and information regarding an electronic product submitted as part of the procedures for obtaining an exemption from notification of a radiation safety defect or failure of compliance with a radiation safety performance standard, described in subpart D of part 1003.

(c) **Clinical investigation** means any experiment that involves a test article and one or more human subjects, and that either must meet the requirements for prior submission to the Food and Drug Administration under section 505(i), 507(d), or 520(g) of the act, or need not meet the requirements for prior submission to the Food and Drug Administration under these sections of the act, but the results of which are intended to be later submitted to, or held for inspection by, the Food and Drug Administration as part of an application for a research or marketing permit. The term does not include experiments that must meet the provisions of part 58, regarding nonclinical laboratory studies. The terms research, clinical research, clinical study, study, and clinical investigation are deemed to be synonymous for purposes of this part.

(d) **Emergency use** means the use of a test article on a human subject in a life-threatening situation in which no standard acceptable treatment is available, and in which there is not sufficient time to obtain IRB approval.

(e) **Human subject** means an individual who is or becomes a participant in research, either as a recipient of the test article or as a control. A subject may be either a healthy individual or a patient.

(f) **Institution** means any public or private entity or Agency (including Federal State, and other agencies). The term facility as used in section 520(g) of the act is deemed to be synonymous with the term institution for purposes of this part.

(g) Institutional Review Board (IRB) means any board committee, or other group formally designated by an institution to review, to approve the initiation of, and to conduct periodic review of, biomedical research involving human subjects. The primary purpose of such review is to assure the protection of the rights and welfare of the human subjects. The term has the same meaning as the phrase institutional review committee as used in section 520(g) of the act.

(h) Investigator means an individual who actually conducts a clinical investigation (i.e., under whose immediate direction the test article is administered or dispensed to or used involving, a subject) or, in the event of an investigation conducted by a team of individuals, is the responsible leader of that team.

(i) Minimal risk means that the probability and magnitude of harm or discomfort anticipated in the research are not greater in and of themselves than those ordinarily encountered in daily life or during the performance of routine physical or psychological examinations or tests.

(j) Sponsor means a person or other entity that initiates a clinical investigation, but that does not actually conduct the investigation, i.e., the test article is administered or dispensed to, or used involving, a subject under the immediate direction of another individual. A person other than an individual (e.g., a corporation or agency) that uses one or more of its own employees to conduct an investigation that it has initiated is considered to be a sponsor (not a sponsor-investigator) and the employees are considered to be investigators.

(k) Sponsor-investigator means an individual who both initiates and actually conducts, alone or with others a clinical investigation, i.e., under whose immediate direction the test article is administered or dispensed to, or used involving, a subject. The term does not include any person other than an individual, e.g., it does not include a corporation or agency. The obligations of a sponsor-investigator under this part include both those of a sponsor and those of an investigator.

(l) Test article means any drug for human use, biological product for human use, medical device for human use, human food additive, color additive, electronic product, or any other article subject to regulation under the act or under sections 351 or 354-360F of the Public Health Service Act.

(m) IRB approval means the determination of the IRB that the clinical investigation has been reviewed and may be conducted at an institution within the constraints set forth by the IRB and by other institutional and Federal requirements.

[46 FR 8975, Jan. 27, 1981, as amended at 54 FR 9038 Mar. 3, 1989; 56 FR 28028, June 18, 1991]

ß 56.103 Circumstances in which IRB review is required.

(a) Except as provided in ßß 56.104 and 56.105, any clinical investigation which must meet the requirements for prior submission (as required in parts 312, 812, and 813) to the Food and Drug Administration shall not be initiated unless that investigation has been reviewed and approved by, and remains subject to continuing review by, an IRB meeting the requirements of this part.

(b) Except as provided in ßß 56.104 and 56.105, the Food and Drug Administration may decide not to consider in support of an application for a research or marketing permit any data or information that has been derived from a clinical investigation that has not been approved by, and that was not subject to initial and continuing review by, an IRB meeting the requirements of this part. The determination that a clinical investigation may not be considered in support of an application for a research or marketing permit does not, however, relieve the applicant for such a permit of any obligation under any other applicable regulations to submit the results of the investigation to the Food and Drug Administration.

(**c**) Compliance with these regulations will in no way render inapplicable pertinent Federal, State, or local laws or regulations.

[46 FR 8975, Jan. 27, 1981; 46 FR 14340, Feb. 27, 1981]

ß 56.104 Exemptions from IRB requirement.

The following categories of clinical investigations are exempt from the requirements of this part for IRB review:

(**a**) Any investigation which commenced before July 27, 1981 and was subject to requirements for IRB review under FDA regulations before that date, provided that the investigation remains subject to review of an IRB which meets the FDA requirements in effect before July 27, 1981.

(**b**) Any investigation commenced before July 27, 1981 and was not otherwise subject to requirements for IRB review under Food and Drug Administration regulations before that date.

(**c**) Emergency use of a test article, provided that such emergency use is reported to the IRB within 5 working days. Any subsequent use of the test article at the institution is subject to IRB review.

(**d**) Taste and food quality evaluations and consumer acceptance studies, if wholesome foods without additives are consumed or if a food is consumed that contains a food ingredient at or below the level and for a use found to be safe, or agricultural, chemical, or environmental contaminant at or below the level found to be safe, by the Food and Drug Administration or approved by the Environmental Protection Agency or the Food Safety and Inspection Service of the U.S. Department of Agriculture.

[46 FR 8975, Jan. 27 1981, as amended at 56 FR 28028, June 18, 1991]

ß 56.105 Waiver of IRB requirement.

On the application of a sponsor or sponsor-investigator, the Food and Drug Administration may waive any of the requirements contained in these regulations including the requirements for IRB review, for specific research activities or for classes of research activities otherwise covered by these regulations.

SUBPART B—ORGANIZATION AND PERSONNEL

ß 56.107 IRB membership.

(**a**) Each IRB shall have at least five members, with varying backgrounds to promote complete and adequate review of research activities commonly conducted by the institution. The IRB shall be sufficiently qualified through the experience and expertise of its members and the diversity of the members, including consideration of race, gender, cultural backgrounds, and sensitivity to such issues as community attitudes, to promote respect for its advice and counsel in safeguarding the rights and welfare of human subjects. In addition to possessing the professional competence necessary to review the specific research activities, the IRB shall be able to ascertain the acceptability of proposed research in terms of institutional commitments and regulations applicable law, and standards of professional conduct and practice. The IRB shall therefore include persons knowledgeable in these areas. If an IRB regularly reviews research that involves a vulnerable category of subjects, such as children, prisoners, pregnant women, or handicapped or mentally disabled persons, consideration shall be given to the inclusion of one or more individuals who are knowledgeable about and experienced in working with those subjects.

(**b**) Every nondiscriminatory effort will be made to ensure that no IRB consists entirely of men or entirely of women, including the institution's consideration of qualified persons of both sexes, so long as no selection is made to the IRB on the basis of gender. No IRB may consist entirely of members of one profession.

(**c**) Each IRB shall include at least one member whose primary concerns are in the scientific area and at least one member whose primary concerns are in nonscientific areas.

(**d**) Each IRB shall include at least one member who is not otherwise affiliated with the institution and who is not part of the immediate family of a person who is affiliated with the institution.

(**e**) No IRB may have a member participate in the IRB's initial or continuing review of any project in which the member has a conflicting interest, except to provide information requested by the IRB.

(**f**) An IRB may, in its discretion, invite individuals with competence in special areas to assist in the review of complex issues which require expertise beyond or in addition to that available on the IRB. These individuals may not vote with the IRB.

[46 FR 8975, Jan. 27, 1981, as amended at 56 FR 28028, June 18, 1991; 56 FR 29756 June 28, 1991]

SUBPART C—IRB FUNCTIONS AND OPERATIONS

ß 56.108 IRB functions and operations.

In order to fulfill the requirements of these regulations, each IRB shall:

(**a**) Follow written procedures: (1) For conducting its initial and continuing review of research and for reporting its findings and actions to the investigator and the institution; (2) for determining which projects require review more often than annually and which projects need verification from sources other than the investigator that no material changes have occurred since previous IRB review; (3) for ensuring prompt reporting to the IRB of changes in research activity; and (4) for ensuring that changes in approved research, during the period for which IRB approval has already been given may not be initiated without IRB review and approval except where necessary to eliminate apparent immediate hazards to the human subjects.

(**b**) Follow written procedures for ensuring prompt reporting to the IRB, appropriate institutional officials, and the Food and Drug Administration of: (1) Any unanticipated problems involving risks to human subjects or others; (2) any instance of serious or continuing non-compliance with these regulations or the requirements or determinations of the IRB; or (3) any suspension or termination of IRB approval.

(**c**) Except when an expedited review procedure is used (see ß 56.110), review proposed research at convened meetings at which a majority of the members of the IRB are present including at least one member whose primary concerns are in nonscientific areas. In order for the research to be approved it shall receive the approval of a majority of those members present at the meeting.

[46 FR 8975, Jan. 27, 1981, as amended at 56 FR 28028, June 18, 1991]

ß 56.109 IRB review of research.

(**a**) An IRB shall review and have authority to approve, require modifications in (to secure approval), or disapprove all research activities covered by these regulations.

(**b**) An IRB shall require that information given to subjects as part of informed consent is in accordance with ß 50.25. The IRB may require that information in addition to that specifically mentioned in ß 50.25, be given to the subjects when in the IRB's judgment the information would meaningfully add to the protection of the rights and welfare of subjects.

(**c**) An IRB shall require documentation of informed consent in accordance with Sec. 50.27 of this chapter, except as follows: (1) The IRB may, for some or all subjects, waive the requirement that the subject, or the subject's legally authorized representative, sign a written consent form if it finds that the research presents no more than minimal risk of harm to subjects and involves no procedures for which written consent is normally required outside the research context; or (2) The IRB may, for some or all subjects, find that the requirements in Sec. 50.24 of this chapter for an exception from informed consent for emergency research are met.

(**d**) In cases where the documentation requirement is waived under paragraph (c)(1) of this section, the IRB may require the investigator to provide subjects with a written statement regarding the research.

(**e**) An IRB shall notify investigators and the institution in writing of its decision to approve or disapprove the proposed research activity, or of modifications required to secure IRB approval of the research activity. If the IRB decides to disapprove a research activity, it shall include in its written notification a statement of the reasons for its decision and give the investigator an opportunity to respond in person or in writing. For investigations involving an exception to informed consent under Sec. 50.24 of this chapter, an IRB shall promptly notify in writing the investigator and the sponsor of the research when an IRB determines that it cannot approve the research because it does not meet the criteria in the exception provided under Sec. 50.24(a) of this chapter or because of other relevant ethical concerns. The written notification shall include a statement of the reasons for the IRB's determination.

(**f**) An IRB shall conduct continuing review of research covered by these regulations at intervals appropriate to the degree of risk, but not less than once per year, and shall have authority to observe or have a third party observe the consent process and the research.

(**g**) An IRB shall provide in writing to the sponsor of research involving an exception to informed consent under Sec. 50.24 of this chapter a copy of information that has been publicly disclosed under Sec. 50.24(a)(7)(ii) and (a)(7)(iii) of this chapter. The IRB shall provide this information to the sponsor promptly so that the sponsor is aware that such disclosure has occurred. Upon receipt, the sponsor shall provide copies of the information disclosed to FDA.

[46 FR 8975, Jan. 27, 1981, as amended at 56 FR 28028, June 18, 1991, and at 61 FR 51497, Oct. 2, 1996]

ß 56.110 Expedited review procedures for certain kinds of research involving no more than minimal risk, and for minor changes in approved research.

(**a**) The Food and Drug Administration has established, and published in the Federal Register, a list of categories of research that may be reviewed by the IRB through an expedited review procedure. The list will be amended, as appropriate through periodic republication in the Federal Register.

(b) An IRB may use the expedited review procedure to review either or both of the following: (1) Some or all of the research appearing on the list **and** found by the reviewer(s) to involve no more than minimal risk, (2) minor changes in previously approved research during the period (of 1 year or less) for which approval is authorized. Under an expedited review procedure the review may be carried out by the IRB chairperson or by one or more experienced reviewers designated by the IRB chairperson from among the members of the IRB. In reviewing the research, the reviewers may exercise all of the authorities of the IRB except that the reviewers may not disapprove the research. A research activity may be disapproved only after review in accordance with the non-expedited review procedure set forth in ß 56.108(c).

(c) Each IRB which uses an expedited review procedure shall adopt a method for keeping all members advised of research proposals which have been approved under the procedure.

(d) The Food and Drug Administration may restrict, suspend, or terminate an institution's or IRB's use of the expedited review procedure when necessary to protect the rights or welfare of subjects. [46 FR 8975, Jan. 27, 1981, as amended at 56 FR 28029, June 18, 1991]

ß 56.111 Criteria for IRB approval of research.

(a) In order to approve research covered by these regulations the IRB shall determine that all of the following requirements are satisfied:

(1) Risks to subjects are minimized: (i) By using procedures which are consistent with sound research design and which do not unnecessarily expose subjects to risk, and (ii) whenever appropriate, by using procedures already being performed on the subjects for diagnostic or treatment purposes.

(2) Risks to subjects are reasonable in relation to anticipated benefits, if any, to subjects and the importance of the knowledge that may be expected to result. In evaluating risks and benefits, the IRB should consider only those risks and benefits that may result from the research (as distinguished from risks and benefits therapies that subjects would receive even if not participating in the research). The IRB should not consider possible long-range effects of applying knowledge gained in the research (for example, the possible effects of the research on public policy) as among those research risks that fall within the purview of its responsibility.

(3) Selection of subjects is equitable. In making this assessment the IRB should take into account the purposes of the research and the setting in which the research will be conducted and should be particularly cognizant of the special problems of research involving vulnerable populations, such as children, prisoners, pregnant women, handicapped, or mentally disabled persons, or economically or educationally disadvantaged persons.

(4) Informed consent will be sought from each prospective subject or the subject's legally authorized representative, in accordance with and to the extent required by part 50.

(5) Informed consent will be appropriately documented, in accordance with and to the extent required by ß 50.27.

(6) Where appropriate, the research plan makes adequate provision for monitoring the data collected to ensure the safety of subjects.

(7) Where appropriate, there are adequate provisions to protect the privacy of subjects and to maintain the confidentiality of data.

(b) When some or all of the subjects, such as children, prisoners, pregnant women, handicapped, or mentally disabled persons, or economically or educationally disadvantaged persons, are likely to be vulnerable to coercion or undue influence additional safeguards have been included in the study to protect the rights and welfare of these subjects.

[46 FR 8975, Jan. 27, 1981, as amended at 56 FR 28029, June 18, 1991]

ß 56.112 Review by institution.

Research covered by these regulations that has been approved by an IRB may be subject to further appropriate review and approval or disapproval by officials of the institution. However, those officials may not approve the research if it has not been approved by an IRB.

ß 56.113 Suspension or termination of IRB approval of research.

An IRB shall have authority to suspend or terminate approval of research that is not being conducted in accordance with the IRB's requirements or that has been associated with unexpected serious harm to subjects. Any suspension or termination of approval shall include a statement of the reasons for the IRB's action and shall be reported promptly to the investigator appropriate institutional officials, and the Food and Drug Administration.

ß 56.114 Cooperative research.

In complying with these regulations, institutions involved in multi-institutional studies may use joint review, reliance upon the review of another qualified IRB, or similar arrangements aimed at avoidance of duplication of effort.

SUBPART D—RECORDS AND REPORTS.

ß 56.115 IRB records.

(a) An institution, or where appropriate an IRB, shall prepare and maintain adequate documentation of IRB activities including the following:

(1) Copies of all research proposals reviewed, scientific evaluations, if any, that accompany the proposals, approved sample consent documents progress reports submitted by investigators, and reports of injuries to subjects.

(2) Minutes of IRB meetings which shall be in sufficient detail to show attendance at the meetings; actions taken by the IRB; the vote on these actions including the number of members voting for, against and abstaining; the basis for requiring changes in or disapproving research; and a written summary of the discussion of controverted issues and their resolution.

(3) Records of continuing review activities.

(4) Copies of all correspondence between the IRB and the investigators.

(5) A list of IRB members identified by name; earned degrees; representative capacity; indications of experience such as board certifications licenses, etc., sufficient to describe each member's chief anticipated contributions to IRB deliberations; and any employment or other relationship between each member and the institution; for example: full-time employee, part-time employee, a member of governing panel or board, stockholder, paid or unpaid consultant.

(6) Written procedures for the IRB as required by ß 56.108(a) and (b).

(7) Statements of significant new findings provided to subjects, as required by ß 50.25.

(b) The records required by this regulation shall be retained for at least 3 years after completion of the research, and the records shall be accessible for inspection and copying by authorized representatives of the Food and Drug Administration at reasonable times and in a reasonable manner.

(c) The Food and Drug Administration may refuse to consider a clinical investigation in support of an application for a research or marketing permit if the institution or the IRB that reviewed the investigation refuses to allow an inspection under this section.

[46 FR 8975, Jan. 27, 1981, as amended at 56 FR 28029, June 18, 1991]

SUBPART E—ADMINISTRATIVE ACTIONS FOR NON-COMPLIANCE

ß 56.120 Lesser administrative actions.

(a) If apparent non-compliance with these regulations in the operation of an IRB is observed by an FDA investigator during an inspection, the inspector will present an oral or written summary of observations to an appropriate representative of the IRB. The Food and Drug Administration may subsequently send a letter describing the non-compliance to the IRB and to the parent institution. The Agency will require that the IRB or the parent institution respond to this letter within a time period specified by FDA and describe the corrective actions that will be taken by the IRB, the institution, or both to achieve compliance with these regulations.

(b) On the basis of the IRB's or the institution's response FDA may schedule a reinspection to confirm the adequacy of corrective actions. In addition, until the IRB or the parent institution takes appropriate corrective action, the Agency may:

(1) Withhold approval of new studies subject to the requirements of this part that are conducted at the institution or reviewed by the IRB;

(2) Direct that no new subjects be added to ongoing studies subject to this part;

(3) Terminate ongoing studies subject to this part when doing so would not subjects; or

(4) When the apparent non-compliance creates a significant threat to the rights and welfare of human subjects notify relevant State and Federal regulatory agencies and other parties with a direct interest in the agency's action of the deficiencies in the operation of the IRB.

(c) The parent institution is presumed to be responsible for the operation of an IRB, and the Food and Drug Administration will ordinarily direct any administrative action under this subpart against the institution. However, depending on the evidence of responsibility for deficiencies, determined during the investigation, the Food and Drug Administration may restrict its administrative actions to the IRB or to a component of the parent institution determined to be responsible for formal designation of the IRB.

ß 56.121 Disqualification of an IRB or an institution.

(a) Whenever the IRB or the institution has failed to take adequate steps to correct the non-compliance stated in the letter sent by the Agency under ß 56.120(a), and the Commissioner of

Food and Drugs determines that this non-compliance may justify the disqualification of the IRB or of the parent institution, the Commissioner will institute proceedings in accordance with the requirements for a regulatory hearing set forth in part 16.

(b) The Commissioner may disqualify an IRB or the parent if the Commissioner determines that:

(1) The IRB has refused or repeatedly failed to comply with any of the regulations set forth in this part, and;

(2) The non-compliance adversely affects the rights or welfare of the human subjects in a clinical investigation.

(c) If the Commissioner determines that disqualification is appropriate, the Commissioner will issue an order that explains the basis for the determination and that prescribes any actions to be taken with regard to ongoing clinical research conducted under the review of the IRB. The Food and Drug Administration will send notice of the disqualification to the IRB and the parent institution. Other parties with a direct interest, such as sponsors and clinical investigators, may also be sent a notice of the disqualification. In addition, the Agency may elect to publish a notice of its action in the *Federal Register.*

(d) The Food and Drug Administration will not approve an application for a research permit for a clinical investigation that is to be under the review of a disqualified IRB or that is to be conducted at a disqualified institution, and it may refuse to consider in support of a marketing permit the data from a clinical investigation that was reviewed by a disqualified IRB as conducted at a disqualified institution unless the IRB or the parent institution is reinstated as provided in ß 56.123.

ß 56.122 Public disclosure of information regarding revocation.

A determination that the Food and Drug Administration has disqualified an institution and the administrative record regarding that determination are disclosable to the public under part 20.

ß 56.123 Reinstatement of an IRB or an institution.

An IRB or an institution may be reinstated if the Commissioner determines upon an evaluation of a written submission from the IRB or institution that explains the corrective action that the institution or IRB plans to take, that the IRB or institution has provided adequate assurance that it will operate in compliance with the standards set forth in this part. Notification of reinstatement shall be provided to all persons notified under ß 56.121(c).

ß 56.124 Actions alternative or additional to disqualification.

Disqualification of an IRB or of an institution is independent of, and neither in lieu of nor a precondition to, other proceedings or actions authorized by the act. The Food and Drug Administration may at any time, through the Department of Justice institute any appropriate judicial proceedings (civil or criminal) and any other appropriate regulatory action, in addition to or in lieu of, and before, at the time of, or after, disqualification. The Agency may also refer pertinent matters to another Federal State, or local government Agency for any action that Agency determines to be appropriate.

INTERNATIONAL GUIDELINES

The Nuremberg Code

THE NUREMBERG CODE

From "Trials of War Criminals Before the Nuremberg Military Tribunals Under Control Council Law No. 10," Vol. 2, Nuremberg, October 1946–April 1949. (Washington, DC: US Government Printing Office, 1949). pp 181–182.

The great weight of the evidence before us is to the effect that certain types of medical experiments on human beings, when kept within reasonably well-defined bounds, conform to the ethics of the medical profession generally. The protagonists of the practice of human experimentation justify their views on the basis that such experiments yield results for the good of society that are unprocurable by other methods or means of study. All agree, however, that certain basic principles must be observed in order to satisfy moral, ethical and legal concepts.

1. The voluntary consent of the human subject is absolutely essential.

    This means that the person involved should have legal capacity to give consent; should be so situated as to be able to exercise free power of choice, without the intervention of any element of force, fraud, deceit, duress, overreaching, or other ulterior form of constraint or coercion; and should have sufficient knowledge and comprehension of the elements of the subject matter involved as to enable him to make an understanding and enlightened decision. This latter element requires that before the acceptance of an affirmative decision by the experimental subject there should be made known to him the nature, duration, and purpose of the experiment; the method and means by which it is to be conducted; all inconveniences and hazards reasonably to be expected; and the effects upon his health or person which may possibly come from his participation in the experiment.

    The duty and responsibility for ascertaining the quality of the consent rests upon each individual who initiates, directs or engages in the experiment. It is a personal duty and responsibility which may not be delegated to another with impunity.

2. The experiment should be such as to yield fruitful results for the good of society, unprocurable by other methods or means of study, and not random and unnecessary in nature.

3. The experiment should be so designed and based on the results of animal experimentation and a knowledge of the natural history of the disease or other problems under study that the anticipated results will justify the performance of the experiment.

4. The experiment should be so conducted as to avoid all unnecessary physical and mental suffering and injury.

5. No experiment should be conducted where there is an a priori reason to believe that death or disabling injury will occur; except perhaps, in those experiments where the experimental physicians also serve as subjects.

6. The degree of risk to be taken should never exceed that determined by the humanitarian importance of the problem to be solved by the experiment.

7. Proper preparations should be made and adequate facilities provided to protect the experimental subject against even remote possibilities of injury, disability, or death.

8. The experiment should be conducted only by scientifically qualified persons. The highest degree of skill and care should be required through all stages of the experiment of those who conduct or engage in the experiment.

9. During the course of the experiment the human subject should be at liberty to bring the experiment to an end if he has reached the physical or mental state where continuation of the experiment seems to him to be impossible.

10. During the course of the experiment the scientist in charge must be prepared to terminate the experiment at any stage, if he has probable cause to believe in the exercise of the good faith, superior skill and careful judgement required of him that a continuation of the experiment is likely to result in injury, disability, or death to the experimental subject.

The Declaration of Helsinki (Edinburgh Revision, 2000)

WORLD MEDICAL ASSOCIATION: DECLARATION OF HELSINKI

Ethical Principles for Medical Research Involving Human Subjects

Adopted by the 18th WMA General Assembly Helsinki, Finland, June 1964 and amended by the 29th WMA General Assembly, Tokyo, Japan, October 1975 35th WMA General Assembly, Venice, Italy, October 1983 41st WMA General Assembly, Hong Kong, September 1989 48th WMA General Assembly, Somerset West, Republic of South Africa, October 1996 and the 52nd WMA General Assembly, Edinburgh, Scotland, October 2000

A. INTRODUCTION

1. The World Medical Association has developed the Declaration of Helsinki as a statement of ethical principles to provide guidance to physicians and other participants in medical research involving human subjects. Medical research involving human subjects includes research on identifiable human material or identifiable data. 2. It is the duty of the physician to promote and safeguard the health of the people. The physician's knowledge and conscience are dedicated to the fulfillment of this duty. 3. The Declaration of Geneva of the World Medical Association binds the physician with the words, "The health of my patient will be my first consideration," and the International Code of Medical Ethics declares that, "A physician shall act only in the patient's interest when providing medical care which might have the effect of weakening the physical and mental condition of the patient." 4. Medical progress is based on research which ultimately must rest in part on experimentation involving human subjects. 5. In medical research on human subjects, considerations related to the well-being of the human subject should take precedence over the interests of science and society. 6. The primary purpose of medical research involving human subjects is to improve prophylactic, diagnostic and therapeutic procedures and the understanding of the aetiology and pathogenesis of disease. Even the best proven prophylactic, diagnostic, and therapeutic methods must continuously be challenged through research for their effectiveness, efficiency, accessibility and quality. 7. In current medical practice and in medical research, most prophylactic, diagnostic and therapeutic procedures involve risks and burdens. 8. Medical research is subject to ethical standards that promote respect for all human beings and protect their health and rights. Some research populations are vulnerable and need special protection. The particular needs of the economically and medically disadvantaged must be recognized. Special attention is also required for those who cannot give or refuse consent for themselves, for those who may be subject to giving consent under duress, for those who will not benefit personally from the research and for those for whom the research is combined with care. 9. Research Investigators should be aware of the ethical, legal and regulatory requirements for research on human subjects in their own countries as well as applicable international requirements. No national ethical, legal or regulatory requirement should be allowed to reduce or eliminate any of the protections for human subjects set forth in this Declaration.

B. BASIC PRINCIPLES FOR ALL MEDICAL RESEARCH

10. It is the duty of the physician in medical research to protect the life, health, privacy, and dignity of the human subject. 11. Medical research involving human subjects must conform to generally accepted scientific principles, be based on a thorough knowledge of the scientific literature, other

relevant sources of information, and on adequate laboratory and, where appropriate, animal experimentation. 12. Appropriate caution must be exercised in the conduct of research which may affect the environment, and the welfare of animals used for research must be respected. 13. The design and performance of each experimental procedure involving human subjects should be clearly formulated in an experimental protocol. This protocol should be submitted for consideration, comment, guidance, and where appropriate, approval to a specially appointed ethical review committee, which must be independent of the investigator, the sponsor or any other kind of undue influence. This independent committee should be in conformity with the laws and regulations of the country in which the research experiment is performed. The committee has the right to monitor ongoing trials. The researcher has the obligation to provide monitoring information to the committee, especially any serious adverse events. The researcher should also submit to the committee, for review, information regarding funding, sponsors, institutional affiliations, other potential conflicts of interest and incentives for subjects. 14. The research protocol should always contain a statement of the ethical considerations involved and should indicate that there is compliance with the principles enunciated in this Declaration. 15. Medical research involving human subjects should be conducted only by scientifically qualified persons and under the supervision of a clinically competent medical person. The responsibility for the human subject must always rest with a medically qualified person and never rest on the subject of the research, even though the subject has given consent. 16. Every medical research project involving human subjects should be preceded by careful assessment of predictable risks and burdens in comparison with foreseeable benefits to the subject or to others. This does not preclude the participation of healthy volunteers in medical research. The design of all studies should be publicly available. 17. Physicians should abstain from engaging in research projects involving human subjects unless they are confident that the risks involved have been adequately assessed and can be satisfactorily managed. Physicians should cease any investigation if the risks are found to outweigh the potential benefits or if there is conclusive proof of positive and beneficial results. 18. Medical research involving human subjects should only be conducted if the importance of the objective outweighs the inherent risks and burdens to the subject. This is especially important when the human subjects are healthy volunteers. 19. Medical research is only justified if there is a reasonable likelihood that the populations in which the research is carried out stand to benefit from the results of the research. 20. The subjects must be volunteers and informed participants in the research project. 21. The right of research subjects to safeguard their integrity must always be respected. Every precaution should be taken to respect the privacy of the subject, the confidentiality of the patient's information and to minimize the impact of the study on the subject's physical and mental integrity and on the personality of the subject. 22. In any research on human beings, each potential subject must be adequately informed of the aims, methods, sources of funding, any possible conflicts of interest, institutional affiliations of the researcher, the anticipated benefits and potential risks of the study and the discomfort it may entail. The subject should be informed of the right to abstain from participation in the study or to withdraw consent to participate at any time without reprisal. After ensuring that the subject has understood the information, the physician should then obtain the subject's freely-given informed consent, preferably in writing. If the consent cannot be obtained in writing, the non-written consent must be formally documented and witnessed. 23. When obtaining informed consent for the research project the physician should be particularly cautious if the subject is in a dependent relationship with the physician or may consent under duress. In that case the informed consent should be obtained by a well-informed physician who is not engaged in the investigation and who is completely independent of this relationship. 24. For a research subject who is legally incompetent, physically or mentally incapable of giving consent or is a legally incompetent minor, the investigator must obtain informed consent from the legally authorized representative in accordance with applicable law. These groups should not be included in research unless the research is necessary to promote the health of the population represented and this research cannot instead be performed on legally competent persons. 25. When a subject deemed legally incompetent, such as a minor child, is able to give assent to decisions about participation in research, the investigator must obtain that assent in addition to the consent of the legally authorized representative. 26. Research on individuals from whom it is not possible to obtain consent, including proxy or advance consent, should be done only if the physical/mental condition that prevents obtaining informed consent is a necessary characteristic of the research population. The specific reasons for involving research subjects with a condition that renders them unable to give informed consent should be stated in the experimental protocol for consideration and approval of the review committee. The protocol should state that consent to remain in the research should be obtained as soon as possible from the individual or a legally authorized surrogate. 27. Both authors and publishers have ethical obligations. In publication of the results of research, the investigators are obliged to preserve the accuracy of the results. Negative as well as positive results should be published or otherwise publicly available. Sources of funding, institutional affiliations and any possible conflicts of interest should be declared in the publication. Reports of experimentation not in accordance with the principles laid down in this Declaration should not be accepted for publication.

C. ADDITIONAL PRINCIPLES FOR MEDICAL RESEARCH COMBINED WITH MEDICAL CARE

28. The physician may combine medical research with medical care, only to the extent that the research is justified by its potential prophylactic, diagnostic or therapeutic value. When medical research is combined with medical care, additional standards apply to protect the patients who are research subjects. 29. The benefits, risks, burdens and effectiveness of a new method should be tested against those of the best current prophylactic, diagnostic, and therapeutic methods. This does not exclude the use of placebo, or no treatment, in studies where no proven prophylactic, diagnostic or therapeutic method exists. 30. At the conclusion of the study, every patient entered into the study should be assured of access to the best proven prophylactic, diagnostic and therapeutic methods identified by the study. 31. The physician should fully inform the patient which aspects of the care are related to the research. The refusal of a patient to participate in a study must never interfere with the patient-physician relationship. 32. In the treatment of a patient, where proven prophylactic, diagnostic and therapeutic methods do not exist or have been ineffective, the physician, with informed consent from the patient, must be free to use unproven or new prophylactic, diagnostic and therapeutic measures, if in the physician's judgement it offers hope of saving life, re-establishing health or alleviating suffering. Where possible, these measures should be made the object of research, designed to evaluate their safety and efficacy. In all cases, new information should be recorded and, where appropriate, published. The other relevant guidelines of this Declaration should be followed. § § § 7.10.2000 09h14

THE BELMONT REPORT

OFFICE OF THE SECRETARY

ETHICAL PRINCIPLES AND GUIDELINES FOR THE PROTECTION
OF HUMAN
SUBJECTS OF RESEARCH

THE NATIONAL COMMISSION FOR THE PROTECTION
OF HUMAN SUBJECTS
OF BIOMEDICAL AND BEHAVIORAL RESEARCH

APRIL 18, 1979

AGENCY: Department of Health, Education, and Welfare.

ACTION: Notice of Report for Public Comment.

SUMMARY: On July 12, 1974, the National Research Act (Pub. L. 93-348) was signed into law, there-by creating the National Commission for the Protection of Human Subjects of Biomedical and Behavioral Research. One of the charges to the Commission was to identify the basic ethical principles that should underlie the conduct of biomedical and behavioral research involving human subjects and to develop guidelines which should be followed to assure that such research is conducted in accordance with those principles. In carrying out the above, the Commission was directed to consider: (i) the boundaries between biomedical and behavioral research and the accepted and routine practice of medicine, (ii) the role of assessment of risk-benefit criteria in the determination of the appropriateness of research involving human subjects, (iii) appropriate guidelines for the selection of human subjects for participation in such research and (iv) the nature and definition of informed consent in various research settings.

The Belmont Report attempts to summarize the basic ethical principles identified by the Commission in the course of its deliberations. It is the outgrowth of an intensive four-day period of discussions that were held in February 1976 at the Smithsonian Institution's Belmont Conference Center supplemented by the monthly deliberations of the Commission that were held over a period of nearly four years. It is a statement of basic ethical principles and guidelines that should assist in resolving the ethical problems that surround the conduct of research with human subjects. By publishing the Report in the *Federal Register,* and providing reprints upon request, the Secretary intends that it may be made readily available to scientists, members of Institutional Review Boards, and Federal employees. The two-volume Appendix, containing the lengthy reports of experts and specialists who assisted the Commission in fulfilling this part of its charge, is available as DHEW

Publication No. (OS) 78-0013 and No. (OS) 78-0014, for sale by the Superintendent of Documents, U.S. Government Printing Office, Washington, D.C. 20402.

Unlike most other reports of the Commission, the Belmont Report does not make specific recommendations for administrative action by the Secretary of Health, Education, and Welfare. Rather, the Commission recommended that the Belmont Report be adopted in its entirety, as a statement of the Department's policy. The Department requests public comment on this recommendation.

National Commission for the Protection of Human Subjects
of Biomedical and Behavioral Research

Members of the Commission

Kenneth John Ryan, M.D., Chairman, Chief of Staff, Boston Hospital for Women.

Joseph V. Brady, Ph.D., Professor of Behavioral Biology, Johns Hopkins University.

Robert E. Cooke, M.D., President, Medical College of Pennsylvania.

Dorothy I. Height, President, National Council of Negro Women, Inc.

Albert R. Jonsen, Ph.D., Associate Professor of Bioethics, University of California at San Francisco.

Patricia King, J.D., Associate Professor of Law, Georgetown University Law Center.

Karen Lebacqz, Ph.D., Associate Professor of Christian Ethics, Pacific School of Religion.

*** David W. Louisell, J.D., Professor of Law, University of California at Berkeley.

Donald W. Seldin, M.D., Professor and Chairman, Department of Internal Medicine, University of Texas at Dallas.

*** Eliot Stellar, Ph.D., Provost of the University and Professor of Physiological Psychology, University of Pennsylvania.

*** Robert H. Turtle, LL.B., Attorney, VomBaur, Coburn, Simmons & Turtle, Washington, D.C.

*** Deceased.

Table of Contents

Ethical Principles and Guidelines for Research Involving Human Subjects
A. Boundaries Between Practice and Research
B. Basic Ethical Principles
1. Respect for Persons
2. Beneficence
3. Justice
C. Applications
1. Informed Consent
2. Assessment of Risk and Benefits
3. Selection of Subjects

Ethical Principles & Guidelines for Research Involving Human Subjects

Scientific research has produced substantial social benefits. It has also posed some troubling ethical questions. Public attention was drawn to these questions by reported abuses of human subjects in biomedical experiments, especially during the Second World War. During the Nuremberg War Crime Trials, the Nuremberg code was drafted as a set of standards for judging physicians and scientists who had conducted biomedical experiments on concentration camp prisoners. This code became the prototype of many later codes(1) intended to assure that research involving human subjects would be carried out in an ethical manner.

The codes consist of rules, some general, others specific, that guide the investigators or the reviewers of research in their work. Such rules often are inadequate to cover complex situations; at times they come into conflict, and they are frequently difficult to interpret or apply. Broader ethical principles will provide a basis on which specific rules may be formulated, criticized and interpreted.

Three principles, or general prescriptive judgments, that are relevant to research involving human subjects are identified in this statement. Other principles may also be relevant. These three are comprehensive, however, and are stated at a level of generalization that should assist scientists, subjects, reviewers and interested citizens to understand the ethical issues inherent in research involving human subjects. These principles cannot always be applied so as to resolve beyond dispute particular ethical problems. The objective is to provide an analytical framework that will guide the resolution of ethical problems arising from research involving human subjects.

This statement consists of a distinction between research and practice, a discussion of the three basic ethical principles, and remarks about the application of these principles.

Part A: Boundaries Between Practice & Research

A. Boundaries Between Practice and Research

It is important to distinguish between biomedical and behavioral research, on the one hand, and the practice of accepted therapy on the other, in order to know what activities ought to undergo review for the protection of human subjects of research. The distinction between research and practice is blurred partly because both often occur together (as in research designed to evaluate a therapy) and partly because notable departures from standard practice are often called "experimental" when the terms "experimental" and "research" are not carefully defined.

For the most part, the term "practice" refers to interventions that are designed solely to enhance the well-being of an individual patient or client and that have a reasonable expectation of success. The purpose of medical or behavioral practice is to provide diagnosis, preventive treatment or therapy to particular individuals.(2) By contrast, the term "research' designates an activity designed to test an hypothesis, permit conclusions to be drawn, and thereby to develop or contribute to generalizable knowledge (expressed, for example, in theories, principles, and statements of relationships). Research is usually described in a formal protocol that sets forth an objective and a set of procedures designed to reach that objective.

When a clinician departs in a significant way from standard or accepted practice, the innovation does not, in and of itself, constitute research. The fact that a procedure is "experimental," in the sense of new, untested or different, does not automatically place it in the category of research. Radically new procedures of this description should, however, be made the object of formal research at an early stage in order to determine whether they are safe and effective. Thus, it is the responsibility of medical practice committees, for example, to insist that a major innovation be incorporated into a formal research project.(3)

Research and practice may be carried on together when research is designed to evaluate the safety and efficacy of a therapy. This need not cause any confusion regarding whether or not the activity requires review; the general rule is that if there is any element of research in an activity, that activity should undergo review for the protection of human subjects.

Part B: Basic Ethical Principles

B. Basic Ethical Principles

The expression "basic ethical principles" refers to those general judgments that serve as a basic justification for the many particular ethical prescriptions and evaluations of human actions. Three basic principles, among those generally accepted in our cultural tradition, are particularly relevant to the ethics of research involving human subjects: the principles of respect of persons, beneficence and justice.

1. Respect for Persons.—Respect for persons incorporates at least two ethical convictions: first, that individuals should be treated as autonomous agents, and second, that persons with diminished autonomy are entitled to protection. The principle of respect for persons thus divides into two separate moral requirements: the requirement to acknowledge autonomy and the requirement to protect those with diminished autonomy.

An autonomous person is an individual capable of deliberation about personal goals and of acting under the direction of such deliberation. To respect autonomy is to give weight to autonomous persons' considered opinions and choices while refraining from obstructing their actions unless they are clearly detrimental to others. To show lack of respect for an autonomous agent is to repudiate that person's considered judgments, to deny an individual the freedom to act on those considered judgments, or to withhold information necessary to make a considered judgment, when there are no compelling reasons to do so.

However, not every human being is capable of self-determination. The capacity for self-determination matures during an individual's life, and some individuals lose this capacity wholly or in part because of illness, mental disability, or circumstances that severely restrict liberty. Respect for the immature and the incapacitated may require protecting them as they mature or while they are incapacitated.

Some persons are in need of extensive protection, even to the point of excluding them from activities which may harm them; other persons require little protection beyond making sure they undertake activities freely and with awareness of possible adverse consequence. The extent of protection afforded should depend upon the risk of harm and the likelihood of benefit. The judgment that any individual lacks autonomy should be periodically reevaluated and will vary in different situations.

In most cases of research involving human subjects, respect for persons demands that subjects enter into the research voluntarily and with adequate information. In some situations, however, application of the principle is not obvious. The involvement of prisoners as subjects of research provides an instructive example. On the one hand, it would seem that the principle of respect for persons requires that prisoners not be deprived of the opportunity to volunteer for research. On the other hand, under prison conditions they may be subtly coerced or unduly influenced to engage in research activities for which they would not otherwise volunteer. Respect for persons would then dictate that prisoners be protected. Whether to allow prisoners to "volunteer" or to "protect" them presents a dilemma. Respecting persons, in most hard cases, is often a matter of balancing competing claims urged by the principle of respect itself.

2. Beneficence.—Persons are treated in an ethical manner not only by respecting their decisions and protecting them from harm, but also by making efforts to secure their well-being. Such treatment falls under the principle of beneficence. The term "beneficence" is often understood to cover acts of kindness or charity that go beyond strict obligation. In this document, beneficence is understood in a stronger sense, as an obligation. Two general rules have been formulated as complementary expressions of beneficent actions in this sense: **(1)** do not harm and **(2)** maximize possible benefits and minimize possible harms.

The Hippocratic maxim "do no harm" has long been a fundamental principle of medical ethics. Claude Bernard extended it to the realm of research, saying that one should not injure one person regardless of the benefits that might come to others. However, even avoiding harm requires learning what is harmful; and, in the process of obtaining this information, persons may be exposed to risk of harm. Further, the Hippocratic Oath requires physicians to benefit their patients "according to their best judgment." Learning what will in fact benefit may require exposing persons to risk. The problem posed by these imperatives is to decide when it is justifiable to seek certain benefits despite the risks involved, and when the benefits should be foregone because of the risks.

The obligations of beneficence affect both individual investigators and society at large, because they extend both to particular research projects and to the entire enterprise of research. In the case of particular projects, investigators and members of their institutions are obliged to give forethought to the maximization of benefits and the reduction of risk that might occur from the research investigation. In the case of scientific research in general, members of the larger society are obliged to recognize the longer term benefits and risks that may result from the improvement of knowledge and from the development of novel medical, psychotherapeutic, and social procedures.

The principle of beneficence often occupies a well-defined justifying role in many areas of research involving human subjects. An example is found in research involving children. Effective ways of treating childhood diseases and fostering healthy development are benefits that serve to justify research involving children—even when individual research subjects are not direct beneficiaries. Research also makes it possible to avoid the harm that may result from the application of previously accepted routine practices that on closer investigation turn out to be dangerous. But the role of the principle of beneficence is not always so unambiguous. A difficult ethical problem remains, for example, about research that presents more than minimal risk without immediate prospect of direct benefit to the children involved. Some have argued that such research is inadmissible, while others have pointed out that this limit would rule out much research promising great benefit to children in the future. Here again, as with all hard cases, the different claims covered by the principle of beneficence may come into conflict and force difficult choices.

3. Justice.—Who ought to receive the benefits of research and bear its burdens? This is a question of justice, in the sense of "fairness in distribution" or "what is deserved." An injustice occurs when some benefit to which a person is entitled is denied without good reason or when some burden is imposed unduly. Another way of conceiving the principle of justice is that equals ought to be treated equally. However, this statement requires explication. Who is equal and who is unequal? What considerations justify departure from equal distribution? Almost all commentators allow that distinctions based on experience, age, deprivation, competence, merit and position do sometimes constitute criteria justifying differential treatment for certain purposes. It is necessary, then, to explain in what respects people should be treated equally. There are several widely accepted formulations of just ways to distribute burdens and benefits. Each formulation mentions some relevant property on the basis of which burdens and benefits should be distributed. These formulations are (**1**) to each person an equal share, (**2**) to each person according to individual need, (**3**) to each person according to individual effort, (**4**) to each person according to societal contribution, and (**5**) to each person according to merit.

Questions of justice have long been associated with social practices such as punishment, taxation and political representation. Until recently these questions have not generally been associated with scientific research. However, they are foreshadowed even in the earliest reflections on the ethics of research involving human subjects. For example, during the 19th and early 20th centuries the burdens of serving as research subjects fell largely upon poor ward patients, while the benefits of improved medical care flowed primarily to private patients. Subsequently, the exploitation of unwilling prisoners as research subjects in Nazi concentration camps was condemned as a particularly flagrant injustice. In this country, in the 1940's, the Tuskegee syphilis study used disadvantaged, rural black men to study the untreated course of a disease that is by no means confined to that population. These subjects were deprived of demonstrably effective treatment in order not to interrupt the project, long after such treatment became generally available.

Against this historical background, it can be seen how conceptions of justice are relevant to research involving human subjects. For example, the selection of research subjects needs to be scrutinized in order to determine whether some classes (e.g., welfare patients, particular racial and ethnic minorities, or persons confined to institutions) are being systematically selected simply because of their easy availability, their compromised position, or their manipulability, rather than for reasons directly related to the problem being studied. Finally, whenever research supported by public funds leads to the development of therapeutic devices and procedures, justice demands both that these not provide advantages only to those who can afford them and that such research should not unduly involve persons from groups unlikely to be among the beneficiaries of subsequent applications of the research.

Part C: Applications

C. Applications

Applications of the general principles to the conduct of research leads to consideration of the following requirements: informed consent, risk/benefit assessment, and the selection of subjects of research.

1. Informed Consent.—Respect for persons requires that subjects, to the degree that they are capable, be given the opportunity to choose what shall or shall not happen to them. This opportunity is provided when adequate standards for informed consent are satisfied.

While the importance of informed consent is unquestioned, controversy prevails over the nature and possibility of an informed consent. Nonetheless, there is widespread agreement that the consent process can be analyzed as containing three elements: information, comprehension and voluntariness.

Information. Most codes of research establish specific items for disclosure intended to assure that subjects are given sufficient information. These items generally include: the research procedure, their purposes, risks and anticipated benefits, alternative procedures (where therapy is involved), and a statement offering the subject the opportunity to ask questions and to withdraw at any time from the research. Additional items have been proposed, including how subjects are selected, the person responsible for the research, etc.

However, a simple listing of items does not answer the question of what the standard should be for judging how much and what sort of information should be provided. One standard frequently invoked in medical practice, namely the information commonly provided by practitioners in the field or in the locale, is inadequate since research takes place precisely when a common understanding does not exist. Another standard, currently popular in malpractice law, requires the practitioner to reveal the information that reasonable persons would wish to know in order to make a decision regarding their care. This, too, seems insufficient since the research subject, being in essence a volunteer, may wish to know considerably more about risks gratuitously undertaken than do patients who deliver themselves into the hand of a clinician for needed care. It may be that a standard of "the reasonable volunteer" should be proposed: the extent and nature of information should be such that persons, knowing that the procedure is neither necessary for their care nor perhaps fully understood, can decide whether they wish to participate in the furthering of knowledge. Even when some direct benefit to them is anticipated, the subjects should understand clearly the range of risk and the voluntary nature of participation.

A special problem of consent arises where informing subjects of some pertinent aspect of the research is likely to impair the validity of the research. In many cases, it is sufficient to indicate to subjects that they are being invited to participate in research of which some features will not be revealed until the research is concluded. In all cases of research involving incomplete disclosure, such research is justified only if it is clear that (**1**) incomplete disclosure is truly necessary to accomplish the goals of the research, (**2**) there are no undisclosed risks to subjects that are more than minimal, and (**3**) there is an adequate plan for debriefing subjects, when appropriate, and for dissemination of research results to them. Information about risks should never be withheld for the purpose of eliciting the cooperation of subjects, and truthful answers should always be given to direct questions about the research. Care should be taken to distinguish cases in which disclosure would destroy or invalidate the research from cases in which disclosure would simply inconvenience the investigator.

Comprehension. The manner and context in which information is conveyed is as important as the information itself. For example, presenting information in a disorganized and rapid fashion, allowing too little time for consideration or curtailing opportunities for questioning, all may adversely affect a subject's ability to make an informed choice.

Because the subject's ability to understand is a function of intelligence, rationality, maturity and language, it is necessary to adapt the presentation of the information to the subject's capacities. Investigators are responsible for ascertaining that the subject has comprehended the information. While there is always an obligation to ascertain that the information about risk to subjects is complete and adequately comprehended, when the risks are more serious, that obligation increases. On occasion, it may be suitable to give some oral or written tests of comprehension. Special provision may need to be made when comprehension is severely limited—for example, by conditions of immaturity or mental disability. Each class of subjects that one might consider as incompetent (e.g., infants and young children, mentally disable patients, the terminally ill and the comatose) should be considered on its own terms. Even for these persons, however, respect requires giving them the opportunity to choose to the extent they are able, whether or not to participate in research. The objections of these subjects to involvement should be honored, unless the research entails providing them a therapy unavailable elsewhere. Respect for persons also requires seeking the permission of other parties in order to protect the subjects from harm. Such persons are thus respected both by acknowledging their own wishes and by the use of third parties to protect them from harm.

The third parties chosen should be those who are most likely to understand the incompetent subject's situation and to act in that person's best interest. The person authorized to act on behalf of the subject should be given an opportunity to observe the research as it proceeds in order to be able to withdraw the subject from the research, if such action appears in the subject's best interest.

Voluntariness. An agreement to participate in research constitutes a valid consent only if voluntarily given. This element of informed consent requires conditions free of coercion and undue influence. Coercion occurs when an overt threat of harm is intentionally presented by one person to another in order to obtain compliance. Undue influence, by contrast, occurs through an offer of an excessive, unwarranted, inappropriate or improper reward or other overture in order to obtain compliance. Also, inducements that would ordinarily be acceptable may become undue influences if the subject is especially vulnerable.

Unjustifiable pressures usually occur when persons in positions of authority or commanding influence—especially where possible sanctions are involved—urge a course of action for a subject. A continuum of such influencing factors exists, however, and it is impossible to state precisely where justifiable persuasion ends and undue influence begins. But undue influence would include actions such as manipulating a person's choice through the controlling influence of a close relative and threatening to withdraw health services to which an individual would otherwise be entitle.

2. Assessment of Risks and Benefits.—The assessment of risks and benefits requires a careful arrayal of relevant data, including, in some cases, alternative ways of obtaining the benefits sought in the research. Thus, the assessment presents both an opportunity and a responsibility to gather systematic and comprehensive information about proposed research. For the investigator, it is a means to examine whether the proposed research is properly designed. For a review committee, it is a method for determining whether the risks that will be presented to subjects are justified. For prospective subjects, the assessment will assist the determination whether or not to participate.

The Nature and Scope of Risks and Benefits. The requirement that research be justified on the basis of a favorable risk/benefit assessment bears a close relation to the principle of beneficence, just as the moral requirement that informed consent be obtained is derived primarily from the principle of respect for persons. The term "risk" refers to a possibility that harm may occur. However, when expressions such as "small risk" or "high risk" are used, they usually refer (often ambiguously) both to the chance (probability) of experiencing a harm and the severity (magnitude) of the envisioned harm.

The term "benefit" is used in the research context to refer to something of positive value related to health or welfare. Unlike, "risk," "benefit" is not a term that expresses probabilities. Risk is properly contrasted to probability of benefits, and benefits are properly contrasted with harms rather than risks of harm. Accordingly, so-called risk/benefit assessments are concerned with the probabilities and magnitudes of possible harm and anticipated benefits. Many kinds of possible harms and benefits need to be taken into account. There are, for example, risks of psychological harm, physical harm, legal harm, social harm and economic harm and the corresponding benefits. While the most likely types of harms to research subjects are those of psychological or physical pain or injury, other possible kinds should not be overlooked.

Risks and benefits of research may affect the individual subjects, the families of the individual subjects, and society at large (or special groups of subjects in society). Previous codes and Federal regulations have required that risks to subjects be outweighed by the sum of both the anticipated benefit to the subject, if any, and the anticipated benefit to society in the form of knowledge to be gained from the research. In balancing these different elements, the risks and benefits affecting the immediate research subject will normally carry special weight. On the other hand, interests other than those of the subject may on some occasions be sufficient by themselves to justify the risks involved in the research, so long as the subjects' rights have been protected. Beneficence thus requires that we protect against risk of harm to subjects and also that we be concerned about the loss of the substantial benefits that might be gained from research.

The Systematic Assessment of Risks and Benefits. It is commonly said that benefits and risks must be "balanced" and shown to be "in a favorable ratio." The metaphorical character of these terms draws attention to the difficulty of making precise judgments. Only on rare occasions will quantitative techniques be available for the scrutiny of research protocols. However, the idea of systematic, nonarbitrary analysis of risks and benefits should be emulated insofar as possible. This ideal requires those making decisions about the justifiability of research to be thorough in the accumulation and assessment of information about all aspects of the research, and to consider alternatives systematically. This procedure renders the assessment of research more rigorous and precise, while making communication between review board members and investigators less subject to misinterpretation, misinformation and conflicting judgments. Thus, there should first be a determination of the validity of the presuppositions of the research; then the nature, probability and magnitude of risk should be distinguished with as much clarity as possible. The method of ascertaining risks should be explicit, especially where there is no alternative to the use of such vague categories as small or slight risk. It should also be determined whether an investigator's estimates of the probability of harm or benefits are reasonable, as judged by known facts or other available studies.

Finally, assessment of the justifiability of research should reflect at least the following considerations: (i) Brutal or inhumane treatment of human subjects is never morally justified. (ii) Risks should be reduced to those necessary to achieve the research objective. It should be determined whether it is in fact necessary to use human subjects at all. Risk can perhaps never be entirely eliminated, but it can often be reduced by careful attention to alternative procedures. (iii) When research involves significant risk of serious impairment, review committees should be extraordinarily insistent on the justification of the risk (looking usually to the likelihood of benefit to the subject — or, in some rare cases, to the manifest voluntariness of the participation). (iv) When vulnerable populations are involved in research, the appropriateness of involving them should itself be demonstrated. A number of variables go into such judgments, including the nature and degree of risk, the condition of the particular population involved, and the nature and level of the anticipated benefits. (v) Relevant risks and benefits must be thoroughly arrayed in documents and procedures used in the informed consent process.

3. Selection of Subjects.—Just as the principle of respect for persons finds expression in the requirements for consent, and the principle of beneficence in risk/benefit assessment, the principle of justice gives rise to moral requirements that there be fair procedures and outcomes in the selection of research subjects.

Justice is relevant to the selection of subjects of research at two levels: the social and the individual. Individual justice in the selection of subjects would require that researchers exhibit fairness: thus, they should not offer potentially beneficial research only to some patients who are in their favor or select only "undesirable" persons for risky research. Social justice requires that distinction be drawn between classes of subjects that ought, and ought not, to participate in any particular kind of research, based on the ability of members of that class to bear burdens and on the appropriateness of placing further burdens on already burdened persons. Thus, it can be considered a matter of social justice that there is an order of preference in the selection of classes of subjects (e.g., adults before children) and that some classes of potential subjects (e.g., the institutionalized mentally infirm or prisoners) may be involved as research subjects, if at all, only on certain conditions.

Injustice may appear in the selection of subjects, even if individual subjects are selected fairly by investigators and treated fairly in the course of research. Thus injustice arises from social, racial, sexual and cultural biases institutionalized in society. Thus, even if individual researchers are treating their research subjects fairly, and even if IRBs are taking care to assure that subjects are selected fairly within a particular institution, unjust social patterns may nevertheless appear in the overall distribution of the burdens and benefits of research. Although individual institutions or investigators may not be able to resolve a problem that is pervasive in their social setting, they can consider distributive justice in selecting research subjects.

Some populations, especially institutionalized ones, are already burdened in many ways by their infirmities and environments. When research is proposed that involves risks and does not include a therapeutic component, other less burdened classes of persons should be called upon first to accept these risks of research, except where the research is directly related to the specific conditions of the class involved. Also, even though public funds for research may often flow in the same directions as public funds for healthcare, it seems unfair that populations dependent on public healthcare constitute a pool of preferred research subjects if more advantaged populations are likely to be the recipients of the benefits.

One special instance of injustice results from the involvement of vulnerable subjects. Certain groups, such as racial minorities, the economically disadvantaged, the very sick, and the institutionalized may continually be sought as research subjects, owing to their ready availability in settings where research is conducted. Given their dependent status and their frequently compromised capacity for free consent, they should be protected against the danger of being involved in research solely for administrative convenience, or because they are easy to manipulate as a result of their illness or socioeconomic condition.

(1) Since 1945, various codes for the proper and responsible conduct of human experimentation in medical research have been adopted by different organizations. The best known of these codes are the Nuremberg Code of 1947, the Helsinki Declaration of 1964 (revised in 1975), and the 1971 Guidelines (codified into Federal Regulations in 1974) issued by the U.S. Department of Health, Education, and Welfare Codes for the conduct of social and behavioral research have also been adopted, the best known being that of the American Psychological Association, published in 1973.

(2) Although practice usually involves interventions designed solely to enhance the well-being of a particular individual, interventions are sometimes applied to one individual for the enhancement of the well-being of another (e.g., blood donation, skin grafts, organ transplants) or an intervention may have the dual purpose of enhancing the well-being of a particular individual, and, at the same time, providing some benefit to others (e.g., vaccination, which protects both the person who is vaccinated and society generally). The fact that some forms of practice have elements other than immediate benefit to the individual receiving an intervention, however, should not confuse the general distinction between research and practice. Even when a procedure applied in practice may benefit some other person, it remains an intervention designed to enhance the well-being of a particular individual or groups of individuals; thus, it is practice and need not be reviewed as research.

(3) Because the problems related to social experimentation may differ substantially from those of biomedical and behavioral research, the Commission specifically declines to make any policy determination regarding such research at this time. Rather, the Commission believes that the problem ought to be addressed by one of its successor bodies.

National Institutes of Health
Bethesda, Maryland 20892

Additional Resources

International Conference on Harmonisation (ISH), Guidelines for Good Clinical Practice
http://www.ich.org/ich5e.html

Council for International Organizations of Medical Sciences (CIOMS), International Ethical Guidelines for Biomedical Research Involving Human Subjects (revised Aug. 2002)
http://www.cioms.ch/frame_guidelines_nov_2002.htm

The World Health Organization (WHO), Operational Guidelines for Ethics Committees That Review Biomedical Research (Geneva, 2000)
http://www.who.int/tdr/publications/publications/pdf/ethics.pdf

Index

A

Abbreviated New Drug Application (ANDA), 353
Abuse. *See* Fraud and abuse
Access: to documentation, 308; to inspection information, 318; to source date, 243
Accountability, evaluation plans and, 89
Accreditation, in clinical trials, 404, 407–409
Acculturation, 102
Advance directives, 171–172
Adverse events: anticipating, 168–169; compliance issues, 265; documenting, 422–423; DSMBs and, 328; FWA recommendations, 372; high-risk areas for compliance, 458; investigator responsibilities, 228; patient safety and, 327, 331; reporting, 296, 334–341; risk management and, 410, 423–425
Advertising: IRBs and, 270; research documentation, 251–252; for research participants, 249–250
Agency for Health Care Policy and Research, 99
Agency for Healthcare Research and Quality (AHRQ), 15, 450
Agency for International Development, 17
Agency for Toxic Substances and Disease Registry (ATSDRO), 450
Agreements: model for sponsors, 469; NIH Guidelines element, 81, 88; research documentation, 251–252
Allegations: defined, 472, 489; not made in good faith, 485; research integrity officer and, 461; responding to, 476, 491–492
Alzheimer's disease. *See* Decisionally incapable subjects
American Medical Association, 3
Americans with Disabilities Act (ADA): emergency research and, 172; informed consent and, 167; screening healthcare professionals, 416–417
Animals: Animal Welfare Act, 3; organ transplant studies, 265; product metabolism in, 246; violation of regulations, 493
Anti-Kickback Statute, 291, 447–448
Anticipated benefits, 298–299

Approvals: conditional study approval, 305; exemptions from, 271–272; marketing approval, 347–348; masked studies, 272; study approval, 295–298
Assessment process: allegations and, 476, 495–496; anticipated benefits, 298–299; research protocols, 242; understanding study population, 84–85
Assimilation, 102
Association for the Accreditation of Human Research Protection Programs, Inc. (AAHRPP), 404, 408–409, 536
Association of American Medical Colleges (AAMC), 226, 291, 408
Association of American Universities (AAU), 408
Assumption of the risk, 395
Assurances: of compliance, 318–319; defined, 271, 274–275; international institutions and, 376; IRBs and, 272, 286; multisite and collaborative studies, 366–368; regulatory oversight and, 317; reporting requirements and, 308; sufficient knowledge mandate, 281–283; types of, 367–368
Authorization: HIPAA and, 15–16, 212; waivers, 16, 214–215
Authorized Institutional Official, 276
Autonomy, respect for, 525

B

Battery, 392
Behavioral research: FDA and Common Rule comparison, 12; HIV and, 364; information disclosure, 363; IRBs considerations, 362; state statutes, 28–29; techniques, 361
The Belmont Report: Assurances and, 274; baseline regulation, 2; behavioral research and, 363; contents, 617–627; ethical principles, 94; as guideline, 527; normative ethics and, 524
Beneficence, 94, 524–525
Benefits: anticipated benefits, 298–299; favorable risk-benefit ratio, 240; risk/benefit analysis, 298, 301, 529

Bioethics, 2, 7, 165, 217, 540
Biologics: emergency use, 171; FDA usage regulations, 352–353; vaccine trial term, 260
Bioresearch Monitoring Programs (FDA), 234–235
Breach of confidentiality, 392
Breach of contract, 393
Burden of proof, 492

C

Case-control studies, 99, 255–256
Case Report Forms (CRF), 250
Casuistry, 526
Center for Biologic Evaluation and Research (CBER), 272, 318
Center for Devices and Radiological Health (CDRH), 318, 356
Center for Drug Evaluation and Research (CDER), 272, 317
Center for Medicare and Medicaid Services (CMS), 8, 464. *See also* Health Care Financing Administration
Centers for Disease Control and Prevention (CDC), 15, 99, 449
Central Intelligence Agency, 2
Chief financial officer (CFO), 446
Chief Privacy Officer (CPO), 218
Chief Risk Officer (CRO), 413
Children. *See* Minors
Civil law, 234, 237, 393–395
Civil Rights Act (1964), 66, 167
Claims management process, 424–425
Class I devices, 351
Class II devices, 351
Class III devices, 351
Clinical investigators: adverse events and, 296; Certificate of Confidentiality, 400; conflict-of-interest, 226–227, 279–280; corrective actions against, 231–237; FDA Emergency Consent Regulation, 170; FWAs and, 370; GCP guidance, 250–251; General Services Administration list, 233; indemnification of, 399–400; international research and, 376, 535–536, 539; IRBs and, 96–97, 279–280, 307; lawsuit defenses, 394–395; LEP guidance, 167; managing non-compliance, 462; need for specialized training, 64, 67; NIH Guidelines, 119; patient safety and, 327; qualifications, 222–227; regulatory oversight and, 317–318; reporting study completion, 295; responsibilities of, 227–231; risk management and, 416–418; standard of care, 397–398; waivers for limiting liability and, 399
Clinical Laboratory Improvement Act of 1976 (CLIA), 240
Clinical trials: compliance plan elements, 454–457; confidentiality exemptions, 209–210; controversial issues outside U.S., 538–539; defined, 120; issues in, 122; NIH definition, 134–137; phases of, 257–258; table of state statutes, 25–56; various phases and considerations, 258–259. *See also* Randomized clinical trials

Clinical trials, phase I, 258–259. *See also* Investigational New Drug Application
Clinical trials, phase II, 258–259
Clinical trials, phase III: defined, 102, 258–259; NIH definition, 135–137; NIH Guidelines issues, 122–123; patient safety and, 330; peer reviews and, 147
Clinical trials, phase IV, 258–259
Code of Ethics, 1, 3
Code of Federal Regulations (CFR): consent documentation methods, 174–175; human research and, 10; informed consent, 156–157; informed consent checklist, 178–179; 21 CFR Part 50, 590–600; 21 CFR Part 56, 601–611. *See also* Common Rule
Collaborative studies, 366–373
Commercial value material, 169, 291
Common Rule: adoption of, 7; Assurances and, 366–368; in clinical trials, 10; confidentiality and, 209–212; criteria for research approval, 297–298; departments and agencies list, 17–20; FDA regulation comparison, 11–12; 45 CFR 46 contents, 562–589; HSS and, 2–3; human research and, 344–347; informed consent and, 156–157; international research, 535–536; IRBs and, 269–271; primary elements of, 10; prisoners as research subjects, 161; regulatory framework, 9; suspending/terminating study approvals, 295–296; waivers of informed consent, 303
Communication: adverse event treatment, 340–341; clinical research compliance plan, 456; defined, 102; due diligence checklist, 467; emergency research notification, 171; literacy and, 167–168; NIH Guidelines element, 81, 92–93; OPRR informed consent recommendations, 185; risk management and, 410; self-assessment and, 405; between sponsor and IRBs, 296; understanding study population, 85
Community: community-based organizations, 102; emergency research notification, 171; methods for understanding, 99; recruitment involvement, 65; study design evaluations, 65; understanding study population, 82, 84
Comparative negligence, 395
Compassionate use, 354
Compensation: benefits and, 299; for injuries, 399; IRB members, 286; risks and, 300
Competitive continuation (type 2) applications, 143
Complaints (importance of documentation), 63
Compliance. *See* Corporate compliance; Regulatory compliance
Conditional study approval, 305
Conditions of Participation for Hospitals in Medicare and Medicaid, 168–169, 327
Confidentiality: breach of confidentiality, 392; certificate of confidentiality, 217, 400; of clinical trials information, 207–219; as ethical principle, 529; FDA and Common Rule comparison, 12; HIV studies and,

263; informed consent and, 157; QI Program and, 406; research misconduct and, 232, 491
Conflict-of-interest: clinical investigators and, 226–227, 279–280; commercial value material and, 169; defined, 472; ethical issues, 530–531; investigator disclosures, 225–226; IRB composition and, 279; non-compliance, 462; risk management and, 410; standards dealing with, 291
Consentless research, 169–172
Consequentialism (Utilitarianism), 525
Consumer Product Safety Commission, 17
Continuous quality improvement (CQI), 405
Contractual considerations: breach of contract, 393; Common Rule and, 11; due diligence checklist, 466, 468; FWA recommendations, 372–373; risk management and, 410; sample language, 469
Contributory negligence, 395
Cooperative Project Assurances (CPAs), 367
Cooperative Research Protocol Programs (CRPPs), 367
Corporate compliance: clinical trials and, 447–454; federal agencies and, 446–447; non-compliance, 460–463; research compliance plan, 454–460; structure, 444–446
Corporate compliance officer, 455, 457–458
Corrective action, 470–486
Costs: charging study participants, 259; routine costs, 14
Council for International Organizations of Medical Sciences (CIOMS), 536
Covered entity, 211–212
Credentialing: criteria for, 418–419; due diligence checklist, 467; risk management and, 416–418
Criminal law: FDCA, 237; research misconduct, 234; violation of, 493
Cultural competence, 102
Cultural considerations: informed consent and, 166–168; study population and, 82–83; subject recruitment and retention, 65–66
Cultural diversity, 138–141, 278

D

Damages, 397
Data Safety Monitoring Board (DSMB), 304, 327–330
Debarment, 319, 469–486
Deciding official, 472, 475, 489
Decision-making, IRBs and, 297–306
Decision trees: avoiding gender bias, 61–62; NIH Guidelines, 78–80, 137; substantiating documentation, 460
Decisionally incapable subjects: evaluation checklist, 191; informed consent and, 164–166
Declaration of Helsinki: Assurances and, 274; contents, 614–616; as guideline, 527; human rights, 1; international research, 536
Declaration of Human Rights, 1
Deemed trials, 15
Denial of coverage, 172
Deontology, 525–526
Department Appeals Board (DAB), 450

Department of Agriculture, 18
Department of Commerce, 18
Department of Defense (DOD), 15, 18
Department of Education, 18
Department of Energy, 2, 18
Department of Health and Human Services (HHS): absence of clear guidelines, 60; Assurances and, 274–275; children as research subjects, 158–159, 180–181; Common Rule, 2–3; ethically appropriate financial incentives and, 67; FWA forms for domestic institutions, 376–382; FWA forms for international institutions, 383–390; human research under FDCA, 346; informed consent, 156–157; investigator disclosures, 225; IRBs, 286, 355; Limited English Proficiency guidance, 167; Office of Civil Rights, 16; Office of Minority Health, 63–64; policies and procedures on financial interests, 290–291; protecting research participants, 2; regulatory oversight, 318–319; research misconduct and, 13; tracking FDA Emergency Consent Regulation, 171
Department of Homeland Security, 3, 260
Department of Housing and Urban Development, 19
Department of Justice, 19
Department of Labor, 19
Department of Transportation, 19
Department of Veterans Affairs (VA): accreditation and, 407; accreditation models, 404; Common Rule and, 19; deemed trials, 15; DHHS FWA forms, 381–382
Depression, behavioral research and, 363
Determination: equitable selection, 301; of informed consent, 302; IRB formats, 291–292; of minimized risk, 300; reasonable risks, 301
Disabilities: developmentally disabled, 25–56, 66, 279; informed consent and, 167; mentally ill, 25–56, 279
Disclosure: of adverse events, 339–341; behavioral research and, 363; clinical investigators and, 225–226; confidentiality and QI Program, 406; financial interests of IRB members, 286; included with informed consent, 168–169
Discrimination, emergency research and, 172
Disqualification, of investigators, 236
Division of Assurances and Quality Improvement (DAQI), 405–406
Documentation: adverse events and, 335–336, 422–423; avoiding gender bias in selection process, 62–63; confidentiality pledges, 216–217; due diligence checklist, 467; high-risk areas for compliance, 459; included in reviews, 289; independent IRBs and, 277; informed consent, 174–175, 179, 186, 197–201, 302; investigator responsibilities, 229; Investigator's Brochure, 290; IRBs and, 306–308; permission and assent, 159–160; record management, 421–425; research protocols and, 243, 250–253; risk management and, 410; sponsor access to, 308; substantiating through compliance, 459–460. *See also* Reporting
Double billing, 463

Double dipping, 8
Drug Amendments (1962), 2
Due diligence, 466–468
Durable medical equipment, 444

E

E-recruiting considerations, 66–67
Education: avoiding gender bias through, 61; clinical
    research compliance plan, 455; due diligence
    checklist, 467; investigators and, 64, 67, 223–225;
    maintaining confidentiality through, 217–218;
    patient safety and, 334; requirements for IRB
    members, 285–286; risk management and, 410.
    See also Training
Efficacy, 242, 247, 351
Emergency Medical Treatment and Active Labor
    Act (EMTALA), 172
Emergency research, 169–172, 302–303
Emergency treatment (adverse events), 340–341
Emergency use: conditions for, 355–356; informed consent
    and, 357; of investigational drugs or biologics, 171;
    IRB reviews and, 272–273
Emotional distress, infliction of, 392
Employees: cooperation from, 492; defined, 489;
    as research participants, 273; scientific
    misconduct and, 469; understanding study
    population, 84
Environmental Protection Agency, 20
Epidemiologic studies, 255
Errors and omissions (E&O), 420
Ethical issues: behavioral research, 362; bioethics, 2, 7,
    165, 217, 540; Code of Ethics, 1, 3; framework for,
    528–530; frequently used theories, 524–526;
    guidelines, 526–527; international research and,
    374, 539; investigator disclosures, 225–226; NIH
    Guidelines, 94–95; normative ethics, 524–525;
    organ transplant studies, 264–265; placebos,
    531–532; research protocols and, 240, 243;
    risk/benefit analysis, 529
Ethnic considerations: categories defined, 121; NIH
    application guidelines, 141; NIH exclusions/
    justifications, 145–146; NIH Guidelines policy
    Q&A, 133–134; Office of Minority Health, 63–64;
    steps to avoid discrimination, 64–65; study
    population and, 82; subject recruitment or
    selection, 63
Ethnographic research, 363
Evaluation plans: impact evaluation, 103; IRB
    self-evaluation tool, 310–317; NFC evaluations, 405;
    NIH Guidelines element, 81, 89–92; outcome
    evaluation, 103; substantiating documentation,
    459–460
Evidentiary standards, 492–493
Executive Memorandum (June 2000), 14
Experimentation. *See* Human research
Experts: as information source, 98; negligence
    lawsuits and, 397
Extended care facilities, 25–56, 444

F

Fair participant selection, 240, 528–529
False Claims Act, 447, 461
Falsified research: compliance issues, 265; corporate
    compliance and, 447; ORI and, 16; research
    misconduct, 230–232
FDA-483 (Inspectional Observations), 235
FDA Emergency Consent Regulation, 170–172
FDA Modernization Act of 1997, 9
Feasibility, evaluation plans and, 89
Federal agencies: Common Rule list, 17–20; corporate
    compliance, 446–447, 452–454; human
    experimentation regulation, 7–9; international
    research and, 536; overseeing IRBs, 317–319;
    qualified immunity, 395; rectifying medical errors,
    326; research misconduct and, 232–234; sovereign
    immunity, 395
Federal Coordinating Council for Science, Engineering,
    and Technology, 7–8
Federal Register: Emergency Rule, 170; as information
    source, 99; misconduct findings, 450; NIH
    Guidelines, 115–123; publishing common rule, 8
Federal regulations/statutes: adverse event reporting,
    338–339; Assurances, 366–367; behavioral research
    exemptions, 362; billing and coding practices, 8;
    Certificate of Confidentiality, 400; clinical trials and,
    17; consentless research, 169–172; due diligence
    checklist, 468; foreign clinical studies and, 9; fraud
    and abuse and, 16; human research and, 3; informed
    consent, 156–157, 166–167; investigators on
    IRBs, 279–280; IRB size and mixture, 278–279;
    liability to military personnel, 395–396; patient
    safety, 327; proving standard of care and, 398;
    reporting non-compliance, 310; selection and
    recruitment of subjects, 60; state statutes and,
    23–24; venues for filing lawsuits, 394; waivers
    and, 174, 399–400
Federal Trade Commission, 66
Federalwide Assurance (FWA): defined, 274–275, 367;
    domestic institutions, 376–382; educational
    requirements, 285–286; international institutions,
    374–377, 383–390; IRB registration and, 273;
    multisite and collaborative studies, 368–373
Federation of American Societies for Experimental
    Biology, 408
Feedback mechanisms, 89, 93
Feres doctrine, 395–396
Fetal research: informed consent, 161–164; table of state
    statutes, 25–56
Fieldwork, behavioral research and, 363
Final National Coverage of Clinical Trials Program, 464
Financial interests: applicant disclosures, 225–226;
    clinical investigators and, 226–227; conflict-of-
    interest and, 530; disclosure by IRB members, 286;
    IRB composition and, 279; policies and procedures
    on, 290–291
Fiscal intermediaries, 14, 464
Focus groups, as information sources, 99

Food, Drug, and Cosmetic Act (FDCA): Drug Amendments of 1962, 2; FDA actions for research misconduct, 236–237; human research under, 343–359; private cause of action and, 394; radioactive drugs and, 261

Food and Drug Administration (FDA): advertising for participants, 249–250; clinical trials, 134–135; Common Rule and, 9, 11–12; compensation for participant injuries, 399; consentless research, 170; deemed trials, 15; Division of Scientific Investigations, 318; DSMBs and, 328–329; emergency care and, 273, 302–303; emergency use, 171, 355–356; GCP and, 536; gender issues for clinical trials, 353–354; general controls, 352; human research regulations, 8, 344; information sheets, 3, 60; informed consent and, 2; international research and, 539–540; investigators and, 225–226, 228–231, 234–235; Investigator's Brochure and, 290; IRB self-evaluation tool, 311–317; IRBs and, 269–270, 274, 292, 355; ORA, 449; organ transplant studies, 265; primary reviewer system, 289–290; RDRC, 261; regulatory oversight, 317–318, 448; research misconduct, 236–237; sponsor and IRB communication, 296; SR/NSR devices, 350; suspending/terminating study approvals, 295–296; 21 CFR Part 50, 590–600; vaccine trials, 260; violation of regulations, 494

Foreign research. *See* International research

Formative evaluation, 102

45 CFR 46. *See* Common Rule

Fraud and abuse: clinical trials and, 16–17; compliance enforcement, 447; corporate compliance, 453; federal requirements and, 8; financial fraud, 8, 494; institutional responsibilities, 232; lawsuits and, 392–393, 396; research and children subject of, 159; study funding arrangements and, 291

Fraud and Abuse Control Program, 447

Freedom of Information Act (FOIA), 318, 406

Funding: fraud and abuse, 291; NIH Guidelines and, 149; research misconduct and, 232; research protocols, 243; state regulations and, 24

G

Gender considerations: avoiding bias in research subjects, 61–63; clinical trials for FDA studies, 353–354; cultural issues, 66; disparity in selection and recruitment, 60–61; NIH application guidelines, 140; NIH exclusions/justifications, 143–144; NIH Guidelines issues, 122; NIH inclusion policy and, 148. *See also* Men; Women

General controls, 352

General Services Administration (GSA), 233, 450

Geographic regions, cultural diversity and, 140–141

Good Clinical Practice (GCP): International Conference on Harmonization, 3; international research, 536; outline, 240–243; study documentation, 250–253

Good faith allegation, 472, 489

Government Accounting Office, 318

Grants, compliance guidelines, 464

Grievances, patient rights, 168–169, 327

Group C drugs, 357

H

Handicapped. *See* Disabilities

Health Care Financing Administration (HCFA): deemed trials, 15; as information source, 99; National Coverage Policy, 14. *See also* Center for Medicare and Medicaid Services

Health Insurance Portability and Accountability Act (HIPAA): clinical trials and, 15–16; compliance enforcement, 447; confidentiality and, 8; e-recruiting concerns, 66–67; HIPAA Privacy Rule, 16, 208, 211; Privacy Boards, 212–215

Health Maintenance Organizations (HMOs), 14, 464

Health Resources and Services Administration (HRSA), 99, 449–450

Historical study, 254

HIV-related research protocols: behavioral research and, 364; controversial issues, 538; Parallel Track program and, 358; special concerns, 263–264

Home health care, 41

Homeland Security Act, 3

Hospice, compliance guidelines, 444

Hospitals: adverse event treatment, 340–341; as communities, 82; compliance guidelines, 444; IRB reviews and, 277; risk identifiers and, 410–411; state statutes, 41

Human research: defined, 120; due diligence checklist, 466–468; ethical issues in, 523–533; evolution of, 1–5; FDCA and, 343–359; federal agencies and, 7–9; human subjects defined, 271; issues, 121–122; medical malpractice liability in, 391–401; NIH definition, 137; OPRR decision chart, 194; state regulation of, 23–56; violation of regulations, 493. *See also* Research participants

Human Research Protection Accreditation Program (HRPAP), 408

Human Subjects Research Subcommittee, 9

I

Immunity, 395

Impact evaluation, 103

In vitro procedures: scientific research and, 344; table of state statutes, 25–56

Incentives: benefits and, 299; cautions using, 86; considering, 302; IRBs ensuring ethically appropriate, 67–68; QI Program, 405; recruitment and, 58–59

Indemnification, of clinical investigators, 399–400

Independent Ethics Committee (IEC), 270–271, 375

Indian Health Service (HIS), 450

Individually identifiable information, 209, 330

Infliction of emotional distress, 392

Information Sheets, 3, 60

Informed consent: checklists, 178–179, 192–193; clinical trials and, 155–206; common concerns to address, 202–206; confidentiality disclosure and, 210; consent as lawsuit defense, 394; consentless research, 169–172; decisionally incapable subjects, 164–166; determination of, 302; documentation, 174–175, 251; emergencies, 302–303, 357; experimental therapy and, 25; federal regulations, 156–157, 166–167; fetal research, 161–164; first statute, 2; FWAs and, 369–370; high-risk areas for compliance, 458; HIPAA research authorization, 212; human research under FDCA, 347; international institutions and, 375; IRBs and, 270; lack of informed consent, 392, 398; minors and, 158–160, 180–181; modifications and waivers of, 173–174, 179–180, 196; OHSR documentation guidelines, 197–201; OPRR, 177, 182–186; patient safety and, 331; pregnant women, 161–164; prisoners, 161; radioactive materials and, 262; recruitment practices and, 59; research protocol and, 240; risks and, 300, 410; state statutes, 24, 26–29, 31, 46, 53; suggestions for obtaining, 175–176; template, 187–190; topics for disclosure, 168–169; withdrawing, 172–173

Initial review groups (IRGs), 146, 148

Inquiries: conducting, 476–479, 496–505; defined, 473, 489

Inspections: FDA and Common Rule comparison, 12; regulatory oversight and, 317–318; research misconduct, 234–236

Institute of Medicine (IOM), 218, 326, 409

Institutional counsel, 489

Institutional Radiation Safety Committee (IRSC), 262

Institutional review boards (IRBs): accreditation programs, 407–409; activities of, 286–296; beginning of, 2; behavioral research and, 362; children as research subjects, 158–160; Common Rule and, 9, 12, 269; composition of, 278–286; confidentiality and, 210; conflicts of interest and, 531; current effectiveness of, 310; decision-making by, 297–306; decisionally incapable persons, 165–166; documentation, 252, 306–308; DSMBs and, 328–330; e-recruiting concerns, 66; ethical principles and, 94, 524; FDA Emergency Consent Regulation, 170–171; FDA Information Sheets, 3; FDA misconduct notification procedure, 237; federal guidelines for recruitment, 60; financial incentives, 67–68; FWAs and, 368–370; gender bias, 61–63; HIV studies and, 263–264; human research under FDCA, 346–347; IND/IDE requirements, 345; informed consent, 157, 173–175; innovative practices, 296; international research and, 375, 539; investigators and, 223, 227–231; LEP guidance, 167; neonate research, 162–163; NIH and, 119, 148, 150; non-compliance, 308–309, 462–463; observational studies, 254–256; organ transplant studies, 264–265; overview, 270–277; Parallel Track program and, 358; patient safety and, 327; points of consideration for, 96–97; policies and procedures, 287–289; pregnant women and fetuses, 161; protocol issues/considerations, 248–253; QA Self-Assessment Tool, 406–407, 427–442; quality assurance, 308–317; radioactive material studies, 261–263; recruitment practices, 59; regulatory oversight of, 317–319; resource adequacy considerations, 227; reviews, 256–257; risk management and, 413–414; self-evaluation of, 310–317; specialized training needs, 64; sponsors and, 296; SR and NSR study differences, 348–351; study population considerations, 83–84; sufficient knowledge mandate, 281–283; 21 CFR Part 56, 601–611; waivers and, 179–180, 210–211, 214–215; workloads, 306. *See also* IRB members; IRB reviews

Institutions: Certificate of Confidentiality, 400; common examples of non-compliance, 309; DHHS forms for, 376–382; FWAs and, 368–373; IRBs and, 275–277, 286, 295, 307; potential lawsuit defenses, 394–395; research misconduct responsibilities, 231–232; vicarious liability and, 393

Insurance: clinical research and, 400; denial of coverage, 172; financial incentives for subjects and, 67; research documentation, 251; research protocols, 243; risk management and, 409–410, 419–421

Intellectual property, 218

Interagency Human Subjects Coordinating Council, 8

InterInstitutional Amendment (IIA), 367–368

International Conference on Harmonisation (ICH): FDA and, 9; Good Clinical Practice, 3, 240–243; international research and, 536

International Ethical Guidelines for Biomedical Research Involving Human Subjects, 527, 536–538

International research: Common Rule and, 9; considerations, 535–541; DHHS FWA forms for, 383–390; due diligence checklist, 468; FDA and Common Rule comparison, 11; FWAs and, 371, 374–377; NIH and, 120, 149; regulations and, 9. *See also* Declaration of Helsinki; The Belmont Report; The Nuremberg Code

Interviews: adverse events and, 336; features, 254; as information sources, 99

Investigational Device Exemption (IDE): adverse events and, 228; applicant disclosures, 225–226; consentless research and, 170; human research under FDCA, 345; international research and, 539–540; Treatment IND/IDE, 354–355

Investigational drugs: control responsibilities, 229; controversial issues outside U.S., 538; emergency use, 171; Group C drugs, 357; Investigator's Brochure and, 290; IRB review, 2; pharmacists and, 358

Investigational New Drug Application (IND): adverse events and, 228; applicant disclosures, 225–226; consentless research and, 170; deemed trials, 15; FDA and Common Rule comparison, 11; human research under FDCA, 344–345; international research, 9, 539–540; IRB review waivers, 272; open protocol IND, 353; patient safety and, 327; radioactive materials and, 262; scientific research steps and, 344; Treatment IND/IDE, 354–355; vaccine trials and, 260

Investigational use, 352

Investigations: of adverse events, 422; adverse events and, 335–336; conducting, 479–483, 505–517; defined, 222, 473, 490

Investigators. *See* Clinical investigators

Investigator's Brochure, 243–248, 251, 290

IRB Guidebook: financial recruitment incentives and, 67; issuance of, 3; racial and ethnic minorities, 63; types of research, 271

IRB members: alternates for, 283–284; educational requirements, 285–286; financial interests disclosure, 286; high-risk areas for compliance, 459; potential liability of, 393–394; required information about, 306–307; risk management and, 416–418

IRB reviews: collecting follow-up data and, 294–295; consequences if not conducted, 294; emergencies and, 272–273; FDA waiver *vs.* HHS regulations, 355; joint reviews, 277; 510(k) devices and, 348; proposed changes, 305–306; regulatory oversight, 292; responsibilities, 270; Treatment IND/IDE, 355; waivers for, 272

J

Joint Commission on Accreditation of Healthcare Organizations (JCAHO), 404, 408

Justice: defined, 525; ethical issues, 94; HIV studies and, 263

K

510(k) devices, 347–348

L

Lack of informed consent, 392, 398

Language considerations: feedback mechanisms, 93; informed consent and, 166–168; patient safety and, 332; sample informed consent form, 177; study population and, 82, 85; subject recruitment and retention, 65–66

Lawsuits: negligence lawsuits, 396–398; potential defenses, 394–395; theories of law that may arise, 392–393; time periods for filing, 396; venues for filing, 394

Learned intermediary, 395

Liability: government to military personnel, 395–396; IRB members and, 393–394; limiting, 399–400; product liability, 393; vicarious liability, 393

"Limited English Proficiency" (LEP), 66

Literacy, effective communication and, 167–168

Literature searches, 98

Long-term facilities, 25–56, 444

Loss exposures, 410, 412–413

M

Mainstream, 103

Majority groups, 121

Marketing: FDA usage regulations, 352–353; off-label and investigational use, 273; PMA and 510(k) differences, 347–348

Masked studies, 272

Medic-Alert bracelets, 330, 332–333

Medicaid: Center for Medicare and Medicaid Services, 8, 464; Conditions of Participation for Hospitals in Medicare and Medicaid, 168–169, 327; fraud and abuse, 447; Stark Self-Referral provisions, 448

Medical Device Amendments (1976), 351–352

Medical devices, 345, 351–353

Medical malpractice liability, 391–401

Medicare: clinical trials and, 13–15; Conditions of Participation for Hospitals in Medicare and Medicaid, 168–169, 327; corporate non-compliance and, 463–464; fraud and abuse, 447; human research regulations and, 8; Stark Self-Referral provisions, 448

Medicare+Choice, 14, 444, 464

Meetings: documenting, 307; frequency of, 289; minutes of, 462–463; quorums at, 284–285; substitutes for IRB members, 283–284

Men, 141, 143–144

Mentally ill, 25–56, 279

Military personnel, 395–396

Minimal risk, 300

Minority groups: NIH Guidelines Appendix A, 113–123; NIH Guidelines Outreach Notebook, 73–112; NIH Guidelines Q&A, 125–153

Minors: informed consent and, 158–160, 180–181; research involving pregnant women, 162; special requirements for wards, 160; table of state statutes, 25–56

Misconduct. *See* Research misconduct; Scientific misconduct

Modified Single Project Assurance, 367

Monitoring: clinical research compliance plan, 456–457; confidentiality and, 218; documentation access, 251; FWA recommendations, 372; investigators by FDA, 234–235; IRBs and, 303–304; NIH DSMB guidelines, 330; research documentation, 253; risk management, 300, 410; vaccine trials, 260

Moral factors, prioritizing, 525

Multicenter studies: DSMBs and, 328; NIH application guidelines, 142; state regulations and, 24

Multiple Project Assurances (MPAs), 274–275, 367

Multisite and collaborative studies, 366–373

N

National Aeronautics and Space Administration, 20

National Associate of State Universities and Land Grant Colleges, 408

National Bioethics Advisory Commission (NBAC), 165, 217, 540

National Center for Health Statistics, 99

National Commission for the Protection of Human Subjects of Biomedical and Behavioral Research, 2

National Committee for Quality Assurance (NCQA), 404, 407–408

National Council for Radiation Protection and Measurement (NCRPM), 262

National Coverage Policy, 14

National Health Interview Survey (NHIS), 98

National Institutes of Health (NIH): Certificate of Confidentiality, 400; clinical trial oversight, 448; deemed trials, 15; DSMB guidance, 329–330; investigator requirements, 223–224; minority inclusion guidelines, 63–64; OER, 449; OPERA, 449; protection of human subjects, 2; Regulatory Burden Advisory Group, 305–306

National Office of Human Research Oversight (NOHRO), 452

The National Research Act (1974), 2

National Science and Technology Council, 9

National Science Foundation, 20

National Standard for Privacy of Medical Information, 16, 208, 211

National Standards on Culturally and Linguistically Appropriate Services in Health Care, 66

Need to know access, 217

Neglect, children subject of, 159

Negligence: contributory negligence, 395; defined, 397; *Feres* doctrine, 395–396; IRB member liability, 393–394; limiting liability through waivers, 399; professional negligence, 396–398; statute of limitations for filing lawsuits, 396

Neonatal research, 161–164

New Drug Application (NDA), 344

NIH Guidelines on inclusion of women and minorities as subjects in clinical research: Appendix A, 113–123; Outreach Notebook, 73–112; Questions and Answers, 125–153

NIH Revitalization Act (1993), 13, 131–132

Nonaffiliated members: attendance by, 284; DSMB composition and, 329; FWAs and, 370; IRB and, 280–281

Noncompliance. *See* Regulatory non-compliance

Nonmaleficence, 524

Nonscientists, 280

Nonsignificant risk (NSR) study, 348–351

Normative ethics, 524–525

Not-for-cause (NFC) evaluations, 405

Notice of Initiation of Disqualification Proceedings and Opportunity to Explain, 235–236

Notice of Opportunity for Hearing, 236

Notification: of adverse events, 422; non-compliance and QI Program, 406; of previous study disapproval, 295; research misconduct and, 232

Nuclear Regulatory Commission, 261–262

The Nuremberg Code: contents, 612–613; formation of, 1; as guideline, 527; international research, 536

O

Observational study, 253–256

Observations: as information source, 99; IRB obligations, 303–304

Occupational Safety and Health Administration (OSHA), 423

Off-label use, 273, 352

Office of Civil Rights (OCR), 16

Office of Extramural Research (OER): clinical trials oversight, 449; decisionally incapable persons, 165–166; policy statement, 64

Office of Human Research Protection (OHRP): Assurances and, 367; clinical trials, 15, 450–451; Common Rule and, 17; creation of, 2; credentialing and, 418; Division of Compliance, 218; DSMB and, 327; educational requirements for IRBs, 285–286; high-risk areas for compliance, 458–459; IRB considerations for research protocols, 248–253; IRB monitoring obligations, 303–304; IRB policies and procedures, 287–289; IRB registration, 273–274; ongoing research reviews, 293; patient safety, 326; primary reviewer system, 289–290; quality improvement and, 404–407; regulatory oversight and, 317–319; reporting, 308, 310; review defined, 292; role of, 12–13; self-assessment tool, 427–442

Office of Human Subjects Research (OHSR), 197–201

Office of Inspector General (OIG): Common Rule, 10; compliance guidelines, 444–446; DSMBs and, 328; financial incentives and, 67; IRB membership categories, 280; IRB monitoring obligations, 304; IRB self-evaluation, 310–311; IRB size and mixture, 278–279; low-volume IRBs, 275–276; ongoing research reviews, 292–293; *Recruiting Human Subjects*, 57; research oversight, 2

Office of Management Administration (OMA), 448–449

Office of Minority Health, 63–64, 66

Office of Policy for Extramural Research Administration (OPERA), 449

Office of Protection from Research Risks (OPRR): Assurance/agreement distinctions, 368; creation of, 2; decision charts, 194–196; educational requirements for investigators, 223; ethical considerations, 94; HIV studies and, 263; informed consent, 166–167, 177, 182–185; IRBs and, 3, 96–97, 270; NIH inclusion policy, 150; patient safety, 326; protecting privacy, 305; regulatory oversight, 317–319

Office of Regulatory Affairs (ORA), 235, 449

Office of Research Integrity (ORI): clinical trials oversight, 449–450; compliance guidelines, 462–463; educational requirements for investigators, 224; oversight responsibilities, 505; plagiarism and, 16; reporting requirements, 483–484, 494–495; research integrity officer, 458; research misconduct defined, 231; review of scientific misconduct, 518–520; role of, 13; whistleblower protections, 230–231

Omnibus Reconciliation Act (1993), 447

On-call protocols, 333

Open label protocols, 353
Open protocol IND, 353
Organ transplant studies, 264–265
Outcome evaluation, 103
Outreach: elements for NIH Guidelines, 81–93; NIH application guidelines, 142; NIH Guidelines, 120
Outreach Notebook, 73–112
Oversight. *See* Regulatory oversight

P

Parallel Track program, 358
Parental consent, 158–163, 180–181
Part 16 Hearing, 236
Partnership for Human Research (PHRP), 404, 408–409, 536
Patient safety: assessment of, 242; in clinical research, 325–341; considerations for, 301; creating environment, 330–334; investigator responsibilities, 227–231; Investigator's Brochure, 247; IRB monitoring obligations, 304; medical devices and, 351; organ transplant studies, 265
Patient's bill of rights: experimental subjects and, 27–28; filing grievances, 168–169, 327; state statutes, 30
Peer Review Organizations (PROs), 14, 405–406
Peer reviews: NIH Guidelines, 119, 146–149; regulatory oversight and, 319
Percentile ranking, NIH funding and, 149
Permission. *See* Informed consent; Parental consent
Pharmacists, investigational drugs and, 358
Pharmakinetics, 246
Physicians: compliance guidelines, 444; conflicts in roles, 530–531; emergency use exceptions, 355–357; FDA regulated products, 277; informed consent and, 302–303; as learned intermediaries, 395; recruitment practices, 58–59; sovereign immunity, 395; test articles in emergencies, 272–273; understanding study population, 84
Pilot tests, 91
Placebos: clinical trials and, 257; controversial issues outside U.S., 538; ethics of, 531–532; HIV studies and, 264; participant understanding of, 95
Plagiarism, 16, 230–232
Policies and procedures: adverse events, 334–337; compliance plan, 454–460; DSMB activities, 330; on financial interests, 290–291; international institutions and, 375; IRBs and, 287–289; NIH Guidelines, 131–137; for patient safety, 327; research documentation, 252–253; risk management and, 414–416; scientific misconduct, 470–522; self-evaluation tool, 311–317
Pregnant women, 25–56, 161–164
Premarket Approval (PMA), 347–348
President's Commission on Bioethics, 2, 7
Primary reviewer system, 289–290, 293–294
Principle-based ethics, 524–525
Priority scores, NIH inclusion policy and, 148–149
Prisoners: informed consent, 161; minimal risk and, 300; table of state statutes, 25–56

Privacy: e-recruiting concerns, 66; HIPAA and, 15–16; HIV studies and, 263; individually identifiable information, 209; intellectual property and, 218; IRB obligations, 304–305; Privacy Boards, 212–215
Private cause of action, 394
Private information, 304
Privileging, risk management and, 416–417
Products: charging for, 259; FDA regulated, 275, 277; liability and, 393; marketed products, 273, 352–353; metabolism in research participants, 246–247
Professional negligence, 396–398
Prospective study, 256
Protected health information (PHI), 66
Protection: AAHRPP approach, 408; accreditation and, 407; behavioral research and, 362; of human subjects, 2–3, 404–407, 590–600; Parallel Track program and, 358; of whistleblowers, 230–231, 475–476, 485, 491
Protocols. *See* Research protocols
Proximate cause, 397
Public Health Service Act, 230–231, 451
Public Health Service (PHS): clinical trials oversight, 448, 451–452; education for research staff, 286; NIH Policy reinforcement, 64; ORI, 449–450; regulatory oversight, 318–319; Tuskegee Study, 2, 63, 86
Public Law 104–191. *See* Health Insurance Portability and Accountability Act (HIPAA)
Public Law 105–115, 9
Public Research in Medicine and Research (PRIM&R), 408
Punitive damages, 397
Purity, 260

Q

QA Self-Assessment Tool (OHRP), 406–407, 427–442
Qualified immunity, 395
Quality assurance: IRBs and, 297, 308–317; research protocols and, 240, 243
Quality improvement, in clinical trials, 404–407
Quality Improvement Organizations (QIOs), 14, 464
Quality Improvement (QI) Program, 405–406
Questionnaires, 254
Qui tam action, 460–462
Quorums, IRBs and, 284–285

R

Race, 103
Racial considerations: avoiding discrimination, 64–65; categories defined, 121; NIH application guidelines, 141; NIH exclusions/justifications, 145; Office of Minority Health, 63–64; study population and, 82; subject recruitment or selection, 63. *See also* Minority groups
Radiation experimentation, 2, 393
Radioactive Drug Research Committee (RDRC), 261
Radioactive materials, 261–263
Radiopaque contrast agents, 261

Randomized clinical trials (RCT): DSMBs and, 328; HIV studies and, 264; IRB considerations, 256–257; participant understanding of, 95

Record keeping. *See* Documentation

Record management, 421–425

Recruitment and selection: equitable nature of, 301; HIV studies and, 263–264; NIH Guidelines Appendix A, 113–123; NIH Guidelines Outreach Notebook, 73–112; NIH Guidelines Q&A, 125–153; of research subjects, 57–69

Registration: IRB with FDA, 274; IRB with OHRP, 273–274

Regulatory compliance: FWAs and, 370, 372; international institutions and, 374–375; investigator responsibilities, 228; language assistance, 167; manufacturers and, 273; NIH and, 148–149; peer reviewers and, 146–148; regulatory oversight and, 318–319; research protocols and, 240, 265; risk management and, 412; state/federal regulations, 24

Regulatory non-compliance: clinical research compliance plan, 457; common examples, 308–309; confidentiality and QI Program, 406; corporations and, 460–463; examples of, 229; FDA and Common Rule comparison, 12; regulatory oversight and, 318–319; response to, 309–310; risk management and, 410

Regulatory oversight: for clinical trials, 448–451; due diligence checklist, 468; IRB reviews of ongoing research, 292; of IRBs, 317–319; OIG and, 2; ORI responsibilities, 505

Rehabilitation Act (1973), 167, 172, 416–417

REM (Roentgen Equivalent in Man), 261

Reporting: adverse events, 296, 328, 334–341; in clinical trials, 421–425; compliance issues, 265; DSMBs and, 328–330; as ethical issue, 530; FDA and Common Rule comparison, 12; inquiry results, 478–479, 504–505; investigation results, 481–484, 511–517; investigator responsibilities, 229; non-compliance, 310; OHRP requirements, 308; ORI requirements, 483–484, 494–495; patient safety and, 327; when study is completed, 295. *See also* Documentation

Request for Proposals (RFPs), 149

Research bracelets, 330, 332–333

Research integrity officer: defined, 473, 490; monitoring allegations, 461; ORI definition, 458; reporting requirements, 495; responsibilities, 474

Research misconduct: corrective actions and, 231–237; defining, 230; HHS authority over, 13

Research participants: adverse event disclosure, 339–341; advertising considerations, 249–250; charging for study products, 259; compensation for injuries, 399; confidentiality assurances to, 216; consentless research and, 169–172; covered entity, 211–212; ensuring safety of, 228; equitable selection, 301; HIPAA and, 15–16; HIV studies and, 263–264; IRBs and, 271; privacy of, 304–305; product metabolism in, 246–247; protecting, 2–3; questions to ask of research team, 192–193; risk and, 300, 412. *See also* Human research; Patient safety; Recruitment and selection; specific categories

Research protocols: approving, 297–298, 355; conditional approval, 305; elements of, 240–248; general issues/considerations, 248–253; investigator responsibilities, 227–231; IRBs and, 269, 295, 297; proving standard of care, 397–398; response to non-compliance, 309–310; reviewing, 302; selection criteria, 62; suspending, 335; types of studies/issues, 254–265

Research record, 473, 490

Resource considerations, 227, 306

Respect for participants, 94, 240, 529

Respondents: defined, 473, 490; protecting, 476, 491; responsibilities, 475

Retaliation: defined, 473–474, 490; whistleblower protection and, 230–232

Retention policies: IRB records, 307; record management, 421–422; scientific misconduct inquiries, 485, 520; study documents, 251

Reviews: cooperative research protocol, 302; defined, 292; documents included in, 289; due diligence checklist, 468; expedited reviews, 300, 305; frequency of, 294, 307–308; high-risk areas for compliance, 458; independent, 240, 529; IRB obligations, 292, 297, 303–304; joint reviews, 277; multi-review matrix, 11; NIH criteria, 100–101; peer reviews, 119, 146–149, 319; primary reviewer system, 289–290, 293–294; protocol selection criteria, 62–63; record review, 254; specialized tools, 65. *See also* IRB reviews

Right to information, 41

Risk/benefit analysis, 240, 298, 301, 529

Risk management: adverse events and, 423–425; assumption of the risk, 395; considering potential harms, 299; corporate compliance and, 458–459; credentialing and, 416–418; defined, 299; determination of minimized, 300; FWA recommendations, 372; insurance and, 409–410, 419–421; policies and procedures, 414–416; risk identifiers, 410–411; risk transfer and, 412–413; roles of risk managers, 413–414

Routine costs, 14

S

Safety. *See* Patient safety

Sample selection, 61–62

Scientific misconduct, 470–522

Scientific theory, 240, 249

Scientific validity, 528

Scientists: conflicts in roles, 530–531; distinguishing IRB members as, 280; DSMB composition and, 329; international research and, 540

Screening: healthcare professionals, 416; patient safety and, 330–331; state statutes, 43

Selection. *See* Recruitment and selection

Self-assessment: AAHRPP approach, 408; OHRP tool, 406–407, 427–442; quality improvement and, 405

Signage, patient safety and, 332

Significant difference, 121

Significant risk (SR) study, 348–351

Single Patient use, 357–358
Single Project Assurances (SPAs), 367
Site of intervention, 103
Social Security Act, 67, 447
Socioeconomic considerations, 82
Sovereign immunity, 395
Sponsors: accessing information, 308, 318; DSMBs and, 328–329; indemnifying investigators, 399–400; international research and, 539; investigator agreement, 250–251; Investigator's Brochure, 243–248; IRBs and, 296; lawsuit defenses, 394–395; misconduct notification procedure, 237; model agreement, 469; non-compliance and, 462–463; patient safety and, 327; risk identifiers and, 410–411; SR/NSR device studies, 349–350; vicarious liability and, 393
Stakeholders, 218
Standard Guidelines and Assessment Tool (SGAT), 408
Standard of care: controversial issues outside U.S., 538–539; negligence lawsuits and, 396–398; proving, 397–398
Standard of proof, 493
Stark Self-Referral provisions, 291, 447–448
State regulations/statutes: adverse event reporting, 338–339; confidentiality and, 215–216; of human research, 23–56; informed consent, 156; NRC and, 262; standard of care and, 398; statute of limitations for filing lawsuits, 396; venues for filing lawsuits, 394
Statistics, research protocols and, 243
Statute of limitations, 394, 396
Sterility, 260
Study population, 81–85
Subjects. *See* Research participants
Subpopulations, 121–123
Subsequent use, 272
Substance Abuse and Mental Health Services Administration (SAMHSA), 449
Sufficient knowledge mandate, 281–283
Suicidal patients, 363
Surveillance, maintaining confidentiality through, 218
Surveys: features, 254; as information sources, 99
Suspension: adverse events and, 335; regulatory oversight and, 319; reporting requirements, 308; of studies, 295, 423

T

Termination: regulatory oversight and, 319; reporting requirements, 308; of studies, 295
Test articles: IRB reviews and, 272–273; Treatment IND/IDEs and, 355
Theoretical equipoise, 257
Theories of law, 392–393

Title VI (Civil Rights Act), 66, 167
To Err Is Human, 326
Toxicology, 246
Training: clinical research compliance plan, 455; FWAs and, 370–371; international institutions and, 376–377; risk management and, 418; state statutes, 56. *See also* Education
Translational ethics, 526
Treatment IND/IDE, 354–355
Tuskegee Study, 2, 63, 86
21 CFR Part 50, 590–600
21 CFR Part 56, 601–611

U

U.S. Congress, 2
U.S. Postal Service, 448
Utilitarianism, 525

V

Vaccine trials, 259–260
Valid analysis, 120–121, 136
Validity, research protocol and, 240
Value, research protocol and, 240
Veterans Affairs Human Research Protection Accreditation Program (VAHRPAP), 404, 407–409
Vicarious liability, 393
Virtue ethics, 526
Vulnerable subject populations, 273, 278–279

W

Waivers: for authorization, 16, 214–215; confidentiality and, 210–211; consentless research, 169–172; of informed consent, 302–303; IRBs and, 272, 303; limiting liability with, 399–400; OPRR decision chart, 196; requirements, 173–174, 179
Wards, special requirements for, 160
Web sites: e-recruiting concerns, 66; patient safety and, 333
Whistleblowers: corporate compliance and, 460–462; defined, 474–475, 491; protections for, 230–231, 475–476, 485, 491
Women: NIH Guidelines Appendix A, 113–123; NIH Guidelines Outreach Notebook, 73–112; NIH Guidelines Q&A, 125–153; study population considerations, 83
World Health Organization, 539

X

X rays, 261–263
Xenografts, 265

Printed in the United States
86151LV00001B/43-50/A